Obesity Surgery
Principles and Practice

To my parents, brothers, and to my fiancé for always understanding that dedication and responsibility inevitably lead to absence.

Cid Pitombo

To my wife, Anne, for believing in and supporting my career-long involvement in Bariatric Surgery, especially in the early days, when our small group of pioneers were looked upon by so many as eccentric opportunists.

Kenneth B. Jones, Jr.

To my wife and children for their understanding and compassion.

Kelvin D. Higa

To my wife, son, and daughter.

José Carlos Pareja

Obesity Surgery
Principles and Practice

Cid Pitombo, MD, PhD, TCBC (Editor-in-Chief)
General and Bariatric Surgery
Minimally Invasive Surgery
Campinas State University (UNICAMP)
Rio de Janeiro/Campinas, Brazil

Kenneth B. Jones, Jr., MD (Co-Editor)
Clinical Assistant Professor, Department of Surgery
Louisiana State University Health Sciences Center
Former President, American Society of Bariatric Surgery
Shreveport, Louisiana

Kelvin D. Higa, MD, FACS (Co-Editor)
President Elect, American Society for Metabolic and Bariatric Surgery
Clinical Professor of Surgery
University of California, San Francisco
Private Practice
Fresno, California

José Carlos Pareja, MD, PhD (Co-Editor)
Professor, Department of Surgery, Head of Pancreas, Biliary, and Obesity Surgery
Campinas State University (UNICAMP)
President, Scientific Committee, Brazilian Society for Bariatric Surgery
Campinas, Brazil

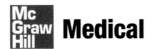

New York   Chicago   San Francisco   Lisbon   London   Madrid   Mexico City   Milan
New Delhi   San Juan   Seoul   Singapore   Sydney   Toronto

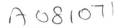
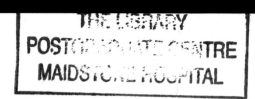
Obesity Surgery: Principles and Practice

1 2 3 4 5 6 7 8 9 0   CTP/CTP   0 9 8 7

Set: ISBN 978-0-07-148281-3; MHID 0-07-148281-4
Book: ISBN 978-0-07-149492-2; MHID 0-07-149492-8
CD: ISBN 978-0-07-149491-5; MHID 0-07-149491-X

This book was set in Minion by Aptara Inc.
The editors were Marsha S. Loeb and Joe Rusko.
The production supervisor was Catherine H. Saggese.
Project management was provided by Aptara Inc.
The designer was Janice Bielawa.
The indexer was Coughlin Indexing Services, Inc.
China Translation & Printing Services, Ltd., was printer and binder.

This book is printed on acid-free paper.

Cataloging-in-Publication Data is on file with the Library of Congress.

Contents

Contributors

Aniceto Baltasar, MD
Clínica San Jorge y Hospital "Virgen de los Lirios"
Alicante, Spain
Laparoscopic Biliopancreatic Diversion: Duodenal Switch

Mitiku Belachew, MD
Professor, Department of Surgery Centre Hospitalier
    Regional de Huy, Belgium,
Honorary Professor of Surgery,
Addis Ababa University,
Addis Ababa, Ethiopia,
Huy, Belgium
Restrictive Procedures: Adjustable Gastric Band

Simon Biron, MD, MSc
Professor and Head, Department of Surgery, Laval University
Laval Hospital
Quebec, Canada
Malabsorptive Procedures: Duodenal Switch

Camilo Boza, MD
Department of Surgery
Hospital Clínico, Pontificia
Universidad Católica de Chile
Santiago, Chile
*Laparoscopic Restrictive Procedures: Sleeve Gastrectomy;
    Two-Stage Approach for High-Risk Patients*

Stacy A. Brethauer, MD
Fellow, Advanced Laparoscopic and Bariatric Surgery
Department of General Surgery, Cleveland Clinic
Cleveland, Ohio
*Physiology and Metabolism in Obesity Surgery: Roux-en-Y
Gastric Bypass*

Jay B. Brodsky, MD
Professor of Anesthesiology, Stanford University School of
    Medicine, Medical Director of Perioperative Services
Stanford University Medical Center
Stanford, California
Anesthetic Concerns

Henry Buchwald, MD, PhD
Professor of Surgery and Biomedical Engineering
    Owen H. and Sarah Davidson Wangensteen Chair in
    Experimental Surgery Emeritus
Department of Surgery, University of Minnesota
Minneapolis, Minnesota
Evolution of Surgery for Morbid Obesity

Jane N. Buchwald, MA
CEO and Director of Publications
MEDWRITE Medical Communications
Maiden Rock, Wisconsin
Evolution of Surgery for Morbid Obesity

Cynthia K. Buffington, PhD
Florida Hospitals Celebration Health Celebration, Florida
*Laparoscopic Gastric Bypass: Evolution, Safety, and Efficacy of
the Banded Gastric Bypass*

Molly J. Carlson, MD
Fellow, Division of Metabolism, Endocrinology,
    and Nutrition
Department of Medicine, University of Washington
VA Puget Sound Health Care System
Seattle, Washington
*Possible Hormonal Mechanisms Mediating the Effects of
Bariatric Surgery*

J.K. Champion, MD
Clinical Professor of Surgery
Mercer University School of Medicine
Director of Bariatric Surgery
    Emory Dunwoody Medical Center
Videoscopic Institute of Atlanta
Marietta, Georgia
Laparoscopic Gastric Bypass: Linear Technique

Contributors

Venita Chandra, MD
Resident, Department of Pediatric Surgery,
Stanford University, Stanford, California
Adolescent Bariatric Surgery

Leonardo Claros, MD
Assistant Professor of Surgery, Tufts University
    Medical School, Co-Director, Center for Weight Control
Caritas Saint Elizabeth's Medical Center
Boston, Massachusetts
Late Complications: Ulcers, Stenosis, and Fistula

Robert N.L. Corprew, Jr.
Brody School of Medicine at East Carolina University
Greenville, North Carolina
Nutritional Consequences and Management

David E. Cummings, MD
Associate Professor of Medicine, Division of Metabolism
Endocrinology, and Nutrition, University of Washington
VA Puget Sound Health Care System
Seattle, Washington
*Possible Hormonal Mechanisms Mediating the Effects of
Bariatric Surgery*

Roger A. de la Torre, MD
Associate Professor, Deptarment of Surgery
University of Missouri School of Medicine
Director of Minimally Invasive Surgery
DePaul Weight Loss Institute, DePaul Health Center
Columbia, Missouri
Laparoscopic Gastric Bypass: Transgastric Circular Stapler

Lucinéia Bernardes de Lima, MD
Belo Horizonte, Brazil
Laparoscopic Biliopancreatic Diversion: Approach

Raymond L. Drew, MD
Adjunct Assistant Professor, Department of Surgery
University of Minnesota, Minneapolis, Minnesota
The Learning Curve

Sanjeev Dutta, MD, MA, FRCSC
Assistant Professor of Surgery and Pediatrics
Lucile Packard Children's Hospital
Stanford University Medical Center
Stanford, California
Adolescent Bariatric Surgery

Álvaro Antônio Bandeira Ferraz, MD, PhD
Associte Professor, Department of Surgery
Federal University of Pernambuco
Hospital das Clínicas
Recife, Brazil
Infection in Obesity Surgery

Edmundo Machado Ferraz, MD, PhD, FACS
Chief, Professor, and Chairman, Department of Surgery
Pernambuco Federal University (UFPE)
Recife, Brazil
Infection in Obesity Surgery

Fauze Maluf Filho, MD
Associate Professor, Department of Gastroenterology
Gastrointestinal Endoscopy Unit
University of São Paulo Medical School
São Paulo, Brazil
Endoscopic Evaluation and Treatment

Adriana Sales Finizola, MD
Surgeon, Maringá Obesity Center
Maringá, Brazil
Laparoscopic Gastric Bypass: Silastic Ring

Matthew A. Fitzer, MD
Faxton-St. Luke's Healthcare,
New Hartford, New York
Laparoscopic Gastric Bypass: Transgastric Circular Stapler

Karen E. Foster-Schubert, MD
Acting Instructor, Department of Medicine
Division of Metabolism
Endocrinology, and Nutrition
University of Washington School of Medicine
VA Puget Sound Health Care System
Seattle, Washington
*Possible Hormonal Mechanisms Mediating the Effects of
Bariatric Surgery*

Eldo E. Frezza, MD, MBA, FACS
Division of General Surgery, Department of Surgery
Texas Tech University Health Sciences Center
Lubbock, Texas
Cost and Economic Impact of Bariatric Surgery

Daniel J. Gagné, MD
Assistant Professor of Surgery, Temple University School of
Medicine, Director of Bariatric and Minimally Invasive
    Surgery
Western Pennsylvania Hospital
Pittsburgh, Pennsylvania
*Restrictive Procedures: Laparoscopic Revision of Vertical
Banding to Gastric Bypass*

Michel Gagner, MD, FRCSC, FACS
Professor of Surgery, Joan and Stanford I. Weill Medical
    College of Cornell University
Chief of Laparoscopic and Bariatric Surgery
New York-Presbyterian Hospital
New York, New York
*Laparoscopic Restrictive Procedures: Sleeve Gastrectomy;
Two-Stage Approach for High-Risk Patients*

Bruno Geloneze, MD, PhD
Professor of Endocrinology and Medical
    Director of Laboratory of Investigation on Obesity
Metabolism, and Diabetes (LIMED)
University of Campinas (UNICAMP)
Campinas, Brazil
Metabolic Syndrome: Diagnosis, Clinical Presentations, and Surgical Treatment

Carolina G. Goncalves, MD
Clinical Fellow, Department of General Surgery
Division of Advanced Laparoscopic and Bariatric Surgery
Cleveland Clinic
Cleveland, Ohio
Physiology and Metabolism in Obesity Surgery: Roux-en-Y Gastric Bypass

Luiz Henrique de Sousa, MD
Professor, University of São Paulo, Chief of Staff
Division of Obesity Surgery, Hospital Fêmina
Goiânia, Brazil
Requirements of the Clinic and Institution

Luiz Henrique de Sousa Filho, MD
Clinical Staff, Division of Bariatric Surgery
Hospital Fêmina
Goiânia, Brazil
Requirements of the Clinic and Institution

Kelvin D. Higa, MD, FACS
President Elect, American Society for Metabolic and
    Bariatric Surgery
Clinical Professor of Surgery
University of California, San Francisco
Private Practice
Fresno, California
Laparoscopic Gastric Bypass: Hand Sewn

Jennifer Elizabeth Higa
Fresno, California
Laparoscopic Gastric Bypass: Hand Sewn

Frédéric-Simon Hould, MD
Department of Surgery, Laval University, Laval Hospital
Quebec, Canada
Malabsorptive Procedures: Duodenal Switch

Kenneth B. Jones, Jr., MD
Clinical Assistant Professor, Department of Surgery
Louisiana State University Health Sciences Center
Former President, American Society of Bariatric Surgery
Shreveport, Louisiana
Current Role of Open Bariatric Surgery

Julie J. Kim, MD
Center for Minimally Invasive Obesity Surgery
Tufts-New England, Medical Center
Boston, Massachusetts
Late Complications: Ulcers, Stenosis, and Fistula

Ester Labrunie, MD, PhD
Professor, Department of Medicine
Federal University of Rio de Janeiro (UFRJ)
Rio de Janerio, Brazil
Radiographic Evaluation and Treatment; Radiographic Evaluation and Treatment: Intervention

Stéfane Lebel, MD
Department of Surgery, Laval Hospital, Laval University
Quebec, Canada
Malabsorptive Procedures: Duodenal Switch

Luiz Cláudio Lerner, MD
Medical Staff, Department of Anesthesiology
Hospital Universitário
Clementino Fraga Filho
Universidade Federal do Rio de Janeiro
Rio de Janerió, Brazil
Anesthetic Concerns

Odette Lescelleur, MD
Department of Surgery, Laval University, Laval Hospital
Quebec, Canada
Malabsorptive Procedures: Duodenal Switch

Marcelo Simas Lima, MD
Research Fellow, Gastrointestinal Endoscopy Unit
University of São Paulo Medical School
São Paulo, Brazil
Endoscopic Evaluation and Treatment

Angelo Loss, MD, ACBC
Abdominal Surgery Post-graduation School
Rio de Janeiro Federal University
Cid Pitombo Clinic, Member
Brazilian College of Surgeons, Member
Brazilian Society of Laparoscopic Surgery
Rio de Janeiro, Brazil
Intraoperative Issues; Gastric Pacing

Kenneth G. MacDonald, Jr., MD
Professor, Department of Surgery
Brody School of Medicine at East Carolina University
Southern Surgical Associates
Greenville, North Carolina
Early Complications in Bariatric Surgery

Daniéla Magro, PhD
Professor, Researcher, and Collaborator
Department of Preventive and Social Medicine
Medical Science School (FCM)
University of Campinas (UNICAMP)
Campinas, Brazil
Weight Recidivism

José E. Manso, MD
Associate Professor, Department of Surgery
Federal University of Rio de Janeiro, Chief Editor
The Journal of the Brazilian College of Surgeons
Rio de Janeiro, Brazil
Intraoperative Issues

Picard Marceau, MD, PhD, FRCS, FACS
Professor, Department of Surgery, Laval University
Laval Hospital, Quebec, Canada
Malabsorptive Procedures: Duodenal Switch

Simon Marceau, MD
Department of Surgery, Laval University, Laval Hospital
Quebec, Canada
Malabsorptive Procedures: Duodenal Switch

João Batista Marchesini, MD, PhD, FACS
Senior Professor of Surgery
Post Graduate Course in Clinical Surgery,
Associate Professor of Surgery (retired)
Paraná University Medical School
Former President of the Brazilian Society for Bariatric
    Surgery, Certified in General Surgery by the American
    Board of Surgery (USA)
Curitiba, Brazil
*Biliopancreatic Diversion: Duodenal Switch; Intragastric
Balloon*

Edson Marchiori, MD
Professor and Head, Department of Medicine
University Federal Fluminense
Rio de Janeiro, Brazil
*Radiographic Evaluation and Treatment; Radiographic
Evaluation and Treatment: Intervention*

Robert T. Marema, MD, FACS
Medical Director, Division of Bariatric Surgery,
    Flagler Hospital
St. Augustine, Florida
*Laparoscopic Gastric Bypass: Evolution, Safety, and Efficacy of
the Banded Gastric Bypass*

Edward E. Mason, MD, PhD, FACS
Emeritus Professor of Surgery, Roy J. and Lucille A. Carver
College of Medicine, University of Iowa Hospitals and Clinics
Iowa City, Iowa
Restrictive Surgery

CJL. Mendes, MD
Specialist in General Surgery
Member of the Sociedade Brasileira de Cirurgia Bariátrica
ATLS Instructor, the USP Medicine University
Former Professor and Head of Emergency Room
Hospital Escola in the Medicine University of Santo Amaro
São Paulo, Brazil
Laparoscopic Roux-en-Y Banded Gastric Bypass

Pablo R. Miguel, MD
Laparoscopic Surgeon, Mãe de Deus Hospital
Porto Allegre, RS, Brazil
Intragastric Balloon

Marcel Milcent, MD, ACBC
Abdominal Surgery Post-Graduation School
Rio de Janeiro Federal University,
Cid Pitombo Clinic, Brazilian College of Surgeons Member,
IFSO Member, Brazilian Society for Bariatric Surgery
    Member
Brazilian Society for Laparoscopic Surgery Member
Rio de Janeiro, Brazil
Intraoperative Issues; Gastric Pacing

Karl A. Miller, MD, FACS
Associate Professor of Surgery, Head, Department of Surgery,
Ludwig-Boltzmann-Institute for Gastroenterology and
    Experimental Surgery, Hospital Hallein
Obesity Surgery Center, Krakenhaus Hallein
Hallein, Austria
*Laparoscopic Restrictive Procedures: Adjustable Gastric
Banding*

Melodie K. Moorehead, PhD
Drs. Moorehead, Prish, & Associates, P.A.
Fort Lauderdale, Florida
Bariatric Surgery Psychology

Daoud Nasser, MD
Professor of Surgery, Maringá State University
Chief Surgeon, Maringá Obesity Center
Maringá, Brazil
Laparoscopic Gastric Bypass: Silastic Ring

Ninh T. Nguyen, MD
Associate Professor of Surgery, Department of Surgery, Chief
Division of Gastrointestinal Surgery, University of California
Irvine Medical Center
Orange, California
Rationale for Minimally Invasive Bariatric Surgery

Paul E. O'Brien, MD, FRACS
Director, Centre for Obesity Research and Education,
Monash University Medical School
The Center for Obesity Research and Education (CORE)
Melbourne, Australia
*Restrictive Procedures: Utilization of Adjustable Gastric
Banding for Failed Stapled Operations*

Joost Overduin, PhD
Division of Metabolism, Endocrinology, and Nutrition
Department of Medicine, University of Washington
VA Puget Sound Health Care System
Seattle, Washington
*Possible Hormonal Mechanisms Mediating the Effects of
Bariatric Surgery*

Dyker Santos Paiva, MD
Laparoscopic Biliopancreatic Diversion: Approach

José Carlos Pareja, MD, PhD
Professor, Department of Surgery, Head of Pancreas,
Biliary, and Obesity Surgery
Campinas State University (UNICAMP)
President, Scientific Committee, Brazilian Society for
    Bariatric Surgery
Campinas, Brazil
Weight Recidivism

Michael Perez, MD, FACS
U.S. Bariatric
Fort Lauderdale, Florida
*Laparoscopic Gastric Bypass: Evolution, Safety, and Efficacy
of the Banded Gastric Bypass*

Cid Pitombo, MD, PhD, TCBC
General and Bariatric Surgery
Minimally Invasive Surgery
Campinas State University (UNICAMP)
Rio de Janeiro/Campinas, Brazil
*Central Nervous System Regulation and Hormonal Signaling;
Radiographic Evaluation and Treatment; Radiographic
Evaluation and Treatment: Intervention*

Walter J. Pories, MD, FACS
Professor of Surgery, Biochemistry, Exercise, and Sport
    Sciences, Metabolic Institute
Brody School of Medicine at East Carolina University
Chief, Metabolic Institute, Former President ASBS
Greenville, North Carolina
Nutritional Consequences and Management

Robert A. Rabkin, MD, FACS
Pacific Laparoscopy, St. Mary's Medical Center
California Pacific Medical Center
San Francisco, California
Hand-Assisted Laparoscopic Duodenal Switch

Francesco Rubino, MD
Assistant Professor, Department of Surgery
Catholic University, Rome, Italy
Attending Surgeon, European Institute of Technology
    (IRCAD-EITS), University Louis Paster
Strasbourg, France
*Physiology and Metabolism in Obesity Surgery: Roux-en-Y
Gastric Bypass*

Paulo Sakai, MD, PhD
Associate Professor of Gastroenterology
Gastrointestinal Endoscopy Unit
University of São Paulo Medical School
São Paulo, Brazil
Endoscopic Evaluation and Treatment

José A. Sallet, MD
São Paulo, Brazil
Intragastric Balloon

Paulo C. Sallet, MD
São Paulo, Brazil
Intragastric Balloon

Edson Lemes Sardinha, MD
Collaborative Professor of CET-SBA
Federal University of Goiás
Goiânia, Brazil
Requirements of the Clinic and Institution

Philip R. Schauer, MD
Professor of Surgery, Cleveland Clinic Lerner College of
    Medicine
Director, Division of Advanced Laparoscopic and Bariatric
    Surgery, Bariatric and Metabolic Institute
Cleveland, Ohio
*Physiology and Metabolism in Obesity Surgery: Roux-en-Y
Gastric Bypass*

Michael L. Schwartz, MD, PhD
Adjunct Professor of Surgery, University of Minnesota
Minneapolis, Minnesota
The Learning Curve

Nicola Scopinaro, MD, FACS (Hon)
Professor of Surgery, University of Genoa School of Medicine,
Genoa, Italy
*Malabsorptive Procedures: Biliopancreatic
Diversion-Scopinaro Procedure; Biliopancreatic Diversion:
Revisional Surgery*

J. Stephen Scott, MD, FACS
Associate Professor, Department of Surgery
University of Missouri School of Medicine
Medical Director, DePaul Weight Loss Institute
DePaul Health Center, Columbia, Missouri
Laparoscopic Gastric Bypass: Transgastric Circular Stapler

Michael H. Shannon, MD
Senior Fellow, Division of Nedocrinology
Department of Medicine, University of Washington
VA Puget Sound Health Care System
Seattle, Washington
*Possible Hormonal Mechanisms Mediating the Effects of
Bariatric Surgery*

Scott A. Shikora, MD
Professor of Srugery, Tufts University School of Medicine,
Chief of Bariatric Surgery
Center for Minimally Invasive Obesity Surgery
Tufts-New England Medical Center
Boston, Massachusetts
Late Complications: Ulcers, Stenosis, and Fistula

Contributors

Christine Simard, MD, FRCP, CD
Department of Surgery, Laval University, Laval Hospital
Quebec, Canada
Malabsorptive Procedures: Duodenal Switch

Serge Simard, MSc
Biostatistician, Laval University
Laval Hospital Research Center
Quebec, Canada
Malabsorptive Procedures: Duodenal Switch

Harvey J. Sugerman, MD, FACS
Professor Emeritus, Department of Surgery
Virginia Commonwealth University,
Editor-in-Chief, Surgery for Obesity and Related Diseases
    Sanibel, Florida
Pathophysiology of Severe Obesity and the Effects of Surgically Induced Weight Loss

Thomas Szegö, MD, PhD
Albert Einstein Hospital
São Paulo, Brazil
Laparoscopic Roux-en-Y Banded Gastric Bypass

Marcos Tambascia, MD
Professor, University of Campinas
Campinas, Brazil
Preoperative Evaluation of Patients

Michael E. Tarnoff, MD
Assistant Professor, Division of Bariatric and Minimally
    Invasive Surgery, Department of Surgery
Tufts-New England Medical Center
Boston, Massachusetts
Late Complications: Ulcers, Stenosis, and Fistula

Ampadi Thampi, MD, MS, FRCS
Fellow in Bariatric and Laparoscopic Surgery
Division of Gastrointestinal Surgery
Department of Surgery, Brody School of Medicine
    at East Carolina University
Pitt County Memorial Hospital
    Greenville, North Carolina
Nutritional Consequences and Management

Renam Catharina Tinoco, MD, TCBC, FACS
Professor, Department of Surgery
University Rio de Janeiro State
São Jose do Avai Hospital
Itaperuna, Brazil
Laparoscopic Gastric Bypass: Trans-Oral Circular Stapling

Augusto Claudio Tinoco, MD
Professor, Department of General Surgery
São Jose do Avai Hospital
Itaperuna, Brazil
Laparoscopic Gastric Bypass: Trans-Oral Circular Stapling

RoseMarie Toussaint, MD, FACS
Ypsilanti, Michigan
Laparoscopic Gastric Bypass: Evolution, Safety, and Efficacy of the Banded Gastric Bypass

Esteban Varela, MD
Department of Surgery, University of California
Irvine Medical Center
Orange, California
Rationale for Minimally Invasive Bariatric Surgery

Michael D. Williams, MD, FACS
Chief of Surgery, Emory Dunwoody Medical Center
Laparoscopic and Endoscopic Surgery Institute, P.C.
Marietta, Georgia
Laparoscopic Gastric Bypass: Linear Technique

Samuel E. Wilson, MD
Department of Surgery, University of California
Irvine Medical Center
Orange, California
Rationale for Minimally Invasive Bariatric Surgery

Alan Wittgrove, MD
Medical Director, Wittgrove Bariatric Center
Scripps Memorial Hospital
La Jolla, California
Laparoscopic Gastric Bypass: Circular Stapler Technique

Kendi Yamazaki, MD
Senior Resident, Gastrointestinal Endoscopy Unit
Hospital das Clinicas,
University of São Paulo Medical School
São Paulo, Brazil
Endoscopic Evaluation and Treatment

Michael Barker, MD
Brody School of Medicine,
East Carolina University
Greenville
Nutritional Consequences and Management

Georgia Bartholdi, MD
General and Bariatric Surgery
Cid Pitombo Clinic
Rio de Janiero, Brazil
Gastric Pacing

Foreword

Anticipation is warranted in the reading of this book. Obesity surgery has attained wide acceptance. Each author has a different special interest based upon training and background, but all with a common interest and desire to help the severely obese through the use of one or more surgical operations. This monumental effort marks a time of change. We have a rich retrospective view of 100 years of operations on the stomach, used for treatment of so-called peptic ulcer, and 40 years for treatment of severe obesity. In the hands of surgeons with extensive experience, the 30-day operative mortality has decreased to less than one-half percent. Half of the deaths occur after discharge. A low risk combined with increasing numbers of operations can result in unacceptable numbers of deaths. We must find ways to reduce the prevalence of operative mortality. This will probably be by decreasing lethal complications but more importantly involving the patient in his or her postoperative care through greater knowledge of what has been done to anatomy, how it can cause lethal complications, and how to recognize the need for emergency return to the hospital.

Laparoscopic and robotic surgery is so kind to the abdominal wall that patients can often leave the hospital in a few days. There are fewer adhesions, wound infections, and hernias. Between 1980 and 2000 the prevalence of people in the United States with a BMI of 30 doubled. There is increasing awareness that obesity is a disease that can be successfully treated with a surgical operation. There is currently a rapid increase in the number of excellent centers for obesity surgery but this will not provide for the needs of millions of severely obese patients. We should be operating earlier before there are irreversible changes but this increases the demand for limited resources. The more complex operations require more lifelong monitoring and care. Patients need to become the most important member of their care team, able to inform others of their new anatomy and the lifelong complications that need prevention, diagnosis, and treatment.

A well-designed, simple restriction operation would seem to be the logical solution to some of the problems that are a result of radical changes in anatomy and ever-increasing use of surgical operations. In the United States very few patients are offered a simple restrictive operation that has a minimum of foreign material. The history of stomach surgery is one of decreasing complexity and abandonment of surgery, as new and more effective medications become available and as the lifelong side effects and complications increase in prevalence. Prevalence of complications increases with time after an operation and also with increasing use of an operation. There remain many questions about the lifelong effects. Some will be answered in this book and more will be raised. The future of surgical treatment of obesity rests with those who find the best answers for the most patients. Are we making adequate use of the greatest-available and ever-present resource, well-informed and involved patients?

Edward E. Mason, MD, PhD, FACS

Preface

The way modern men lead their lives—or sometimes are led by it—is far different than the way our ancestors did. The speed of this change has not been followed, however, by the natural physiological modifications that would adapt us to less physical effort and more food availability. We ate the necessary, now we eat unnecessarily. We strived for food, now we call for delivery. The advance of obesity (and its well-known consequences) is the most trivial result in this conjuncture.

Bariatric surgery has grown exponentially in recent years, but its contribution has had little impact on the pandemic of morbid obesity. This book goes into some detail of the history, the present day application of our science to the problem, and predictions for the future.

Several bariatric procedures have been developed in the past decades and were diffused throughout the world. Techniques such as the gastric bypass procedure (GBP), the treatment of choice in some countries (i.e., US and Brazil), may not display the same status in others, with different cultural and socioeconomic conditions. Biliopancreatic diversions (BPDs) are the choice in some other places (Italy, Canada) and gain more adepts in the United States every day. The adjustable gastric banding is the preference in most of Europe and in Australia.

The reader will quickly see that this is not a book based solely on technique, pre- and post-op care, minimally invasive surgery, or any other specific entities peculiar to bariatric surgery. It is all the above, and, as a special treat, a number of videos on technique are included. Our purpose is to emphasize the fact that bariatric operations go far beyond being "just an operation." A book a bit different from the usual was then pursued, for being a bariatric (or metabolic) surgeon demands knowledge not only of technical aspects of the procedures accepted to date, but also, and perhaps even more, of the physiological complexities involved in the anatomical modifications imposed by each one of them. These alterations have indeed led us to a wide range of new information that we still begin to assimilate. Today, we bariatric surgeons discuss physiology, hormones, central nervous system (CNS) signaling and interact with a variety of medical specialists.

The physiological understanding of each technique was described by its respective *inventor*. Endocrinologists, psychologists, clinicians, and researchers were also invited to this debate.

We could summarize all this as a great achievement. It is extremely exciting to know that we managed to unite in one publication the most reliable worldwide experience on obesity surgery so far.

Cid Pitombo, MD, PhD
Kenneth B. Jones, Jr., MD
Kelvin D. Higa, MD
José Carlos Pareja, MD, PhD

Basic Principles

Evolution of Surgery for Morbid Obesity

Henry Buchwald, MD, PhD • Jane N. Buchwald, MA

INTRODUCTION

The history of bariatric surgery is relatively short, highly productive, imaginative, and one with tremendous impact on the history of surgery, the development of laparoscopic surgery, and the world epidemic of morbid obesity.

This history extends only slightly longer than 50 years in duration, a post–World War II phenomenon of the late twentieth century. During these 50 years, over 50 operations, or variations of operations, have been proposed to manage morbid obesity. These procedures have involved inducing malabsorption, restricting consumption, combinations of malabsorption and restriction, electrical stimulation, gastric balloons, and extra-gastrointestinal innovations. The nuances proposed within these broad categories are a testimonial to the varied, and often convoluted, thought processes of surgeons and other pioneers in obesity therapy.

There have been few, if any, surgical applications that have so radically changed the field of surgery as has bariatric surgery. From an obscure procedure occasionally performed, often derided by other physicians and even surgeons, bariatric surgery has come to dominate general surgery. In many hospitals and specialty centers, bariatric surgery is the most common class of operations being performed. As laparoscopic techniques have been applied to more and more procedures, nowhere has laparoscopy become more prevalent than in bariatric surgery. This development of laparoscopic bariatric surgery has impacted hospitals and device manufacturers, all eager to offer up-to-date laparoscopic operating room suites, laparoscopic instrumentation, and robotics.

At the turn of the twenty-first century, overweight (body mass index (BMI) ≥ 25 kg/m^2) is a world epidemic involving nearly two billion people, including nearly two-thirds of US citizens, of whom 50–60 million are obese (BMI ≥ 30 kg/m^2) and about 10 million are morbidly obese (BMI ≥ 40 or ≥ 35 with significant comorbidities). This epidemic of obesity affects one out of every four adults in the United States and one out of every five children. The comorbid conditions of morbid obesity are responsible for a decrease in life expectancy of about 9 years in women and of about 12 years in men. Unfortunately, long-term weight loss results with diet therapy, with and without support organizations, has failed in the treatment of this disease. There are currently no truly effective pharmaceutical agents to treat obesity, especially morbid obesity. Bariatric surgery today is the treatment of choice and the only effective therapy in the management of morbid obesity. It is, therefore, incumbent on every surgeon, in particular the bariatric surgeon, as well as the rest of the medical profession, and, to some extent, private and government health-care providers, the public, especially the obese public, to have knowledge of the evolution of surgical procedures for morbid obesity.

Previous publications have traced this history in a linear thematic manner—i.e., the history of malabsorptive procedures, malabsorptive/restrictive procedures, purely restrictive procedures, and other procedures (Figure 1–1).[1] This chapter will look at the bariatric surgery innovations over the past 50 years in cross-section, or horizontally, by decade, in order to provide a chronology of concurrent concepts, at times competitive, at times complementary, and at times oblivious of parallel developments. Table 1–1 provides a chronological overview of the surgical innovations for morbid obesity.

1950s

The first operation specifically performed to induce weight loss was the jejunoileal bypass. This was a strictly malabsorptive procedure. In 1953, Dr. Richard L. Varco of the Department of Surgery at the University of Minnesota probably performed the first jejunoileal bypass.[2] His operation consisted of an end-to-end jejunoileostomy with a separate ileocecostomy for drainage of the bypassed segment (Figure 1–2). Varco did not publish this innovation, and his contribution may well have been preceded by an intestinal resection specifically for the management of obesity by Victor Henriksson of Gothenberg, Sweden.[3]

In 1954, Kremen, Linner, and Nelson published the first citation of jejunoileal bypass as a weight-loss procedure.[4] In the Discussion section of their research article on the nutritional aspects of the small intestine in dogs, they described a patient upon whom they had performed an end-to-end jejunoileal bypass for reduction of body weight.

The 1950s ended with no formal publication on a series of patients undergoing bariatric surgery, reflecting a general lack of interest by surgeons and others in this concept.

1960s

The concept of selective malnutrition did not, however, die out. There were other innovators who asked the question of whether the "short-gut syndrome" could not be harnessed as treatment for the morbidly obese. Surgical-instituted controlled malabsorption would ideally provide for massive weight loss, eventual weight maintenance, minimal short- and long-term side effects and complications, and reversibility. The complications of malabsorptive surgery would determine the cost/benefit ratios of the malabsorptive procedures. Reversibility was essential in order to provide a safe retreat from a potential iatrogenic catastrophe.

About 10 years after its origin, bariatric surgery immerged into its exploratory phase. In 1963, Payne, DeWind, and Commons published the results of the first clinical program with massive intestinal bypass for the management of morbidly obese patients.[5] In a series they had actually initiated in 1956, they described bypassing nearly the entire small intestine, the right colon, and half of the transverse colon in 10 morbidly obese female patients. They restored intestinal continuity by a T-shaped end-to-side anastomosis of the proximal 37.5 cm of jejunum to the mid-transverse colon. Weight loss was dramatic, but electrolyte imbalance, uncontrolled diarrhea, and liver failure proved prohibitive and required eventual reversal of this jejunoileal bypass.[6] Payne and DeWind actually conceived their original procedure to lead to unlimited weight loss, requiring a second operation to restore additional intestinal length and weight equilibrium when ideal body weight was attained. They never achieved body-weight maintenance following their second operation, since their patients regained their lost weight.[7] This proved to be a valuable lesson for the future: If the bariatric procedure is reversed, morbidly obese patients will regain their preoperative weight.

Proceeding in a similar fashion to the original work of Payne and DeWind, Lewis, Turnbull, and Page reported on their series of end-to-side jejunotransverse colostomy bypasses, in which the proximal 75 cm of jejunum was anastomosed to the transverse colon. As in Payne's and DeWind's series, significant complications eventually required reversal of these bypasses.[8]

In the mid-1960s, Sherman et al.,[9] along with Payne and Dewind,[7] proposed abandonment of anastomosis to the colon and, instead, advocated restoration of intestinal continuity proximal to the ileocecal valve by an end-to-side jejunoileostomy. The aim of this less radical bypass was to achieve an eventual balance between caloric intake and body caloric needs, eliminating the necessity for a second operation and minimizing postoperative side effects. In 1966, Lewis, Turnbull, and Page described their second series of jejunoileal bypass patients, 11 individuals in whom they had performed an end-to-side jejunocecostomy.[10] In 1969, in a series of 80 morbidly obese patients, Payne and DeWind established what was to become a standard for the end-to-side jejunoileostomy procedure: Anastomosis of the proximal 35 cm

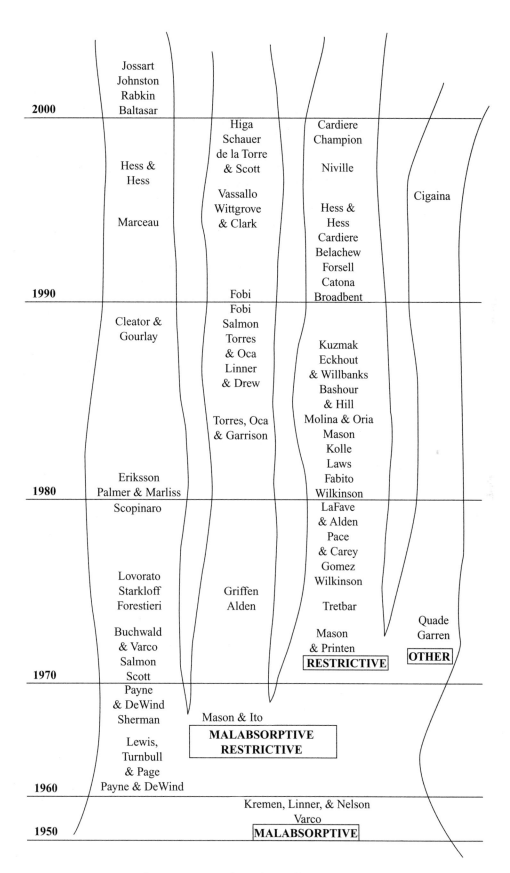

Figure 1–1. Genealogical tree of bariatric surgery.

Table 1–1.

Chronological Overview of Procedures for Morbid Obesity

	Malabsorptive	Malabsorptive/Restrictive	Restrictive	Other
1950s	1953 Varco 1954 Kremen, Linner, Nelson			
1960s	1963 Payne & DeWind 1965 Sherman 1966 Lewis, Turnbull, Page 1969 Payne & DeWind	1966 Mason & Ito		
1970s	1971 Scott 1971 Salmon 1971 Buchwald & Varco 1977 Forestieri 1978 Starkloff 1978 Lavorato 1979 Scopinaro	1977 Alden 1977 Griffen	1971 Mason & Printen 1976 Tretbar 1978 Wilkinson 1979 Gomez 1979 Pace & Carey 1979 LaFave & Alden	1974 Quaade
1980s	1980 Palmer & Marliss 1981 Erikson 1988 Cleator & Gourley	1983 Torres, Oca, Garrison 1986 Linner & Drew 1987 Torres & Oca 1988 Salmon 1989 Fobi	1980 Wilkinson 1981 Fabito 1981 Laws 1982 Kolle 1982 Mason 1983 Molina & Oria 1985 Bashour & Hill 1986 Eckhout & Willbanks 1986 Kuzmak	1985 Garren
1990s	1993 Marceau 1998 Hess & Hess	1991 Fobi 1994 Wittgrove & Clark 1997 Vassallo 1999 de la Torre & Scott 1999 Schauer 1999 Higa	1993 Broadbent 1993 Catona 1993 Forsell 1993 Belachew 1994 Cardiere 1994 Hess & Hess 1998 Niville 1999 Champion 1999 Cadière	1996 Cigaina
2000s	2001 Baltasar 2003 Rabkin 2003 Johnston 2006 Jossart			

(14 inches) of jejunum to the terminal ileum, 10 cm (4 inches) from the ileocecal valve.[7] This operation, known as the "14 + 4," became the most commonly used bariatric operation and version of the jejunoileal bypass in the United States (Figure 1–3). This procedure allowed for significant weight loss with moderate long-term side effects and complications, and did not require a second restorative operation.

In the mid-1960s, a separate genus of bariatric operations evolved independently from the jejunoileal bypass. These procedures combined intestinal malabsorption

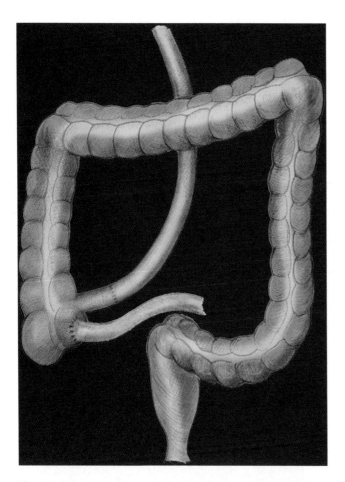

Figure 1–2. 1953 Varco and 1954 Kremen, Linner, Nelson: Jejunoileal bypass—end-to-end jejunoileostomy with ileocecostomy.

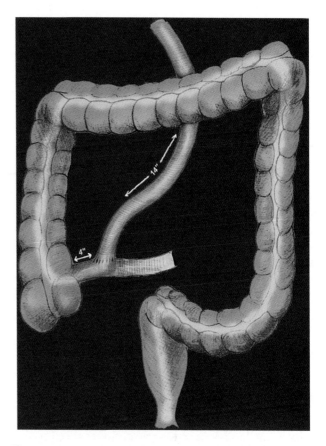

Figure 1–3. 1969 Payne and DeWind: Jejunoileal bypass—classic 14″ + 4″ end-to-side jejunoileostomy.

with gastric restriction, relying primarily on gastric restriction for weight loss. Minimal long-term complications associated with the malabsorptive/restrictive gastric bypass procedures made them preferable to the jejunoileal bypass procedures. Though the jejunoileal bypass was a highly effective weight-reduction operation, it was associated with gas-bloat syndrome, steatorrhea, electrolyte imbalance, nephrolithiasis, hepatic fibrosis, cutaneous eruptions, and impaired mentation.[2] The gastric bypass easily supplanted the jejunoileal bypass but it was not free of problems. Gastric bypass can cause dumping, iron deficiency anemia, vitamin B$_{12}$ malabsorption, and loss of the ability to visualize the distal stomach and duodenum. In addition, bowel obstruction in a patient with a gastric bypass can be catastrophic with reflux into the bypassed gastric remnant, which, without an outlet for decompression, can rupture.

The first gastric bypass was developed by Mason and Ito in 1966.[11] In their original procedure, the stomach was divided horizontally, without the benefit of a stapling device, and a loop (not Roux) gastrojejunostomy was created between the proximal gastric pouch and the proximal jejunum (Figure 1–4). The original upper gastric pouch was 100–150 mL in volume, with a stoma of 12 mm in diameter.

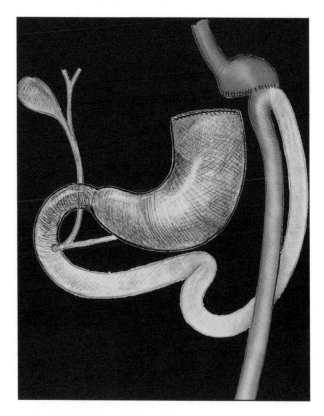

Figure 1–4. 1967 Mason and Ito: Gastric bypass—gastric transection with loop gastrojejunostomy.

Thus, the 1960s closed out with the jejunoileal bypass as the primary bariatric procedure, itself in a state of development, and gastric restrictive surgery making a quiet appearance.

1970s

The 1970s was a decade of high activity in bariatric surgery. Modifications and large series of jejunoileal bypass procedures were published before the decline and essential disappearance of that approach. Its malabsorptive successor—the biliopancreatic diversion—emerged. Gastric bypass was refined and dominated bariatric surgery in the United States. Mason moved on to restrictive bariatric surgery and the development of gastroplasty. Others sowed the seeds for prosthetic gastric restriction. And at least one innovator started to explore entirely extra-gastrointestinal means to treat morbid obesity.

Although Payne and DeWind's classic jejunoileal bypass was widely adopted, nearly 10% of patients did not achieve significant weight loss. It was believed that this might be due to a reflux of nutrients into the bypassed ileum.[6] Thus, Scott et al.,[12] Salmon,[13] and Buchwald and Varco[14] independently returned to the original Varco and Kremen procedure of an end-to-end anastomosis to prevent reflux into the terminal ileum. In all these end-to-end operations, the ileocecal valve was preserved in order to decrease postoperative diarrhea and electrolyte loss, the appendix was removed, and the jejunal stump was attached to the transverse mesocolon or the cecum to avoid intussusception. In 1971, Scott et al. reported 12 morbidly obese patients in whom 30 cm of jejunum was anastomosed to 30 cm of ileum, with the bypassed bowel drained into the transverse or sigmoid colon.[12] Also in 1971, Salmon reported his variation of the end-to-end jejunoileostomy: 25 cm of jejunum was anastomosed to 50 cm of ileum, and the bypassed bowel was drained into the mid-transverse colon.[13] In the same year, 1971, Buchwald and Varco reported a series in which 40 cm of jejunum was anastomosed to 4 cm of ileum, with the bypassed bowel drained into the cecum near the ileocecal valve.[14] In addition to producing significant weight loss, Buchwald and Varco reported that their operation provided marked amelioration of hyperlipidemia. In their series, preoperatively hyperlipidemic patients showed an average decrease in cholesterol of 90% (from 898 to 90 mg/dL), and a reduction in average triglycerides of 96% (from 7,255 to 230 mg/dL).

In other attempts to deal with the ileal reflux problem, a series of modifications were introduced but rarely performed by others than the primary authors. Forestieri et al.,[15] Starkloff et al.,[16] and Palmer and Marliss[17] created various modifications of the end-to-side jejunoileal anastomosis to prevent reflux into the bypassed segment without the necessity of dividing the ileum and separately draining the bypassed segment.

In the 1970s, the modern malabsorptive procedures emerged. These operations share a key trait: No limb of the small intestine is left without flow through it. The enteric limb has the flow of food, and the biliary or biliopancreatic limb contains the flow of either bile or bile and pancreatic juice. In 1978, Lavorato et al. performed a standard end-to-side jejunoileal bypass; however, they anastomosed the proximal end of the bypassed segment of the small intestine to the gallbladder, thereby diverting bile into the bypassed limb.[18] Several years later, actually in the 1980s, a similar operation was published by Eriksson.[19] These biliointestinal bypasses have not been widely performed, and the modern malabsorptive operative era began with Scopinaro et al.'s biliopancreatic diversion, first described in 1979.[20]

Thousands of biliopancreatic diversions have now been performed, particularly in Italy, mainly by Dr. Scopinaro. His current biliopancreatic diversion consists of a horizontal partial gastrectomy (leaving 200–500 mL of proximal stomach) with closure of the duodenal stump, gastrojejunostomy with a 250-cm Roux limb, and anastomosis of the long biliopancreatic limb to the Roux limb 50 cm proximal to the ileocecal valve, creating an extremely short common channel (Figure 1–5).[21]

Even though Mason turned his attention to gastroplasty, others did not. In 1977, Alden performed a

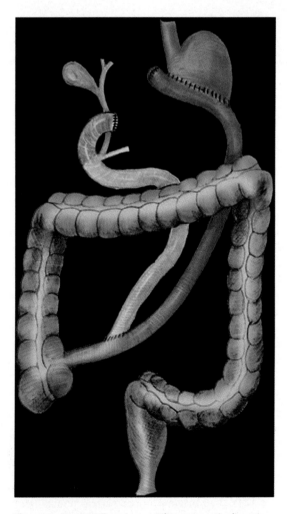

Figure 1–5. 1979 Scopinaro: Biliopancreatic diversion.

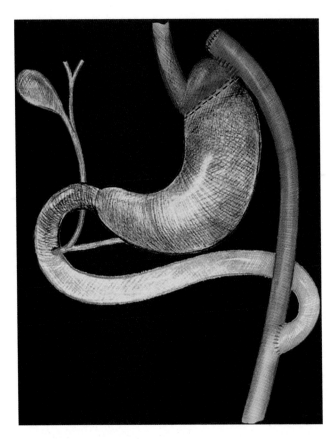

Figure 1–6. 1977 Griffen: Gastric bypass—horizontal gastric stapling with Roux gastrojejunostomy.

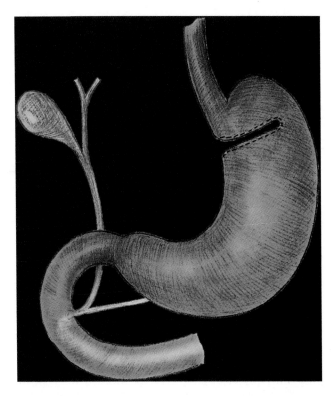

Figure 1–7. 1971 Mason and Printen: Gastroplasty—partial gastric transection, greater curvature conduit.

gastrointestinal bypass consisting of a horizontal staple-line without gastric division and a loop gastrojejunostomy.[22] Also in 1977, Griffen et al. reported on the use of a horizontal gastric bypass, but with a Roux-en-Y gastrojejunostomy rather than a loop gastrojejunostomy (Figure 1–6).[23] This gastrointestinal bypass had the advantage of avoiding tension on the loop and preventing bile reflux into the upper gastric pouch.[24] Both Griffen et al.[23] and Buckwalter[25] reported randomized studies demonstrating that Roux-en-Y gastrointestinal bypass patients were achieving weight loss equivalent to that previously seen after the jejunoileal bypass and associated with far fewer side effects and complications. The simple modifications of Mason's gastric bypass by Alden and Griffen changed the tenor of bariatric surgery and for the next two decades established gastric bypass as the dominant operation in this field.

Very early in the 1970s (1971) Mason and Printen performed the first restrictive bariatric surgery procedure.[26] In their 1971 gastroplasty procedure, they divided the stomach horizontally from lesser curvature to greater curvature, leaving an undivided gastric conduit at the greater curvature (Figure 1–7). In principle, the solely restrictive operations have fewer problems than the gastric bypass, can be performed more rapidly, do not involve entry into the bowel or an anastomosis, and are fundamentally more physiologic, since no part of the gastrointestinal tract is bypassed or rerouted.

The original gastric restrictive procedure of Mason was unsuccessful in maintaining weight loss.[26,27] In 1979, Gomez introduced the horizontal gastric stapling modification of the divided gastroplasty and, in addition, reinforced the greater curvature outlet with a running suture.[27] This, too, did not result in lasting success. Similarly, the gastric partitioning operation of Pace et al., introduced in 1979, was unsuccessful, since the partitioning created by the removal of several staples from the middle of the stapling instrument was followed by widening of the gastrogastrostomy outlet.[28] To overcome this problem, in 1979, LaFave and Alden performed a total gastric cross stapling and a sewed anterior gastrogastrostomy; this operation also had no weight loss in the long term.[29] Thus, at the close of the 1970s, gastroplasty was in its developmental phase and performed horizontally, rather than vertically.

In the productive 70s, the precursors of gastric banding are to be found in the fundoplication procedure of Tretbar et al. (1976)[30] and the mesh wrapping of the entire stomach by Wilkinson (1980).[31] Wilkinson et al., in 1978, actually initiated gastric banding per se.[32] His band was placed during open surgery and was not adjustable.

Finally, for the 1970s, it should be mentioned that, in 1974, Quaade et al. described stereotaxic stimulation and electrocoagulation of sites in the lateral hypothalamus.[33] In three of the five patients receiving unilateral electrocoagulation lesions, there was a statistically significant but transient reduction in caloric intake and a short-term reduction in body weight.

1980s

In the 1980s, malabsorptive procedures were essentially limited to the biliopancreatic diversion of Scopinaro, who brought physiologic understanding in compliance with the technique of his procedure and maintained biliopancreatic diversion on the world stage of bariatric surgery. There was one more attempt, however, by Cleator and Gourlay to modify drainage of the old jejunoileal bypass by use of an ileogastrostomy.[34]

With respect to gastric bypass, there was a flurry of activity. Multiple variations of the Roux gastric bypass were introduced. Torres, Oca, and Garrison stapled the stomach vertically rather than horizontally.[35] Linner and Drew reinforced the gastrojejunal outlet with a fascial band.[36] Torres and Oca reported a modification of the vertical Roux nondivided gastric bypass with the creation of a long Roux limb for individuals who had failed their original procedure.[37] This marked the origin of the long-limb gastric bypass, a decade later popularized as a primary operation for the super obese by Brolin et al.[38] Salmon combined two procedures—a vertical banded gastroplasty and a distal gastric bypass.[39] In 1989, Fobi introduced his first Silastic ring vertical gastric bypass, creating a small vertical pouch drained by a gastrojejunostomy and containing a restrictive Silastic ring proximal to the gastrojejunostomy.[40]

The 1980s was truly the decade of the vertical banded gastroplasty. In 1981, Fabito was the first to perform a vertical gastroplasty by employing a modified TA 90 stapler and reinforcing the outlet with seromuscular sutures.[41] That same year, Laws was probably the first to use a Silastic ring as a permanent, nonexpandable support for the vertical gastroplasty outlet (Figure 1–8).[42] In 1980, Mason performed his last gastroplasty variation—the vertical banded gastroplasty.[43] This vertical banded gastroplasty involved a novel concept, namely, making a window, a through-and-through perforation in both walls of the stomach, with the end-to-end stapling instrument just above the crow's foot on the lesser curvature. This window was used for the insertion of a standard TA-90 stapler to the angle of His to create a small staple vertical pouch. The lesser curvature outlet was banded with a 1.5-cm wide polypropylene mesh collar through the gastric window and around the lesser curvature conduit (Figure 1–9). In 1986, Eckhout, Willbanks, and Moore introduced an innovation of vertical banded gastroplasty that soon rivaled in popularity the Mason procedure.[44] This was the Silastic ring vertical gastroplasty using a specially constructed notched stapler to avoid the window of the Mason procedure. Also, the nonreactive, far narrower (2.5-mm diameter) Silastic ring prevents the formation of granulation tissue at times induced by the polypropylene mesh with subsequent outlet obstruction.

Clinical progress with gastric banding in the 1980s was rather dormant; however, the basic inventions necessary for the popularity of gastric banding were introduced during this decade. Kolle (1982)[45] and Molina and Oria (1983)[46] placed nonadjustable gastric bands during open surgery. An

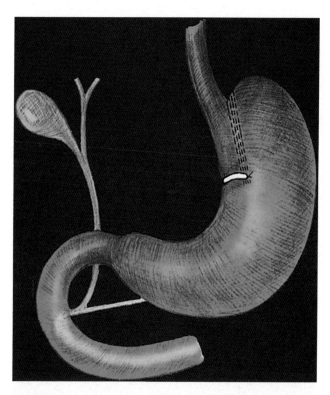

Figure 1–8. 1981 Laws: Gastroplasty—Silastic ring vertical gastroplasty.

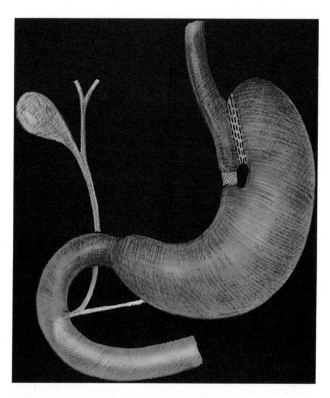

Figure 1–9. 1982 Mason: Gastroplasty—vertical banded gastroplasty.

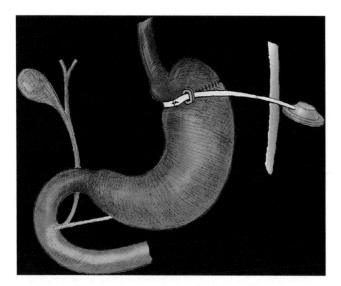

Figure 1–10. 1986 Kuzmak: Gastric band—adjustable Silastic.

interesting device modification of the Pace procedure[28] was introduced by Bashour and Hill with their "gastro-clip."[47] In 1986, Kuzmak introduced the inflatable Silastic band connected to a subcutaneous port, which is used for the percutaneous introduction or removal of fluid to adjust the caliber of the gastric band (Figure 1–10).[48] This first adjustable gastric band was placed during open surgery.

1990s

In the 1990s, the biliopancreatic diversion underwent a modification on this side of the Atlantic with the introduction of the duodenal switch by Hess and Marceau. The Hess and Hess procedure deviated from the Scopinaro procedure by 1) making a lesser curvature gastric tube with a greater curvature gastric resection, rather than performing a horizontal gastrectomy; 2) preserving the pylorus; 3) anastomosing the enteric limb to the proximal duodenum; and 4) dividing the duodenum, with closure of the distal duodenal stump (Figure 1–11).[49] The Marceau et al. version of the duodenal switch, cross-stapled the duodenum distal to the duodenoileostomy, without dividing the duodenum.[50] The duodenum, however, unlike the stomach, does not tolerate cross-stapling and these patients displayed disruption of the staple-line with regaining of weight. The currently popular biliopancreatic diversion/duodenal switch is based on the procedure introduced by Hess and Hess.[49] Hess has been active in organizing standardization of this operation using a 100-mL gastric reservoir. At present, there is no general agreement as to the varying lengths of the enteric and biliopancreatic limbs and the common channel, as well as the method for performing the duodenoileostomy.

In the 1990s, Fobi modified his combination vertical gastric bypass and gastroplasty by dividing the stomach and interposing the jejunal Roux limb between the gastric pouch

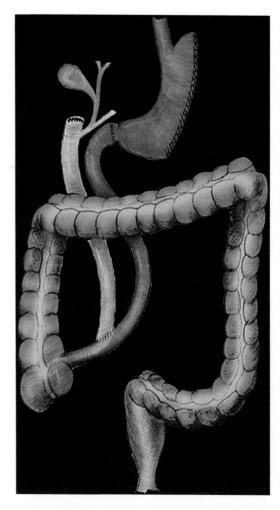

Figure 1–11. 1998 Hess and Hess: Duodenal switch with division of the duodenum.

and the bypassed stomach to ensure maintenance of the gastric division (Figure 1–12).[53] Over the years, the Fobi procedure has gained an ever-increasing following of advocates. Another combined procedure innovation was introduced by Vassallo et al., who performed a distal biliopancreatic diversion with no gastric resection and a transient vertical banded gastroplasty constructed with a polydioxane band that is absorbed within 6 months.[54]

The 1990s became the heyday for gastric bypass and, in particular, laparoscopic gastric bypass. In 1994, Wittgrove, Clark, and Tremblay were the first to report their results with laparoscopic Roux gastric bypass.[55] They performed the gastrojejunostomy by introducing the anvil of an end-to-end stapler endoscopically. This procedure was modified by de la Torre and Scott by the introduction of the anvil of the stapler intra-abdominally to allow greater precision in anvil placement and avoid esophageal complications.[56] Schauer et al. abandoned use of the end-to-end stapler and introduced the intra-abdominal linear endostapler instrument for performing the gastrojejunostomy.[57] Finally, Higa et al., in 1999, to avoid the relatively high incidence of gastrointestinal anastomotic leaks in employing a stapled gastrojejunostomy

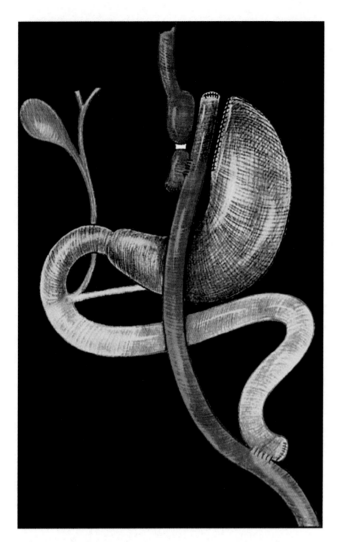

Figure 1–12. 1991 Fobi: Gastric bypass—vertical gastric division with interposed Roux gastrojejunostomy and proximal Silastic ring.

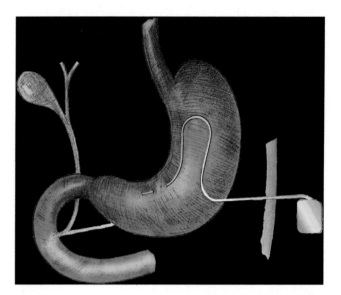

Figure 1–13. 1999 Cigaina: Gastric electrode bipolar pulsation.

anastomosis, described a technique for hand-sewing the gastrojejunostomy laparoscopically.[58]

In 1994, Cadiere[59] and Hess and Hess[60] introduced laparoscopic technique to the vertical banded gastroplasty. Hess and Hess performed the gastroplasty procedure with complete transaction of the staple line.[60] In 1999, Champion et al. reported on doing a laparoscopic vertical banded gastroplasty using a wedge excision of the fundus of the stomach.[61]

Adjustable gastric banding did not become a popular bariatric procedure until its employment laparoscopically and this occurred in the 1990s. In 1992–1993, Broadbent et al.[62] and Catona et al.[63] were probably the first to perform gastric banding laparoscopically and in 1993, Belachew et al.[64] and Forsell et al.[65] were the first to perform adjustable gastric banding laparoscopically. Niville et al. reported placing the posterior aspect of the band at the distal esophagus and constructing an extremely small ("virtual") gastric pouch.[66] Currently, optimized results with laparoscopic adjustable gastric banding have been reported with 1) a high retrogastric tunnel above the lesser sac (pars flaccida approach); 2) a small

gastric pouch of 15 mL; 3) band imbrication anteriorly by at least four gastrogastric sutures; and 4) delaying band inflation until about 4 weeks postoperatively.[67] In 1999, Cadiere et al. reported the world's first laparoscopic adjustable gastric banding executed robotically.[68]

In 1996, Cigaina et al. were the first to report on the use of electrical pacing of the stomach to induce weight loss.[69] In this procedure, and subsequent modifications, electrodes are placed into the wall of the stomach and connected to a pacer in a subcutaneous pocket (Figure 1–13). These systems are still in the experimental phase.

2000s

Fifty years after the introduction of the malabsorptive jejunoileal bypass, the descendants of this operation continue to flourish and evolve. In order to overcome the extreme technical difficulties of performing biliopancreatic diversion/duodenal switch laparoscopically, and the relatively high rate of complications encountered early in the development of the laparoscopic technique, hybrid procedures, combining open and laparoscopic surgery,[70] as well as hand-assisted techniques were developed.[70,71]

The difficulty in mastering the laparoscopic duodenal switch, the ultimate malabsorptive procedure, led to advocacy of the sleeve gastrectomy, a purely restrictive operation. Free-standing gastric sleeve resection is truly a development of the twenty-first century, and today has several advocates notably Jossart.[72] In full fairness, the modern advocates of sleeve gastrectomy owe their thinking not only to the difficulties of performing a duodenal switch laparoscopically but also to the pioneering work done by Johnston et al. with the Magnestrasse and Mill operation.[73]

With respect to gastric bypass and vertical banded gastroplasty there have been few innovative modifications so far in the twenty-first century. Experiments are under way to perform a gastric bypass with the assistance of the endoscope but these efforts are, as yet, experiments.

ADDENDUM

Although it is not a truly surgical procedure, the endoscopic insertion of gastric balloons or other space-occupying devices to create satiety and to induce weight loss should be mentioned. This approach was popularized by the 1985 FDA approval of the Garren-Edwards gastric bubble.[74] The original use of this device was for the most part a failure and associated with serious complications. Currently, the concept of an intraluminal gastric prosthesis, using improved designs, is again gaining popularity as a technique to induce weight loss prior to a standard bariatric procedure or as a free-standing instrument for weight reduction.

CONCLUSION

This chapter has delineated the evolutionary tree of bariatric surgery. In the future, certain branches of this tree will become obsolete, whereas other branches will sprout new and exciting concepts. The richness of ingenuity displayed in the evolution of bariatric surgery gives ample testimony to the ever-increasing need for effective obesity management. Contrary to the expectations of some in the 1980s that bariatric surgery will converge toward a single, "gold standard," procedure, such as the middle-of-the-road gastric bypass, we have seen a divergence of procedures and a plethora of new thought in this field. Currently, there is a trend both toward the least invasive, simplest, and safest restrictive operations, as well as toward the most weight-effective, slightly more risky, complicated malabsorptive operations. Some day, bariatric surgery may be a historical footnote, but it will always be a page in the history of surgery, of which bariatric surgeons can be proud of their record of helping humankind and of providing the first effective therapy for the disease of morbid obesity.

References

1. Buchwald H, Buchwald JN. Evolution of operative procedures for the management of morbid obesity 1950–2000. *Obes Surg* 12:705–717, 2002.
2. Buchwald H, Rucker RD. The rise and fall of jejunoileal bypass. In: Nelson RL, Nyhus LM (eds.): *Surgery of the Small Intestine.* Norwalk, Appleton Century Crofts, 1987; p. 529–541.
3. Henrikson V: Kan tunnfarmsreesektion forsvaras som terapi mot fettsot? *Nordisk Medicin* 47:744, 1952. Translations: Can small resection be defended as therapy for obesity? *Obes Surg* 4:54, 1994.
4. Kremen AJ, Linner LH, Nelson CH: An experimental evaluation of the nutritional importance of proximal and distal small intestine. *Ann Surg* 140:439–444, 1954.
5. Payne JH, DeWind LT, Commons RR: Metabolic observations in patients with jejunocolic shunts. *Obes Res* 4:304–315, 1996.
6. Deitel M: Jejunocolic and jejunoileal bypass: An historical perspective. In: Deitel M (ed.): *Surgery for the Morbidly Obese Patient.* Philadelphia, PA, Lea & Febiger, 1998; p. 81–89.
7. Payne JH, DeWind LT: Surgical treatment of obesity. *Am J Surg* 118:141, 1969.
8. Lewis LA, Turnbull RB, Page LH: "Short-circuiting" of the small intestine. *JAMA* 182:77–79, 1962.
9. Sherman CD, May AG, Nye W: Clinical and metabolic studies following bowel bypassing for obesity. *Ann NY Acad Sci* 131:614–622, 1965.
10. Lewis LA, Turnbull RB, Page LH: Effects of jejunocolic shunt on obesity, serum lipoproteins, lipids, and electrolytes. *Arch Intern Med* 117:4–16, 1966.
11. Mason EE, Ito C: Gastric bypass in obesity. *Surg Clin N Am* 47:1345–1352, 1967.
12. Scott HW, Sandstead HH, Brill AB: Experience with a new technique of intestinal bypass in the treatment of morbid obesity. *Ann Surg* 174:560–572, 1971.
13. Salmon PA: The results of small intestine bypass operations for the treatment of obesity. *Surg Gynecol Obstet* 132:965–979, 1971.
14. Buchwald H, Varco RL: A bypass operation for obese hyperlipidemic patients. *Surgery* 70:62–70, 1971.
15. Forestieri P, DeLuca L, Bucci L: Surgical treatment of high degree obesity. Our own criteria to choose the appropriate type of jejunoileal bypass: A modified Payne technique. *Chir Gastroenterol* 11:401–408, 1977.
16. Starkloff GB, Stothert JC, Sundaram M: Intestinal bypass: A modification. *Ann Surg* 188:697–700, 1978.
17. Palmer JA, Marliss EB: The present status of surgical procedures for obesity. In: Deitel M (ed.): *Nutrition in Clinical Surgery.* Baltimore, MD, Williams & Wilkins, 1980. p. 281–292.
18. Lavorato F, Doldi SB, Scaramella R: Evoluzione storica della terapia chirurgica della grande obesita. *Minerva Med* 69:3847–3857, 1978.
19. Eriksson F: Biliointestinal bypass. *Int J Obes* 5:437–447, 1981.
20. Scopinaro N, Gianetta E, Civalleri D: Biliopancreatic bypass for obesity, II: Initial experiences in man. *Br J Surg* 66:618–620, 1979.
21. Scopinaro N, Adami GF, Marinari GM, et al.: Biliopancreatic diversion: Two decades of experience. In: Deitel M, Cowan SM Jr (eds.): *Update: Surgery for the Morbidly Obese Patient.* Toronto, Canada: FD-Communications, 2000; p. 227–258.
22. Alden JF: Gastric and jejuno-ileal bypass: A comparison in the treatment of morbid obesity. *Arch Surg* 112:799–806, 1977.
23. Griffen WO, Young VL, Stevenson CC: A prospective comparison of gastric and jejunoileal bypass procedures for morbid obesity. *Ann Surg* 186:500–507, 1977.
24. McCarthy HB, Rucker RD, Chan EK, et al.: Gastritis after gastric bypass surgery. *Surgery* 98:68–71, 1985.
25. Buckwalter JA: Clinical trial of jejunoileal and gastric bypass for the treatment of obesity: Four-year progress report. *Am Surg* 46:377–381, 1980.
26. Printen KJ, Mason EE: Gastric surgery for relief of morbid obesity. *Arch Surg* 106:428–431, 1973.
27. Gomez CA: Gastroplasty in morbid obesity. *Surg Clin North Am* 59:1113–1120, 1979.
28. Pace WG, Martin EW, Tetirick CE, et al.: Gastric partitioning for morbid obesity. *Ann Surg* 190:392–400, 1979.
29. LaFave JW, Alden JF: Gastric bypass in the operative revision of the failed jejuno-ileal bypass. *Arch Surg* 114:438–444, 1979.
30. Tretbar LL, Taylor TL, Sifers EC: Weight reduction: Gastric plication for morbid obesity. *J Kans Med Soc* 77:488–490, 1976.
31. Wilkinson LH: Reduction of gastric reservoir capacity. *J Clin Nutr* 33:515–517, 1980.
32. Wilkinson LH, Peloso OA: Gastric (reservoir) reduction for morbid obesity. *Arch Surg* 116:602–605, 1981.
33. Quaade F, Vaernet K, Larsson S: Sterotaxic stimulation and electrocoagulation of the lateral hypothalamus in obese humans. *Acta Neurochir* (Wien) 30:1111–1117, 1974.
34. Cleator IGM, Gourlay RH: Ileogastrostomy for morbid obesity. *Can J Surg* 31:114–116, 1988.

35. Torres JC, Oca CF, Garrison RN: Gastric bypass: Roux-en-Y gastro-jejunostomy from the lesser curvature. *South Med J* 76:1217–1221, 1983.

36. Linner JR, Drew RL: New modification of Roux-en-Y gastric bypass procedure. *Clin Nutr* 5:33–34, 1986.

37. Torres J, Oca C: Gastric bypass lesser curvature with distal Roux-en-Y. *Bariatric Surg* 5:10–15, 1987.

38. Brolin RE, Kenler HA, Gorman JH, et al.: Long-limb gastric bypass in the super obese. A prospective randomized study. *Ann Surg* 21:387–395, 1992.

39. Salmon PA: Gastroplasty with distal gastric bypass: A new and more successful weight loss operation for the morbidly obese. *Can J Surg* 31:111–113, 1988.

40. Fobi MA: The surgical technique of the banded Roux-en-Y gastric bypass. *J Obes Weight Reg* 8:99–102, 1989.

41. Fabito DC: Gastric vertical stapling. Read before the *Bariatric Surgery Colloquium*, Iowa City, IA, June 1, 1981.

42. Laws HL, Piatadosi S: Superior gastric reduction procedure for morbid obesity. A prospective, randomized trial. *Am J Surg* 193:334–336, 1981.

43. Mason EE: Vertical banded gastroplasty. *Arch Surg* 117:701–706, 1982.

44. Eckhout GV, Willbanks OL, Moore JT: Vertical ring gastroplasty for obesity: Five year experience with 1463 patients. *Am J Surg* 152:713–716, 1986.

45. Kolle K: Gastric banding. In: *OMGI 7th Congress, Stockholm*, 1982, Abst No 145:37.

46. Molina M, Oria HE: Gastric segmentation: A new, safe, effective, simple, readily revised and fully reversible surgical procedure for the correction of morbid obesity. In: *6th Bariatric Surgery Colloquium*, Iowa City, IA, 2–3 June 1983, Abst 15.

47. Bashour SB, Hill RW: The gastro-clip gastroplasty: An alternative surgical procedure for the treatment of morbid obesity. *Tex Med* 81:36–38, 1985.

48. Kuzmak LI: Silicone gastric banding: A simple and effective operation for morbid obesity. *Contemp Surg* 28:13–18, 1986.

49. Hess DW, Hess DS: Biliopancreatic diversion with a duodenal switch. *Obes Surg* 8:267–282, 1998.

50. Marceau P, Biron S, Bourque R-A, et al.: Biliopancreatic diversion with a new type of gastrectomy. *Obes Surg* 3:29–35, 1993.

51. de Csepel J, Burpee S, Jossart G, et al.: Laparoscopic biliopancreatic diversion with a duodenal switch for morbid obesity: A feasibility study in pigs. *J Laparoendosc Adv Surg Tech A* 11:79–83, 2001.

52. Ren CJ, Patterson E, Gagner M: Early results of laparoscopic biliopancreatic diversion with duodenal switch: A case series of 40 consecutive patients. *Obes Surg* 10:514–523, 2000.

53. Fobi MA: Why the operation I prefer is Silastic ring vertical banded gastric bypass. *Obes Surg* 1:423–426, 1991.

54. Vassallo C, Negri L, Della Valle A, et al.: Biliopancreatic diversion with transitory gastroplasty preserving duodenal bulb: 3 years experience. *Obes Surg* 7:30–33, 1997.

55. Wittgrove AC, Clark GW, Tremblay, LJ: Laparoscopic gastric bypass, Roux-en-Y: Preliminary report of five cases. *Obes Surg* 4:353–357, 1994.

56. de la Torre RA, Scott JS: Laparoscopic Roux-en-Y gastric bypass: A totally intra-abdominal approach—technique and preliminary report. *Obes Surg* 9:492–497, 1999.

57. Schauer PR, Ikramuddin S, Gourash W, et al.: Outcomes of laparoscopic Roux-en-Y gastric bypass for morbid obesity. *Ann Surg* 232:515–529, 2000.

58. Higa KD, Boone KB, Ho T: Laparoscopic Roux-en-Y gastric bypass for morbid obesity in 850 patients: Technique and follow-up. Poster presented at American Society of Bariatric Surgery, 1999.

59. Cadiere GB, Bruyns J, Himpens J, Favretti F: Laparoscopic gastroplasty for morbid obesity. *Br J Surg* 81:524, 1994.

60. Hess DW, Hess DS: Laparoscopic vertical banded gastroplasty with complete transaction of the staple-line. *Obes Surg* 4:44–46, 1994.

61. Champion JK, Hunt T, DeLisle N: Laparoscopic vertical banded gastroplasty and Roux-en-Y gastric bypass in morbid obesity. *Obes Surg* 9:123, 1999.

62. Broadbent R, Tracy M, Harrington P: Laparoscopic gastric banding: A preliminary report. *Obes Surg* 3:63–67, 1993.

63. Catona A, Gossenberg M, La Manna A, et al.: Laparoscopic gastric banding: Preliminary series. *Obes Surg* 3:207–209, 1993.

64. Belachew M, Legrand M, Jacquet N: Laparoscopic placement of adjustable silicone gastric banding in the treatment of morbid obesity: An animal model experimental study. A video film: A preliminary report [abstract]. *Obes Surg* 3:140, 1993. Abstract 5.

65. Forsell P, Hallberg D, Hellers G: Gastric banding for morbid obesity: Initial experience with a new adjustable band. *Obes Surg* 3:369–374, 1993.

66. Niville E, Vankeirsblick J, Dams A, et al.: Laparoscopic adjustable esophagogastric banding: A preliminary experience. *Obes Surg* 8:39–42, 1998.

67. Belachew M, Legrand MJ, Vincent V ; History of Lap-Band®: From dream to reality. *Obes Surg* 11:297–302, 2001.

68. Cadiere GB, Himpens J, Vertruyen M: The world's first obesity surgery performed by a surgeon at a distance. *Obes Surg* (England) 9:206–209, 1999.

69. Cigaina V, Pinato G, Rigo V: Gastric peristalsis control by mono situ electrical stimulation: A preliminary study. *Obes Surg* 6:247–249, 1996.

70. Rabkin RA, Rabkin JM, Metcalf B, et al.: Laparoscopic technique for performing duodenal switch with gastric reduction. *Obes Surg* 13:263–268, 2003.

71. Baltasar A, Bou R, Bengochea M, et al.: Duodenal switch: an effective therapy for morbid obesity—intermediate results. *Obes Surg* 11:54–58, 2001.

72. Lee CM, Feng JJ, Cirangle PT, et al.: Evolution of the laparoscopic duodenal switch and sleeve gastrectomy procedures. In: Buchwald H, Pories W, Cowan GM Jr (eds.): *Bariatric Surgery*. Philadelphia, PA, Elsevier. In press

73. Johnston D, Dachtler J, Sue-Ling HM, et al.: The Magenstrasse and Mill operation for morbid obesity. *Obes Surg* 13:10–16, 2003.

74. Garren M, Garren L, Giordano F: The Garren gastric bubble: An Rx for the morbidly obese. *Endoc Rev* 2:57–60, 1984.

Pathophysiology of Severe Obesity and the Effects of Surgically Induced Weight Loss

Harvey J. Sugerman, MD

Severe obesity is associated with multiple comorbidities which reduce the life expectancy and markedly impair the quality of life. Obesity-related problems begin at the head and end at the toes, affecting almost EVERY ORGAN in between. Morbidly obese patients can suffer from central (android) obesity or peripheral (gynoid) obesity or a combination of the two. Gynoid obesity is associated with degenerative joint disease and venous stasis in the lower extremities. Android obesity is associated with the highest risk of mortality-related problems due to the "Metabolic Syndrome" or "Syndrome X," as well as increased intra-abdominal pressure (IAP). The metabolic syndrome is associated with insulin resistance, hyperglycemia, and type 2 diabetes mellitus (DM) and this is associated with nonalcoholic liver disease (NALD) or nonal-

coholic steatohepatitis (NASH), polycystic ovary syndrome, nephrotic syndrome of obesity, and systemic hypertension. Increased IAP is probably responsible in part or totally for obesity hypoventilation, venous stasis disease, pseudotumor cerebri, gastroesophageal reflux disease, stress urinary incontinence, and systemic hypertension. Central obesity is also associated with increased neck circumference and sleep apnea. Additional comorbidities include an increased risk of several cancers (uterine, breast, prostate, esophagus, colon, kidney), problems with pregnancy and delivery, and problems with infections (necrotizing panniculitis and pancreatitis) as well as difficulty in diagnosing peritonitis. The encouraging data are that almost all of these comorbidities resolve or improve significantly with surgically induced weight loss.

INTRODUCTION

Severe obesity is associated with a large number of problems that have given rise to the term "morbid obesity" (Table 2–1).

Table 2–1.

Morbidity of Severe Obesity

Central obesity
    Metabolic complications (Syndrome X)
        Non-insulin dependent diabetes (adult onset/Type II)
        Hypertension
        Dyslipidemia: Elevated triglycerides, cholesterol
        Cholelithiasis, cholecystitis
    Increased intra-abdominal pressure
        Stress overflow urinary incontinence
        Gastroesophageal reflux
        Venous disease: Thrombophlebitis, venous stasis ulcers
            Pulmonary embolism
        Obesity hypoventilation syndrome
        Nephrotic syndrome
        Hernias (Incisional, Inguinal)
        Preeclampsia
        Pseudotumor cerebri
Respiratory insufficiency of obesity (Pickwickian syndrome)
    Obesity hypoventilation syndrome
    Obstructive sleep apnea syndrome
Cardiovascular dysfunction
    Coronary artery disease
    Increased complications after coronary bypass surgery
    Heart failure subsequent to
        Left ventricular concentric hypertrophy—hypertension
        Left ventricular eccentric hypertrophy—obesity
        Right ventricular hypertrophy—pulmonary failure
    Prolonged Q-T interval with sudden death
Sexual hormone dysfunction
    Amenorrhea, hypermenorrhea
    Stein-Leventhal or polycystic ovary syndrome: hirsutism, ovarian cysts
    Infertility
    Endometrial carcinoma
    Breast carcinoma
Other carcinomas: colon, renal cell, prostate
Infectious complications
    Difficulty recognizing peritonitis
    Necrotizing pancreatitis
    Necrotizing subcutaneous infections
    Wound infections, dehiscence
Pseudotumor cerebri (idiopathic intracranial hypertension)
Degenerative osteoarthritis
    Feet, ankles, knees, hips, back, shoulders
Psychosocial impairment
Decreased employability, work discrimination

Although some consider this term to be pejorative, severe obesity is often associated with a number of problems that are truly morbid and incapacitating. The medical problems caused by obesity begin with the head and end with the toes and involve almost every organ in between. Several of these problems contribute to the earlier mortality associated with obesity and include coronary artery disease, severe hypertension that may be refractory to medical management, impaired cardiac function, adult onset (type 2) diabetes mellitus, obesity hypoventilation, and sleep apnea syndromes (SASs), cirrhosis, venous stasis, and hypercoagulability leading to an increased risk of pulmonary embolism, and necrotizing panniculitis.[1,2] Morbidly obese patients can also die as a result of difficulties in recognizing the signs and symptoms of peritonitis.[3] There is an increased risk of prostate, uterine, breast, kidney, esophageal, liver, and colon cancer. Premature death is much more common in the severely obese individual; one study noted a 12-fold excess mortality in morbidly obese men in the 25–34 year age group.[4] Increased morbidity and mortality have been noted in several other studies.[5–8]

A number of obesity-related problems may not be associated with death but can lead to significant physical or psychological disability. These include degenerative osteoarthritis, pseudotumor cerebri (idiopathic intracranial hypertension), cholecystitis, skin infections, chronic venous stasis ulcers, stress overflow urinary incontinence, gastroesophageal reflux, sex hormone imbalance with dysmenorrhea, hirsutism, infertility (polycystic ovary syndrome), the nephrotic syndrome, and nonalcoholic liver disease (NALD) or, in its more severe form, nonalcoholic steatohepatitis (NASH). Many morbidly obese patients suffer from severe psychological and social disability, including marked prejudice regarding employment.[9,10]

CENTRAL (ANDROID) VERSUS PERIPHERAL (GYNOID) FAT DISTRIBUTION

It has been noted that central obesity is associated with a higher mortality than is peripheral obesity, commonly referred to as android versus gynoid obesity because of their relative prevalence in men and women, respectively. This has been attributed to metabolically more active visceral adipose tissue than to subcutaneous fat so that there is a greater rate of glucose production, type 2 diabetes, and hyperinsulinism. Increased insulin secretion is thought to increase sodium reabsorption and, thus, cause hypertension.[11–18] Central obesity also is associated with a greater production of cholesterol, primarily in the form of low-density lipoprotein, leading to a higher than normal incidence of atherosclerotic cardiovascular disease, and an increased incidence of gallstones. The increased visceral fat has been related to an increased waist:hip ratio, or in more common terms as the "apple" versus "pear" distribution of fat. Computerized axial tomographic (CAT) scans, however, have noted a much better correlation between anterior–posterior abdominal diameter and visceral fat distribution than with the waist:hip ratio,[19,20] especially in women who may have both central and peripheral obesity. In this situation, the peripheral obesity "dilutes" the central obesity using a W:H ratio, so that either waist circumference alone or sagittal abdominal diameter should be used as a measurement of central obesity.

A recent study documented an increased bladder pressure in morbidly obese women, which was associated with a high incidence of urinary incontinence.[21] It is quite probable that much of the comorbidity of severe obesity is related to an increased intra-abdominal pressure (IAP)[22] secondary to a central distribution of fat (Table 2–1) and that the urinary bladder pressure, a surrogate for IAP, is highly correlated with the sagittal abdominal diameter or waist circumference. In animal studies,[23] a close relationship between urinary bladder pressure and directly measured IAP has been found. In addition to urinary incontinence, this increased IAP is probably responsible for increased venous stasis disease and venous stasis ulcers, gastroesophageal reflux, nephrotic syndrome secondary to increased renal venous pressure, incisional and inguinal hernias, and obesity hypoventilation syndrome (OHS) secondary to a high-riding diaphragm and restrictive lung disease. This can also lead to an increased intrapleural pressure which can then cause increased intracardiac pressures so that severely obese patients with OHS may require high cardiac filling pressures to maintain an adequate cardiac output.[23,24] It is also quite possible that increased IAP is also responsible for the high incidence of systemic hypertension in the morbidly obese, as well as the cause of "idiopathic" intracranial hypertension.[23,25-27]

In a previous study,[22] we noted a much higher IAP in morbidly obese patients at the time of gastric bypass surgery than five nonobese patients who were undergoing colectomy, ileal pouch anal anastomosis (IPAA) for ulcerative colitis. To realize how high these pressures can be in severe obesity, one needs to relate them to the pressures seen in patients with an acute abdominal compartment syndrome[28,29] where it is generally thought that a urinary bladder pressure of $\geq$20–25 cm H_2O is an indication to return the patient to the operating room for emergency laparotomy and abdominal decompression. Many severely obese patients have urinary bladder pressures well above 25 cm H_2O. Surgically induced weight loss was associated with a significant decrease in sagittal abdominal diameter, urinary bladder pressures, and obesity comorbidity.[30]

Hypertension

We hypothesize that obesity-associated hypertension is secondary to an increased IAP rather than to increased insulin-induced sodium reabsorption. The presumed pathophysiology is related to activation of the renin–angiotensin–aldosterone system through one or a combination of three possible renal mechanisms. The first presumed mechanism is due to direct pressure on the renal veins, leading to an increased glomerular capillary pressure, a capillary leak with either a microalbuminuria commonly seen in the morbidly obese or, on occasion, a large protein leak with development

of the nephrotic syndrome.[31,32] The increased glomerular pressure probably stimulates the juxta-glomerular apparatus (JGA) to increased renin secretion.[33] A second mechanism relates to a direct pressure on the renal capsule, leading to a renal compartment syndrome and activation of the renin–angiotensin–aldosterone system. The third possibility relates to the increased pleural pressure secondary to a rising diaphragm, which impedes venous return to the heart, leading to a decrease in cardiac output and renal arterial pressure which again stimulates activation of the JGA to produce renin.[23,34] Increased renin and aldosterone levels are seen in a porcine model of acutely increased IAP.[34] Activation of the renin–angiotensin–aldosterone system leads to salt and water retention, commonly seen in the severely obese, and vasoconstriction. Surgically induced weight loss is associated with a clinically significant, long-lasting improvement in blood pressure with elimination of antihypertensive medications in two-thirds to three-quarters of hypertensive patients or a marked decrease in their use.[35-43] The Swedish Obesity Study (SOS) initially noted a significant improvement in both diabetes and hypertension in the surgically treated patients as compared to matched controls.[36] However, the improvement in hypertension for the overall group was no longer present at 8 years after surgery.[38] Unfortunately, only 6% of the surgical patients in the SOS trial had a gastric bypass, 70% a vertical banded gastroplasty, and 24% a gastric banding. The gastric bypass patients had a significantly greater weight loss than either the gastroplasty or gastric banded patients and also maintained a significant decrease in both systolic and diastolic pressure at 5 years after surgery.[39]

Cardiac Dysfunction and Dyslipidemia

Morbid obesity may be associated with cardiomegaly and impaired left, right, or biventricular function (Table 2–2). Severe obesity may be associated with a high cardiac output and a low systemic vascular resistance leading to left ventricular hypertrophy. Obesity also is associated with hypertension, which leads to concentric left ventricular hypertrophy. This combination of obesity and hypertension with left ventricular eccentric and concentric hypertrophy may lead to left ventricular failure.[44,45] Correction of morbid obesity improves cardiac function in these patients.[24,46-49] Morbid obesity is also associated with an accelerated rate of coronary atherosclerosis. These patients often have hypercholesterolemia and a decreased high-density to low-density lipoprotein (HDL:LDL) ratio. In the Nurses Study, women with a BMI >29 kg/m^2 have a significantly increased incidence of myocardial angina and/or infarction.[50,51] Surgically induced weight loss has been shown in several studies to significantly reduce triglyceride and LDL cholesterol levels while increasing HDL levels.[38,43,52-56] Respiratory insufficiency associated with morbid obesity can result in hypoxemic pulmonary artery vasoconstriction, which in severe cases may lead to right, or biventricular, heart failure associated with tricuspid valvular insufficiency. Correction of hypoxemia and hypercarbia with surgically induced weight loss will correct

Table 2–2.

Obesity Comorbidity "From the Top of the Head to the Tip of the Toes and Almost Every Organ IN BETWEEN"

Head
  Brain
  Stroke
  Headaches
    Hypertension
    Pseudotumor cerebri: Headaches
        I. Optic Nerve: Visual field cuts; blindness
        III. Oculomotor nerve palsy
        V. Trigeminal nerve: Tic Douloureux
        VII. Facial nerve: Bell's palsy
        VIII. Auditory nerve: Pulsatile tinnitus
  Eyes: Diabetic retinopathy + Pseudotumor
    complications
  Mouth/Throat
    Sleep Apnea

Chest
  Breast cancer
  Obesity hypoventilation
    Heavy chest wall
    Elevated diaphragm
    Increased intra-thoracic pressure
    Decreased expiratory reserve volume

Heart
  Left ventricular hypertrophy
    Eccentric: Increased cardiac output
    Concentric: Increased peripheral vascular
      resistance
  Increased cardiac filling pressures (CVP, PAP, WP)
  Right heart failure
    Tricuspid insufficiency

Esophagus
  Acid reflux
  Asthma
  Adenocarcinoma
  Esophageal varices

Abdomen
  Gallbladder
    Cholecystitis
    Adenocarcinoma
  Liver
    Nonalcoholic liver disease (NALD)
    Nonalcoholic steatohepatitis (NASH)
    Cirrhosis
    Type 2 diabetes mellitus
  Spleen
    Splenomegaly (portal hypertension)
    Hypersplenism (portal hypertension)
  Pancreas
    Type 2 diabetes mellitus
    Necrotizing pancreatitis
  Colon
    Adenocarcinoma
    Diverticulitis

General
  Difficulty diagnosing peritonitis
  Hernia
    Incisional
    Inguinal
    Spigelian
  Wound infection
  "Apron"
    Peau d'orange lymphatic stasis

Kidney
  Hypertension
  Proteinuria
  Renal cell carcinoma

Urinary bladder
  Stress incontinence

Ovaries/Uterus
  Increased estradiol, androstenedione
  Polycystic ovary syndrome, Stein-Leventhal syndrome
    Infertility
    Dysmenorrhea
    Hirsutism
  Endometrial carcinoma
  Breast cancer

Prostate: Adenocarcinoma

Anus
  Perianal abscesses
  Necrotzing panniculitis

Integument
  Necrotizing panniculitis
  Hirsutism

Increased risk of operative complications
  Colectomy
  Hysterectomy
  Kidney, liver transplantation

Spine
  Herniated disc

Upper extremities
  Shoulder girdle pain
  Edema

Lower extremities
  Osteoarthritis
    Hip arthralgia
    Knee arthralgia
  Venous stasis
    Edema
    Thrombophlebitis
    Stasis ulcers
    Pulmonary embolism
  Toes
    Diabetic neuropathy
    Diabetic ulcers

the elevated pulmonary artery and wedge pressures within 3–9 months after surgery.[24] Severe obstructive SAS may be associated with prolonged sinus arrest, premature ventricular contractions, and sudden death.

Pulmonary Dysfunction

Respiratory insufficiency of obesity is associated with either OHS, obstructive SAS, or a combination of the two, commonly called the Pickwickian syndrome.[24,57–64]

Obesity Hypoventilation Syndrome: This problem arises primarily from the increased IAP in patients with central, abdominal obesity, which leads to high-riding diaphragm.[22,65] As a result, the lungs are squeezed, producing a restrictive pulmonary defect. A heavy, obese thoracic cage may also contribute to the pathophysiology secondary to a decreased chest wall compliance. These patients have a markedly decreased expiratory reserve volume, leading to alveolar collapse and arteriovenous shunting at end expiration. They also have smaller reductions in all other lung volumes.[59] They have hypoxemia and hypercarbia while awake and a blunted ventilator response to CO_2.

Chronic hypoxemia leads to pulmonary artery vasoconstriction. However, obesity hypoventilation patients often have both markedly elevated pulmonary artery pressures and pulmonary capillary wedge pressures, suggesting both right and left ventricular failures. Despite these high pressures, overt heart failure is unusual, even with pulmonary capillary wedge pressures as high as 40 mm Hg.[24] These pressures are increased as a result of a marked increase in pleural pressures secondary to the high-riding diaphragm and increased IAP, so that the transatrial and transventricular pressures may be, in fact, normal.[23] These findings have been noted in a porcine model of acutely increased IAP. Thus, morbidly obese patients with OHS may not respond well to diuresis and may need these elevated pressures to maintain an adequate cardiac output.

As a result of the increased inferior vena caval and pulmonary artery pressures, obesity hypoventilation patients are at risk for a fatal pulmonary embolism.[57] Thus, right heart catheterization should be considered prior to obesity surgery and a prophylactic inferior vena caval filter inserted at the time of surgery in patients with a mean pulmonary artery pressure ≥40 mm Hg. Surgically induced weight loss[24,59,60,63] corrects hypoxemia, hypercarbia, and increased cardiac filling pressures associated with OHS.

Sleep Apnea Syndrome: SAS is associated with central obesity and is due to both depression of the normal genioglossus reflex, possibly secondary to a large, heavy tongue, and deposition of fat within the hypopharynx with narrowing of the cervical airway.[58] These patients snore loudly while asleep and suffer from severe daytime somnolence with tendencies to fall asleep while driving or at work. The daytime somnolence is probably secondary to impaired stage III, IV, and Rapid Eye Movement (REM) sleep. The diagnosis of obstructive SAS is suggested by a history of severe daytime somnolence, frequent nocturnal awakening, loud snoring, and morning headaches and is confirmed with sleep polysomnography. This technique documents cessation of airflow during sleep associated with persistent respiratory efforts. Most of the apneic episodes are obstructive, but some are central. The latter is seen with central nervous system hypoxemia, analogous to the Cheyne-Stokes respirations seen at high altitude. The severity of sleep apnea is usually determined by the respiratory disturbance index (RDI), which is a combination of apneic episodes (cessation of airflow for ≥10 seconds) and hypopneic episodes (diminution by 50% of airflow for ≥10 seconds) and is divided into mild (RDI ≤ 19), moderate (RDI 20–39), and severe (RDI ≥ 40). Moderate to severe sleep apnea should be treated with nocturnal nasal continuous positive airway pressure (nasal CPAP); if the patient cannot tolerate nasal CPAP and has severe sleep apnea, a tracheostomy should be considered at the time of obesity surgery. All patients with moderate to severe sleep apnea should be managed with intubation and mechanical ventilation in the intensive care unit, and weaned on the morning after surgery. If they also have obesity hypoventilation then they may have to be ventilated for several days until their arterial blood gases return to their preoperative values.

Patients with severe sleep apnea have difficulty staying awake during the day. This syndrome may be associated with sudden death and should always be considered in trauma victims who have fallen asleep while driving. We have seen many patients with severe sleep apnea who are in occupations that are incompatible with this syndrome: taxicab and interstate truck drivers and state prison guards! Surgically induced weight loss corrects or markedly improves SAS, permitting removal of their tracheostomy tube or discontinuation of nasal CPAP.[59–64]

In a series from the Medical College of Virginia, 12.5% of the patients who underwent gastric surgery for morbid obesity had respiratory insufficiency.[59] Of the affected individuals, 51% had SAS alone, 12% had OHS alone, and 37% had both. Of these, 64% were men in contrast to only 14% of the entire group of patients who underwent surgery for obesity. Patients with respiratory insufficiency were significantly more obese than those without pulmonary dysfunction. However, obesity is not the only factor causing respiratory embarrassment, since many patients who underwent surgery for morbid obesity and did not have a clinically significant pulmonary problem, weighed more than the patients with respiratory insufficiency. Most of the obese patients with respiratory dysfunction had an additional pulmonary problem, such as sarcoidosis, heavy cigarette use, recurrent pulmonary embolism, myotonic dystrophy, or idiopathic pulmonary fibrosis. Obstructive SAS and OHS are associated with a high mortality and serious morbidity; weight reduction will correct both.[24,59−64]

Diabetes

Obesity is a frequent etiologic factor in the development of type 2 adult onset diabetes mellitus. Morbidly obese patients can be very resistant to insulin due to the marked down-regulation of insulin receptors. The tendency toward hyperglycemia manifested by obese patients is another risk factor for coronary artery disease as well as for fatal subcutaneous infections. Gastric-surgery-induced weight loss, performed both open and laparoscopically, is associated with resolution of the diabetes[38,40,42,66−79] in 85% of patients and this effect is long-lasting (Table 2–3). Pories and colleagues have found that the earlier the patients with type 2 diabetes

mellitus undergo weight reduction gastric bypass surgery, the greater is their likelihood to have complete resolution of their diabetes.[67,68] In another study, it was noted that patients without diabetes or hypertension are significantly younger by 5 years than those with either diabetes or hypertension and are significantly younger by another 5 years than those with both diabetes and hypertension.[42] Furthermore, patients were more likely to correct their diabetes and hypertension, the more weight they lost.[42] These data support earlier operations in morbidly obese diabetic patients before their diabetic-related complications develop (neuropathy, retinopathy, renal insufficiency). Peripheral insulin resistance, primarily in skeletal muscle, is present in morbidly obese patients and may resolve with surgically induced weight loss. There are data suggesting that type 2 diabetes mellitus could be a disease of the foregut.[69] The gastric bypass operation has been found to decrease the progression and mortality of non-insulin-dependent diabetes mellitus when compared to a matched control group of patients who either chose not to have surgery or were unable to obtain insurance coverage.[70]

Table 2–3.

Decreases in Obesity Comorbidity After Weight-Loss Surgery

Comorbidity	Reference
Type 2 diabetes mellitus	38, 40, 42, 66–79
Systemic hypertension	35–43
Obstructive sleep apnea	59–64
Obesity hypoventilation	24, 59, 60, 63
Cardiac dysfunction	24, 45–49
Pseudotumor cerebri	27, 110
Venous stasis disease	81
Gastroesophageal reflux	90–92
Asthma	98, 99
Dyslipidemia	38, 43, 52–56
Stress urinary incontinence	21
Polycystic ovary syndrome	102
Pregnancy outcomes	104–107
Fatty liver disease	122–125
Musculoskeletal pain	85–87
Health-related quality of life	126–130
Psychological status	131–136
Mortality	70, 137

Venous Stasis Disease

Morbidly obese patients have an increased risk for deep venous thrombosis, venous stasis ulcers, and pulmonary embolism. Low levels of antithrombin III may increase their risk of blood clots.[80] The increased weight within the abdomen raises the IAP and, therefore, the inferior vena caval pressure with an increased resistance to venous return, leading to the pretibial bronze edema, lower extremity venous stasis ulcers, and tendency to deep venous thrombosis. A similar mechanism may be responsible for the increased risk of pulmonary embolism in patients with right heart failure secondary to hypoxemic pulmonary artery vasoconstriction. Venous stasis ulcers can be incapacitating and extremely difficult to treat in the morbidly obese; weight reduction may be the critical factor, as skin grafts, pressure stockings, medicated rigid compression boots, and wound care are often ineffective. Surgically induced weight loss reduces IAP and permits healing of these stasis ulcers.[81]

Degenerative Joint Disease

The increased weight in the morbidly obese leads to early degenerative arthritic changes of the weight-bearing joints, including the knees, hips, and spine. Many orthopedic surgeons refuse to insert total hip or knee prosthetics in patients weighing over 250 pounds because of an unacceptable incidence of prosthetic loosening.[82] There is a high risk of complications in obese patients following intramedullary nailing of femoral fractures.[83] Severe obesity is a common problem in patients requiring intervertebral disc surgery.[84] Weight reduction following gastric surgery for obesity permits subsequent successful joint replacement[85] and is associated with decreases in musculoskeletal and lower back pain.[86,87] In some instances, the decrease in pain following weight loss obviates the need for joint or intervertebral disc surgery.

Gastroesophageal Reflux and Asthma

Morbidly obese patients frequently suffer from gastro-esophageal reflux disease (GERD). Although one study did not find a relationship to severe obesity,[88] others have.[89] This is also probably secondary to an increased IAP. The lower esophageal sphincter may be normal in these patients, but the increased IAP can overcome a normal sphincter pressure. Surgically induced weight loss has corrected this problem.[90-92] GERD resolves promptly following gastric bypass for obesity as neither acid nor bile can reflux into the esophagus after this procedure. Some studies have noted an increased GERD following vertical banded gastroplasty,[93-95] which resolves following conversion to gastric bypass.[94,95] An antireflux procedure (e.g., Nissen fundoplication) is probably inappropriate in a severely obese patient, as gastric surgery induced weight loss not only corrects acid and bile reflux but also improves additional comorbidity usually present in these individuals. The increase risk of GERD in obese individuals increases their risk of esophageal adenocarcinoma and the epidemic of obesity may be one explanation for the marked increase in the incidence of this cancer.[96,97] Two studies have documented improvement in asthma following surgically induced weight loss, presumably due to prevention of nocturnal gastroesophageal reflux and tracheobronchial aspiration or spasm.[98,99]

Urinary Incontinence

Severely obese women often have stress overflow urinary incontinence. Some men with central obesity also complain of urinary urgency, although incontinence in men is rare. Significantly increased urinary bladder pressures have been noted in women with this problem.[21] Surgically induced weight loss is associated with correction of urinary incontinence in 95% of patients, often within a few months of surgery, and this is associated with a significant decrease in urinary bladder pressure when measured 1 year after surgery. The rapid resolution of this vexing problem, often within 1–2 months after surgery, may be related to a rapid decrease in intra-abdominal and urinary bladder pressures following obesity-surgery-induced weight loss as a result of the relationship between wall tension and volume of a sphere according to LaPlace's Law, where pressure is proportional to the radius to the fourth power. This is best thought of as a tense balloon that rapidly loses tension when a small amount of air escapes.

Female Sexual Hormone Dysfunction

Women often suffer from sexual dysfunction due to excessive levels of both the virilizing hormone, androstenedione, and the feminizing hormone, estradiol. These may produce infertility, hirsutism, ovarian cysts (Stein-Leventhal or polycystic ovary syndrome), hypermenorrhea, and a significantly increased risk of breast and endometrial carcinoma. Polycystic ovary syndrome has also been found to be associated with type 2 diabetes and, in mild cases, may improve with metformin treatment.[100,101] Surgically induced weight loss often returns sex hormone levels to normal, increasing fertility and menstrual regularity.[102] It is thought that there may be a higher incidence of neural tube defects in infants born to women during the rapid weight loss that occurs after surgery,[103] probably due to deficient folic acid levels. Thus, birth control is strongly recommended for 1 year after surgically induced weight loss procedures. Surgery has permitted pregnancies in previously infertile morbidly obese women. Increased weight also increases the risk of complications of pregnancy, including the higher incidence of preeclampsia seen in obese women, problems with delivery, and an increased risk of venous thrombosis and pulmonary embolism. Surgically induced weight loss is associated with decreased pregnancy-related complications, including preeclampsia, and reduces the frequency of cesarean section.[104-107]

Pseudotumor Cerebri

Pseudotumor cerebri, also known as idiopathic intracranial hypertension, may be associated with morbid obesity. The problem is almost always seen in women. Symptoms include severe headache, which is usually worse in the morning, bilateral pulsatile auditory tinnitus, and visual field cuts. Severely increased intracranial pressure (ICP) can lead to permanent blindness. Additional cranial nerves that can be involved include the Vth (Tic Douloureux), the VIth (oculomotor nerve paralysis), and the VIIth (Bell's palsy). Studies suggest that pseudotumor cerebri is secondary to an increased IAP leading to an increased pleural pressure and decreased venous drainage from the brain with a consequent cerebral venous engorgement and an increased ICP. Increased ICP occurs in a porcine model of acutely increased IAP, which is prevented by median sternotomy.[25,26] Patients with impending blindness should undergo emergent optic nerve fenestration.[108] In the past, pseudotumor cerebri has been treated with ventriculo-peritoneal or lumboperitoneal cerebrospinal fluid (CSF) shunts. There is a high incidence of shunt occlusion[109] and in some instances patients can have continued headache and auditory tinnitus despite a patent shunt. These failures are probably secondary to shunting from a high-pressure system to another high-pressure system. Patients may also develop major neurological complications following insertion of ventriculo-peritoneal or lumboperitoneal shunts. Surgically induced weight loss decreases CSF pressures, relieves headache and tinnitus,[27,110] and is the procedure of choice rather than CSF-peritoneal shunting. The rapid resolution of headache, tinnitus, and other pseudotumor cerebri symptoms is probably a result of the rapid decrease in IAP. It is difficult to understand, however, why this syndrome is almost entirely restricted to women since men with central obesity also have increased intra-abdominal and pleural pressures.

Malignancy Risk with Obesity

In addition to uterine carcinoma, there is also a significantly increased risk of breast, prostate, kidney, and esophageal and colon cancer in the morbidly obese.[96,97,111-114] The increased risk of breast, uterine, and prostate cancers are probably secondary to the high levels of sex hormones seen in these patients. As previously mentioned, the increased incidence of GERD in the morbidly obese, a probable consequence of increased IAP, is probably responsible for the increased incidence of esophageal adenocarcinoma. The causes for the increased colon and renal cell cancer incidence are unknown.

Hernia Risk with Obesity

Severe obesity is also associated with a significantly increased risk of all types of hernias. This is also probably secondary to the increased IAP associated with central obesity. A significantly higher incidence of incisional hernia has been noted following open gastric bypass surgery for morbid obesity than after total colectomy, proctectomy, and stapled IPAA for ulcerative colitis, of whom 60% were taking approximately 30 mg of prednisone and their incisions were lower midabdomen to above the umbilicus, both of which are thought to increase the risk of hernia.[115] Reduced risk of incisional hernias and other wound-related complications are significant advantages of the laparoscopic approach for obesity surgery. We have seen bilateral spigelian hernias in one of our morbidly obese patients who also developed an incisional hernia. Repair of incisional hernias in morbidly obese patients has a high risk of recurrence and should probably be reinforced with a polypropylene mesh.[115]

Infectious Problems Associated with Morbid Obesity

There is a higher incidence of fulminant diverticulitis,[116,117] necrotizing pancreatitis,[118] and necrotizing panniculitis[119] in severely obese patients. This is probably due to the increased retroperitoneal and subcutaneous fat, as well as diabetes, which provides an ideal growth medium for bacteria.

Nonalcoholic Liver Disease/Nonalcoholic Steatohepatitis

NALD is also associated with type 2 diabetes mellitus. The exact pathophysiology is unknown. It is presumably secondary to the increased glycogen deposition in the liver with subsequent conversion to fat.[120] Increased fatty infiltration produces markedly enlarged livers which can make bariatric surgery much more difficult and dangerous, and may prevent a successful laparoscopic procedure because of the difficulty in elevating the left lobe of the liver from the gastroesophageal tissues. The increased fat in the liver may be metabolized to free fatty acids, which may be quite toxic to tissues and be responsible for the development of NASH and the subsequent development of severe cirrhosis.[88] There is a serious concern that NASH may overtake a combination of hepatitis A, B, and C and the primary cause for liver failure and the need for liver transplantation if the epidemic of severe obesity remains unchecked.[121] Surgically induced weight loss has been found to significantly decrease the severity of hepatic steatosis.[122–125]

Quality of Life

Severe obesity is associated with a marked reduction in the quality of life. Several studies have documented an improvement in the quality of life following surgically induced weight loss.[126–130] Psychological profiles document significant psychological impairment in the morbidly obese which also improves following surgically induced weight loss.[10,131–136] However, there may also be an increased risk of suicide if the individual believes that severe obesity was the total cause of their emotional impairment, which does not resolve following major weight loss after surgery. Lastly, the morbidly obese are at risk for prejudice in many areas, including physicians, but more economically important, with regards to employment.[137,138]

Mortality

Two studies have documented a decrease in mortality following bariatric surgery. One noted a significantly decreased mortality (1% vs 4.5%) in diabetic patients who underwent gastric bypass as compared to diabetic patients who for insurance or personal reasons did not undergo surgery for obesity.[70] The other study from Canada noted a significantly lower long-term mortality (0.7% vs 6.2%, $p < 0.001$) in patients who underwent surgery for obesity from 1983 to 2002 [194 vertical banded gastroplasty (35% subsequently converted to gastric bypass) and 841 gastric bypass] when compared to an age and sex matched nonoperated cohort.[139] Furthermore, the surgical patients also had a significantly decreased rate of developing new medical conditions (cardiovascular, cancer, endocrine, infectious diseases, psychiatric, and digestive). The SOS has not yet reported a significantly decreased mortality in the surgical patients as compared to the control cohort, but 94% of the surgical patients in this study underwent a purely gastric restrictive procedure and have not lost as much weight as the 6% of patients who underwent a gastric bypass operation and could be a reason for the absence of a mortality benefit to date.[41]

References

1. Sjöström LV: Morbidity of severely obese subjects. *Am J Clin Nutr* 55:508S–515S, 1992.
2. Sjöström LV: Mortality of severely obese subjects. *Am J Clin Nutr* 55:516S–523S, 1992.
3. Mason EE, Printen KJ, Barron P, et al.: Risk reduction in gastric operations for obesity. *Ann Surg* 190:158–165, 1979.
4. Drennick EJ, Bale GS, Seltter F, et al.: Excessive mortality and causes of death in morbidly obese men. *JAMA* 243:443–445, 1980.
5. Folsom AR, Kaye SA, Sellers TA, et al.: Body fat distribution and 5-year risk of death in older women. *JAMA* 269:483–487, 1993.
6. VanItalie TB: Obesity: Adverse effects on health and longevity. *Am J Clin Nutr* 32:2723–2733, 1979.
7. Lew EA, Garfinkel L: Variations in mortality by weight among 750,000 men and women. *J Chronic Dis* 32:563–568, 1979.

8. Kral JG: Morbid obesity and health related risks. *Ann Intern Med* 103:1043–1046, 1985.

9. Sarlio-Lahteenkorva S, Stunkard A, Rissanen A: Psychosocial factors and quality of life in obesity. *Int J Obes Relat Metab Disord* 19:1S–5S, 1995.

10. Stunkard AJ, Wadden TA: Psychological aspects of severe obesity. *Am J Clin Nutr* 55:532S–534S, 1991.

11. Kissebah A, Vydelingum N, Murray R, et al.: Relation of body fat distribution to metabolic complications of obesity. *J Clin Endocrinol Metab* 54:254–257, 1982.

12. Reaven GM: Syndrome X: 6 years later. *J Intern Med Suppl* 736:13–22, 1994.

13. Kvist A, Chowdhury B, Grangard U, Tylen U, Sjostrom L: Total and visceral adipose tissue volumes derived from measurements with computed tomography in adult men and women: Predictive equations. *Am J Clin Nutr* 48:1351–1361, 1988.

14. Gillum RF: The association of body fat distribution with hypertension, hypertensive heart disease, coronary heart disease, diabetes and cardiovascular risk factors in men and women aged 18–79 years. *J Chronic Dis* 40:421–428, 1987.

15. Micciolo R, Bosello O, Ferrari P, Armellini F: The association of body fat location with hemodynamic and metabolic status in men and women aged 21–60 years. *J Clin Epidemiol* 44:591–608, 1991.

16. Björntorp P: Abdominal obesity and the metabolic syndrome. *Ann Med* 24:465–468, 1992.

17. Johnson D, Prud'homme D, Després JP, Nadeau A, Tremblay A, Bouchard C: Relation of abdominal obesity to hyperinsulinemia and high blood pressure in men. *Int J Obes* 16:881–890, 1992.

18. Mauriege P, Després JP, Marcotte M, et al.: Abdominal fat cell lipolysis, body fat distribution, and metabolic variables in premenopausal women. *J Clin Endocrinol Metab* 71:1028–1035, 1990.

19. Sjöström L: A computer-tomography based multicompartment body composition technique and anthropometric predictions of lean body mass, total and subcutaneous adipose tissue. *Int J Obes* 15 (Suppl 2):19–30, 1991.

20. Lemiuex S, Prud'homme D, Tremblay A, Bouchard C, J-P Després: Anthropometric correlates to changes in visceral adipose tissue over 7 years in women. *Int J Obes* 20:618–624, 1996.

21. Bump RC, Sugerman HJ, Fantl JA, et al.: Obesity and lower urinary tract function in women: Effects of surgically induced weight loss. *Am J Obstet Gynecol* 167:392–397, 1992.

22. Sugerman H, Windsor A, Bessos M, Wolfe M: Abdominal pressure, sagittal abdominal diameter and obesity co-morbidity. *J Int Med* 241:71–79, 1997.

23. Ridings PC, Bloomfield GL, Blocher CR, Sugerman HJ: Cardiopulmonary effects of raised intra-abdominal pressure before and after volume expansion. *J Trauma* 39:1071–1075, 1995.

24. Sugerman HJ, Baron PL, Fairman RP, Evans CR, Vetrovec GW: Hemodynamic dysfunction in obesity hypoventilation syndrome and the effects of treatment with surgically induced weight loss. *Ann Surg* 207:604–613, 1988.

25. Bloomfield GL, Ridings PC, Blocher CS, Marmarou A, Sugerman HJ: Effects of increased intra-abdominal pressure upon intracranial and cerebral perfusion pressure before and after volume expansion. *J Trauma* 40:936–943, 1996.

26. Bloomfield GL, Ridings PC, Blocher CR, Sugerman HJ: Increased pleural pressure mediates the effects of elevated intra-abdominal pressure upon the central nervous and cardiovascular systems. *Crit Care Med* 25:496–503, 1997.

27. Sugerman HJ, Felton WL, Sismanis A, Salvant JB, Kellum JM: Effects of surgically induced weight loss on pseudotumor cerebri in morbid obesity. *Neurology* 45:1655–1659, 1995.

28. Harman PK, Kron IL, McLachlan HD, et al.: Elevated intra-abdominal pressure and renal function. *Ann Surg* 196:594–599, 1982.

29. Iberti TJ, Lieber CE, Benjamin E: Determination of intra-abdominal pressure using a transurethral bladder catheter: Clinical validation of the technique. *Anesthesiology* 70:47–50, 1989.

30. Sugerman H, Windsor A, Bessos M, Kellum J, Reines H, DeMaria E: Effects of surgically induced weight loss on urinary bladder pressure, sagittal abdominal diameter and obesity co-morbidity. *Int J Obes Relat Metab Disord* 22:230–235, 1998.

31. Valensi P, Assayag M, Busby M, Paries J, Lormeau B, Attali J-R: Microalbuminuria in obese patients with or without hypertension. *Int J Obes Relat Metab Disord* 20:574–579, 1996.

32. Weisinger JR, Kempson RL, Eldridge FL, Swenson RS: The nephrotic syndrome: A complication of massive obesity. *Ann Intern Med* 81:440–447, 1974.

33. Doty JM, Saggi BH, Sugerman HJ, et al.: The effect of increased renal venous pressure on renal function. *J Trauma* 47:1000–1004, 1999.

34. Bloomfield GL, Blocher CR, Sugerman HJ: Elevated intra-abdominal pressure increases plasma renin activity and aldosterone levels. *J Trauma* 42:997–1004, 1997.

35. Alaud-din A, Meterissian S, Lisbona R, MacLean LD, Forse RA: Assessment of cardiac function in patients who were morbidly obese. *Surgery* 108:809–818, 1990.

36. Foley EF, Benotti PN, Borlase BC, Hollingshead J, Blackburn GL: Impact of gastric restrictive surgery on hypertension in the morbidly obese. *Am J Surg* 163:294–297, 1992.

37. Carson JL, Ruddy ME, Duff AE, Holmes NJ, Cody RP, Brolin RE: The effect of gastric bypass surgery on hypertension in morbidly obese patients. *Ann Int Med* 154:193–200, 1994.

38. Sjostrom CD, Lissner L, Wedel H, et al.: Reduction in incidence of diabetes, hypertension and lipid disturbances after intentional weight loss induced by bariatric surgery: The SOS Intervention Study. *Obes Res* 7:477–484, 1999.

39. Ben-Dov I, Grossman E, Stein A, Shachor D, Gaides M: Marked weight reduction lowers resting and exercise blood pressure in morbidly obese subjects. *Am J Hypertens* 13:251–255, 2000.

40. Sjostrom CD, Peltonen M, Wedel H, et al.: Differentiated long-term effects of intentional weight loss on diabetes and hypertension. *Hypertension* 36:20–25, 2000.

41. Sjostrom CD, Peltonen M, Sjostrom L: Blood pressure and pulse pressure during long-term weight loss in the obese: The Swedish Obese Subjects (S0S) Intervention Study. *Obes Res* 9:188–195, 2001.

42. Sugerman HJ, Wolfe LG, Sica DA, Clore JN: Diabetes and hypertension in severe obesity and effects of gastric bypass-induced weight loss. *Ann Surg* 237:751–756, 2003.

43. Frigg A, Peterli R, Peters T, Ackermann C, Tondelli P: Reduction in co-morbidities 4 years after laparoscopic adjustable gastric banding. *Obes Surg* 14:216–223, 2004.

44. Messerli FH, Sundgaard-Riise K, Reisin ED, et al.: Disparate cardiovascular effects of obesity and arterial hypertension. *Am J Med* 74:808–811, 1983.

45. Alpert MA, Terry BE, Kelly DL: Effect of weight loss on cardiac chamber size, wall thickness and left ventricular function in morbid obesity. *Am J Cardiol* 55:783–786, 1985.

46. Alpert MA, Lambert CR, Panayiotou H, et al.: Relation of duration of morbid obesity to left ventricular mass, systolic function, and diastolic filling, and effect of weight loss. *Am J Cardiol* 76:1194–1197, 1995.

47. Karason K, Wallentin I, Larsson B, Sjostrom L: Effects of obesity and weight loss on left ventricular mass and relative wall thickness: Survey and intervention study. *Br Med J* 315:912–916, 1997.

48. Karason K, Wallentin I, Larsson B, Sjostrom L: Effects of obesity and weight loss on cardiac function and valvular performance. *Obes Res* 6:422–429, 1998.

49. Kanoupakis E, Michaloudis D, Fraidakis O, Parthenakis F, Vardas P, Melissas J: Left ventricular function and cardiopulmonary performance following surgical treatment of morbid obesity. *Obes Surg* 11:552–558, 2001.

50. Manson JE, Colditz GA, Stampfer MJ, et al.: A prospective study of obesity and risk of coronary heart disease in women. *N Engl J Med* 322:882–889, 1990.

51. Manson JE, Willett WC, Stampfer MJ, et al.: Body weight and mortality among women. *N Engl J Med* 333:677–685, 1995.

52. Gleysteen JJ: Results of surgery: Long-term effects on hyperlipidemia. *Am J Clin Nutr* 55:591S–593S, 1992.

53. Buffington CK, Cowan GS Jr, Smith H: Significant changes in the lipid-lipoprotein status of premenopausal morbidly obese females following gastric bypass surgery. *Obes Surg* 4:328–335, 1994.

54. Wolf AM, Beisiegel U, Kornter B, Kuhlmann HW: Does gastric restriction surgery reduce the risks of metabolic diseases? *Obes Surg* 8:9–13, 1998.

55. Busseto L, Pisent C, Rinaldi D, et al.: Variation in lipid levels in morbidly obese patients operated with Lap-Band® adjustable gastric banding system: Effects of different levels of weight loss. *Obes Surg* 10:569–577, 2000.

56. Brolin RE, Bradley LJ, Wilson AC, Cody RP: Lipid risk profile and weight stability after gastric restrictive operations for morbid obesity. *J Gastrointest Surg* 4:464–469, 2000.

57. MacGregor MI, Block AJ, Ball WC: Topics in clinical medicine. Serious complications and sudden death in the Pickwickian syndrome. *Hopkins Med J* 189:279–295, 1970.

58. Guilleminault C, Partinen M, Quera-salva MA, Hayes B, Dement WC, Nino-Murcia G: Determinants of daytime sleepiness and obstructive sleep apnea. *Chest* 94:32–37, 1986.

59. Sugerman HJ, Fairman RP, Baron PL, Kwentus JA: Gastric surgery for respiratory insufficiency of obesity. *Chest* 90:82–91, 1986.

60. Sugerman HJ, Fairman RP, Sood RK, et al.: Long-term effects of gastric surgery for treating respiratory insufficiency of obesity. *Am J Clin Nutr* 55:597S–601S, 1992.

61. Charuzi I, Ovnat A, Peiser J, et al.: The effect of surgical weight reduction on sleep quality in obesity-related sleep apnea syndrome. *Surgery* 97:535–538, 1985.

62. Charuzi I, Lavie P, Peiser J, Peled R: Bariatric surgery in morbidly obese sleep-apnea patients: Short and long-term follow-up. *Am J Clin Nutr* 55:594S–596S, 1992.

63. Boone KA, Cullen JJ, Mason EE, Scott DH, Doherty C, Maher JW: Impact of vertical banded gastroplasty on respiratory insufficiency of severe obesity. *Obes Surg* 6:454–458, 1996.

64. Rasheid S, Banasiak M, Gallagher SF, et al.: Gastric bypass is an effective treatment for obstructive sleep apnea in patients with clinically significant obesity. *Obes Surg* 13:58–61, 2003.

65. Hackney JD, Crane MG, Collier CC, Rokaw S, Griggs DE: Syndrome of extreme obesity and hypoventilation: Studies of etiology. *Ann Intern Med* 51:541–552, 1959.

66. Herbst CA, Hughes TA, Gwynne JT, et al.: Gastric bariatric operation in insulin-treated adults. *Surgery* 95:201–204, 1984.

67. Pories WJ, MacDonald KG, Morgan EJ, et al.: Surgical treatment of obesity and its effect on diabetes: 10-y follow-up. *Am J Clin Nutr* 55:582S–585S, 1992.

68. Pories WJ, Swanson MS, MacDonald KG, et al.: Who would have thought it? An operation proves to be the most effective therapy for adult-onset diabetes mellitus? *Ann Surg* 222:339–350, 1995.

69. Hickey MS, Pories WJ, MacDonald KG Jr, et al.: A new paradigm for type 2 diabetes mellitus: Could it be a disease of the foregut? *Ann Surg* 227:637–643, 1998.

70. MacDonald KG Jr, Long SD, Swanson MS, et al.: The gastric bypass operation reduces the progression and mortality of non-insulin dependent diabetes mellitus. *J Gastrointest Surg* 1:213–220, 1997.

71. Pories WJ, Albrecht RJ: Etiology of type II diabetes mellitus: Role of the foregut. *World J Surg* 25:527–531, 2001.

72. Neve HJ, Soulsby CT, Whiteley GS, Kincey J, Taylor TV: Resolution of diabetes following vertical gastroplasty in morbidly obese patients. *Obes Surg* 3:75–78, 1993.

73. Castagneto M, De Gaetano A, Mingrone G, et al.: Normalization of insulin sensitivity in obese patients after stable weight reduction with biliopancreatic diversion. *Obes Surg* 4:161–168, 1994.

74. Luyckx FH, Scheen AJ, Desaive C, Dewe W, Gielen JE, Lefebvre PJ: Effects of gastroplasty on body weight and related biological abnormalities in morbid obesity. *Diabetes Metab* 24:355–361, 1998.

75. Sjostrom CD, Lissner L, Wedel H, Sjostrom L: Reduction in incidence of diabetes, hypertension and lipid disturbances after intentional weight loss induced by bariatric surgery: The SOS Intervention Study. *Obes Res* 7:477–484, 1999.

76. Dixon JB, O'Brien PE: Health outcomes of severely obese type 2 diabetic subjects 1 year after laparoscopic adjustable gastric banding. *Diabetes Care* 25:397–398, 2002.

77. Schauer PR, Burguera B, Ikramuddin S, et al.: Effect of laparoscopic Roux-en-Y gastric bypass on type 2 diabetes mellitus. *Ann Surg* 238:467–484, 2003.

78. Polyzogopoulou EV, Kalfarentzos F, Vagenakis AG, Alexandrides TK: Restoration of euglycemia and normal acute insulin response to glucose in obese subjects with type 2 diabetes following bariatric surgery. *Diabetes* 52:1098–1103, 2003.

79. Giusti V, Suter M, Heraief E, Gaillard RC, Burckhardt P: Effects of laparoscopic gastric banding on body composition, metabolic profile and nutritional status of obese women: 12-months follow-up. *Obes Surg* 14:239–245, 2004.

80. Chan P, Lin TH, Pan WH, Lee YH: Thrombophilia associated with obesity in ethnic Chinese. *Int J Obes Relat Metab Disord* 19:756–759, 1995.

81. Sugerman HJ, Kellum JM, DeMaria EJ: Risks and benefits of gastric bypass in morbidly obese patients with severe venous stasis disease. *Ann Surg* 234:41–46, 2001.

82. Winiarsky R, Barth P, Lotke P: Total knee arthroplasty in morbidly obese patients. *J Bone Joint Surg Am* 80(12):1770–1774, 1998.

83. McKee MD, Waddekk JP: Intramedullary nailing of femoral fractures in morbidly obese patients. *J Trauma* 36:208–210, 1994.

84. Bostman OM: Body mass index and height in patients requiring surgery for lumbar intervertebral disc herniation. *Spine* 18:851–854, 1993.

85. Parvizi J, Trousadale RT, Sarr MG: Total joint arthroplasty in patients surgically treated for morbid obesity. *J Arthroplasty* 15(8):1003–1008, 2000.

86. Peltonen M, Lindroos AK, Torgerson JS: Musculoskeletal pain in the obese: A comparison with the general population and long-term changes after conventional and surgical obesity treatment. *Pain* 104:549–557, 2003.

87. Melissas J, Volakakis E, Hadjipavlou A: Low-back pain in morbidly obese patients and the effect of weight loss following surgery. *Obes Surg* 13:389–393, 2003.

88. Zacchi P, Mearin F, Humbert P, et al.: Effect of obesity on gastroesophageal resistance to flow in man. *Dig Dis Sci* 36:1473–1480, 1991.

89. Rigaud D, Merrouche M, LeMod G, et al.: Facteurs de reflux gastro-oesophagien acide dans l'obesite severe. *Gastroenterol Clin Biol* 19:818–825, 1995.

90. Deitel M, Khanna RK, Hagen J, Ilves R: Vertical banded gastroplasty as an antireflux procedure. *Am J Surg* 155:512–514, 1988.

91. Smith SC, Edwards CB, Goodman GN: Symptomatic and clinical improvement in morbidly obese patients with gastroesophageal reflux disease following Roux-en-Y gastric bypass. *Obes Surg* 7:479–484, 1997.

92. Frezza EE, Ikramuddin S, Gourash W, et al.: Symptomatic improvement in gastroesophageal reflux disease (GERD) following laparoscopic Roux-en-Y gastric bypass. *Surg Endosc* 16:1027–1031, 2002.

93. Naslund E, Granstrom L, Melcher A, Stockeld D, Backman L: Gastro-oesophageal reflux before and after vertical banded gastroplasty in the treatment of obesity. *Eur J Surg* 162:303–306, 1996.

94. Kim CH, Sarr MG: Severe reflux esophagitis after vertical banded gastroplasty for treatment of morbid obesity. *Mayo Clin Proc* 67:33–35, 1992.

95. Sugerman HJ, Kellum JM Jr, DeMaria EJ, Reines HD: Conversion of failed or complicated vertical banded gastroplasty to gastric bypass in morbid obesity. *Am J Surg* 171:263–269, 1996.

96. Wei JT, Shaheen N: The changing epidemiology of esophageal adenocarcinoma. *Semin Gastroinetest Dis* 14:112–127, 2003.

97. Macgregor A, Greenberg RA: Effect of surgically induced weight loss on asthma in the morbidly obese. *Obes Surg* 3:15–21, 1993.

98. Engel LS, Chow WH, Vaughan TL, et al.: Population attributable risks of esophageal and gastric cancers. *J Natl Cancer Inst* 17:1404–1413, 2003.

99. Dixon JB, Chapman L, O'Brien P: Marked improvement in asthma after Lap-Band® surgery for morbid obesity. *Obes Surg* 9:385–389, 1999.

100. Nestler JE, Jakubowicz DJ, Evans WS, Pasquali R: Effects of metformin on spontaneous and clomiphene-induced ovulation in the polycystic ovary syndrome. *N Eng J Med* 338:1876–1880, 1998.

101. Nestler JE, Jakubowicz DJ, Reamer P, Gunn RD, Allan G: Ovulatory and metabolic effects of D-chiro-inositol in the polycystic ovary syndrome. *N Engl J Med* 340:1314–1320, 1999.

102. Deitel M, Toan BT, Stone EM, et al.: Sex hormone changes accompanying loss of massive excess weight. *Gastroenterol Clin N Am* 16:511–515, 1987.

103. Robert E, Francannet C, Shaw G: Neural tube defects and maternal weight reduction in early pregnancy. *Reprod Toxicol* 9:57–59, 1995.

104. Friedman D, Cunco S, Valenzano M, et al.: Pregnancies in an 18-year follow-up after biliopancreatic diversion. *Obes Surg* 5:308–313, 1995.

105. Wittgrove AC, Jester L, Wittgrove P, Clark GW: Pregnancy following gastric bypass for morbid obesity. *Obes Surg* 8:461–464, 1998.

106. Dixon JB, Dixon ME, O'Brien PE: Pregnancy after Lap-Band surgery: Management of the band to achieve health weight outcomes. *Obes Surg* 11:59–65, 2001.

107. Skull AJ, Slater GH, Duncombe JE, Fielding GA: Laparoscopic adjustable banding in pregnancy: Safety, patient tolerance and effect on obesity-related pregnancy outcomes. *Obes Surg* 14:230–235, 2004.

108. Liu GT, Volpe NJ, Schatz NJ, Galetta SL, Farrar JT, Raps EC: Severe sudden visual loss caused by pseudotumor cerebri and lumboperitoneal shunt failure. *Am J Ophthalmol* 122:129–131, 1966.

109. Rosenberg ML, Corbett JJ, Smith C, et al.: Cerebrospinal fluid diversion procedures in pseudotumor cerebri. *Neurology* 43:1071–1072, 1993.

110. Sugerman HJ, Felton WL 3rd, Sismanis A, et al.: Gastric surgery for pseudotumor cerebri associated with severe obesity. *Ann Surg* 21:682–685, 1999.

111. Bayderdorffer E, Mannes GA, Ochsenkuhn T, Kopcke W, Wiebecke B, Paumgartner G: Increased risk of 'high-risk' colorectal adenomas in overweight men. *Gastroenterol* 104:137–144, 1993.

112. Garfinkel L: Overweight and cancer. *Ann Int Med* 103:1034–1036, 1985.

113. Snowdon DA, Phillips R, Choi W: Diet, obesity, and risk of fatal prostate cancer. *Am J Epidemiol* 120:244–250, 1984.

114. Yu MC, Mack TM, Hanisch R, Cicioni C, Henderson BE: Cigarette smoking, obesity, diuretic use, and coffee consumption as risk factors for renal cell carcinoma. *JNCI* 77:351–356, 1986.

115. Sugerman HJ, Kellum JM Jr, Reines HD, DeMaria EJ, Newsome HH, Lowry JW: Greater risk of incisional hernia with morbidly obese than steroid-dependent patients and low recurrence with prefascial polypropylene mesh. *Am J Surg* 171:80–84, 1996.

116. Schauer PR, Ramos R, Ghiatas AA, Sirinek KR: Virulent diverticular disease in young obese men. *Am J Surg* 164:443–448, 1992.

117. Konvolinka CW: Acute diverticulitis under age forty. *Am J Surg* 167:562–565, 1994.

118. Funnell IC, Bornman PC, Weakley SP, Terblanche J, Marks IN: Obesity: An important prognostic factor in acute pancreatitis. *Br J Surg* 80:484–486, 1993.

119. Nauta RJ: A radical approach to bacterial panniculitis of the abdominal wall in the morbidly obese. *Surgery* 107:134–139, 1990.

120. Harrison SA, Kadakia S, Lang KA, Schenker S: Nonalcoholic steatohepatitis: What we know in the new millennium. *Am J Gastroenterol* 97:2714–2724, 2002.

121. Hui JM, Kench JG, Chitturi S, et al.: Long-term outcomes of cirrhosis in nonalcoholic steatohepatitis compared with hepatitis C. *Hepatology* 38:420–427, 2003.

122. Ranlov I, Hardt F: Regression of liver steatosis following gastroplasty or gastric bypass for morbid obesity. *Digestion* 47:208–214, 1990.

123. Silverman EM, Sapala JA, Appelman HD: Regression of hepatic steatosis in morbidly obese persons after gastric bypass. *Am J Clin Pathol* 104:23–31, 1995.

124. Luyckx FH, Desaive C, Thiry A, et al.: Liver abnormalities in severely obese subjects: Effect of drastic weight loss after gastroplasty. *Int J Obes Relat Metab Disord* 22:222–226, 1998.

125. Kral JG, Thung SN, Biron S, et al.: Effects of surgical treatment of the metabolic syndrome on liver fibrosis and cirrhosis. *Surgery* 135:48–58, 2004.

126. Rand CS, Macgregor A, Hankins G: Gastric bypass surgery for obesity: Weight loss, psychosocial outcome, and morbidity one and three years later. *South Med J* 79(12):1511–1514, 1986.

127. Kral JG, Sjostrom LV, Sullivan MB: Assessment of quality of life before and after surgery for severe obesity. *Am J Clin Nutr* 55(Suppl 2):611S–614S, 1992.

128. Schauer PR, Ikramuddin S, Gourash W, et al.: Outcomes after laparoscopic Roux-en-Y gastric bypass for morbid obesity. *Ann Surg* 232(4):515–529, 2000.

129. Nguyen NT, Goldman C, Rosenquist CJ, et al.: Laparoscopic versus open gastric bypass: A randomized study of outcomes, quality of life, and costs. *Ann Surg* 234:279–291, 2001.

130. Dixon JB, O'Brien PE: Changes in comorbidities and improvements in quality of life after LAP-BAND placement. *Am J Surg* 184:51S–54S, 2002.

131. van Gemert WG, Severijas RM, Gree JW, Groenman N, Soeters PB: Psychological functioning of morbidly obese patients after surgical treatment. *Int J Obes Relat Metab Disord* 22:393–398, 1998.

132. Wadden TA, Sarwer DB, Womble LG, Foster GB, McGuckin BG, Schimmel A: Psychological aspects of obesity and obesity surgery. *Surg Clin North Am* 81:1001–1024, 2001.

133. Maddi SR, Fox SR, Khoshaba DM, Harvey RH, Lu JL, Persico M: Reduction in psychopathology following bariatric surgery for morbid obesity. *Obes Surg* 11:680–685, 2001.

134. Papageorgiou GM, Papakonstantinou A, Mamplekou E, Terzis I, Melissas J: Pre- and postoperative psychological characteristics in morbidly obese patients. *Obes Surg* 12:534–539, 2002.

135. Dixon JB, Dixon ME, O'Brien PE: Depression in association with severe obesity: Changes with weight loss. *Arch Intern Med* 163:2058–2065, 2003.

136. Herpertz S, Kleimann R, Wolf AM, Langkafei M, Scaf W, Hebebrand J: Does obesity surgery improve psychosocial functioning? A systematic review. *Int J Obes Relat Metab Disord* 27:1300–1314, 2003.

137. Klesges RC, Klem ML, Hanson CL, et al.: The effects of applicant's health status and qualifications on simulating hiring decisions. *Int J Obes* 14:527–535, 1990.

138. Pingitore R, Dugoni BL, Tindale RS, Spring B: Bias against overweight job applicants in a simulated employment interview. *J Appl Psychol* 79:909–917, 1994.

139. Christou NV, Sampalis JS, Lieberman M, et al.: Surgery decreases long-term mortality, morbidity and health care use in morbidly obese patients. *Ann Surg* 240:416–23, 2004; discussion 423–4.

3

Rationale for Minimally Invasive Bariatric Surgery

Ninh T. Nguyen, MD • Esteban Varela, MD • Samuel E. Wilson, MD

BACKGROUND

Bariatric surgery is increasing in North America. In a population-based study, Pope et al.[1] reported that the number of bariatric procedures performed in the United States increased from 4,925 operations in 1990 to 12,541 operations in 1997, then increased sharply to 70,256 procedures in 2002.[2] Although the first case series of laparoscopic gastric bypasses (GBPs) was reported in 1994, the dissemination of the laparoscopic approach did not occur until 1999.[2,3] The subsequent growth of bariatric surgery in 1999 was similar to the expansion of antireflux surgery in 1993 after introduction of the laparoscopic Nissen fundoplication technique.[4]

The impact of laparoscopy on bariatric surgery has been even greater with bariatric operations, including GBP and other procedures, estimated to reach more than 120,000 procedures in 2005.

Despite acceptance of laparoscopic bariatric surgery by both surgeons and the public, some third-party payers are reluctant to provide insurance coverage for the laparoscopic method. In September 2003, the Blue Cross and Blue Shield Association's Technology Evaluation Center indicated that there was insufficient evidence to form conclusions about the relative efficacy and morbidity of the laparoscopic approach to GBP.[5] The high demand for minimally invasive bariatric surgery combined with increase in surgeons who are skilled in the technique demands a clear understanding of the evidence-based data on which the safety of minimally invasive bariatric surgery is based. This chapter reviews the current scientific rationale for the use of minimally invasive technique in bariatric surgery.

RATIONALE FOR MINIMALLY INVASIVE BARIATRIC SURGERY

At the onset, it is important to consider why laparoscopic bariatric surgery was introduced as an alternative to open bariatric surgery. No doubt, open bariatric surgery can be performed with a good outcome, but the wound-related complications such as infection and late incisional hernia can be troublesome. Postoperative wound infections occur in as many as 15% of morbidly obese patients and late incisional hernias occur in up to 20% of patients.[6–8] Accordingly, bariatric surgery would be improved by minimizing the morbidity of the access incision. In addition, morbidly obese patients undergoing the laparoscopic approach benefit from a reduction in postoperative pain, shorter length of hospital stay, and faster recovery. These attributes have all been well-documented from several laparoscopic intra-abdominal operations including cholecystectomy, antireflux surgery, and removal of solid organs. The minimally invasive technique is a reasonable approach in the morbidly obese as these patients have many comorbidities that can magnify the likelihood for postoperative complications. In essence, minimally invasive bariatric surgery was initiated to improve the perioperative outcomes—primarily a reduction in postoperative complications arising directly or indirectly from the abdominal wall incision.

TRIALS OF LAPAROSCOPIC VERSUS OPEN BARIATRIC SURGERY

The ideal model for evaluating the safety and efficacy of minimally invasive bariatric surgery is a trial of the laparoscopic versus open GBP. Gastric bypass is a complex bariatric operation that can be associated with certain perioperative and long-term morbidity. The laparoscopic approach to GBP was designed to achieve the same intra-abdominal procedure as the open GBP but through multiple small access incisions. Large clinical series have demonstrated the safety and efficacy of laparoscopic GBP; however, there have been only three prospective, randomized trials comparing laparoscopic versus open GBP.[9–11] The first randomized trial reported by Westling et al.[9] involved 51 patients (laparoscopic = 30, open = 21). The results of this small trial are difficult to interpret because of the author's high conversion rate from laparoscopic to open procedures (23%), which probably reflects data accrued during the learning curve for the laparoscopic procedure. A comparison between laparoscopic and open GBP is valid only if (1) the anatomic and metabolic principles of the laparoscopic operation are similar to those of the open

operation and (2) the surgeon has completed the learning curve of the laparoscopic approach. The second prospective, randomized trial was published by Nguyen et al. in 2001 and the last trial was published by a group from Murcia, Spain, in 2004.[10,11] The results from these two trials will be considered in detail in the following sections.

OUTCOMES OF LAPAROSCOPIC VERSUS OPEN GASTRIC BYPASS

Postoperative Pulmonary Function

By reducing the size of the access incision and therefore operative trauma to the host, minimally invasive bariatric surgery has physiological advantages over open bariatric surgery. This concept has been demonstrated for other minimally invasive procedure such as cholecystectomy, antireflux surgery, and colectomy.[12] In a study examining changes in pulmonary function after laparoscopic and open gastric, Nguyen and colleagues[13] demonstrated significantly less impairment of postoperative pulmonary function after the laparoscopic procedure. The forced expiratory volume at 1 second was 38% higher on the first postoperative day after laparoscopic than after open GBP.[13] There was also a lower rate of segmental atelectasis after laparoscopic GBP.[13] Less pulmonary impairment after laparoscopic GBP represents an objective measure of the physiologic advantage of the laparoscopic approach.

Postoperative Pain

The magnitude of postoperative pain is often a reflection of the extent of the surgical incision and operative trauma associated with the procedure. Postoperative pain is significantly less after laparoscopic GBP, as demonstrated by a lower utilization of intravenous morphine sulfate on the first postoperative day.[13] Despite utilizing greater dosages of narcotics, open GBP patients still reported higher visual analog pain scores.[13]

Weight Loss

Theoretically, long-term weight loss after minimally invasive bariatric surgery should not differ from that of open bariatric surgery as the primary difference between the two techniques is in the method of access and not the gastrointestinal (GI) anatomic construction. Short-term weight loss, however, appears to be better if the patient has had a minimally invasive approach. In Nguyen's randomized trial of laparoscopic versus open GBP, a higher percentage of excess body weight was lost at 6 months after laparoscopic compared to open GBP (54% vs 45%, respectively, $p < 0.05$) but not at 1 year (68% for laparoscopy vs 62% for open).[10] Similar results were reported by Courcoulas et al.,[14] who found that excess body weight loss at 6 months was higher after laparoscopic GBP than after open GBP (52% vs 45%, respectively) but similar weight loss was observed at 1 year (69% for laparoscopy vs 65% for open). Greater weight loss in patients who underwent minimally invasive bariatric surgery within the first 6 months postoperatively is probably due to the earlier resumption of physical activities and initiation of an exercise program as these patients experienced a shorter recovery time. Long-term weight loss appears to be similar after laparoscopic and open bariatric surgery. Wittgrove and Clark[15] reported that 78% of patients who underwent laparoscopic GBP had lost greater than 50% of their excess body weight at 4-year follow-up. In a randomized trial of laparoscopic versus open GBP, Lugan et al.[11] reported similar weight loss between the two groups at 3 years.

COMPLICATIONS OF LAPAROSCOPIC VERSUS OPEN GASTRIC BYPASS

Minimally invasive bariatric surgery, particularly laparoscopic GBP, is technically challenging, as it requires skill in intestinal dissection and reconstruction techniques coupled with advanced suturing and intracorporeal knot-tying techniques. Therefore, the development of any new laparoscopic operations can be associated with a "learning curve."[16] Mastering the technique of laparoscopic GBP often requires between 75 and 100 cases.[17,18] Results of minimally invasive bariatric surgery are more fairly compared to that of open bariatric surgery after the learning curve of the laparoscopic operation has been achieved.

Leak

In a review of the literature on studies reporting outcome of laparoscopic and open GBP published between 1994 and 2002, Podnos et al.[19] reported that the rate of anastomotic leak was 1.7% for open GBP (range, 0.5%–6.1%) and 2.1% for laparoscopic GBP (range, 0.9%–4.3%). The higher reported leak rate after laparoscopic GBP may represent the "learning curve" of the laparoscopic procedure. Wittgrove and Clark[15] reported 9 anastomotic leaks (3.0%) in their first 300 laparoscopic GBP procedures and only 2 leaks (1.0%) in their last 200 laparoscopic GBP procedures. Similarly, See et al.[20] reported a 20% leak rate in a small cohort of 20 laparoscopic GBP patients during their first-year experience. In contrast, Higa et al.[21] reported a 0.3% incidence of anastomotic leak in 1,500 laparoscopic GBP procedures, demonstrating that anastomotic leak can be low when performed by an experienced surgical team.

Wound Complications

The incidence of wound infection after minimally invasive bariatric surgery is lower than that of open bariatric surgery.[19] Additionally, abdominal wall infection after open bariatric surgery is often complex requiring opening of a large wound, which results in a protracted course of wound care. Conversely, trocar-site infection after minimally invasive bariatric surgery can be managed with short courses of local wound care. In a randomized trial of laparoscopic versus open GBP,

the rate of wound infection was significantly less after laparoscopic GBP (1.3% vs 10.5%).[10] Another clinical advantage of minimally invasive bariatric surgery is the reduced incidence of late incisional hernia, which can be as high as 20% after open bariatric surgery.[6–8] Podnos et al.[19] confirmed that incisional hernia formation after open GBP was higher than that after laparoscopic GBP (8.6% vs 0.5%, respectively). In addition, wound dehiscence and evisceration have been completely eliminated in minimally invasive bariatric surgery. In a matched cohort analysis of laparoscopic versus open GBP, Courcoulas et al.[14] reported a 7.5% incidence of wound dehiscence after open GBP compared to none after laparoscopic GBP.

Retained Foreign Body

An unappreciated benefit of the minimally invasive bariatric surgery is the reduced risk for retained foreign body. Morbidly obese patients undergoing bariatric surgery are at high risk for retained intra-abdominal instrumentation and laparotomy sponges. Gawande and colleagues[22] reported that the risk for a retained foreign body after surgery increases in emergency operations, unplanned changes in procedure, and patients with a high body mass index. The excessive intra-abdominal fat in morbidly obese individual may conceal operative instruments and laparotomy sponges and manual palpation may not detect the presence of an intra-abdominal foreign body. The risk of retained instruments and sponges is essentially eliminated with the laparoscopic approach as it is impossible to insert these items through the trocar. However, small foreign objects such as a Penrose drain or the spike from the circular stapler can still be inadvertently left intra-abdominally during laparoscopic GBP. In Nguyen's randomized trial of laparoscopic versus open GBP, a retained laparotomy sponge occurred in one patient in the open group.[10]

Bowel Obstruction

One of the potential benefits of minimally invasive bariatric surgery is the reduction of adhesions, but has not been realized as a clinical reduction in postoperative bowel obstruction. Podnos et al.[19] reported that the frequency of both early and late postoperative bowel obstruction was higher after laparoscopic GBP. The reason for the higher rate of early bowel obstruction after laparoscopic GBP appears to be a technical factor relating to the construction of the jejunojejunostomy. Use of a linear stapler to close the jejunojejunostomy anastomotic defect can narrow the afferent aspect of the Roux limb resulting in an early bowel obstruction. In addition, angulation of the afferent aspect of the Roux limb at the level of the jejunojejunostomy may occur because of failure in placement of the antiobstruction suture. The majority of early bowel obstructions after laparoscopic GBP are technically preventable by making the appropriate changes in technique. The frequency of late bowel obstruction is also reported to be higher after laparoscopic compared to open GBP (3.1% vs 2.1%, respectively).[19] The higher frequency of late bowel obstruction is a result of internal herniation, which can occur at the jejunojejunostomy, transverse mesocolon, or at the Petersen mesenteric defect. In a large series of laparoscopic GBP ($n = 2,000$), Higa et al.[23] reported an incidence of 3.1% for postoperative bowel obstruction.

Gastrointestinal Hemorrhage

Gastrointestinal hemorrhage is not an infrequent complication after laparoscopic GBP. The presentation consists of hematemesis, bright red blood per rectum, and/or hypotension. The source of postoperative GI bleeding is from the gastric remnant, gastrojejunostomy, or the jejunojejunostomy staple-lines. The frequency of postoperative GI hemorrhage is higher after laparoscopic than after GBP (1.9% vs 0.6%), which may be related to the aggressive use of anticoagulants for deep venous thrombosis prophylaxis, the frequent use of a stapled gastrojejunostomy, and less frequent oversewing of staple-lines.[19] Intraoperative measures to prevent postoperative GI hemorrhage include the use of shorter staple height stapler (3.5 mm for stomach tissue and 2.5 mm for small bowel tissue), routine oversewing of staple-line edges, or the use of staple-line reinforcement products.

Anastomotic Stricture

Stricture at the gastrojejunostomy anastomosis is a frequent complication after both open and laparoscopic GBP. In a comparative study of laparoscopic versus open GBP, DeMaria and colleagues[24] reported no significant difference in stomal stenosis rate (24% vs 20%) between the two techniques. Factors contributing to development of anastomotic stricture include technical factors such as tension or ischemia and the techniques for construction of the anastomosis such as the use of mechanical stapler versus hand-sewn. In a study comparing the rate of stenosis between the three techniques for creation of the gastrojejunostomy, Gonzalez et al.[25] reported that the circular stapler technique has the highest rate of stricture (31%) compared to hand-sewn (3%) or linear stapler (0%) technique.

Mortality

The mortality after minimally invasive bariatric surgery appears to be similar or lower than that of open bariatric surgery. Podnos et al.[19] reported a lower rate of mortality after laparoscopic compared to open GBP (0.23% vs 0.87%, respectively). In a large cohort of patients ($n = 1,035$) who underwent open GBP, Christou et al.[26] reported a 0.4% perioperative mortality rate. Using multivariate analysis, Fernandez et al.[27] reported that patient characteristics (preoperative weight and hypertension) and complications (leak and pulmonary embolism) were independent risk factors for perioperative death, and the access methods (open vs laparoscopic) were not independently predictive of death. In their series, the mortality rates after open GBP ($n = 1,431$) and laparoscopic GBP ($n = 580$) were 1.9% and 0.7%, respectively.[26] Whether laparoscopic

GBP will ultimately result in lower operative mortality than would open GBP remains to be seen; however, there is now sufficient evidence from the literature to refute the claim that laparoscopic GBP is associated with a higher mortality rate.

CONCLUSIONS

The fundamental differences between minimally invasive bariatric surgery and open bariatric surgery are the methods of abdominal wall access and operative exposure. By reducing the size of the surgical incision and the trauma associated with the operative exposure, the physiologic insult is less in minimally invasive bariatric surgery. Advantages of minimally invasive bariatric surgery include less impairment of postoperative pulmonary function and pulmonary atelectasis. Other advantages of the laparoscopic approach include lower operative blood loss, a shorter hospital stay, reduction in postoperative pain, and faster recovery. The main disadvantage of the laparoscopic approach is the steep learning curve, which may require experience in as much as 100 operations to overcome. Minimally invasive bariatric surgery does not differ from open bariatric surgery with respect to long-term weight loss and improvement of comorbidities. Surgeons experienced in minimally invasive bariatric surgery may confidently offer the minimally invasive approach to their patients undergoing surgical treatment for morbid obesity, realizing significant clinical advantage.

References

1. Pope GD, Birkmeyer JD, Finlayson SR: National trends in utilization and in-hospital outcomes of bariatric surgery. *J Gastrointest Surg* 6:855–861, 2002.
2. Nguyen NT, Root J, Zainabadi K, et al.: Accelerated growth of bariatric surgery with the introduction of minimally invasive surgery. *Arch Surg* 140:1198–1202, 2005.
3. Wittgrove AC, Clark GW, Tremblay LJ: Laparoscopic gastric bypass, Roux-en-Y: Preliminary report of five cases. *Obes Surg* 4:353–357, 1994.
4. Finlayson SRG, Laycock WS, Birkmeyer JD: National trends in utilization and outcomes of antireflux surgery. *Surg Endosc* 17:864–867, 2003.
5. Newer techniques in bariatric surgery for morbid obesity: Blue Cross and Blue Shield Association's Technology Evaluation Center. Assessment Program, 2003;18. Available at: www.bluecares.com.
6. Kellum JM, DeMaria EJ, Sugerman HJ: The surgical treatment of morbid obesity. *Curr Probl Surg* 35:791–858, 1998.
7. Pories WJ, Swanson MS, MacDonald KG, et al.: Who would have thought it? An operation proves to be the most effective therapy for adult-onset diabetes mellitus. *Ann Surg* 222:339–350, 1995.
8. Oh CH, Kim HJ, Oh S: Weight loss following transected gastric bypass with proximal Roux-en-Y. *Obes Surg* 7:142–147, 1997.
9. Westling A, Gustavsson S: Laparoscopic vs open Roux-en-Y gastric bypass: A prospective, randomized trial. *Obes Surg* 11:284–292, 2001.
10. Nguyen NT, Goldman C, Rosenquist CJ, et al.: Laparoscopic versus open gastric bypass: A randomized study of outcomes, quality of life, and costs. *Ann Surg* 234:279–289, 2001.
11. Lugan JA, Frutos D, Hernandez Q, et al.: Laparoscopic versus open gastric bypass in the treatment of morbid obesity: A randomized prospective study. *Ann Surg* 239:433–437, 2004.

12. Schwenk W, Bohm B, Witt C, et al.: Pulmonary function following laparoscopic or conventional colorectal resection. *Arch Surg* 134:6–12, 1999.

13. Nguyen NT, Lee SL, Goldman C, et al.: Comparison of pulmonary function and postoperative pain after laparoscopic versus open gastric bypass: A randomized trial. *J Am Coll Surg* 192:469–476, 2001.

14. Courcoulas A, Perry Y, Buenaventura P, Luketich J: Comparing the outcomes after laparoscopic versus open gastric bypass: A matched paired analysis. *Obes Surg* 13:341–346, 2003.

15. Wittgrove AC, Clark GW: Laparoscopic gastric bypass, Roux-en-Y 500 patients: Technique and results, with 3–60 month follow-up. *Obes Surg* 10:233–239, 2000.

16. Oliak D, Ballantyne GH, Weber P, et al.: Laparoscopic Roux-en-Y gastric bypass: Defining the learning curve. *Surg Endosc* 17:405–408, 2003.

17. Nguyen NT, Rivers R, Wolfe BM: Factors associated with operative outcomes in laparoscopic gastric bypass. *J Am Coll Surg* 197:548–557, 2003.

18. Schauer PR, Ikramuddin S, Hamad G, et al.: The learning curve for laparoscopic Roux-en-Y gastric bypass is 100 cases [abstract]. *Surg Endosc* 16:S190, 2002.

19. Podnos YD, Jimenez JC, Wilson SE, Stevens M, Nguyen NT: Complications after laparoscopic gastric bypass. *Arch Surg* 138:957–961, 2003.

20. See C, Carter PL, Elliott D, et al.: An institutional experience with laparoscopic gastric bypass complications seen in the first year compared with open gastric bypass complications during the same period. *Am J Surg* 183:533–538, 2002.

21. Higa KD, Ho T, Boone KB: Laparoscopic Roux-en-Y gastric bypass: Technique and 3-year follow-up. *J Laparoendosc Adv Surg Tech* 11:377–382, 2001.

22. Gawande AA, Studdert DM, Orav EJ, et al.: Risk factors for retained instruments and sponges after surgery. *N Engl J Med* 348:229–235, 2003.

23. Higa KB, Ho T, Boone KB: Internal hernias after laparoscopic Roux-en-Y gastric bypass: Incidence, treatment and prevention. *Obes Surg* 13:350–354, 2004.

24. DeMaria EJ, Schweitzer MA, Kellum JM, Sugerman HJ: Prospective comparison of open versus laparoscopic Roux-en-Y proximal gastric bypass for morbid obesity [abstract]. *Obes Surg* 10:131, 2000.

25. Gonzalez R, Lin E, Venkatesh KR, Bowers SP, Smith CD: Gastrojejunostomy during laparoscopic gastric bypass: Analysis of 3 techniques. *Arch Surg* 138:181–184, 2003.

26. Christou NV, Sampalis JS, Liberman M, et al.: Surgery decreases long-term mortality, morbidity, and health care use in morbidly obese patients. *Ann Surg* 240:416–424, 2004.

27. Fernandez AZ, Demaria EJ, Tichansky DS, et al.: Multivariate analysis of risk factors for death following gastric bypass for treatment of morbid obesity. *Ann Surg* 239:698–703, 2004.

4

Current Role of Open Bariatric Surgery

Kenneth B. Jones, Jr, MD, FACS

Open bariatric surgery in the age of the laparoscope? You've got to be joking. Certainly I must be a dinosaur or an old dog who refuses to learn new tricks. Maybe I am afraid of the "learning curve." Or just maybe I know something others may not, or are reluctant to acknowledge for one reason or another. How do we define "minimally invasive"? Smaller (or less morbid) incisions, quicker recovery, and less pain are the impressions most would have. Is the laparoscope absolutely required in this definition?

The biggest advantage of the laparoscopic approach to bariatric surgery compared to standard open procedures is the "vast improvement" in wound morbidity. As a matter of fact, in the American Society for Bariatric Surgery (ASBS) and the Society of American Gastrointestinal Endoscopic Surgeons (SAGES) guidelines for laparoscopic and conventional surgical treatment of morbid obesity, under Surgical Techniques, it is mentioned that "...wound complications such as infections, hernias, and dehiscenses appear to be significantly

reduced."[1] This statement is made based on the assumption that we are comparing laparoscopic to open bariatric surgery via an upper midline incision.

Since we are not making one large incision, the assumption is that multiple small incisions produce less pain, a less expensive and shorter hospital stay, and a more rapid return to work and one's usual activities. However, I will demonstrate from my own experience and with the support of published data, that if one simply alters the open incision, that part of the question becomes moot, and other aspects of the "open" postoperative recovery period are at least equal, if not superior, to laparoscopic Roux-en-Y gastric bypass (LRYGBP). Note that my remarks are directed toward Roux-en-Y gastric bypass (RYGBP), not malabsorptive or restrictive procedures considered elsewhere in this book.

I begin my argument by presenting my data concerning primary open RYGBP (ORYGBP). In a series of over 2,400 cases over a 17-year period, the excess weight loss at 10 years postop was 62%, comparable to several other published series.[2–5] The leak rate was 0.5% in primary (1°) RYGBP and the mortality rate was 0.2%.[5] A more recent report[6] plus over 700 gastroplasty procedures beginning in 1979 now totals over 3,800 primary and revision bariatric procedures. Reoperations in this series of 1° RYGBP procedures has been 1.4%[33] due to leaks, staple-line failures, incisional hernias, wound dehiscence, and definitive surgery for peptic ulcer disease. I have excluded many dermatopanniculectomies, which were done following successful weight loss, as well as a few cholecystectomies. I have used the following criteria for cholecystectomy at the time of bariatric surgery: (1) gallstones, symptomatic or not, (2) a strong family history of gallbladder disease, (3) a relatively strong family history of American Indian or Latin American heritage, or (4) cholesterolosis of the gallbladder at the time of surgery. Using these criteria, the handful of patients who have returned for laparoscopic cholecystectomy at a later date is about what one would expect from the normal population.[7]

With this vast experience in bariatric surgery, why do I continue to prefer the procedure open? To put it simply, there is an increased incidence of complications using the laparoscopic approach compared to my open approach, especially during the "learning curve," as well as a higher cost. When you combine this with significantly less wound morbidity of the left subcostal incision (LSI), there is simply no real advantage in doing the minimally invasive RYGBP laparoscopically.

I instigated a study along with 15 other seasoned, "open" bariatric surgeons with a combined total of 25,759 cases representing over 200 surgeon years' experience, who pooled their ORYGBP data and compared the results to the leading LRYGBP papers in the literature.[6]

In the overall series, our incisional hernia rate was 6.4%, using the standard midline incision and only 0.3% with the LSI. Return to surgery in less than 30 days was 0.7%, deaths 0.25%, leaks 0.4%. The average length of stay (LOS) was 3.4 days and return to usual activity was 21 days. Small bowel obstruction (SBO) was significantly higher with the LRYGBP, and surgical equipment costs averaged approximately $3,000 less for open cases, with an added expense for longer operative time. This more than makes up for the shorter LOS with the laparoscopic approach (Table 4–1.)[6] These data compared quite favorably in comparison to the leading published series in the world literature.[8–12]

Table 4–1.

Complete Data, Orlando 2005 Group of Open Bariatric Surgeons[6]

	No.	Staple-line failure or gastro-gastric fistula (%)	Incisional hernias (%)	Return to SX 30 d.	Mortality	Leaks	ALOS	Return to work (days)
Jaroch	1106	0	210/19	17	6	1	4	21
Flanagan	1413	0	141/10	33	9	7	3.3	28
Benotti	858	58/7	?	8	5	6	4.5	7
Afram	2076	80/4	207/10	16	8	16	2.5	12
Capella	3648	40/1	73/2	8	7	4	3	10
Wood, Kole, Schuhknecht, Hendrick, Sapala	7033	1/<.02	281/4	10	15	10	2.5	21
Cooper	984	20/2	20/2	16	2	3	4	17
Shapiro	782	1/<0.13	63/8	14	0	14	3.1	42
Lorio	619	3/0.5	93/15	0	1	0	3	28
Sweet	994	0	20/2	24	5	12	3	21
Howell	3500	11/0.3	535/15	33	2	8	4.75	28
Jones	2746	20/0.7	8/0.3	13/0.5%	5/0.2%	13/0.5%	3.2	17
	25,759	234/0.9%	1641/6.6%	176/0.7%	65/0.25%	94/0.36%	3.4	21

LEAKS

If one looks at the data from Schauer,[8] DeMaria and Sugerman,[9] and Wittgrove and Clark[10] in their published series, we see that their leak rate is almost 3%. However, Champion,[11] who does gastroscopy on all of his patients during surgery, has a leak rate very similar to mine, 0.4%. Higa,[12] who does a double-layer, hand-sewn anastomosis without staples at the gastrojejunostomy, had only 12 leaks in his first 1,040 cases (Table 4–2). We compared our leak data to this group and noted a significant difference favoring our open technique: 2% vs 0.4%, a 500% difference ($p < .001$).[6] We also compared our mean leak rate to three other large, combined lap versus open retrospective combined review series with rates of 2%,[14] 2%,[15] and 1.9%,[16] all statistically significantly inferior to our experience of 0.36% ($p < .001$).

LRYGBP requires stomach transection, which has a significantly higher incidence of leaks compared to stapling in continuity. Kirkpatrick and Zapas in 212 patients in primary divided ORYGBP had 13 leaks, or 6%.[4] Suter et al. in 107 patients in primary divided LRYGBP had a leak rate of 5%.[13] Smith, Goodman, and Edwards[17] doing divided ORYGBP had a leak rate of 1.8% compared to the combined experience of Linner,[18] Yale,[19] and this author of 0.6%.[20] However, in our 2005 Orlando series, the pouch transectors' leak rate was 0.3% compared to the stapled in continuity rate of 0.6% ($p = $ NS).[6] Although not of clinical significance, this likely indicates the advantages of experience or perhaps that the open linear cutting instruments are more efficient than laparoscopic surgery.

Why the higher incidence of leaks with LRYGBP? In my own experience, I have always tried to adhere to the "one-centimeter rule," meaning that if the anastomosis is made incorporating the staple line, there will be some element of ischemia. If staple lines are crossed at approximately 90° angle, the risk of ischemia will be less, and if staple lines are parallel and less than 1-cm apart (the "one-centimeter rule"), or as the crossing staple lines approach parallel, there will be a higher risk of leakage.[21,22] In addition to the above, if one transects a hollow viscus, cut ends must heal and seal. However, when stapling in continuity with no transection, sealing takes place immediately and healing will occur, as there is no compromise of blood supply to the tissue. In my entire experience, I have had only one patient who has had a perforation along the upper/lower pouch staple line in a 1° ORYGBP. This was an individual who had a previously undiagnosed insulinoma and a seizure on her fourth postop day, which ripped holes in the proximal and distal pouches at the staple line, as well as causing a 180° disruption at the gastrojejunostomy. At reexploration, there was no evidence of ischemia, with good bleeding of the edges that had perforated.

Technical error at surgery is a rare cause of postop leaks since "leak tests" are standard prior to completion of our operations. Therefore, leaks are primarily caused by ischemia and/or excess tension at the anastomoses, plain and simple. Do laparoscopic surgeons ignore the "one-centimeter rule," causing more ischemia and necrosis? Does the abandonment of the retrocolic approach to the gastrojejunostomy to decrease SBOs increase tension at the anastomosis? These are questions needing answers before the safer, time-tested open technique can be legitimately abandoned.

COST

The laparoscopists argue that patients get out of the hospital sooner. In several published series,[6,8,10] this appears to be the case, that is, about 2 rather than 3 days, saving approximately $1,000. However, I have never seen a leak that was clinically manifested in the first 72 hours after surgery. Should the patient be released in 1 or 2 days to return home several hundred miles away, a leak could be catastrophic. I compared equipment costs with laparoscopic versus open RYGBP in one of my two hospitals, and found that laparoscopic equipment costs approximately $5,200 versus the open stapling equipment of about $1,700, or a $3,500 difference. Two other contributing surgeons in our Orlando 2005 study[6] compared their open experience to LRYGBP relative to cost: Howell in North Dakota (+$2,900) and Sapala in New York City (+$3,400). Hospitals will probably double that cost to make a profit, making a difference to the patient of about $6,000. Subtracting $1,000 for one less hospital day, and adding the additional OR time at $1,250 per hour, the total charge to the patient is going to be about $7,000 more for LRYGBP. Assuming that at least half of the 140,000 bariatric cases in 2004 were LRYGBP (ASBS estimate), at an added hospital cost of $7,000/case multiplied by 70,000, this results in one half billion dollars in added overall cost in the United States, which has reduced surgical access due to third-party reimbursement backlash. It is no wonder the insurance carriers are balking and adding nuisance red tape, like mandatory preoperative 6–12 month MD-supervised dieting, which we know is only a delay tactic

Table 4–2.

Leaks in lap vs open RYGBP

	# Cases	Leaks	%
Schauer[2]	275	12	4.4
DeMaria & Sugerman[9]	281	11	5.1
Wittgrove & Clark[4]	500	13	2.5
Champion[5]	825	3	0.4
Higa[6]	1,040	12	1.2
	2,921	51	1.75
('04)			
Jones [open][7]	2,421	13	0.5% $p < .001$
2005 Orlando group [open]	25,759	94	0.36% $p < .001$

to deny access, and enhance their bottom lines. This becomes a stewardship issue for us.

OR TIME AND LENGTH OF STAY

Paxton and Matthews found that LRYGBP requires an extra one and a half hours in the OR compared to ORYGBP. They also noted an average LOS of two and a half days for LRYGBP compared to our 3.4 days. It is also interesting to note that in the ORYGBP group, the patients averaged 20 pounds heavier, indicating that the more technically difficult, higher BMI patients undergo open surgery more frequently than laparoscopic surgery.[16] From a strictly practical standpoint, if I am going to spend less time per case in the OR as the laparoscopic group, and since there is little difference in reimbursement for either approach, time will allow higher volume with a significantly positive effect on my reimbursement compared to the laparoscopic group.

SMALL BOWEL OBSTRUCTION

Higa[23] and Podnos'[14] studies totaling 4,887 patients revealed a postop SBO rate of 3%. Capella in the Orlando 2005 study compared 483 LRYGBP patients to 739 ORYGBP patients and found a return to surgery for SBO rate of 7.45% in the former group, 0 in the latter.[6] However, in a previous published report of 1,174 patients I found 7 (0.6%) in my patient population, with only one due to an internal hernia (<0.1%), three due to retrograde intussusception, two from adhesions of previous surgery, and one from a spontaneous bowel wall hematoma.[24] All of these results are statistically significant ($p \leq .001$) (Table 4–2).

OPERATIVE MORTALITY RATES

Comparing our group of 25,759 open cases[6] to Podnos' 3,464 LRYGBP cases, and the International Bariatric Surgery Registry (IBSR) 2002 pooled data of 13,554 cases, mortality rate results were virtually the same: 0.25%, 0.23%, 0.27%, respectively ($p = $ NS). Podnos' open cases revealed a significantly higher mortality rate (0.87%). IBSR data had an LRYGBP mortality rate of only 0.15%, lower than the four studies mentioned above.

LEFT SUBCOSTAL INCISION

Again, when we compare LRYGBP to open, the traditional assumption is that open procedures are being done through midline incisions. However, when one compares my results as well as those of Alvarez-Cordero, using the LSI, and several other published series, our incidence of incisional hernia is 38 times less than those series done through a large midline incision (Table 4–3).[25–29] Also, simply stated, muscle has a much better blood supply and heals considerably better than relatively thin midline fascia.

Table 4–3.

Incisional Hernias, Vertical vs LSI[29]

	No. of procedures	Hernias
Mason, Amoral, Sugerman, Alvarez-Cordero, [vertical: midline]	1,147	87 (7.6%) [38× more]
Alvarez-Cordero, Jones [LSI]	2,200	4 (0.2%)

Why is my incisional hernia rate so low when traditional bariatric surgical patient follow-up is so poor? I use a sampling technique. For instance, all bariatric patients seen for a 4-month period in 1996 who came to the clinic for a variety of reasons, primarily follow-up RYGBP anywhere from 1–10 years, were "spot checked" for hernias. We examined 173 consecutive patients and found no hernias. In another study, the incisional hernia rate was 5/1,367 (0.4%).[5] Our wound morbidity was 2.2%.[29] More recently, examining my data from November 2003 through November 2004, 720 consecutive patients were checked during routine visits, with 5 hernias (0.7%) found.

If one compares the wound morbidity of several of the LRYGBP series to my ORYGBP–LSI experience, it is easy to see that the rate of hernias and other wound morbidity is actually less than with the laparoscopic approach.[8–10] I frequently tell my patients that in addition to the higher complication rate and cost of LRYGBP, you may choose a procedure done through a single 7-inch incision, or several incisions equaling 7 inches, take your choice. Both heal equally well.

It is interesting that in the pre-laparoscopic era, incisional hernias were rarely mentioned, were considered almost totally harmless with rare incarcerations, and although unsightly, they could afford an opportunity for the patient to return to the operating room for a repair and have a relatively inexpensive panniculectomy done at the same time, which ordinarily would be covered by the third-party insurance payer. In the present day laparoscopic era, an incisional hernia is considered to be very undesirable, as the absence of same justifies LRYGBP's almost negligible incisional morbidity rates. For these reasons, the LSI has not achieved widespread popularity.

As a preceptor for the ASBS, two of my preceptees were quite accomplished laparoscopic bariatric surgeons. Their combined series of 476 cases demonstrated an incisional hernia rate with the LSI of 1.5% compared to 7.6% when one looks at the combined series mentioned above.[25–28]

PAIN CONTROL

At our Bariatric Surgery Center of the Mid South at CHRISTUS Schumpert Medical Center in Shreveport, LA, the pain control staff has indicated there is no real difference in the pain endured by either approach—an anecdotal conclusion, but what subjective studies are not?

TECHNIQUE

My procedure is a modification of the Oca–Torres procedure,[30] with the following changes: (1) an LSI, (2) the TA-90B four row Autosuture stapler fired two times, reinforced proximally and distally with ligaclips, (3) a vertical pouch, with no short gastric vessels being taken down and no transection of the pouch, stapled in continuity, (4) a retrocolic antegastric gastrojejunostomy, hand-sewn in two layers, utilizing a #38 Mercury bougie (13 mm in diameter) for accurate stoma sizing, and (5) an enteroenterostomy that is done utilizing linear cutting and stapling instruments, a gastrojejunal limb of 75–150 cm, and biliopancreatic limb of 60–100 cm, depending on the patient's BMI according to the recommendations of Brolin.[31]

I pay particular attention to the following: (1) "one-centimeter rule," (2) care in transection and freeing up of jejunum and the need for adequate length and freedom of the distally transected jejunum to avoid tension at the gastrojejunostomy, (3) care in freeing up the EG junction to avoid perforation and ischemia, (4) a leak test (I prefer the "air bubble" test), and (5) I frequently use gastrostomy tubes in the bypassed stomach: in apple-shaped men; in long, difficult revisions; in patients with diabetes mellitus to avoid problems with diabetic gastroparesis; frequently with BMI's greater than 50 and always when greater than 60; in all JI bypass conversions; and in patients with marginal pulmonary status.

Because of the higher incidence of SBO that has been reported with the laparoscopic approach compared to open,[6,12,23,32] I always take special care to make an adequate transverse colonic mesenteric opening and secure it to the Roux limb prior to closure to prevent herniation. I also do an adequate closure of Peterson's hernia as well as the potential hernia associated with the enteroenterostomy, which may be much more difficult or even ignored laparoscopically. The lack of significant adhesion formation may have an effect on the lack of sealing after laparoscopic closure. Following discharge from the hospital, I insist that the patients stay on a semi-soft "gooey" liquid diet for 6 weeks postop. In addition to the above, I try to preserve all blood supply possible, and avoid usage of the electrocautery near hollow viscera and staple-lines, as necrosis and leaks may follow several days later.

If one feels that it is necessary to transect the stomach in order to get adequate freedom of the proximal gastric pouch to reduce tension at the gastrojejunostomy, I instead use the "Jones stitch" from the lower end of the staple-line to the lower lip of the LSI fascia, which effectively and safely pulls the pouch into the operative field. However, transection is sometimes necessary to get adequate length of the proximal pouch, especially with revision procedures.[21,22]

Relative to pouch transection, many felt about 15 years ago that this was always necessary because of the inordinately high incidence of staple-line disruption and secondary gastrogastric fistulae. Capella[33] noted that when stapled in continuity with no transection, disruption of the staples occurred in as much as 23% of the patient population. However, Pories' group[34] demonstrated that there was a 6% gastro-gastric fistula rate when dividing pouches, while Capella noted 2% in his series.

One might ask, "How do I know that my staple line failure rate is less than 1%?" In a study done several years ago, in 650 patients, my assumption was that my staple-line failure rate at that time was 0.6% with the double application of the TA-90B four row Autosuture stapling instrument. I came to this conclusion by UGI series examination of 160 voluntary asymptomatic post-ORYGBP patients and found one staple-line failure. In 19 symptomatic patients (GERD or rapid weight regain) during this period of time, their UGIs revealed four staple-line failures.[35] When patients have problems, they come back. I revisited this again from November 1999 to April 2003 in a series of 724 patients, in whom we did UGI series on 62 symptomatic patients and found only five staple-line failures. Again, this sampling technique indicated the staple-line failure rate was less than 0.7% (5/724).

DISCUSSION

"Lap RYGBP ... is the most technically demanding of all laparoscopic operations. Consequently, many programs reserve LRYGBP procedures for surgical attendings and fellows, while ORYGBP procedures are more frequently performed or assisted by surgical residents. Undoubtedly, this plays a role in the variation between open and lap complication rates ... therefore, there is a significant (learning curve) ... attributed to (one's first) 200 LRYGBP."[16] I could not say it any better. Podnos, in a retrospective review of the literature, compared all reported series greater than 50 cases of lap or open RYGBP at the time. Age and BMI were similar, in the 8 open and 10 laparoscopic series studied. He found significant differences favoring the open technique in gastrointestinal hemorrhage, SBO, and stomal stenosis. Wound problems were significantly greater in the open approach via the standard upper midline incision. There was no significant difference, although a trend toward fewer leaks with the open technique.[14] This discussion adds to the argument that ORYGBP still stands the test of time quite well.

There is a perception that laparoscopic bariatric surgery is patient driven, but would a patient opt to have a procedure done by a new bariatric surgeon during his or her "learning curve," if they knew the significantly higher risk? Higa,[12] Wittgrove,[10] and Schwarz and Drew (see Chapter 17 in this volume) confirm better results with an increase in experience. We therefore should not succumb to the pressure of our patients and industry and their perception that laparoscopic bariatric surgery is always easier and better, for I have demonstrated that there is indeed a higher complication rate and greater cost, with the anticipated end point virtually the same.

The three large comparative studies mentioned in this chapter[14-16] are at best level III laparoscopic versus open gastric bypass combined series, very much like comparing apples to oranges. In these principally retrospective comparisons with no controls in which there is considerable bias, as most bariatric surgeons would agree that open gastric bypass is easier than laparoscopic, the more difficult cases were frequently reserved for the open technique, that is, males, patients with high BMIs, and revisions. Subsequently there were higher complication rates in the open group. This considerably reduces the credibility of these comparative studies and their conclusions that LRYGBP is superior to ORYGBP.

The primary justification for the laparoscopic approach to any type of surgery is based on the assumption that there is much less wound morbidity than in the open technique. This experiment has been going on for over 15 years with inguinal hernias, and there appears to be no difference in efficacy if one does lap or open, and also long-term studies indicate that recurrences in laparoscopic repairs are at a higher rate than in the open.[36]

Colectomies are done laparoscopically, but the trend now appears to be shifting to indicate that it may be best to do them utilizing hand-assisted techniques, as an incision about the size of a human fist is necessary in order to remove the resected colonic lesion from the abdomen, so why not take advantage of better tactile feeling?[37,38]

Nguyen and associates are champions for LRYGBP, with the primary argument that wound morbidity will be virtually avoided. There are no comparative studies in the literature comparing LRYGBP to open RYGBP–LSI until recently.[6] They agree that there is a significantly higher incidence of internal hernias associated with SBO utilizing LRYGBP, as well as gastrointestinal hemorrhage and stricture requiring further intervention, and that the cost is greater while utilizing the lap technique, with no real difference in the ultimate quality of life.[39] While participating in the ACS Bariatric Surgery Primer in October 2004 (New Orleans), Dr. Nicola Scopinaro, the father of biliopancreatic diversion (BPD), stated, "I predict that in Italy we will soon cease doing laparoscopic BPD and RYGBP in favor of open, due to the added cost, which can't be made up in shorter hospital lengths of stay" [paraphrased] [(personal communication)].

Revisions can be done laparoscopically, but should they? I reviewed the literature for a paper on revisions recently and it appears feasible, but is it practical? The Emory group's experience is an example of this. Thirty-nine revisions were done, 18 open. Twenty one were begun laparoscopically, but 10 converted to open due to technical problems. Of the 11 remaining lap cases, one died (9%). No deaths were seen in the open cases.[40] In three other laparoscopic series (64 patients), only 9% experienced major complications, but the average OR time was four and a half hours.[41-43] Is it worth the even greater learning curve for laparoscopic revisions, if the LSI takes wound morbidity out of the equation? Lap revisions are being done more frequently (see Chapter 15), but why struggle so hard to achieve the same or inferior results (more leaks, etc.)?

Why are we so rapidly adopting laparoscopic RYGBP, when we know that there is a higher risk of leaks, a greater learning curve with a higher risk of medical malpractice exposure, earlier discharge in less than 3 days when leaks are rarely manifested before that time, and when there is an added expense of about $7,000 per case? We also know that our patients' return to work is directly proportional to their motivation,[6] as a very small percentage actually do such vigorous labor that they must be off for 6 weeks.

In spite of these arguments, I am not so naïve to believe the horse is not out of the barn. So, if one feels compelled to do exclusively LRYGBP, I would recommend the following: (1) a basic background with considerable experience in advanced laparoscopic surgery; (2) be exposed to at least 10 open bariatric procedures, preferably RYGBP, (3) take a laparoscopic bariatric surgery mini-fellowship if one has not had considerable residency training in same, and (4) use the Schwarz-Drew philosophy (see Chapter 11): They had a vast experience with open gastric bypass, then took a short course in laparoscopic bariatric surgery, operated on several pigs, then did open RYGBP using laparoscopic instruments before they did their first LRYGBP, and their results have been comparable to their previous open experience.

On the basis of above comparative data, the usual arguments suggesting the superiority of the LRYGBP appear flawed. If we take the vertical incision out of the equation, assuming no difference in wound morbidity, we have in the LRYGBP significantly more leaks, GI hemorrhage, SBO, and stomal stenosis, markedly increasing the reoperation rate. This along with the higher cost and a higher learning curve, all contributes to higher medical malpractice risks. I question the wisdom of discharge at 2.5 days or less, as most leaks are not apparent until 3+ days postop. Well-motivated open patients return to work or normal activities in 3 weeks or less.[6] If we sincerely believe it is truly in our patients' best interest to use LRYGBP technique, it is an acceptable modality. If we do so merely to get ahead of our competition across town in spite of our knowledge of greater LRYGBP morbidity, and we have not made the effort to get the proper skills and experience, then we need to reexamine our priorities and motivations.

In conclusion, these data indicate no real advantage of laparoscopic over open RYGBP, and really quite the opposite. If the incision is really the issue, we should change it to either the LSI or mini-midline. Then we would have a safer, less expensive, MUCH EASIER, equally effective procedure; and truly "minimally invasive." In spite of all the evidence I have presented herein, I know that many, if not most, of us will be compelled by our patients, competition, referring MDs, and industry to abandon open in favor of lap RYGBP. Because the ORYGBP–LSI is easier to do, especially in the more difficult cases, including heavier patients, males, and revisions, it must always be available as a reasonable option. Above all, remember the (Dr. Eddie) Reddick Rule: "If you are making no progress laparoscopically for 15 minutes, OPEN; and get 'r done" [paraphrased].

References

1. *Guidelines for Laparoscopic and Open Surgical Treatment of Morbid Obesity.* (Document adopted by the American Society for Bariatric Surgery and the Society of American Gastrointestinal Endoscopic Surgeons, June 2000). *Obes Surg* 10:378–379, 2000.

2. Pories WJ, Swanson JS, MacDonald KG, et al.: Who would have thought it? An operation proves to be the most effective therapy for adult onset diabetes mellitus. *Ann Surg* 222:339–350, 1995.

3. DeMaria EJ, Sugerman HJ, Kellum JM, et al.: Results of 281 consecutive total laparoscopic Roux-en-Y gastric bypasses to treat morbid obesity. *Ann Surg* 235:640–647, 2002.

4. Kirkpatrick JR, Zapas JL: Divided gastric bypass: A fifteen-year experience. *Am Surg* 64 (1):62–66, 1998.

5. Jones KB: Experience with the Roux-en-Y gastric bypass, and commentary on current trends. *Obes Surg* 10:183–185, 2000.

6. Jones KB, Afram JD, Benotti PN, et al.: Open Roux-en-Y gastric bypass versus laparoscopic: A comparative study of over 25,000 open cases and the major laparoscopic bariatric reported series. In press.

7. Jones KB: Simultaneous cholecystectomy: to be or not to be. *Obes Surg* 5:52–54, 1995.

8. Schauer PR, Ikramuddin S, Gourash W, et al.: Outcomes after laparoscopic Roux-en-Y gastric bypass for morbid obesity. *Ann Surg* 232:515–529, 2000.

9. Sugerman HJ, Kellum JM, Engle KM: Gastric bypass for treating severe obesity. *Am J Clin Nutr* 55(Suppl 12):560S–566S, 1992.

10. Wittgrove AC, Clark GW: Laparoscopic gastric bypass, Roux-en-Y—500 patients: Technique and results, with 3–60 month follow-up. *Obes Surg* 10:233–239, 2000.

11. Champion JK, Hunt T, DeLisle N: Role of routine intraoperative endoscopy in laparoscopic bariatric surgery. *Surg Endosc* 16(12):1663–1665, 2002.

12. Higa KD, Bone K, Ho T: Complications of the laparoscopic Roux-en-Y gastric bypass: 1,040 patients—what have we learned? *Obes Surg* 10:509–513, 2000.

13. Suter M, Giusti V, Heraif E: Laparoscopic Roux-en-Y gastric bypass: Initial 2-year experience. *Surg Endosc* 17(4):603–609, 2003.

14. Podnos YD, Jimenez JC, Wilson SE, et al.: Complications after laparoscopic gastric bypass—a review of 3464 cases. *Arch Surg* 138:957–961, 2003.

15. Baker RS, Foote J, Kemmeter P, et al.: The Science of stapling and leaks. *Obes Surg* 14:1290–1298.

16. Paxton JH, Matthews JB: The cost effectiveness of laparoscopic versus open gastric bypass surgery. *Obes Surg* 15:24–34, 2005.

17. Smith SC, Goodman GN, Edwards LB: Roux-en-Y gastric bypass: A seven year retrospective review of 3,855 patients. *Obes Surg* 5:314–318, 1995.

18. Linner JH: *Surgery for Morbid Obesity.* New York, Springer-Verlag, 1984; p. 97.

19. Yale CE: Gastric surgery for morbid obesity. *Arch Surg* 124:941–946, 1989.

20. Jones KB: The double application of the TA-90B four row stapler and pouch formation: Eight rows are safe and effective in Roux-en-Y gastric bypass. *Obes Surg* 3:262–268, 1994.

21. Jones KB: Revisional bariatric surgery—potentially safe and effective. *Surg Obes Relat Disord* 1(6):599–603, 2005.

22. Jones KB: Revisional bariatric surgery—safe and effective. *Obes Surg* 11:183–189, 2001.

23. Higa KD, Ho T, Boone K: Internal hernias after laparoscopic Roux-en-Y gastric bypass: Incidence, treatment and prevention. *Obes Surg* 13:350–354, 2003.

24. Jones KB: Biliopancreatic limb obstruction in gastric bypass at or proximal to the jejuno-jejunostomy: A potentially deadly, catastrophic event. *Obes Surg* 6:485–493, 1996.

25. Mason EE: *Surgical Treatment of Obesity.* London, WB Saunders, 1981; pp. 340–341.

26. Sugerman HJ, McNeill PM: Continuous absorbable vs. interrupted non-absorbable suture for mid line fascial closure. In: *Proceedings of the Second Annual Meeting of the American Society for Bariatric Surgery,* Iowa City, IA, 1985; pp. 153–154.

27. Amaral JF, Thompson WR: Abdominal closure in the morbidly obese. In: *Proceedings of the Third Annual Meeting of the American Society for Bariatric Surgery,* Iowa city, IA, 1986; pp. 191–202.

28. Alvarez-Cordero R, Aragon-Virvette E: Incisions for obesity surgery: A brief report. *Obes Surg* 1:409–411, 1991.

29. Jones KB: The left subcostal incision revisited. *Obes Surg* 8:225–228, 1998.

30. Torres JC, Oca CF, Garrison RN: Gastric bypass Roux-en-Y gastrojejunostomy from the lesser curvature. *Sou Med J* 76:1217–1221, 1983.

31. Brolin RE, La Marca LB, Kenler HA, et al.: Malabsorptive gastric bypass in patients with super obesity. *J Gastrointest Surg* 6(2):195–205, 2002.

32. Courcoulas A, Perry Y, Buenaventuro P, et al.: Comparing the outcomes after laparoscopic versus open gastric bypass: A matched paired analysis. *Obes Surg* 13:341–346, 2003.

33. Capella JF, Capella RF: Staple disruption and marginal ulceration in gastric bypass procedures for weight reduction. *Obes Surg* 1:44–49, 1996.

34. Cucchi SGD, Pories WJ, MacDonald KG, et al.: Gastro-gastric fistulas, a complication of divided gastric bypass surgery. *Ann Surg* 221:387–391, 1995.

35. Jones KB, Homza W, Peavy P, et al.: Double application of the TA-90B four-row autosuture® stapling instrument: A safe, effective method of staple-line production indicated by follow-up GI series. *Obes Surg* 6:494–499, 1996.

36. Grunwaldt LJ, Schwaitzberg SD, Rassner DW: Is laparoscopic inguinal hernia repair an operation of the past? *J Am Coll Surg* 200(4):616–620, 2005.

37. Rivadeneira DE, Marcello PW, Roberts PL, et al.: Benefits of hand-assisted laparoscopic restorative proctocolectomy: A comparative study. *Dis Colon Rectum* 77:1371–1376, 2004.

38. Chang YJ, Marcello PW, Rusin LC: Hand-assisted laparoscopic sigmoid colectomy: Helping hand or hindrance? *Surg Endosc* 19:656–661, 2005.

39. Nguyen NT, Ho HS, Palmer LS, et al.: A comparison study of laparoscopic versus open gastric bypass for morbid obesity. *J Am Coll Surg* 191(2):149–157, 2000.

40. Khaitan L, Van Sickle K, Gonzalez R, et al.: Laparoscopic revision of bariatric procedures: Is it feasible? *Am Surg* 71(1):6–10, 2005.

41. Weber M, Muller MK, Michel JM, et al.: Laparoscopic Roux-en-Y gastric bypass, but not rebanding, should be proposed as a rescue procedure for patients with failed laparoscopic gastric banding. *Ann Surg* 238(6):827–833, 2003.

42. Gagner M, Gentileschi P, de Csepel J, et al.: Laparoscopic reoperative bariatric surgery: Experience from 27 consecutive patients. *Obes Surg* 12:254–260, 2002.

43. McCormick JT, Papasavas PK, Caushaj PF, Gagne DJ: Laparoscopic revision of failed open bariatric procedures. *Surg Endosc* 77(3):413–415, 2003.

The author acknowledges the contributions of Ms. Kimberly King for technical preparation of the manuscript and Ms. Sue Wainwright and Ms. Donna Foshee for data retrieval and analysis.

5

Central Nervous System Regulation and Hormonal Signaling

Cid Pitombo, MD, PhD, TCBC

INTRODUCTION

It is essential that we understand the normal physiological mechanism that makes us feel the hunger and the mechanisms of absorption and control of ingested food amounts as well as the consequences produced by weight gain as adipose tissues increase and the development of many kinds of diseases. The need to eat involves a sequence of control mechanisms. Eating is necessary for a variety of our organs' functions, be it growth or absorption of micronutrients like vitamins and minerals and macronutrients like carbohydrates, fat, proteins, and water. Obesity surgery radically modifies this entire system, and understanding the consequences of these modifications is essential.

What do we know today?

We understand that our body has several mechanisms to control food ingestion and absorption. We also know that basically the central nervous system (CNS), through the hypothalamus, fatty tissue, and the signals produced by a variety of hormones in our digestive system, provides this control.

Table 5–1.

Afferent Signals

Signals coming from digestive tract
  Ghrelin
  GLP-1
  GIP
  PYY3-36
  CCK

Afferent signals descendant from fat tissue
  Lepitin
  Adiponectin

Afferent signals descendant from pancreas
  Insulin

The majority of obesity surgery techniques involve a radical alteration in the digestive tract, therefore resulting in a totally different way of intestinal hormone stimulation and production. With weight loss, there is a complete modification in the morphology and physiology of the adipose tissues, be it visceral or parietal (it is now well-known that this tissue is a powerful "endocrine organ"). The CNS, obviously, will also receive and produce these signals differently. In other words, obesity surgery is not merely a surgery technique, but a metabolic surgery that also implicates a variety of undiscovered mysteries.

The system that controls these mechanisms has both afferent and efferent signals. The afferent ones will be determined by many stimuli beyond the need or surplus of energy accumulation and may or may not work together (see Tables 5–1 and 5–2). The CNS and, specifically, the hypothalamus will manage the efferent signs, mainly the need or not for us to accumulate or burn more energy, as well as our hunger (this topic will be discussed in detail below).

Since survival is more acutely threatened by starvation than obesity, it should come as no surprise that this system is more robustly organized to galvanize in response to deficient energy intake and stores than to excess energy.[1] Since this complex protection system will only engage after obe-

Table 5–2.

Efferent Signals

Appetite

Energy expenditure

Food intake

Satiety effects

Glucose levels

sity surgery, it is essential that we continue to increase our understanding of it.

Today we are aware of, and also study, a huge diversity of mechanisms produced in consequence of many varied techniques, (these will be discussed in specific chapters). Here we will discuss the historical factors and current research lines that are being developed in the bariatric surgery field, divided basically into understanding intestinal hormones and their many functions, fat tissue metabolism and weight loss consequences, interaction of the diabetes "cure" and the effects of bariatric surgery, and, finally, CNS control.

HISTORY

In 1902, William M. Bayliss and Ernest H. Starling[2] published their paper "The mechanism of pancreatic secretion." This was the bird hour of gastrointestinal endocrinology. Moore et al.[3] describe that Starling had already considered the possibility that the duodenum does also supply a chemical excitant for the internal secretion of the pancreas. Not until the discovery of insulin by Banting and Best in 1921, a systematic search for a gut hormone influencing carbohydrate metabolism took place. Different groups published the results of animal experiments, in which the effect of extracts of duodenal mucosa on fasting blood glucose levels or hyperglycemia induced by glucose ingestion or injection had been investigated.

In 1932, La Barre[4] published for the first time the name "incrétine" (incretin) for the substance extracted from the upper gut mucosa, which produces hypoglycemia and does not stimulate pancreatic exocrine secretion. He introduced an idea that considered the use of incretin for the treatment of human diabetes for the years to come. Since several groups demonstrated that the plasma insulin level increased after the injection of an extract of intestinal mucosa, all known gastrointestinal hormones were considered either alone or in combination as possible incretin candidates. In 1970, John C. Brown discovered a new peptide which he named gastric inhibitory polypeptide (GIP) because of its inhibitory effect on gastric acid secretion in *Heidenhain* pouch dogs.[5]

Dr. Joel Habener discovered the glucagon-like peptide-1 (GLP-1) in 1980. The interest in GLP-1 and the other preproglucagon derived peptides has risen almost exponentially, as seminal papers in the early 1990s proposed to use GLP-1 agonists as therapeutic agents for the treatment of type 2 diabetes.

In 1994, the *ob* gene was discovered by Zhang et al.,[36] and the leptin receptor, first reported in *Cell,* was discovered in 1995 by Tartaglia.[37] These discoveries have initiated a great hope in the development of anti-obesity drugs.

Obesity surgery has also been around for a long time. Since the fifties, techniques to approach this population have been known and over four decades many approaches have been "experimented" (see Chapter 1), but very little was studied or understood in relation to their real physiologic effects. Twenty years following jejunoileal bypass, patients had significant intestinal hormonal changes. These findings therefore support a role for gut hormones as important mediators in the hypophagia and weight-reducing effects of bariatric surgery.[6–8] The surprise came in 1982, in the early days of bariatric surgery, when our diabetic morbidly obese patients were relieved, yes, fully relieved, from their insulin requirements in a matter of days.[9]

In 1991, after a National Institutes of Health (NIH) consensus,[10] the surgical techniques were standardized and the indications were organized. From that moment, a great increase in the number of procedures occurred and, consequently, a more refined development of the effects they caused. But what does 15 years mean to Medicine? Very little. About 10 years after the NIH, Dr. Cummings described the Ghrelin peptides (see Chapter 15). It is the only intestinal hormone known to circulate orexigen (appetite stimulant). And now, it is five years later. The effects from obesity surgery on reversing important diseases such as diabetes led to the development of several techniques that take advantage of these studies to try to promote a cure for this population.

CNS REGULATION

Gastrointestinal signals that influence the brain to stop an ongoing meal are collectively called satiety signals because when they are administered exogenously, animals behave as if they are sated, i.e., they eat smaller meals and engage in behaviors that normally occur when meals end.[11,12] Humans given the same compounds also eat smaller meals and report that they are more sated.[13–15]

During the last 10 years, great progress has been achieved in the characterization of the molecular mechanisms involved in the control of food ingestion and energy wastage. The hypothalamus is the region that integrates and coordinates the signals influencing the energy balance. In addition to signals from neuropeptides and neurocytokines, hypothalamic centers involved in energy homeostasis can also be influenced by metabolic substrates. Neurons that receive signals from regulators such as leptin may also sense changes in the levels of glucose and free fatty acids. Hypothalamic neurons that sense both low and high levels of glucose have been identified.[16] Many genetic studies have been trying to demonstrate the circuit action that delivers this operation. Many signs coming from the digestive tract through incretins, GLP-1, and glucose-dependent insulinotropic peptide (GIP), and intestinal hormones like peptide YY_{3-36} (PYY_{3-36}) and ghrelin, as from the fat tissue by leptin, resistin, and adiponectin, besides organs like pancreas and by insulin, promote a variety of responses (efferent signs) by hypothalamus (see Tables 5–1 and 5–2). Each one of these signals has a response from the hypothalamus and will be detailed next. Several surgical techniques have promoted a true short circuit in this signalization. All procedures resulting in induced weight loss reduce the parietal fat and visceral fat, leading to a modification on signalization produced by leptin, adiponectin, and resistin.

An important component of the body weight regulatory systems is melanocortin receptors (MR). The ligands for these receptors' signaling result in weight gain, e.g., agouti mice are obese because of decreased melanocortin signaling.[17] Analogous to the situation with Leptin,[18] Qi et al. found that agouti mice were insensitive to the actions of adiponectin in the brain. This suggests that leptin and adiponectin share common mediators in the CNS.[19] However, leptin and adiponectin elicit different changes in gene expression for ligands of MR.[19] Consistent with this difference, leptin decreases food intake and increases energy expenditure, whereas adiponectin seems to only affect energy expenditure (Figure 5–4).

Cholecystokinin (CCK) is liberated by the small intestine into the circulation in response to the contact with nutrients such as fatty acids, and influences satiety by actions on CCK receptors located on peripheral vagal afferent terminals, which transmit neural signals to the brainstem.[20] The true effects of this hormone in patients submitted to surgeries that promote duodenal bypass are still unknown. The absence of nutrient passage through the duodenum and, therefore, the lack of stimulus to its production apparently markedly decrease its effects after these surgeries.

The surgeries that involve duodenal exclusion, like Roux-en-Y gastric bypass (RYGB) (Figure 5–1) and biliopancreatic diversion (BPD) (Figure 5–2), lead to an early signalization of distal intestinal hormones like GLP-1 and PYY_{3-36}, with this being one of the most studied and defended factors as responsible for the best results in diabetes

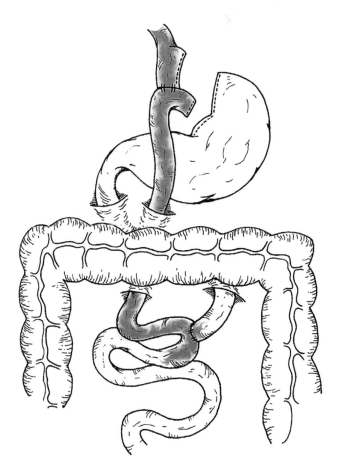

Figure 5–1. Roux-en-Y gastric bypass.

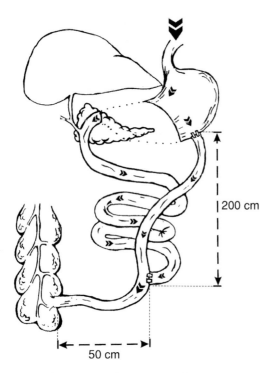

Figure 5–2. Biliopancreatic diversion.

200 cm

50 cm

resolution and weight loss in the long term, when compared to purely restrictive methods. Ghrelin modifies its signaling, especially after RYGB, since it is mostly produced in the gastric fundus, which is excluded from the digestive tract in this case.

What really happens and what are or will be the consequences of that situation in the hypothalamus signalization still remain unknown. Is any neurological alteration shown by this population perhaps related to this signalization? How many more afferent and efferent signals will be produced after obesity surgery? Does the hypothalamus perhaps interpret and answer the "new" signals produced after the surgery in the same way?

GASTROINTESTINAL HORMONES AND FOOD INTAKE

The many techniques in obesity surgery, which involve modification in the digestive tract, like the RYGB and BPD lead, consequently, to a true short circuit in the production of intestinal hormones as well as the signalization to the CNS. Understanding the good and bad consequences of this fact is a priority for us. Finding out what we are really doing with this population is our duty as doctors.

The contemporarily most commonly performed surgery in the United States and Brazil, the RYGB, involves both restrictive and malabsorptive features. A considerable segment of small intestine is bypassed, resulting in a much shorter gastrointestinal tract (Figure 5–1). Well, it is fundamental to understand that, each time we eat, we produce a variety of stimuli, both mechanical and chemical in the enteroendocrine cells, and as a consequence, the production of substances, be they hormones, enzymes, vitamin absorption factors, etc., lead to many effects in the signals to the CNS, as well as in the food digestion and absorption of substances fundamental to our existence, like vitamins, iron, etc. (see Chapter 39). The surgeries that modify this "natural" passage obviously confound this entire system. What really does happen? What effects are produced? We are starting to answer some of these questions, but the more we study, the more questions appear. We will try to explain a little of what we already understand about intestinal hormones (Figure 5–3).

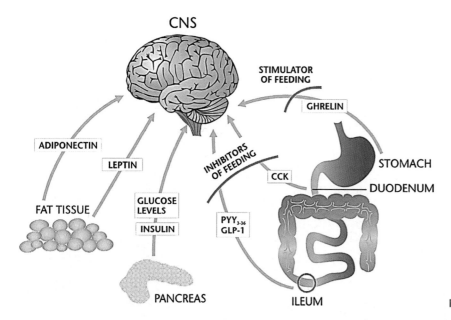

CNS

STIMULATOR OF FEEDING

GHRELIN

ADIPONECTIN

LEPTIN

INHIBITORS OF FEEDING

CCK

STOMACH

DUODENUM

GLUCOSE LEVELS

INSULIN

PYY_{3-36} GLP-1

FAT TISSUE

PANCREAS

ILEUM

Figure 5–3. Normal afferent signals.

Digestion and absorption of nutrients are time-intensive processes needed to protect against malabsorption and metabolic disturbances during the postprandial period. This includes the fine-tuned interaction of gastrointestinal nutrient transit, endocrine and exocrine secretion, and gut–brain responses like the induction of satiety or the feeling of fullness, bloating, or nausea. The interplay between gastrointestinal transit and endocrine pancreatic secretion plays a key role in order to optimize nutrient digestion and absorption.[21] The most studied intestinal hormones in obesity surgery today are ghrelin, CCK, GIP, GLP1, PYY_{3-36}, and oxytomodulin (OXM).

Cholecystokinin

This is one of the most studied hormones. It is a powerful satiation trigger and is secreted primarily in two forms: CCK-33, also known as alimentary (CCK-A or CCK-1), from duodenum and jejunum cells, and CCK-8, the cerebral (CCK-B or CCK-2) made in the CNS. That produced in the duodenum has very well defined functions in the digestive process, like stimulating gallbladder emptying, pancreatic enzyme secretion, gastric emptying, and acid production in the stomach.[22,23]

Surgeries like bypass and the BPD exclude the duodenum, and the true effects in all this signalization will be altered (but, until this moment, is very little understood). There is a discussion on the idea, for example, that the high cholecystopathy incidence in the postoperative period of surgeries like bypass is related to CCK.

Ghrelin

This is a peptide recently discovered by Dr. Cummings (see Chapter 15). Ghrelin is unique among gut hormones in stimulating food intake, and its chronic administration to rats causes obesity.[24] However, its levels have been shown to be smaller in the obese when compared to people of normal weight.[25] The place with the highest ghrelin concentration is the gastric fundus. When this gastric segment is disconnected and isolated, there is a hypothesis that a fatigue in this hormone production exists, which stops acting.

In humans, the serum concentration levels of ghrelin increase before meals and decrease after them.[26] In patients submitted to gastric bypass, its circulating levels do not vary in relation with food and are much lower when compared to nonoperated obese patients, despite massive weight loss. Geloneze et al. has demonstrated that the ghrelin levels decrease dramatically in patients that have undergone gastric bypass.[27] The physiologic and anatomic modification and subsequent effect on ghrelin levels are probably the factors responsible for better, long-term weight loss when we compare bypass methods to banding procedures.

Oxytomodulin

Oxytomodulin decreases intake. Its receptors seem to be related also with GLP-1.[39] At present some studies that involve synthetic OXM infusion in humans, observing the appetite suppressing effects. Long-standing treatments in rats have demonstrated a decrease in weight gain and progressive decrease of food intake.[28] Some view this with hope for obesity treatment.

Glucagon-Like Peptide-2

This has a composition similar to GLP-1 and is also secreted by the ileum cells. Therefore, it is thought that GLP-2 also functions in "alimentary control." However, current studies involving humans have not demonstrated changes.[29,30] Up to now, neither of the hormones appears to have a significant role postoperative to bypass surgery.

Peptide Tyrosine-Tyrosine$_{3-36}$

PYY is a member of the pancreatic polypeptide family, which also includes the pancreatic polypeptides (PPs) and the neuropeptides (NPYs). There are many NPY receptors that feel the PYY effects. It is secreted by terminal ileum and colon cells. Many cells that secrete GLP-1 also secrete PYY. PYY_{1-36} is broken down into PYY_{3-36} by the depeptidil peptidase IV(DPP-IV) enzyme. When the PYY3-36 is produced, the CNS Y2 receptors selectively absorb it, resulting in reduced food intake.[31] The PYY secretion by the gut is proportional to the caloric density of food intake. The presence of carbohydrates and lipids is the first factor to stimulate its production. PYY is also involved in "ileal brake" (see GLP-1).

We suppose that this hormone plays an important part in the weight loss in bypass surgeries, because the promoted deflect leads to a shortened distance in which the food will travel to the ileum, resulting in quicker contact of the nutrients with these cells and, consequently, the PYY will be more rapidly produced, will affect faster, leading to faster satiation. Besides its effects on "ileal brake," there is a hypothesis that the PYY influences the food intake when interacts with Y2 receptors in the hypothalamic arcuate nucleus, which is the control center for food intake.[32,33]

Apolipoprotein A-IV

This is a peptide produced by small intestine cells during lipid digestion, but not in response to carbohydrates. It is also secreted in the arcuate nucleus. Its injection in rat brains reduces ingestion.[34] As it is not affected by carbohydrates, it may have an important role in short- and long-term control of corporal fat. Surgeries like RYGB and BPD exclude the duodenum and a segment of the small intestine, thereby altering the true effects of this peptide. Until now, very little of this mechanism has been understood.

INCRETIN

Glucose-Dependent Insulinotropic Peptide (GIP)

This is released from intestinal K cells. It stimulates insulin secretion and increases β-cell production, inhibiting apoptosis. Different from GLP-1, it does not inhibit gastric emptying in humans.[35] Its action in CNS is also unknown. In surgeries involving gastric bypass, theoretically due to stimulus absence, the GLP-1 does not appear to be a significant factor. (We will study the incretins later in this chapter.) Besides the important function of GLP-1 as GIP over food intake and its anorexigenic mechanisms, it is inescapable to separate incretins from their intimate relation over diabetic effects after obesity surgery.

Glucagon-like-peptide-1 (GLP-1)

- Is an insulinotropic peptide-glucose dependent;
- is an incretin that stimulates insulin secretion in the presence of enteral nutrients;
- slows gastric emptying (which results in reduced food intake);
- is derived from the proglucagon large precursor after modified translation.

This proglucagon is synthesized by enteroendocrine intestinal cells in the ileum and colon. It is an incretin and stimulates insulin secretion in alimentation. In about 2 minutes, the major part of plasmatic GLP-1 is broken down by the enzyme DPP-IV. GLP1 receptors are found in the brain and pancreas.

What GLP-1 does: It decreases intestinal motility and gastric emptying and improves the β-cell function. It is the peptide primarily responsible for the "ileal brake," which is the negative feedback mechanism that regulates nutrient traffic through the digestive tract.

Central and periphery GLP-1 receptors are sensitive to its action and produce reduced food intake. Because of the effect of reducing ingestion and insulin secretion, it is a strong candidate in the treatment of diabetes. The problem is how to extend its "life" and, with it, effects.

The L-cell is an endocrine cell with a triangular form and a long cytoplasm a tic process reaching the gut lumen. This process is equipped with microvilli that protrude into the lumen.[74] Maybe through these microvilli the L cell can sense the presence of nutrients in the lumen and transform this information into a stimulation of secretion.

Several studies have shown that infusions of GLP-1 significantly and dose dependently enhance satiety and reduce food intake in normal subjects.[75] The concentration of intact GLP-1 does rise after meal intake and rises more the larger the meal is.[74] One of the main functions of GLP-1 is to act as one of the hormones of the so-called "ileal brake," a mechanism by which the presence of nutrients in the distal small intestine causes inhibition of upper gastrointestinal motor and secretors' activity. Therefore, besides its effects over glucose metabolism, like PYY, the early production of GLP-1 leads to an incipient satiating effect. Nutrients in the ileum are thought to have satiating effect, curtailing food intake and GLP-1 is released simultaneously.[75] GLP-1 is secreted, along with he other intestinal product of the proglucagon gene, GLP-2 from the L cells, which are found in highest density in the distal ileum. However, the L cells are also found throughout the rest of the small intestine and in high density in the large intestine.[76,77] More recently, a population of cells has been described, in which GLP-1 and GIP are colocalized.[78] What we see is that this variety of places where GLP-1 and GIP are produced makes us wonder that each time we modify the digestive tract position, with the "innovation" of new techniques, new information will present for our discovery.

Because GLP-1 co-exists with GLP-2 and OXM in ascending neurons of the nucleus of the solitary tract, it has been speculated that OXM and GLP-2 also contribute to the regulation of energy homeostasis including satiety. But after gastric bypass, until now, we really do not know what is happening. While peptide YY (PYY) coexpressed with GLP-1 and released from L cells within the ileocolonic junction in parallel to ileal nutrient perfusion is suggested as a humoral mediator of the ileal brake.

Five publications studying a total of 3,568 patients submitted to bypass surgery have demonstrated that diabetics showed a complete remission of the disease in 82%–98% and the majority of the studies show a resolution in about 83%.[79] The most impressive observation is that patients previously diabetic, in many cases, stopped using medication almost immediately after the surgery.[79] The logical mechanism is that with the weight loss insulin sensibility improves. This occurs basically by hormonal action, triggered by adipocytic products, which we will describe later.

Patients with important weight loss have increased adiponectin levels (which also improves insulin sensibility) and muscle receptors for insulin concentration as well as reduced lipids and fatty coenzyme A concentrations in muscle cells, which are known to cause insulin resistance (Figure 5–6).

The bypass benefits to diabetes cannot be measured only with weight loss. What is the mechanism that can explain the dramatic diabetes regression? The most logical idea is the patient ingests practically no food in the postoperative period. Therefore, the pancreatic β-cells are not stimulated. Some days after, the patient starts to feed, but also starts to lose weight and have a negative energy balance, a condition that improves glucose tolerance.

The most interesting possibilities, however, are the intestinal modifications promoted by bypass, improving insulin secretion and action. Ghrelin disturbs insulin secretion and action; therefore, if the ghrelin effects are anti-incretins, worsening the glucose peripheral use, the ghrelin suppression promoted by the bypass can modify glucose availability. Concomitantly, the bypass leads to an earlier stimulus of GLP-1 production and its effects lead to precocious remission of diabetes (Figure 5–6).

ADIPOSE TISSUE

We have already discussed the mechanisms of intestinal hormones and their importance in weight control and the changes that occur after obesity surgery. We also know that fatty tissue is a powerful endocrine organ, i.e., producer of many factors like leptin, adiponectin, resistin, etc., which are involved in weight loss and resolution of comorbidities such as diabetes in obese population.

Leptin

Besides fatty tissue, other locations have been identified as leptin-producing sites, such as the placenta, skeletal muscles, and the stomach. Leptin is produced by the stomach in the fundic cells (pepsinogen secretors cells). Currently, it is estimated that about 25% of circulating blood leptin comes from the stomach. It also has the capacity of reducing food intake.

The biological role of leptin continues to be actively explored. Leptin was initially viewed as an adipocyte-derived signal that functions primarily to prevent obesity, and this was the basis for the name leptin—from the Greek word *leptos* for *thin*.[38] Today, we know that it is an important indicator of fatty tissue for the brain—informing the brain, by its suppression, that the body is starving, and this function is likely to be as important, or more important, as its antiobesity role. In the absence of leptin, the brain senses starvation despite massive obesity.[39]

Today we know that the gut produces a variety of signals that influence hunger and, particularly, signals that limit food amounts. The leptin levels do not alter after food intake, making it clear that it does not participate in this mechanism. On the other hand, leptin deficiency nullifies the efficacy of meal-related signals, since individuals lacking leptin have little or no satiety in response to meals.[40]

The identification of the product of the *ob* gene as the hormone/cytokine leptin led to the understanding of some of the principles of hormone-controlled anorexigenic inputs.[39] Leptin is produced by the white adipose tissue in direct relation to the total body fat mass. An increase of blood leptin levels leads to the activation of the ObRb (leptin receptor) located in neuron bodies at the arcuate nucleus. NPY/AGRPergic neurons are inhibited, while POMC/CARTergic neurons are activated by leptin.[41] These events will ultimately lead to satiety and increased thermogenesis. Thus, increased fat deposition in white adipose tissue exerts a direct effect on the control of hunger and energy wastage.[40,41] Besides, leptin offers a robust anorexigenic signal to the hypothalamus, insulin, which is secreted by the pancreatic β-cells in response to glucose and other nutrient and neural signals, and participates in the central control of feeding and energy conservation.[40] (Figures 5–4 and 5–5). Recent evidence indicates that progressive impairment of insulin and leptin signaling to the hypothalamus may exert a central role in the development of

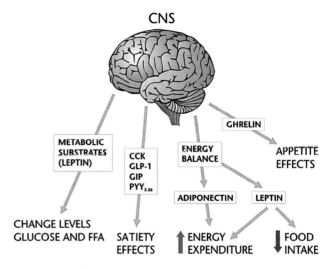

Figure 5–4. Normal efferent signals.

obesity.[42,43] Little is known about the reasons and the mechanisms that lead to central resistance to insulin and leptin action.[39,40]

Adiponectin

Following the characterization of leptin, a series of studies have demonstrated that the adipose tissue produces and secretes several other hormones and cytokines that participate in the control of metabolic events. One striking example is the capacity of tumor necrosis factor α (TNF-α) and interleukin 6 (IL-6), which are produced by adipose tissue proportionally to the total body mass of fat, to impair insulin signal transduction in muscle and liver, by promoting the activation of serine kinases such as Jun N-terminal kinase (JNK) and p38-MAP.[44–46]

Another, and also exciting, example is the protein adiponectin, a 30 kDa protein, which is the product of the

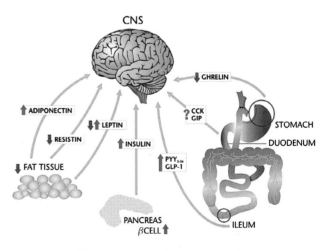

Figure 5–5. Signalization after RYGB.

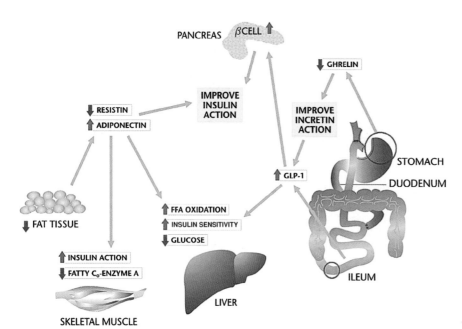

Figure 5–6. Hypothesis of diabetes resolution after RYGB.

most abundant gene transcript of the white adipose tissue, the *apM1* gene.[47] Interestingly, adiponectin is secreted in inverse relation to the total body mass of fat. Low blood levels of adiponectin are found in obese humans and animal models of obesity. Moreover, low levels of adiponectin have been implicated in the development of insulin resistance.[48] According to recent studies, adiponectin improves insulin action in the liver, reducing the expression of the gluconeogenic enzymes PEPKC and G6Pase[49] (Figures 5–5 and 5–6).

The induction of weight loss by dieting leads to significant improvement of most metabolic parameters in insulin resistant and diabetic patients.[50] During weight loss the levels of adiponectin increase significantly and this increase is paralleled by improved responsiveness to insulin[51] (Figures 5–5 and 5–6). Weight loss achieved after bariatric surgery also leads to impressive amelioration of several metabolic parameters.[52] Thus, reduction of blood insulin and leptin levels, reduction of glycated hemoglobin index (HbA1c), and improved insulin action as determined by the clamp method, by the HOMA and by the minimal model, has been reported. Molecular transduction of the insulin signal is also significantly improved after surgery-induced weight loss.[53,54] Finally, the blood levels of adiponectin increase by 40% after weight loss.[52,55]

Resistin

This is another adipoctye-secreted protein. Initial studies suggested that resistin was induced in obesity and might be in part responsible for systemic insulin resistance. The effect of recombinant resistin to induce hepatic insulin resistance has been confirmed,[56] although data on its expression in obesity are conflicting and its cellular mechanism of action remains unknown.[39]

Visceral Fat's Relationship with Comorbidities

Today, there is a truly large population of patients undergoing obesity surgeries daily all around the world. Along with the weight loss there is consequently a great loss of fat, both parietal and visceral, and the resulting effects are generally beneficial.

Visceral adiposity is one of the main risk factors for the development of insulin resistance, diabetes mellitus, hypertension, and cardiovascular disease.[56,57] The mechanisms involved in these common clinical associations are not completely known but include the impaired suppression of hepatic glucose production,[58] increased portal release of free fatty acids,[59] increased visceral production of glycerol,[60] and abnormal production of adipose tissue—derived hormones and cytokines such as TNF-α, IL-1α, IL-6, leptin, adiponectin, and resistin.[61,62]

Recent studies have shown that the removal of visceral fat reverses insulin resistance in two models of obesity[63,65] and one model of aging.[66] The metabolic consequences of visceral fat removal were associated with improved hepatic insulin action[63,65] and with reduced adipose tissue expression of pro-inflammatory cytokines.[65]

Acting on insulin sensitive tissues, pro-inflammatory cytokines can impair insulin signal transduction by promoting the serine phosphorylation of key elements of the insulin signaling pathway.[67] This inhibitory effect is dependent on the activation of serine kinases such as JNK and IKK.[67,68] Once serine phosphorylated, proteins such as the insulin receptor, IRS-1, and IRS-2 can no longer be appropriately tyrosine phosphorylated in response to an incoming insulin signal. As a result, the activation of downstream effectors of the insulin signaling pathway is hampered.[67,69]

Pitombo and Velloso[70] described an animal model with swiss mice. A study shows that removal of visceral fat improves insulin signal transduction and glucose homeostasis in an animal model of diet-induced obesity and diabetes mellitus and these metabolic and molecular outcomes are accompanied by the restoration of adipokine levels.

The worldwide increased incidence of obesity has resulted in various consequences to human health, diabetes among them. At the same time of this epidemic, a great growth in the knowledge of mechanisms involved in obesity and its diseases have arisen and a lot of this is due to the wise observation and studies of groups involved with obesity surgery.

SURGERY EFFECTS ON INTESTINAL HORMONES

These effects prove the powerful effect of intestinal hormones as mediators in hypophagia and weight loss after bypass surgery and bileopancreatic derivations. The increased secretion of primarily GLP-1 and the effects from visceral fat after obesity surgery are mainly responsible for glycemic normalization after surgery. The ileal "transposition" produced by the surgery increases the secretion and distal hormone synthesis like PYY and GLP-1. (This has been proven by jejuno/ileal transposition surgeries in rats.) This verifies the hypothesis that an increase in the independent intestinal hormones control weight and food intake.

Diabetes and morbid obesity have always had a close relationship since weight increase is one of the greatest villains in the production of insulin resistance and diabetes. Diabetes mellitus is a chronic disease of epidemic proportions and new treatments are required for the effective treatment of both type 1 and type 2 diabetes mellitus. Whereas type 1 diabetes is characterized by β-cell failure due to autoimmune insulitis, type 2 diabetes arises as a result of β-cell failure often in the setting of concomitant insulin resistance. Since patients with insulin resistance do not develop hyperglycemia until the β cell is unable to meet the demand for insulin, enhancement of insulin secretion from the islet β cell is an important goal for treatment of patients with type 2 diabetes mellitus.

Glucagon-like-peptide-1 (GLP-1) secretion is clearly meal-related. In the fasting state, the plasma concentrations are very low. Meal intake causes a rapid increase in L-cell secretion, most evident when measured with C-terminal assays.

It has been suggested that the purpose of having two incretin hormones is related to their location with one, GIP, being predominantly secreted from the upper small intestine, and the other mainly secreted from the lower small intestine where the density of the L cells is higher. Therefore, in surgeries that involve the duodenum bypass, the non-contact of nutrients with the duodenal cells can explain the minimal effect on GIP and the great response in GLP-1 secretion. The various techniques in the bariatric surgery field have become a true laboratory for us to study how these mechanisms function and affect this population.

OBESITY SURGERY AND ADVANCES IN DIABETES TREATMENT

Today we discuss whether there is a type of surgery that uses the benefits of bariatric ones and which may be utilized on nonobese diabetic population with BMI < 35. Diabetes is a chronic disease and normally progressive and incurable, with severe consequences on individuals' life quality and longevity. In this case, we surgeons will have not 200,000 or 300,000 patients to be operated on each year, but about 150 million.

In Asian countries, which culturally have vegetarian and rural workers' population and as a consequence small caloric intake and huge energy waste, over thousands of years, have shown a population with no serious obesity problems. Today with globalization and commercial expansion, many countries that had this feature before are showing a changing in life habits, with high calorie food and reduced physical activities, and as a result the obesity epidemic has been increasing day by day. However, due to the specific peculiarity of this population, being obese "during the millennium" is not something expected for these bodies. In response, the obese in these areas develop severe comorbidities like diabetes, hypertension, etc., in a more serious and early way. Its habitual patients with BMI between 30 and 35 with severe diabetes in countries like China and India. In which criteria should we indicate surgery in this population? What would be the most adequate technique? Suddenly, it is more important to reverse the comorbidities than weight loss itself. Pure restrictive surgeries may reduce weight, modify fat tissue signalization, but would not modify incretins' signalization. In this case, probably, we should think about duodenal exclusion surgeries and early activation of incretins.

Rubino and Marescaux[80] have developed an experimental animal model with duodenal exclusion. A surgery with only two anastomoses was performed on rats of the Goto-Kakizaki species, the most widely used animal model of nonobese type 2 diabetes[81] (Figure 5–7). A duodenal exclusion and a simple entero-entero anastomosis was performed, preserving the gastric volume. The obvious purpose was not counting on an expressive weight loss and possible effects over diabetes, but to demonstrate that duodenal exclusion and "pathway" promoted in the distal hormones activation would lead to diabetes reversion without counting on weight loss. The aim was reached.

CONCLUSIONS

In the NIH of 1991, more than a decade ago, only gastric bypass and the vertical banded gastroplasty had been approved. However, today, many other techniques, like bileopancreatic diversion and adjustable gastric band, are accepted by the medical community. All the different groups defend their position and try to claim their technique as the best.

There are many works showing different short- and long-term results according to the country/area being studied.

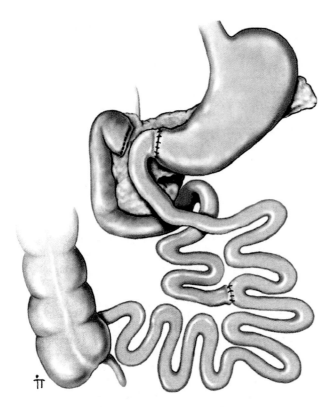

Figure 5–7. *Rubino* procedure.

Today, we live in a world with a massive exchange of communication through the international computer network. Countries such as the United States promote meetings which attract surgeons from all over the world. The conception of results must be minutely studied by the events' participants.

In Brazil, like in the United States, the "gold standard" surgery is the bypass, maybe by the great habit similarity and, as we say, an easier access to the health system. In European countries like Belgium and France, the restrictive surgeries occupy a huge space, maybe due to easier control and doctor follow-up, as well as a less rebellious and more conservative culture. But is there a worldwide surgery? I do not think so. The pattern of the so-called "gold-standard" surgery must be discussed regionally.

Would countries like India and China, for example, with a population habitually vegetarian and mostly with low purchasing power have good results with BPD surgeries? In the same way, could countries where access to the health system is precarious have good results with surgeries that need vitamin replacement, regular laboratory exams, as well as proper image studying like, for example, a late obstruction of the long biliopancreatic channel of a BPD, in which the air absence denotes the need of a CT for diagnosis? Would the execution of malabsorbtive procedures be a safe surgical option? How many hospitals have CT in Africa?

Over the years, extremely effective techniques have been developed in the treatment of this population, using what we call open access. When we see the world as a whole, the majority of surgeons are more adapted to the open access.

How many surgeons have training in advanced laparoscopic surgery? How many hospitals own video laparoscopy equipment and appropriated instruments to safely attend this population? We have also learned that new technology is an excellent instrument, which we can and shall use when available, but we are happy to know we have an instrument less modern technologically, but extremely effective, which is the open approach (see Chapter 4). We can compare the modern American spacecrafts with the Russian spaceships, which serve cosmonautics in the same safe and effective way since the beginning of the space era. The regional logistics must be evaluated along with safety and efficacy. We are talking about lives and not about vanity.

Today, we have learned, after years of effort by the bariatric surgery "dinosaurs," that adequate training (see Chapter 13) leads the surgeon to perform any technique with security. This is what we can call an "operator's formation." Obesity surgery needs surgeons.

What is the difference?

Operators are basically technicians, not necessarily physicians, who learn tasks mechanically and execute them. Surgeons are those who execute the technique with the responsibility of consequences and perception of risks and benefits. We have learned that, in this field, there is no place for operators. Being obesity surgeons requires technical ability and extensive medical knowledge because without which, the results will be drastic. Based on this, adapting the kind of technique to the population to be attended is a must. Like any other field, in medicine we look for cheap methods and safe and secure results.

Educational and historical experience in the bariatric surgery field have led us to a wonderful universe. Today, we have surgeries with a high degree of safety. By reversing obesity, we have decreased enormously the cost that this population caused to the health system. We have learned mechanisms of disease resolution which could be used in the healing of diabetes, for example. But, concomitantly, we have mixed several findings and there remain questions still far away from final answers.

Medical history has always shown us that technical advance makes progress only with accurate clinical observation and logical, scientific studies. We all still have work to do, if we believe that obesity surgery is the right course for our patients.

References

1. Ahima RS, et al.: Role of Leptin in the neuroendocrine response to fasting. *Nature* 382, 250–252, 1996.
2. Bayliss WM, Starling EH: The mechanism of pancreatic secretion, *J Physiol* 28:325–353, 1902.
3. Moore B, Edie ES, Abram JH: On the treatment of diabetes mellitus by acid extract of duodenal mucous membrane. *Biochem J* 1:28–38, 1906.
4. La Barre J: Sur les possibilités dún traitement du diabéte par líncretine. *Bull Acad R Med Belg* 12:620–634, 1932.
5. Brown JC, Mutt V, Pederson RA: Further purification of a polypeptide demonstrating enterogastrone activity. *J Physiol* 209:57–64, 1970.

6. Naslund E, Gryback P, Hellstrom PM, et al.: Gastrointestinal hormones and gastric emptying 20 years after jejunoileal bypass for massive obesity. *Int J Obes Relat Metab Disord* 21:387–392, 1997.

7. Kellum JM, Kuemmerle JF, O'Dorisio TM, et al.: Gastrointestinal hormone responses to meals before and after gastric bypass and vertical banded gastroplasty. *Ann Surg* 211:763–771, 1990.

8. Wilson P, Welch NT, Hinder RA, et al.: Abnormal plasma gut hormones in pathologic duodenogastric reflux and their response to surgery. *Am J Surg* 165:169–177, 1993.

9. Pories WJ: Editorial *Ann Surg* 239(1).

10. National Institute of Health (NIH) Consensus Statements. 84. *Gastroint. Surg. Severe Obes.* 9(1):1–20, 1991.

11. Antin J, Gibbs J, Young RC, et al.: Cholecystokinin elicits the complete behavioral sequence of satiety in rats. *J Comp Physiol Psychol* 89:784–790, 1975.

12. Strubbe JH, Van DG: Temporal organization of ingestive behaviour and its interaction with regulation of energy balance. *Neurosci Biobehav Rev* 26:485–498, 2002.

13. Smith GP, Gibbs J: The development and proof of the cholecystokinin hypothesis of satiety. In: Dourish CT, Cooper SJ, Iversen SD, Iversen LL (eds.): *Multiple Cholecystokinin Receptors in the CNS.* Oxford, Oxford Univ. Press, 1992; pp.166–182.

14. Kissileff HR, Pi-Sunyer FX, Thorton J, Smith GP: Cholecystokinin decreases food intake in man. *Am J Clin Nutr* 34:154–160, 1981.

15. Pi-Sunyer, et al.: C-terminal octapeptide of cholecystokinin decreases food intake in obese men. *Physiol Behav* 29:627–630, 1982.

16. Dunn-Meynell, et al.: Glucokinases is the likely mediator of glucosensing in both glucose-excited and glucose-inhibited central neurons. *Diabetes* 51, 2056–2065, 2002.

17. Olmann M, et al.: Antagonism of Central Melanocortin Receptors in Vitro and in Vivo by Agouti-Related Protein. *Science* 278:135–138, 1997.

18. Halaas JL, et al.: Physiological response to long-term peripheral and central leptin infusion in lean and obese mice. *Proc Natl Acad Sci U S A* 94:8878–8883, 1997.

19. Seeley RJ, D'Alessio DA, Woods SC: Fat hormones pull their weight in the CNS. *Nature* 454–455, 2004.

20. Moram TH: Cholecystokinin and satiety: Current perspective. *Nutrition* 16:858–865, 2000.

21. Schirra J, Göke B: The physiological role of GLP-1 in human: Incretin, ileal brake or more? *Regul Pept* 128:109–115, 2005.

22. Schwartz GJ, Moran TH, White WO, et al.: Relationships between gastric motility and gastric vagal afferent response to CCK and GRP in rats differ. *Am J Physiol* 272:R1726–R1733, 1997.

23. Grider JR: Role of cholecystokinin in the regulation of gastrointestinal motility. *J Nutr* 124:1334S–1339S, 1994.

24. Tschop M, Smiley DL, and Heiman ML: Ghrelin induces adiposity in rodents. *Nature* 407, 908–913, 2000.

25. Metab Tschöp et al., Diabetes 2001; Shiiya et al *J Clin Endocrin Metab*.

26. Cummings 2001; Diabetes.

27. Geloneze B, Tambascia MA, Pareja JC, et al.: Ghrelin: A gut-brain hormone. Effect of gastric bypass surgery. *Obes Surg* 13:17–22, 2003.

28. Cohen MA, Ellis SM, Le Roux CW, et al.: Oxyntomodulin suppresses appetite and reduces food intake in humans. *J Clin Endocrinol Metab* 88:4696–4701, 2003.

29. Sorense LB, Flint a, et al.: No effect of physiological concentrations of glucagons-like peptide-2, on appetite and energy intake in normal weight subjects. *Int J Obes Relat Metab Disord* 27:450–456, 2003.

30. Schmidt PT, Naslund E, et al.: Peripheral administration of GLP-2 to humans has no effect on gastric emptying or satiety. *Regul Pept* 116:21–25, 2003.

31. Sarson DL, Scopinaro N, Bloom SR: Gut hormone changes after jejunoileal (JIB) or Biliopancreatic (BPD) bypass surgery for morbid obesity. *Int J Obes* 5:471–480, 1981

32. Woods Sc, Seeley RJ, Porte DJ, et al.: Signals that regulate food intake and energy homeostasis. *Science* 280:1378–1383, 1998.

33. Schwartz MW, Woods Sc, Porte DJ, et al.: Central nervous system control of food intake. *Nature* 404:661–671, 2000.

34. Atkinson RL, Brent EL: Appetite suppressant activity in plasma of rats after intestinal bypass surgery. *Am J Physiol* 243:R60–R64, 1982.

35. Meier JJ, Goetze O, Asstipp J, et al.: Gastric inhibitory polypeptide does not inhibit gastric emptying in humans. *Am J Physiol Endocrinol Metab* 2 86:E621–E625, 2004.

36. Zhang, et al.: Positional cloning of the mouse obese gene and its human homologue. *Nature* 372: 425–432, 1994.

37. Tartaglia, et al.: Identification and expression cloning of a leptin receptor, OB-R. *Cell* 83:1263–1271, 1995.

38. Halaas, et al.: Weight reducing effects of the plasma protein encoded by the obese gene. *Science* 269:543–546, 1995.

39. Flier JS, et al.: Obesity wars: Molecular progress confronts an expanding epidemic. *Cell* 116:337–350, 2004.

40. Schwartz MW, Kahn SE: Insulin resistance and obesity. *Nature* 402:860–861, 1999.

41. Friedman JM, Halaas JL: Leptin and the regulation of body weight in mammals. *Nature* 395:763–770, 1998.

42. Carvalheira JB, Ribeiro EB, Araujo EP, et al.: Selective impairment of insulin signaling in the hypothalamus of obese Zucker rats. *Diabetologia* 46:1629–1640, 2003.

43. Torsoni MA, Carvalheira JB, et al.: Molecular and functional resistance to insulin in hypothalamus of rats exposed to cold. *Am J Physiol Endocrinol Metab* 285:E216–E223, 2003.

44. Uysal KT, Wiesbrock SM, Marino MW, Hotamisligil, GS: Protection from obesity-induced insulin resistance in mice lacking TNF-alpha function. *Nature* 389:610–614, 1997.

45. Fujishiro M, Gotoh Y, Katagiri H, et al.: Three mitogen-activated protein kinases inhibit insulin signaling by different mechanisms in 3T3-L1 adipocytes. *Mol Endocrinol* 17:487–497, 2003.

46. Rotter V, Nagaev I, Smith U: Interleukin-6 (IL-6) induces insulin resistance in 3T3-L1 adipocytes and is, like IL-8 and tumor necrosis factor-alpha, over expressed in human fat cells from insulin-resistant subjects. *J Biol Chem* 278:45777–45784, 2003.

47. Arner P: The adipocyte in insulin resistance: key molecules and the impact of the thiazolidinediones. *Trends Endocrinol Metab* 14:137–145, 2003.

48. Chandran M, Phillips SA, Ciaraldi T, Henry RR: Adiponectin: More than just another fat cell hormone? *Diabetes Care* 26:2442–2450, 2003.

49. Combs TP, Berg AH, Obici S, Scherer PE, Rossetti L: Endogenous glucose production is inhibited by the adipose-derived protein Acrp30. *J Clin Invest* 108:1875–1881, 2001.

50. Nicklas BJ, Dennis KE, Berman DM, Sorkin J, Ryan AS, Goldberg AP: Lifestyle intervention of hypocaloric dieting and walking reduces abdominal obesity and improves coronary heart disease risk factors in obese, postmenopausal, African-American and Caucasian women. *J Gerontol A Biol Sci Med Sci* 58:181–189, 2003.

51. Esposito K, Pontillo A, Di Palo C, et al.: Effect of weight loss and lifestyle changes on vascular inflammatory markers in obese women: A randomized trial. *JAMA* 289:1799–1804, 2003.

52. Guldstrand M, Ahren B, Adamson U: Improved beta-cell function after standardized weight reduction in severely obese subjects. *Am J Physiol Endocrinol Metab* 284:E557–E565, 2003.

53. Geloneze B, Tambascia MA, Pareja JC, Repetto EM, Magna LA: The insulin tolerance test in morbidly obese patients undergoing bariatric surgery. *Obes Res* 9:763–769, 2001a.

54. Geloneze B, Tambascia MA, Pareja JC, Repetto EM, Magna LA, Pereira SG: Serum leptin levels after bariatric surgery across a range of glucose tolerance from normal to diabetes. *Obes Surg* 11:693–698, 2001b.

55. Pender C, Goldfine ID, Tanner CJ, et al.: Muscle insulin receptor concentrations in obese patients post bariatric surgery: Relationship to hyperinsulinemia. *Int J Obes Relat Metab Disord* 28:363–369, 2004.

56. Rajala MW, Obici S, et al.: Adipose-derived resistin and gut-derived resistin-like molecule-beta selectively impair insulin action on glucose production. *J Clin Invest* 111:225–230, 2003.

57. Ferrannini E, Natali A, Capaldo B, Lehtovirta M, Jacob S, Yki-Jarvinen H: Insulin resistance, hyperinsulinemia, and blood pressure: Role of age and obesity. European Group for the Study of Insulin Resistance (EGIR). *Hypertension* 30:1144–1149, 1997.

58. Fujimoto WY, Bergstrom RW, Boyko E, et al.: Visceral adiposity and incident coronary heart disease in Japanese-American men. The 10-year follow-up results of the Seattle Japanese-American Community Diabetes Study. *Diabetes Care* 22:1808–1812, 1999.

59. O'Shaughnessy IM, Myers TJ, Stephniakowski K, et al.: Glucose metabolism in abdominally obese hypertensive and normotensive subjects. *Hypertension* 26:186–192, 1995.

60. Bjorntorp P: "Portal" adipose tissue as a generator of risk factors for cardiovascular disease and diabetes. *Arteriosclerosis* 10:493–496, 1990.

61. Williamson JR, Kreisberg RA, Felts PW: Mechanism for the stimulation of gluconeogenesis by fatty acids in perfused rat liver. *Proc Natl Acad Sci U S A* 56:247–254, 1966.

62. Hotamisligil GS, Peraldi P, Budavari A, Ellis R, White MF, Spiegelman BM: IRS-1-mediated inhibition of insulin receptor tyrosine kinase activity in TNF-alpha- and obesity-induced insulin resistance. *Science* 271:665–668, 1996.

63. Barzilai N, She L, Liu BQ, et al.: Surgical removal of visceral fat reverses hepatic insulin resistance. *Diabetes* 48:94–98, 1999.

64. Barzilai N, She L, Liu BQ, et al.: Surgical removal of visceral fat reverses hepatic insulin resistance. *Diabetes* 48:94–98, 1999.

65. Kim YW, Kim JY, Lee SK: Surgical removal of visceral fat decreases plasma free fatty acid and increases insulin sensitivity on liver and peripheral tissue in monosodium glutamate (MSG)-obese rats. *J Korean Med Sci* 14:539–545, 1999.

66. Gabriely I, Ma XH, Yang XM, et al.: Removal of visceral fat prevents insulin resistance and glucose intolerance of aging: an adipokine-mediated process? *Diabetes* 51:2951–2958, 2002.

67. Hotamisligil GS: Inflammatory pathways and insulin action. *Int J Obes Relat Metab Disord* 27(Suppl 3):S53–S55, 2003.

68. Barreiro GC, Prattali RR, Caliseo CT, et al.: Aspirin inhibits serine phosphorylation of IRS-1 in muscle and adipose tissue of septic rats. *Biochem Biophys Res Commun* 320:992–997, 2004.

69. Hotamisligil GS: Molecular mechanisms of insulin resistance and the role of the adipocyte. *Int J Obes Relat Metab Disord* 24(Suppl 4):S23–S27, 2000.

70. Pitombo C, Velloso L, et al.: Amelioration of diet-induced diabetes mellitus by removal of visceral fat. *J Endocrinol* 191(3): 699–706, 2006.

71. Bonny C, Oberson A, Negri S, et al.: Cell-permeable peptide inhibitors of JNK: Novel blockers of beta-cell death. *Diabetes* 50:77–82, 2001.

72. Hotamisligil GS, Spiegelman BM: Tumor necrosis factor α: a key component of the obesity-diabetes link. *Diabetes* 43:1271–1278, 1994.

73. Hotamisligil GS, Murray DL, Spiegelman BM, et al.: Tumor necrosis factor α inhibits signaling from the insulin receptor. *Proc Natl Acad Sci U S A* 91:4854–4858, 1994.

74. Eissele R, Gke R, et al.: Glucagon-like peptide-1 cells in the gastrointestinal tract and pancreas of rat, pig and man. *Eur J Clin Invest* 22:283–291, 1992

75. Verdich C, et al.: A meta-analysis of the effect of glucagons-like peptide-1(7-36) amide on ad libitum energy intake in humans. *J Clin Endocrinol Metab* 86:4382–4389, 2001.

76. Damholt AB, Kofod H, Bucham AM: Immunocytochemical evidence for a paracrine interaction between GIP and GLP-1 producing cells in canine small intestine. *Cell Tissue Res* 298:287–293, 1999.

77. Eissele R, et al.: Glucagon-like peptide-1 cells in the gastrointestinal tract and pancreas of rat, pig and man. *Eur J Clin Invest* 22(4):283–291, 1992

78. Mortensen K, et al.: GLP-1 and GIP are localized in a subset of endocrine cells in the small intestine. *Regul Pept* 114:189–196, 2003.

79. Rubino F, Marescaux J: Effect of duodenal-jejunal exclusion in a non-obese animal model of type 2 diabetes. *Ann Surg* 239(1):1–11, 2004.

80. Galli J, Li LS, Glasser A, et al.: Genetic analysis of non-insulin dependent diabetes mellitus in the GK rat. *Nat Genet* 12:31–37, 1996.

Operative Issues

6

Requirements of the Clinic and Institution

Luiz Henrique de Sousa, MD • Edson Lemes Sardinha, MD • Luiz Henrique de Sousa Filho, MD

INTRODUCTION

In the last 10 years the growth of the prevalence of obese people worldwide has influenced society as a whole and various sectors of the medical community which are adapting physically to offer necessary comfort to this segment of the population which, in one way or another, has come to influence considerably all aspects of life in society.

In the United States, for example, the number of obese people currently represents about 18%–38% of the population, in France about 12%–15%, in Australia 18%–20%, in Germany about 18%–27%, and in Brazil, about 15%–30%.

The specific characteristics of the disease of obesity and its comorbidities demand that a multidisciplinary team of specialists function in the preoperative preparation as well as in the postoperative phase. Thus, the physical adaptations necessary for the preoperative phase must include all the places where these professionals who are part of the multidisciplinary team do their work. In addition, there must be a well-defined schedule of service, from the moment the patients seek out the endocrinologist to hear his/her opinion regarding surgical treatment, where there was no previous success with clinical, dietary, or medicinal treatments.

Often patients go directly to a surgeon to get information as to whether or not surgery would be indicated for them, what techniques would be most appropriate, what is the surgical risk, what form of surgery would be used (laparoscopy or open surgery), length of time in the hospital and before returning to routine activities, as well as how much weight they will lose after the procedure and in what time frame the weight loss will occur.

This multidisciplinary team must know the fundamental steps of laparoscopic surgery, the risks, costs, and especially the advantages of this procedure as compared to open surgery, such as less postoperative pain, lack of protracted ileus problem, early food and movement recuperation with less incidence of pulmonary complications and embolic thrombosis, less incidence of infection in the abdominal wall and incisional hernias, and a postoperative recuperation that is much faster, thus resulting in an improved quality of life beginning with the immediate postoperative phase.

QUALIFICATIONS AND TRAINING FOR BARIATRIC SURGEONS

The qualifications for a surgeon to perform bariatric surgeries follow the norms adopted by the International Federation for the Surgery of Obesity (IFSO) approved in Cancun in 1997.[1]

"The Cancun IFSO Statement on Bariatric Surgeon Qualifications: 04-10-1997"

This IFSO Statement is made with the intent to guide those surgeons interested in, or engaged in the practice of, bariatric surgery to understand what qualifications are considered acceptable to the international community of bariatric surgeons (IFSO). This is based upon the IFSO's dedication to optimizing the overall safety and long-term effectiveness of bariatric surgical procedures for those patients who qualify for this surgery.

The IFSO acknowledges that an average, formally certified, general surgeon may be technically capable of performing most primary bariatric surgical procedures. However, like any other area of surgery, the techniques that improve each surgical procedure's safety and effectiveness are exemplified by experienced and frequent practitioners of each particular type of bariatric surgery. The IFSO also acknowledges that the proper patient selection and education as well as short-, intermediate-, and long-term management of primary bariatric surgery patients is extremely complex. This requires considerable experience and judgment, which should best be learned from a preceptor(s) with in-depth experience in bariatric surgery.

IFSO, therefore, strongly recommends that, prior to independently performing primary bariatric surgery, each surgeon meet the following minimal standards:

1. Be a fully trained, qualified, certified general or gastrointestinal surgeon who has completed a recognized general/gastrointestinal surgery program.
2. Has completed a preceptorship in all aspects of bariatric surgery, including patient education, support groups, operative techniques, and postoperative follow-up with an IFSO or IFSO Affiliate Society-designated bariatric surgeon or one who has performed at least 200 bariatric surgical procedures and has five or more years of experience in the field of bariatric surgery.
3. Has received a written approval from his preceptor of his/her satisfactory bariatric surgical abilities (*Preceptor-*

ship or certification is not required of already established, practicing bariatric surgeons as of October 4th, 1997).

4. Maintains a well-informed, up-to-date knowledge of bariatrics and bariatric surgery literature such as contained in the journal Surgery for Obesity and Related Diseases (SOARD).
5. Holds, or has applied for, membership in an Adhering Body of IFSO or, if no such national body is available to him/her, to IFSO directly;
6. Has attended at least one meeting of IFSO or one of its Adhering Bodies or one of its bariatric surgery courses.
7. Is personally committed to strongly encouraging the necessary education and lifelong follow-up of his/her bariatric surgery patients.
8. Performs bariatric surgery in institutions where he/she has made every reasonable effort to obtain equipment, facilities, and support systems adequate for the comfort and safety of bariatric surgery patients.

IFSO also acknowledges that reoperative bariatric surgery is an even more complex and demanding area requiring considerable primary bariatric surgical experience, as well as knowledge of surgical options, precautions, risks, benefits, possible complications, and implications. This requires considerable experience and judgment, which should best be learned from one or more colleagues with in-depth experience of reoperative bariatric surgery. It therefore recommends that the bariatric surgeon, at least early in his/her reoperative bariatric surgical practice, refer back to, confer with, or otherwise work with one or more bariatric surgical colleagues who have extensive experience in reoperative bariatric surgery, ideally 60 or more such cases.

The American Society for Bariatric Surgery and the Society of American Gastrointestinal Endoscopic Surgeons have jointly prepared "Guidelines for Granting Privileges in Bariatric Surgery."[2]

Courses in the United States offer audio-visual classes, training on animals and cadavers, as well as surgical accompaniment in the actual surgical center.[3] The Brazilian Society for Bariatric Surgery's requirements for a bariatric surgeon are that a professional be certified in general or gastrointestinal surgery and has proved the performance of 50 bariatric surgeries. To be certified in laparoscopic surgery, it is necessary to pass the certification exams of the Brazilian College of Gastrointestinal Surgery or the Brazilian College of Surgeons.

There are private and university courses in Brazil that allow the practice of and training in laparoscopic surgery. In the training center under our coordination in the city of Goiânia, we offer an immersion experience where, besides seeing various films with technical details, surgeons perform all the current procedures on animals (gastric banding, gastroplasty with ring bypass, Duodenal Switch procedure, biliopancreatic diversion type Scopinaro). Each surgeon participates in 25 surgeries during 1 week of training. The training may be repeated as often as necessary or desired. After the surgeries on animals, the surgeons assist in performing surgeries with experienced professors in hospital surgical centers (Figure 6–1).

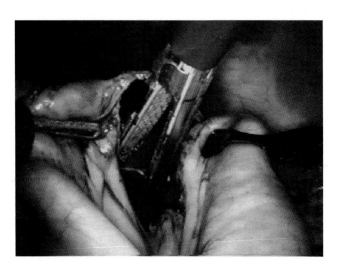

Figure 6–1. Experiment training. Roux-en-Y in dog.

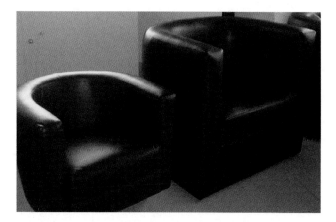

Figure 6–2. Normal-sized chairs and large-sized chairs for obese patients.

NECESSARY ADAPTATIONS FOR PREOPERATIVE EVALUATIONS IN CLINICS AND EXAMINING ROOMS OF THE MULTIDISCIPLINARY TEAM

Obesity and its comorbidities are diagnosed and evaluated in the preoperative phase by the multidisciplinary team guided by a defined schedule in almost all the services associated with bariatric surgery (Table 6–1). This preoperative service program for patients who are candidates for laparoscopic bariatric surgery follows the same system as that of open surgery; therefore, all the sectors involved in this phase necessarily require human and infrastructure adaptations.

The principal adaptations in the clinics of each specialist on the multidisciplinary team involve the physical space. In the clinic, access to the reception area should be easy, and the clinic be pleasant and preferably connected with a garage, since the transportation of some patients is necessarily by car. The reception area access must avoid having steps, the floor should be level and antiskid, and there should be handrails for better patient safety and movement. If the clinics/doctor's offices are located in buildings, access should include wide elevators such as those in hospitals, to allow for the

Table 6–1.

Principal Comorbities That Accompany Obese Patients

Arterial hypertension, diabetes, sleep apnea

Cholelithiasis, umbilical hernia, osteoarthritis

Gastro-esophageal reflux disease, hepatic steatosis, dyslipidemia

Psychological–social disturbances

movement of hospital beds/carts made for extremely obese patients.

The doors of the reception area, the restrooms, the doctor's office, and the physical examining room should be sufficiently wide (with a width of 1.20 m) to allow for the passing of transport carts adequate for the extremely obese patient. All corridors should have handrails firmly secured on the floor, for a greater weight tolerance. These areas, without exception, should be air-conditioned, to provide safety and comfort, since patients in the preoperative preparation phase spend a great deal of their time in the doctor's office and examining rooms.

There should be enough chairs/seats in the reception area and doctor's offices to accommodate all the family members involved in the preparatory phase of the patient who will undergo surgical treatment. These chairs should be made to sustain weight of above 300 kg, measuring approximately 1 m in width by 80 cm in depth, to offer the comfort necessary for prolonged appointment times, which can last up to 2 hours (Figure 6–2). Employees should be trained to offer the best care possible to these patients, starting with the receptionist who is the first point of contact, to the specialized nursing staff.

The weighing scales should be appropriate to weigh patients of up to 300 kg or more, with a practical height measurement rod to facilitate calculating the body mass index (Figure 6–3). Wheelchairs should be available for patients, with the same measurements as the chairs, and sufficiently strong enough to transport patients weighing as much as 300 kg or more. The toilets in the restrooms should be reinforced with supports directly secured to the floor, in order to support the weight of the patients who will use them (Figure 6–4).

The attending doctor must arrange the furniture in his office/clinic, including tables, chairs, bookcases, etc., in such a way that they do not interfere with the movement of people within the room and, if necessary, the passing of a transport cart.

This doctor should be a good listener and attend the patient in an objective, serious and scientific manner, using accessible language to explain and orient family members

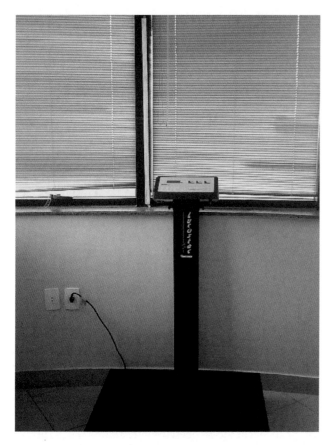

Figure 6–3. Scale for 500 kg and measuring rod to measure height.

and patients about all the aspects involved in this complex disease and its surgical treatment. He can make use of practical computer software, geared to obesity, to collect thorough information about each particular case, filling in relevant

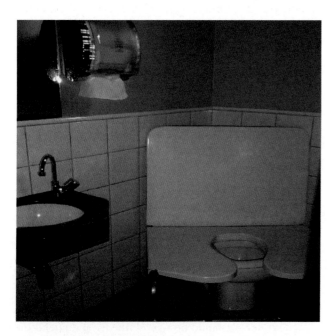

Figure 6–4. Reinforced toilet with handrail supports.

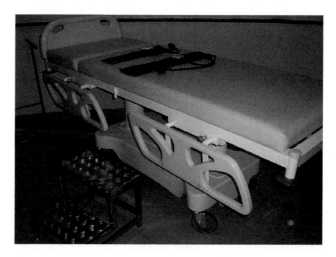

Figure 6–5. Examining table. Two meters length by one-meter width, with a capacity for more than 300 kg.

information about patients including the results of the physical examination, complementary examinations, and requests for opinions and evaluations. Creating an Internet site for patients helps to impart basic knowledge about the surgical techniques, their appropriateness, risks, and complications.

The physical examining table should measure 2.2 m in length and 1.0 m in width, and be able to withstand adequately up to 300 kg. It should have wheels with breaks easily releasable to transport patients from one place to another when necessary (Figure 6–5). The physical examination should be accompanied by a specialized nursing staff who knows how to use equipment specifically designed for the obese patient, for example, the sphygmomanometer with a large cuff for these patients. The equipment and instruments used for preoperative evaluation of obese patients, in the great majority of cases, are the same as that used with nonobese patients. However, for some specialists on the multidisciplinary team, the preoperative evaluation also demands special equipment (Figure 6–6).

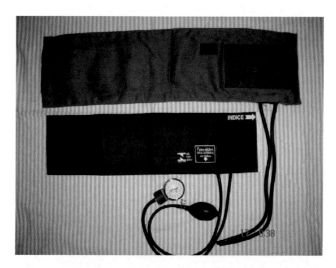

Figure 6–6. Cuffs for arterial pressure of normal size and special size for obese patients.

Also, the preoperative examination rooms for ultrasonography, x-rays, endoscopy, cicloergometry, echocardiography, laboratory tests, catheterization, etc., should have adequate measurements, air conditioning, be comfortable, and have large chairs, examination tables, transport carts, and reclining chairs for postsedation repose especially designed for obese patients.

Computerized tomography examinations are rare in the preoperative period; however, in the postoperative phase they are frequently necessary especially to facilitate the diagnosis of complications and the necessity for reinterventions. The tomography equipment for the obese patient must be larger than the common equipment and also should be included in the radiology departments of the hospitals where bariatric surgery is practiced (see Chapter 20).

Polysomnography clinics also require adaptation, with beds specially designed for obese patients, as the great majority of them suffer from sleep disturbances, the most serious being sleep apnea.

The preanesthetic evaluation is particularly important for obese patients, not only because of the high level of anxiety present, but also due to the comorbidities associated with obesity (Chapter 9).

The patients in the preoperative preparatory phase should participate in meetings which explain and clarify the scientific–ethical issues regarding their disease and its comorbidities. These meetings, which include patients who have already had this surgery as well as those in the preoperative phase, should be held in an appropriate setting which is comfortable and which has chairs for the obese as well as nonobese. In these meetings, the patients are oriented and can talk among themselves in a relaxed atmosphere, accompanied by the multidisciplinary team that has the goal of helping the patients with whatever questions might arise after the classes or conferences with each specialist.

ADAPTATIONS NECESSARY FOR ACCOMMODATION AND PREOPERATIVE HOSPITAL ADMITTANCE

The staff responsible for admitting procedures needs training and basic knowledge sufficient to enable them to understand the psychological conditions of the patients and their families at the time of admittance.

Patients should be taken to their rooms in a reasonable time, since they have already been informed by the anesthesiologist about the necessity of premedication. These rooms should have wide doors, and oversized hospital beds with electronic controls to accommodate the obese patient, restrooms with wide doors which open from the outside, a sufficiently large shower area that can be accessed by wheelchairs strong enough for transporting, and other chairs adequate for bathing, as well as for intestinal and vesicular exoneration.

Hospital clothing should be specifically designed with measurements appropriate for the obese patient, which can be easily put on and removed while on the surgical table. The nursing staff should have specific training in preoperative care such as how to help with bathing, personal hygiene, tricotomy, venous punction, and psychic comfort. The transport carts used in the pre- and postoperative phase must be able to support weight above 350 kg, and be easily moveable in the corridors, elevators, and wide spaces.

If there is premedication, it should be administered intravenously or orally. The attempt to use the intramuscular technique generally results in injecting adipose tissue instead of muscle tissue, with unpredictable results. In the morbidly obese patient, the effects of depressant drugs on the central nervous system are unpredictable and in view of the high prevalence of respiratory disease, premedication should not be administered until the patient is in a setting monitored for safety. This is particularly important for patients with cardiovascular and respiratory diseases, especially because of the risk of obstruction of airways and hypoxemia.

Since the risk of gastric regurgitation is elevated in obese patients, specific measures and care must be taken to prevent this. In certain cases, the preoperative administration of metoclopramide and H_2 receptor blockers is advisable to reduce the volume and increase the pH of gastric content.[6,7] Suggested doses are 10 mg of metoclopramide and 150 mg of ranitidine 1 hour before the administration of the anesthesia. Regarding the preanesthetic medication to reduce anxiety, we use bromazepam 3–6 mg VO the night before and 7.5–15 mg of midazolam 1 hour before surgery with the minimum amount of water necessary to swallow the medicine. This can be given venous also, administered with doses of 0.05 mg/kg light weight, with the patient being monitored in the admission area of the operating room, taking care to avoid possible difficulties such as the obstruction of airways and its consequences.

ADAPTATIONS NECESSARY IN THE SURGICAL CENTER

The doors of the surgical center should be wide with sufficient space for the movement of transport carts for obese patients. The operating room should be equipped with a system for transference from the cart to the operating table and vice versa, which offers easy management without excessive strain on the team.

The principal anesthetic and surgical implications of surgery for the extremely obese patient begin with technical difficulties: Having adequate equipment in the surgical room appropriate for the measurements of the patient, venous access, and tracheal intubations.

Surgical tables should be specifically designed for obese patients, and should be x-ray transparent, and possess accessories such as padded supports on the right/left and end sides, which open easily, permitting electronic table movements in various positions, especially lying on one's side, the *Trendelenburg* position, raised head position, and others. As the heels, buttocks, and shoulders of obese people are at risk for developing ulcerated sores, all the vulnerable areas should be padded and protected. The distribution of body fat can make a common operating table dangerous for the obese patient. For example, excessive posterior extension of the shoulder, with the potential risk of lesions of the brachial plexus, can happen when a patient is put in a supine position with the arms at a 90° angle with the body. Electronic and ultrasound cauterizing instruments are used in the same surgical action, and their pedals should be in strategic positions at the surgeon's feet.

With regard to laparoscopic bariatric surgery, the ideal is to possess two laparoscopes, and obviously two monitors, for better comfort of the team, principally when, in the case of extremely obese patients, it is necessary to use two insufflators (see Chapter 7).

With respect to the instruments used, there should be available short and long scopes of 30°–45°, short graspers (45 cm), and long graspers (80 cm) as, for example, bowel clamps, needle drivers, auxiliary graspers for knots, in order to alternate with facility in the upper and lower abdominal cavity at the time of surgery. In morbidly obese patients, extra-long trocars are necessary, disposable or not, since regular trocars are not able to reach the abdominal cavity, thus impeding the surgical procedure and allowing the leakage of carbon dioxide gas causing a reduction of pneumoperitoneum.

Indispensable equipment for any operating room is a defibrillator, for treatment of critical situations of fatal arrhythmias, such as ventricular fibrillation. As obese patients have more tendency to lose heat during surgery, central body temperature should be monitored by a thermometer connected to the multiparametric monitor and maintained with heat by forced air, which is effective in the obese patient as well as infusion with heated fluids, during the entire surgery and the immediate postoperative phase by means of the system of heating fluids.[10] It is best to avoid postoperative trembling in obese patients, because this could result in more hypoxia, venous, and arterial, in borderline patients at risk of myocardial ischemia. Special care should be continued during the patient's stay in the anesthetic recovery room or in the intensive care unit.

It is important to have in the operating room and the recovery room a monitor to evaluate blood sugar levels, considering the elevated index of diabetes mellitus among morbidly obese patients. We also need to give consideration to specific material for urinary catheterization, especially in long surgeries, as well as catheterization of the gastric pouch, in restrictive gastroplasty.

The prophylaxis of deep vein thrombosis initially is done with elastic stockings connected to equipment that inflates compression intermittently, which also should be available in the operating room and the recovery room. Another helpful method is the use of low-molecular-weight heparin, initiated at the end of surgery, and maintained for 10 days. Immediate physical therapy and early ambulatory recovery are supportive measures for the prevention of Deep Venous Thrombosis (DVP)/Pulmonary Thromboembolism (DTE)[6] (Figure 6–7).

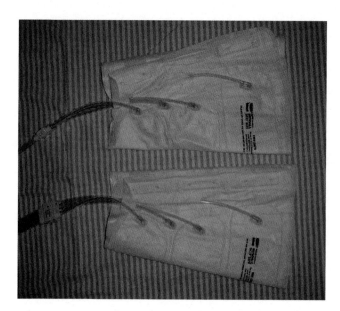

Figure 6–7. Pneumatic compression stockings. Prophylaxis of deep vein thrombosis.

All these structural and technological modifications are extremely necessary, and thus indispensable for services which propose to treat surgically this complex disease that is obesity.

References

1. The Cancun IFSO statement on bariatric surgeon qualifications, Cancun, Mexico. October 4,1997.
2. SAGES/ASBS guidelines for laparoscopic and conventional surgical treatment of morbid obesity. American Society for Bariatric Surgery. May 2000. Available at: http://www.asbs.org/html/quidelines.html. Accessed June 26, 2003.
3. SAGES Endorsed courses. Society of American Gastrointestinal Endoscopic Surgeons. June 12, 2003. Available at: http://www.sages.org/endorsed.html. Accessed July 5, 2003.
4. Sousa LH. Cirurgia videolaparoscópica em obesidade mórbida. Técnicas de Fobi/Capella e Scopinaro 2000 March 10, 2006. Available at: www.imersao.ccdo.com.br.
5. Herron D. Weight loss surgery using minimally invasive surgical techniques. SurgicallySlim July 3, 2003; http://www.surgicalltslim.com.
6. Wilson SL, Manaltea NR, Malvesa JD: Effects of atropine, glycopyrrolate and cimetidine on gastric secretions in markedly obese patients. *Anesth Analg* 60:37, 1981.
7. Manchikanti L, Roush JR, Colliver JR: Effect of preanesthetic ranitidine and metoclopramide on gastric contents of morbidly obese patients. *Anesth Analg* 65:195, 1986.
8. Ogunnaike BO, MD, Jones SB, MD, et al: Anesthetic considerations for bariatric surgery. *Anesth Analg* 95:1793–1805, 2002.
9. Viana PTG, Carraretto AR, de Almeida AV, et al.: Hemodynamic and ventilatory effects of volume or pressure controlled ventilations in dogs submitted to pneumoperitoneum. Comparative study. *Rev Bras Anestesiol* 55(6) 639–654, 2005.
10. Bergalp B, Cesur V, Corapcioglu D, et al.: Obesity and left ventricular diastolic function. *Int J Cardiol* 52:23, 1995.
11. Buckley FP, Martay K: Anestesia e obesidade e doenças gastrintestinais, In: Barash, PG, Cullen, BF, Stoelting, RK (eds.): Anestesia Clínica, 4th ed. São Paulo, Editora Manole, 2004; p 1.035–1.049.
12. Mason DS, Sapaal JA, Wood MH, et al.: Influence of forced air warming on morbidly obese patients undergoing Roux-en-Y gastric bypass. *Obes Surg* 8:453, 1998.

7

Preoperative Evaluation of Patients

Marcos Tambascia MD, PhD

INTRODUCTION

Success of a bariatric surgery will always depend on a series of factors. To be an effective and safe procedure requires a great dedication and a complete understanding of how to manage obese patients. The clinical and surgical team should consider morbid obesity as a disease and not a concern regarding moral failing. When a medical team decides to be involved with a bariatric surgery program, all must be prepared to care for critically ill bariatric surgical patients with regards to cardiopulmonary failure, serious wound problems, and ventilatory and nutritional support. Besides doctors it is necessary to have a complex team prepared to give support, such as nurses, social workers, dieticians, and physical therapists. The infrastructure of the hospital must have beds, wheelchairs, stretchers, chairs, and image and surgical equip-ment capable of managing very obese patients. The great majority of patients have clinical problems that are poorly controlled and also a number of cardiovascular risks that certainly should be treated and established before surgery. The active participation of all patients in both preoperative and postoperative periods is mandatory. This is an opportunity for patients and family to understand the necessity of modifications in life habits for all life. The patients' understanding of the future consequences of bariatric surgery is a precondition for the success.[1] The list of comorbid diseases associated with obesity is long and all of them must be documented and controlled to decrease the risk of the procedure. The preoperative period should involve patient education and behavior modification, wide-approach medical evaluation for risk assessment, and intensive care for its reduction.

Expert anesthesiology support, knowledgeable in the specific problems of the bariatric patient, is certainly necessary (*see* Chapter 10). The anesthesiology support includes an understanding of patient positioning, blood volume and cardiac output changes, airway maintenance, and drug pharmacokinetics in the morbidly obese. It is advisable to have preoperative, intraoperative, and postoperative written protocols. The bariatric surgeon must be able to manage, and have coverage to manage, the postoperative patient and any problems and complications that may occur.

Patients eligible for surgical correction of obesity must be aware that this procedure is only an option for severely obese patients who fail to maintain weight loss after trying medical weight loss strategies, such as modifications in diet, behavior, and exercise, and medically supervised weight loss regimens. Most importantly, only those patients, who are willing to make this complete modification a way of life, should be considered for surgery. Psychiatric disorders, drugs, and alcohol abuse and important organ failure are contraindications for surgery. Considering all these particulars, the mortality rate will be less than 1% and acceptable for bariatric surgery.

The education for patients and family must include the rationale for surgical treatment of obesity. This will consist of information about health risks of obesity by itself and all medical hazards associated with treatment. Certainly, the improvement of quality of life must be the base for discussion, and all the risks and limitations secondary to surgery will be considered as the price to pay for it. The low probability of long-term weight control using conservative methods will be the rationale for undergoing this complete nonreturnable evolution. The improvement of quality of life and the impact on all risk factors associated with obesity must be reviewed as also the possible complications associated with each type of surgical technique. The problems of noncompliance with life-style modification should not be addressed as a difficulty but as part of a new style of life. The mechanisms of weight loss induced by surgery should be very well explained as the differences of gastric restriction or malabsorption or both in any case. It is necessary for all patients to understand that some large amount intake, like alcohol or sweet foods, will prevent weight loss with any surgical procedure.

Morbid obese patient candidates for surgical procedures should be aware of the differences of any technique, especially the advantages and disadvantages of it and why such procedure was chosen for them.[2] Late complications and especially the nutritional issues derived from decreased food intake should be understood and accepted by the patient. This fact is essential for emphasizing the necessity for long-term follow-up and for the use of vitamin and mineral supplementations for life.

CLINICAL EXAMINATION

Obese patient candidates for bariatric surgery usually have an increased risk for perioperative complications related to comorbidities associated with obesity and the excess weight by itself. All comorbidities should be identified prior to surgery. Some patients are not aware of all morbidities they have and are informed just before surgery. Comorbidities like sleep apnea and related disorders, like snoring or somnolence and also hypoventilation syndrome with shortness of breath or tiredness, can be diagnosed in the preoperative period. A great difficulty with such extremely obese patients is the examination of lung and heart, which can be very poor, as well as that of the abdomen. X-ray, CT scan, and EKG are less informative in such patients than in normal weight persons (see Chapter 20). A careful peripheral examination can reveal venous stasis ulcers or hyperpigmentation and edema, suggesting potential risk to deep venous thrombolysis or congestive heart failure. The laboratory evaluation should analyze iron, B_{12}, minerals and especially calcium levels, due to malabsorption of these elements by the surgical procedure and this situation must be corrected. Baseline deficiency can identify preexisting problems and a prompt correction must occur, not a lengthy period of observation to identify the possible deficiency.

CARDIOVASCULAR RISK FACTORS

Morbid obese patients have a cluster of cardiovascular risk factors like hypertension, dyslipidemia, and type 2 diabetes mellitus. The main cause of death among these patients is related to macrovascular diseases like myocardial infarction, cerebrovascular accident, congestive heart failure, and cardiac arrhythmias. Left ventricular hypertrophy resulting from increased blood volume and cardiac output demands by hemodynamic overload, secondary to increased body mass index and hypertension, is a usual feature.[3] Decreased ejection fraction by ventricular dilatation is an important risk factor and a careful examination should exclude or indicate necessary treatment prior to surgery. Right ventricular hypertrophy may also develop and these conditions predispose patients to arrhythmias and heart failure. EKG should be performed on all candidates for surgery and especially for bariatric procedures. All patients with cardiac complaints, old-aged patients, or those with extremely limited physical activity must be submitted to stress testing or dobutamine stress echocardiography[4] or even to a stress thallium scan. Patients with history of previous use of anorectic drugs like dexfenfluramine, fenfluramine, or even serotonin agonist drugs must be submitted to echocardiography to exclude valvular abnormalities.

HEMATOLOGIC ABNORMALITIES

To avoid deep venous thrombosis, patients should be submitted to prophylaxis with anticoagulation due to the high risk for secondary pulmonary embolism.[5] Although there is no guideline to the prophylactic anticoagulation, the use of low-molecular-weight heparin and unfractionated heparin is equally effective. The use of calf compressive device and early mobilization is also recommended.[6,7] To patients with BMI over 60 or those suffering of pulmonary hypertension or even with previous history of deep venous thrombosis, a prophylactic vena cava filter placement should be considered. For all patients with high risk for thrombosis a lower extremity duplex ultrasonography and arterial blood gas evaluation should be done.

PULMONARY FUNCTION

Respiratory function is impaired in morbid obese patients. Large chest wall and increased abdominal pressure contribute to respiratory insufficiency. As a result, patients usually have a decreased functional reserve capacity and tendency to desaturation. Preoperative evaluation for pulmonary problems should include questionnaire for sleep apnea symptoms. All closely associated with the patient, like wife or other relative, should be asked about sleep apnea or snoring.[8] The incidence of obstructive sleep apnea and related comorbidities are very high in morbid obese patients. The evaluation prior to surgery can dictate whether continuous positive airway pressure or nasal oxygen are indicated. This procedure usually will recommend patients to use this device prior and in the postoperative period. Postoperative pulmonary complications are the most common morbidity in major surgeries and unfortunately preoperative evaluation usually tends to focus more on cardiac problems. The major pulmonary complications that should be diminished through proper preoperative evaluation and intervention include pneumonia, prolonged mechanical ventilation or respiratory failure, atelectasis, bronchospasm, and exacerbations of chronic obstructive pulmonary disease. Patients who develop a postoperative pulmonary complication are more common than patients who develop a postoperative cardiovascular complication. Chronic obstructive pulmonary disease, besides general health status and older age, is the factor most frequently associated to postoperative pulmonary complications. Physical examination findings can be helpful in assessing risk magnitude and decreased breath sounds as well as prolonged expiration, rales, and wheezes, or rhonchi. These are associated with an increase in pulmonary complications compared with the absence of any of these findings. Preoperative arterial blood gases should be a base for potential postoperative hypoxia or hypercapnia. All patients with significant preoperative abnormalities of arterial oxygenation are at risk for pulmonary complications and should be submitted to continuous monitoring of arterial oxygen saturation. Some patients will require home oxygen prior and after surgery.

RENAL FUNCTION

There is no contraindication of renal insufficiency in the consideration for bariatric surgery, although such patients should be evaluated for coexisting medical problems, like cardiac or pulmonary diseases. The treatment of obesity should benefit in maintaining and preserving kidney function, regardless of whether weight reduction is achieved by diet and exercise or by bariatric surgery. Weight loss will reduce hypertension and improve type 2 diabetes control, the two main risk factors for development of end stage renal disease. In patients with well-established renal insufficiency, particularly in those with creatinine levels above 2 mg/dL, the preoperative evaluation of the causes of this insufficiency is mandatory to treat the coexisting medical problems like diabetes and hypertension. In such patients, good care should be given to avoid episodes of hypotension or hypovolemia. Acute postoperative renal failure is usually more associated with bad prognosis than prior chronic renal insufficiency.

HEPATIC FUNCTION

Nonalcoholic steatotic hepatitis (NASH) has a high probability to occur in morbidly obese patients.[9] The incidence of this comorbidity can be around 60% or 80% in previous studies using liver biopsy at the time of surgery. Most of these patients were asymptomatic prior surgery with any major increases in perioperative mortality. Patients with the combination of diabetes, hypertension, and dyslipidemia, all components of metabolic syndrome, and diagnosed to be NASH should have a liver biopsy during surgery to observe fibrosis or the evolution to cirrhosis.[10] Rarely a micronodular cirrhosis of the liver will be detected, but the great majority of services prefer to conduct the gastric restrictive operation safely and not interrupt it. Patients with known hepatic disease must be carefully evaluated for hepatic function preoperatively. Certainly, a patient with hypoalbuminemia secondary to hepatic failure would be at a very high risk for exacerbation of the hypoalbuminemia after surgery, by the relative restriction of normal oral protein intake.[11] Active chronic viral hepatitis has a potential risk to the operative personnel and should be considered.

GASTROINTESTINAL FUNCTION

Obese patients are prone to suffer from a number of gastrointestinal disorders and the most common condition is gastroesophageal reflux disease. Usually this comorbidity will improve or disappear after surgery. Patients with known history of gastroesophageal reflux disease should undergo an evaluation for peptic ulcer disease, *Helicobacter pylori*, gastric ulcerations, and polyps and should be properly treated. Cholelithiasis is frequently found in morbidly obese patients, placing them at risk for biliary complications. The extremely common occurrence of cholelithiasis and cholecystitis supports the argument for routine cholecystectomy during bariatric surgery. Other gastrointestinal complications are ventral hernias associated to morbid obesity, and the decision to repair it during the bariatric surgery or after that will depend on the surgeon's experience.

ENDOCRINE FUNCTION

A preoperative laboratorial evaluation should include thyroid function and if the patients are hypothyroid, replacement therapy is indicated and the surgery should only be realized when a steady euthyroid state is achieved. Hyperthyroidism, although rare in obese patients, similarly needs to achieve a euthyroid condition prior the surgery. If there is clinical suspicion of Cushing's disease, a careful evaluation should exclude it before the procedure, or indicate appropriate therapy.

DIABETES MELLITUS

It will be very probable that a morbidly obese patient will present with diabetes mellitus. Poor glucose control has been associated with poor wound healing, decreased resistance to infections, and increased mortality in critically ill patients. Bariatric surgery offers a highly successful way of curing or ameliorating diabetes mellitus. Among morbidly obese patients undergoing weight loss surgery there is an approximately 80%–98% cure of the diabetes mellitus.[16] Preoperative testing usually includes serum glycated hemoglobin, fasting, and postprandial glucose. Optimization of glucose control should be encouraged to reduce intraoperative complications and A1c levels should be under 7%. Some of the patients will be on oral therapy but the majority will be using insulin to control the disease. When admitted to hospital, all patients on insulin, including those who were on insulin at home and the glucose level well controlled, should receive their usual insulin regimen until the surgery day; for patients on oral drugs, insulin requirements vary widely from individual to individual. Type II diabetic patients, who by definition are insulin resistant, may have insulin requirements severals fold higher than usual nonobese patients. The goal for glucose control is to avoid the undesirable short-term effects of hypo- and hyperglycemia and this means that glucose should be between 100–200 mg/dL. Glucose under 200 mg/dL should decrease the short-term diabetes complications that may occur during a hospitalization, while lower glucoses (with a HgA1c goal of about 7%) are desired for the long-term prevention of microvascular and macrovascular disease. The preferred method of managing a diabetic patient who is not eating is an intravenous insulin drip.[17] The key features are a fixed dextrose drip and an algorithm allowing patients to receive the amount of insulin required to maintain their glucose level from 120 to 180 mg/dL. Diabetic patients should be brought under strict control prior to surgery because of the risk of infection and to avoid the interactions of hyperglycemia and the immune system. Usually on the morning of surgery, patients need to decrease their insulin dose to half, and during the surgical procedure hypoglycemia must be avoided by glucose monitorization and proper glucose infusion, if necessary, to prevent counterregulatory-hormone-induced cardiovascular complications.

PSYCHOLOGIC EVALUATION

All patients considered for bariatric surgery should be analyzed for a comprehensive psychological review.[18] The examination performed by an individual with expertise in the management of bariatric patients must evaluate patients' personal and social history, eating habits, history of psychiatric disorders, personality profiling, and level of compliance. This evaluation can exclude some patients of surgical indication or indicate those who may benefit from preoperative and postoperative psychotherapy. Noncompliance with previous medical care, untreated depression, personality disorders, and schizophrenia can be a contraindication for surgery in such patients.

CONCLUSION

The clinical and surgical team should always keep in mind the importance of careful evaluation and care of surgical candidates, before, during, and after bariatric surgery, in order to afford them the best opportunity to alleviate their comorbidities, thereby allowing them an integration to a new longer, healthier, happier life.

References

1. Harvey EL, Glenny AM, Kirk SF, Summerbell CD: A systematic review of interventions to improve health professionals' management of obesity. *Int J Obes* 23:1213–222, 1999.
2. Balsiger BM, Luque deLeon EL, Sarr MG: Surgical treatment of obesity: Who is an appropriate candidate? *Mayo Clin Proc* 72:551–57, 1997.
3. Karason K, Lindroos AK, Stenlof K, Sjostrom L: Relief of cardiorespiratory symptoms and increased physical activity after surgical induced weight loss: Results from the Swedish Obese Subjects Study. *Arch Intern Med* 160:1797–1802, 2000.
4. Madu EC: Transesophageal dobutamine stress echocardiography in the evaluation of myocardial ischemia in morbidly obese patients subjects. *Chest* 117:657–61, 2000.
5. Wu EC, Barba CA: Current practices in the prophylaxis of venous thromboembolism in bariatric surgery.*Obes Surg* 10:7–13, 2000.
6. Heit JA, Silverstein MD, Mohr DN, Petterson TM, O'Fallon WM, Melton L: Risk factors for deep thrombosis and pulmonary embolism: A population-based case-control study. *Arch Intern Med* 160:809–15, 2000.
7. Mismetti P, Laporte S, Darmon JY, Buchmuller A, Decousus H: Meta-analysis of low molecular weight heparin in the prevention of venous thromboembolism in general surgery. *Br J Surg* 88:913–30, 2001.
8. Benumoff JL: Obstructive sleep apnea in the adult obese patient: Implication for airway management. *J Clin Anesth* 13:144–56, 2001.
9. Moretto M, Kupski C, Mottin CC, Repetto G, Gprcia Toneto M, Rizzolli J, Berleze D, de Souza Brito CL, Casagrande D, Colossi: Hepatic steatosis in patients undergoing bariatric surgery and its relationship to body mass index and co-morbidities. *Obes Surg* 13: 622–24, 2003.
10. Dixon JB, Bhathal PS, O'Brich PE: Nonalcoholic fatty liver disease: Predictors of nonalcoholic steatohepatitis and liver fibrosis in the severely obese. *Gastroenterology* 121:91–100, 2001.

11. Beymer C, Kowdley KV, Larson A, Edmonson P, Dellinger EP, Flum DR: Prevalence and predictors of asymptomatic liver disease in patients undergoing gastric bypass surgery. *Arch Surg* 138:1240–244, 2003.

12. Amaral JF, Thompson WR: Gallbladder disease in the morbidly obese. *Am J Surg* 149:551–557, 1985.

13. Shiffman ML, Sugerman HJ, Kellum JH, Brewer WH, Moore EW: Gallstone formation after rapid weight loss: A prospective study in patients undergoing gastric bypass surgery for treatment of morbid obesity. *Am J Gastroenterol* 86:1000–1005, 1991.

14. Cucchi SG, Pories WJ, MacDonald KG, Morgan EJ: Gastrogastric fistulas, a complication of divided gastric bypass surgery. *Ann Surg* 221:387–391, 1995.

15. MacLean LD, Rhode BM, Nohr C, Katz S, McLean AP: Stomal ulcer after gastric bypass. *J Am Coll Surg* 185:1–7, 1997.

16. Pories WJ, MacDonald KG, Flickenger EG, Dohm GL, Sinha MK, Barkat HA, May HJ, Khazanie P, Swamson MS, Morgan E: Is type II diabetes mellitus (NIDDM) a surgical disease? *Ann Surg* 215:633–643, 1992.

17. Van den Berghe G, Wouters P, Weekers F, Verwaest C, Bruyninckx F, Schetz M, Vlasselaers D, Ferdinande P, Lauwers P, Bouillon R: Intensive insulin therapy in critically ill patients. *N Engl J Med* 345:1359–1367, 2001.

18. Beck AT, Steer RT. *Manual for the Beck Depression Inventory (MBDI)*. San Antonio, TX: Psychological Corporation, 1993.

8

Intraoperative Issues

Marcel Milcent, MD • Angelo Loss, MD • José E. Manso, MD, PhD

INTRODUCTION

Laparoscopic surgery is quite dependent on specific material and instruments. This relation gets even closer in laparoscopic bariatric procedures. The characteristics of the patients associated with the complexities of the different techniques require nothing less than the best designed and properly working tools.[1] The constant development of new instruments makes laparoscopic bariatric interventions easier and safer,[2] minimizing complications and reducing costs.[3]

When considering the material part of laparoscopy in bariatrics, there is a conjunct of environments that surround the patient and relate with each other: (1) the operating room settlement; (2) the laparoscopy kit (equipments in the set); (3) the instruments that get in direct contact with the patient

(trocars, graspers, etc.); and (4) the tubes and cables that interface group 2 with group 3.

OPERATING ROOM

The surgical room should be wide, in order to have all equipment fit comfortably, and permit easy transit of personnel. The surgical table should be able to take excess weight, as well as move in accordance with the surgeon's needs, preferably remote-controlled. In addition, the table's design ought to enable concomitant procedures, such as cholangiographies during associated cholecystectomies. For fixing the patient, comfortable and self-adhering bands should be applied around the arms, legs, and over the

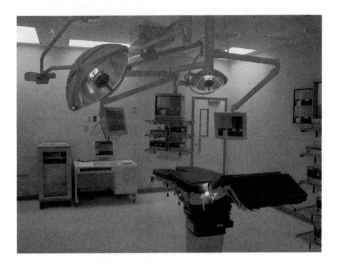

Figure 8–1. Modern surgical suite.

hips. (For material specific to anesthesia, please refer to Chapter 10.)

Electric outlets should be evenly distributed to obviate the need for crossing wires. CO_2 supply coming from the wall pipes discards space-demanding gas canisters and the need to replace them when empty. In modernly designed operating rooms, most of the outlets and gas tubes come from ceiling booms; these can also accommodate the entire laparoscopic set and video recording devices (Figure 8–1). If the institution is involved with teaching programs, i.e., university hospitals, there should be video and voice live transmission for education; this feature also provides with the capability of intraoperative consultation. The nurse's desk should contain all room controls, such as lighting, video recording, video signal switchers, still-image recorder/printer, overhead boom motor controls, and sound system. Considering ergonomics, the use of additional, opposite-side placed monitors in the operating room during laparoscopic bariatric procedures facilitates the assistants' work, mostly for the one at the same side as the laparoscopy kit (Figure 8–1). A smaller monitor dedicated to the anesthesia helps the anesthesiologist follow the procedure and perform tasks (such as bougie insertion) without leaving the head of the table.[4]

The use of calf-length pneumatic compression hose, along with low-weight heparin, short operative time, and early postoperative ambulation, reduces the risk of deep venous thrombosis and its consequences.[5,6]

After finishing the operation, the patient should be moved to the transport bed with aid of a sliding device or air mattress so as to avoid arm or back lesions, which may occur when OR staff moves a noncooperative, heavy, somnolent person.

OPEN SURGERY

The likelihood to proceed to open surgery can never be forgotten, even if the team has enough experience. The rate of

conversion to open procedure ranges from 0.5% to 4.2% in larger series.[7–12] Sometimes, difficulty comes just when one does not exercise prevention. Long instruments (clamps, needle holders) and proper autostatic retractors must be in stand by, especially if the surgeon foresees any trouble possibility. Among the factors identified as predictors of a greater possibility of conversion to open operation are steatohepatitis, diabetes mellitus, adhesions from various causes, previous bile leaks, BMI, weight,[9] large waist size,[9,11] increased waist/hip ratio, and male gender.[11]

LAPAROSCOPIC SET

The laparoscopic set is comprised of the apparatuses that provide illumination, receive the images from inside the patient, process them into visual images, and sustain the peritoneal cavity dilated by gas. Usually, the kit is composed of parts from the same manufacturer, as they function better this way. The hospital surgical unit should have one complete stand-by laparoscopic set, to attend to unpredicted material failure without imposing unnecessary conversion to open surgery.

Light Source

This device must provide light as white as possible, not to disturb color perception from inner organs and tissues. It also has to be powerful enough to brighten the focus object and the scope surroundings. A xenon gas bulb is the one that best fits this profile so far. Moreover, the xenon gas bulb has a longer lifetime, about 500 hours, while the halogen lasts about 250 hours. After the lifetime (which the manufacturer informs) of the bulb expires, the bulb should be replaced, for even the still functioning bulbs tend to cause narrowing of visual field.[13]

Light Cable

The fiber-optic cable must be chosen having in mind that the thicker the cable, more units of light transmitting optic fibers it has, hence more brightness.[13] The difference in cable length should not be important in this specific case.

Insufflation

The insufflator is a device that provides carbon dioxide (CO_2) flow at a determined rate, in liters per minute (L/min), until the intraperitoneal pressure achieves an also predetermined value, in centimeters of water (cm H_2O). The intraabdominal pressure of morbidly obese patients is already elevated as a consequence of the enlarged visceral and parietal fat, one of the accepted causes for the metabolic syndrome affecting this group (Chapter 11). Not surprisingly, it is not unusual to measure initial pressures (just after the gas is turned on) as high as 15 cm H_2O. Thus, the insufflation apparatus has to function with high-pressure levels; the authors believe that 20 cm H_2O is enough for most bariatric

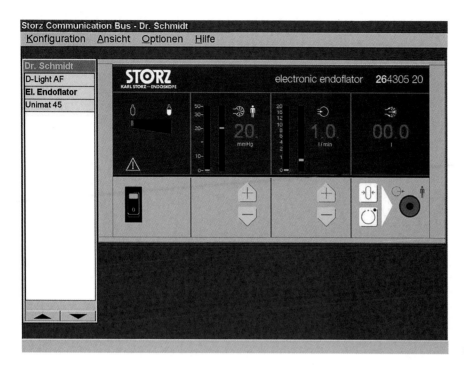

Figure 8–2. On-screen insufflator controls.

operations carried out by laparoscopy, and this can be increased with the advice of an anesthesiologist. Furthermore, as surgical exposition depends on sustained abdominal distension, the flow capacity has to be high too (20–30 L/min maximum flow rate), since the amount of gas to propel into a larger abdominal cavity to reach a fixed pressure is bigger. The insufflator is to respond quickly and "strongly" after suctions or gas leaks, especially in the event of bleeding. In the absence of such material, two insufflators may be connected to two trocars with separate gas tubes, or a Y tube (with two trocar ends) may be used to minimize the flow-limiting effect of the trocar connection. In addition, warming of the injected gas prevents endoscope fading; there is no evidence, however, that it helps to avoid hypothermia unless the gas is humidified too.[14] Automatic exsufflation is an important security feature, as it diminishes the probability of hyperpressure states.[14] Coupling with the monitor may display the insufflator parameters on the screen, facilitating the capture of information and ergonomics (Figure 8–2).[14]

Camera Body

Clear image is a cornerstone of videolaparoscopic surgery. The video unit should reproduce with fidelity what happens inside. The camera has to be precise in signal capturing and have trustful transmitting capability to the monitors, such as tri-chip (RGB) or digital connections (depending on the monitor used). Automatic white balancing is also useful.

Microcamera

The camera head, being the piece held by the surgeon, has to be easy to grab and contain simple but essential controls, like zoom and focus. It may as well have other options like still-image capturing and recording start/stop buttons. Its at-

taching to the endoscope must be facilitated and firm. It is inside the camera head where lies the charge-coupled-device (CCD) complex; this tool is responsible for converting photons into electrical signals.[15] The tri-chip cameras are so called for having three CCDs compounding their optic system, each capturing one different primary color (red, green, blue) and transmitting them separately to the camera body. In the analog tri-chip cameras, the video information is also passed to the monitor separately, one cable for each primary color. The digital camera, on its turn, after receiving the signals from the CCDs, converts them to digital image and passes them to the monitor via a digital cable, diminishing signal loss.

Monitors

The most commonly used monitors nowadays are the cathode-ray tube (CRT) ones. They receive analog signals from the video camera and transduce them into electron beams divided into the three primary colors (red, green, blue). These beams hit a phosphor plate that lies in the screen, and the amount of each color beam will result in different colors on the dots in the screen, building the respective image.[16] The CRT monitors are consequently best exploited when the camera signaling comes separately, one cable for each primary color (RGB).

The development of digital television has brought this kind of screen into the operating room, and among the types of digital monitors, liquid crystal display (LCD) is currently used in laparoscopy. In its screen every dot is controlled by one transistor. This kind of monitor gains more preference everyday because of its light weight and higher possibility of faster resolution improvement. Being a digital screen, it has to be connected to the camera by a digital video interface cable, or equivalent, i.e.,15 pin RGB-S. It should be stated that LCDs have shorter lifetimes, about 4–5 years, while CRTs operate in good conditions for decades.

Monitor Resolution

Monitors resolution is a product of the vertical versus horizontal-line distribution along the screen. The vertical-line arrangement is dictated by the color system used (PAL, NTSC, HDTV-PAL, HDTV-NTSC). The horizontal-line capacity may be adjusted during the manufacturing. A monitor with capacity for 800–900 horizontal lines provides good image. CRT monitors still provide the best resolutions, while LCDs try to keep up by improving fast. Larger screens (19 inches or more) facilitate the viewing, but it is important to mention that an increase in size does not necessarily mean a gain in resolution, and that bigger screens should be viewed from longer distances, keeping a range of about 4 to 5 times the size of the screen, for the surgeon's eyes comfort. Also, it is useless to have a high-definition monitor if the camera does not generate such images, or the cables do not transmit them faithfully.

Three-Dimensional Vision

There are many ways developed to date to enhance surgeon's vision and sense of depth in laparoscopy, including modifications in the endoscope, camera, monitors, and eye pieces that decode specially created images from the monitors. Most of these features add costs to the procedure, without resulting in better image quality when comparing to the conventional two-dimensional devices. Further improvement is needed before routine adoption of 3D imaging in laparoscopic surgery.[17]

INSTRUMENTS

Access to Peritoneal Cavity

Veress's Needle

Closed access to peritoneal cavity is attained with this device. Usually, the puncture site is at the left upper quadrant in the morbidly obese. The puncture part length has to overcome these patients' thick subcutaneous fat layer.

Trocars

> *Size*: For the same reason described above, for some patients (the experienced surgeon will notice it is not always necessary), trocars must be longer.
> *Retractile blades*: These are useful when puncturing the abdominal cavity, mostly for the first port acquisition, to avoid injury to internal organs as the cutting tip recoils just after entering the cavity.
> *Optical Tip*: This specially designed trocar has a transparent plastic tip, through which the maneuvers can be visualized when the scope is inside the trocar. It is particularly helpful when dealing with adhesions.[18]

> *Hasson*: Should the open technique be used, the Hasson's trocar aids in avoiding air leak through the larger abdominal wall orifice.

Optic Scopes

The endoscope, in order to provide good exposition, should have an angled tip, at least 30°. Although it is sometimes difficult to show structures distant from the endoscope port in wider abdominal cavities, it should be kept in mind that longer endoscopes tend to lose image quality because of the more intricated lens conjunct.[19]

Laparoscopic Instruments

Liver Retractors

The way of exposing the angle of His junction by retracting the liver left lobe varies according to the surgeon preferences. Some use specific retractors, while others prefer to clamp the right crux during the dissection of the angle of His. We consider it important to provide steadiness to whatever instrument is applied in retracting the liver so as to avoid inadvertent hepatic lesions. For this reason, we use an autostatic instrument-grabbing arm attached to operating table that holds the retractor firm and frees one assistant's hand, bringing utility and comfort together (Figure 8–3).

Graspers

Laparoscopic grasping clamps may serve the surgeon's preferences as long as they are as atraumatic as possible, i.e., fenestrated graspers. Harsh manipulation of digestive segments may cause injuries, occasionally hard to notice during the procedure. For some graspers it is important to have mechanisms to hold the closed position (Figure 8–4).[20]

Staplers

> *Linear staplers*: The stapler applier must be thin enough to fit the trocar, the 12-mm one being the thinner

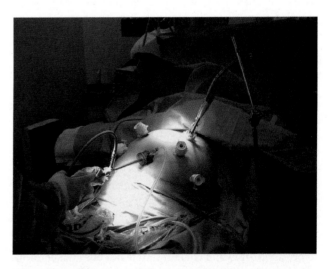

Figure 8–3. Autostatic grabbing arm holding liver retractor during gastric bypass.

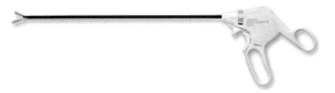

Figure 8–4. Endoscopic grasper.

to date. The length does matter in this case, as distant places must be reached to acquire safe and precise stapling/cutting. Also, it has to be prone to attachment with the different stapling loading units (Figure 8–5).

Loading units: The stapling loading units are the parts that actually staple and cut the tissues. They vary according to length (30, 45, and 60 mm) and staple size (2.5, 3.5, 4.5, and 5.5 mm). Thicker wall organs should be stapled with longer staple (4.5 mm up) units (Figure 8–6). The smallest staple cartridges (2.5 mm) are vascular-targeted and are used when there is hemostatic concern. We prefer to disconnect the stomach with blue loads (3.5 mm) and use the white ones (2.5 mm) to divide the small bowel and make the jejunojejunostomy.

Circular staplers: Two of the gastric bypass techniques employ open surgery circular staplers (Figure 8–7) to perform the gastrojejunostomy. The stapler anvil is put in the recently constructed pouch whether by pulling in by a nasogastric tube or by a gastrotomy (see Chapter 14), and the stapler is inserted in one of the ports and passed through the edge of the Roux limb. The anvil is then connected to the stapler and then fired, forming the anastomosis.

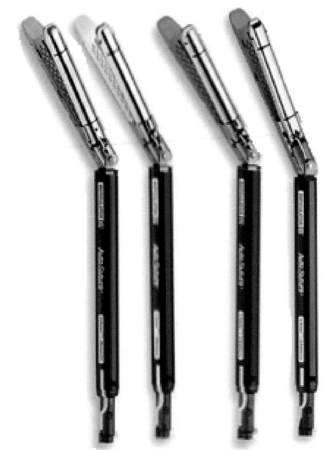

Figure 8–6. Loading units.

Staple-Line Reinforcements

Mechanisms of reinforcement of the staple-line have emerged with the intent to lower the rates of stapling-related bleeding and fistulas derived from staple-line failure. A publication stated that the use of bovine pericardial strips to buttress the staple-line during laparoscopic gastric bypass has been shown to reduce bleeding and operative time in humans[21]; the same product increases staple-line burst pressure in animal models, suggesting that pericardial strips strengthen the staple-lines.[22] Reinforcement with absorbable glycolide copolymer was also found to decrease bleeding, either during laparoscopic sleeve gastrectomy with or without duodenal switch (which may

have contributed to shorter hospital stay, decreased costs, and lower morbidity)[23] or during laparoscopic gastric bypass.[24] The application of fibrin sealant is also object of study as an adjunct to laparoscopic suturing.[25] Should these data be confirmed in larger series, the cost of these products would be easily justified by their benefits.[22]

Clip Appliers

This instrument's use not only relies on its obvious hemostatic characteristics, but serves to set important surgical references too, such as proximal/distal ends of bowel loops; it is also useful in possibly associated cholecystectomy.

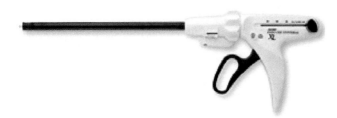

Figure 8–5. Endoscopic stapler (applier).

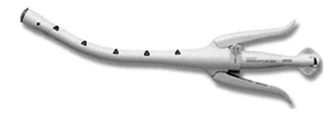

Figure 8–7. Circular stapler.

Suction and Irrigation

Good suction and irrigation are essential for endoscopic bariatric surgery, as for laparoscopy in general. Blood not only hampers exposition, but also steals brightness from the optic system, and should be promptly aspirated. Digestive secretions that escape from opened bowel segments should also be evacuated at once, for septic reasons. Irrigation allows cleansing of clotted blood and fibrin in the complication scenario, as well as confirming hermeticism of anastomoses by water-bubble tests.

Suturing

Even with the advent of stapling/cutting instruments, hand sewing is still required for orifice closure (stapling openings, mesenteric defects), bowel fixation, staple-line reinforcement, or even the main anastomoses (see Chapter 25). Thus, one should be familiar with laparoscopic suturing, as this can be inexcusably time-consuming.

Needle holders: Long needle drivers are almost always required in the surgical treatment of obesity—not only in bariatric surgery, but also in general laparoscopic surgery performed in morbid obese individuals, as this population grows every day and is affected by other surgical conditions. Being usually a 5-mm-thickness instrument, making it longer increases the possibility of it getting deformed by the strength necessary to manipulate it inside the abdominal cavity of a person with a thick abdominal wall (wall torque)—reason for which it should be delicate, yet resistant. Disposable needle holders that have an alternating side needle are some surgeons' preference, as they may facilitate needle handling and knot tying.

Energy Instruments

The importance of energy conducting devices resides in their capability to cut, coagulate, or do both at the same time with hemostatic ends. Monopolar and bipolar energies have been extensively used in surgical procedures and can be applied to laparoscopic surgery, namely bariatrics, as long as the instruments have proper connections for them. The development of ultrasonic dissectors, which contain a more than 55,000-Hz vibrating blade, has allowed cutting and coagulation without the hazard of heat dispersion to surrounding structures.[26]

ROBOTIC SURGERY

Usage of robotic-assisted surgery has taken place in the performance of the most common bariatric operations, namely gastric bypass, gastric banding, and biliopancreatic diversion with duodenal switch.[27,28] Although frequently applied in the most technically demanding parts, such as gastrojejunal and duodenojejunal anastomoses, and retrogastric dissection, there has been report of totally robotic gastric bypass.[29] Its advantages comprise 3-dimensional view, motion scaling for precise hand movement, mechanical forces that counteract the abdominal wall torque, and articulated wrists that facilitate manipulation in small working areas.[27] It is still an uncommon feature in surgical units, mainly due to costs[30]; this poses delay on the publication of larger series, necessary at present. So far, results have been encouraging; longer operative time has been noted with laparoscopic gastric banding.[27]

Robotic arms for the camera have also been used. These may be voice-commanded or guided by optoelectronic tracking systems that use light-emitting diodes in the instruments' tips, whose light is followed by a sensitive camera.[30]

References

1. Carbonell AM, Joels CS, Sing RF, et al.: Laparoscopic gastric bypass surgery: Equipment and necessary tools. *J Laparoendosc Adv Surg Tech A* 13(4):241–245, 2003.
2. Parikh MS, Shen R, Weiner M, et al.: Laparoscopic bariatric surgery in super-obese patients (BMI > 50) is safe and effective: A review of 332 patients. *Obes Surg* 15(6):858–863, 2005.
3. Nguyen NT, Goldman C, Rosenquist CJ, et al.: Laparoscopic versus open gastric bypass: A randomized study of outcomes, quality of life, and costs. *Ann Surg* 234(3):279–291, 2001.
4. Herron DM, Gagner M, Kenyon TL, et al.: The minimally invasive surgical suite enters the 21st century. *Surg Endosc* 15:415–422, 2001.
5. Gonzalez QH, Tishler DS, Plata-Munoz JJ, et al.: Incidence of clinically evident deep venous thrombosis after laparoscopic Roux-en-Y gastric bypass. *Surg Endosc* 18(7):1082–1084, 2004.
6. Prystowsky JB, Morasch MD, Eskandari MK, et al.: Prospective analysis of the incidence of deep venous thrombosis in bariatric surgery patients. *Surgery* 138(4):759–763, 2005; discussion: 763–765.
7. Alami RS, Morton JM, Sanchez BR, et al.: Laparoscopic Roux-en-Y gastric bypass at a veterans affairs and high-volume academic facilities: A comparison of institutional outcomes. *Am J Surg* 190:821–825, 2005.
8. Olbers T, Fagevik-Olsén M, Maleckas A, et al.: Randomized clinical trial of laparoscopic Roux-en-Y gastric bypass versus laparoscopic vertical banded gastroplasty for obesity. *Br J Surg* 92:557–562, 2005.
9. Schwartz ML, Drew RL, Chazin-Caldie M: Factors determining conversion from laparoscopic to open Roux-en-Y gastric bypass. *Obes Surg* 14(9):1193–1197, 2004.
10. Felix EL, Swartz DE: Conversion of laparoscopic Roux-en-Y gastric bypass. *Am J Surg* 186:648–651, 2003.
11. Schwartz ML, Drew RL, Chazin-Caldie M: Laparoscopic Roux-en-Y gastric bypass: Preoperative determinants of prolonged operative times, conversion to open gastric bypasses, and postoperative complications. *Obes Surg* 13(5):734–738, 2003.
12. Schauer PR, Ikramuddin S, Gourash W, et al.: Outcomes after laparoscopic Roux-en-Y gastric bypass for morbid obesity. *Ann Surg* 232(4):515–529, 2000.
13. Mutter D, Garcia A: All technologies for equipment: Cold light source. Online. 2003. Available at: http://www.websurg.com/tableofcontents/index.php?spec=5mla. Accessed February 15, 2006.
14. Garcia A, Mutter D, Jourdan I: All technologies for equipment: The insufflator in laparoscopy. Online. 2005. Available at: http://www.websurg.com/tableofcontents/index.php?spec=5. Accessed February 15, 2006.
15. Garcia A, Mutter D, Jourdan I: All technologies for equipment: Video camera. Online. 2003. Available at: http://www.websurg.com/tableofcontents/index.php?spec=5. Accessed February 15, 2006.
16. Garcia A, Mutter D: All technologies for equipment: Video monitor. Online. 2003 Available at: http://www.websurg.com/tableofcontents/index.php?spec=5. Accessed February 15, 2006.
17. Garcia A, Mutter D, Jourdan I: All technologies for equipment: 3D vision. Online. 2005. Available at: http://www.websurg.com/tableofcontents/index.php?spec=5. Accessed February 15, 2006.

18. Leroy J, Dutson E, Henri M: All technologies for equipment: Access and trocar complications. Online. 2005. Available at: http://www.websurg.com/tableofcontents/index.php?spec=5. Accessed February 15, 2006.

19. Mutter D, Garcia A, Jourdan I: All technologies for equipment: Endoscopes. Online. 2005. Available at: http://www.websurg.com/tableofcontents/index.php?spec=5. Accessed February 15, 2006.

20. Mutter D, Garcia A, Jourdan I: All technologies for equipment: Laparoscopic instruments. Online. 2005. Available at: http://www.websurg.com/tableofcontents/index.php?spec=5. Accessed February 15, 2006.

21. Angrisani L, Lorenzo M, Borrelli V, et al.: The use of bovine pericardial strips on linear stapler to reduce extraluminal bleeding during laparoscopic gastric bypass: Prospective randomized clinical trial. *Obes Surg* 14(9):1198–1202, 2004.

22. Shikora SA: The use of staple-line reinforcement during laparoscopic gastric bypass. *Obes Surg* 14(10):1313–1320, 2004.

23. Consten ECJ, Gagner M, Pomp A, et al.: Decreased bleeding after laparoscopic sleeve gastrectomy with or without duodenal switch for morbid obesity using a stapled buttressed absorbable polymer membrane. *Obes Surg* 14(10):1360–1366, 2004.

24. Nguyen NT, Longoria M, Welbourne S, et al.: Glycolide copolymer staple-line reinforcement reduces staple site bleeding during laparoscopic gastric bypass: A prospective randomized trial. *Arch Surg* 140(8):773–778, 2005.

25. Lee MM, Provost DA, Jones DB: Use of fibrin sealant in laparoscopic gastric bypass for the morbidly obese. *Obes Surg* 14(10):1321–1326, 2004.

26. Mutter D: All technologies for equipment. Basic principles: Electrocautery and high-frequency currents in surgery. Online. 2001. Available at: http://www.websurg.com/tableofcontents/index.php?spec=5. Accessed February 15, 2006.

27. Moser F, Horgan S: Robotically assisted bariatric surgery. *Am J Surg* ;88(Suppl):38S–44S, 2004.

28. Jacobsen G, Berger R, Horgan S: The role of robotic surgery in morbid obesity. *J Laparoendosc Adv Surg Tech A* 13:279–283, 2003.

29. Mohr CJ, Nadzam GS, Curet MJ: Totally robotic Roux-en-Y gastric bypass. *Arch Surg* 140(8):779–786, 2005.

30. Camarillo DB, Krummel TM, Salisbury JK: Robotic technology in surgery: Past, present, and future. *Am J Surg* 188(Suppl):2S–15S, 2004.

Bariatric Surgery Psychology

Melodie Moorehead, PhD

Bariatric surgery psychology is a specialty area of psychology, requiring specialized training for mental health experts. This training would have a parallel to what would be required of general surgeons obtaining the specialized training to enable them to perform safe and effective bariatric surgery. In numerous bariatric surgery forums, such as The American Society for Bariatric Surgery (ASBS), the International Federation for the Surgery of Obesity (IFSO), and the American College of Surgeons (ACS), the bariatric surgery healthcare field has demonstrated recognition of the valued role of the bariatric mental health provider.

The discussions in this chapter focus on both theoretical and applied aspects for psychological assessment and care of the morbidly/super obese patient presenting for surgery. The primary purpose of this chapter is to briefly highlight and elucidate the "Who, What, Where, When, and Why" regarding the role and benefits of bariatric surgery psychology. The clinical data and observations presented are gleaned from a biomedical literature review and 20 plus years of clinical experience in the design and implementation of the psychological standardized protocol presented at both the ASBS and

IFSO. The chapter is designed to be a user-friendly document that can help sensitize any interested party to obtain a better understanding of the strengths and challenges faced by the bariatric surgery patient. Another goal is to support the consideration, awareness, and decision to integrate the bariatric surgery mental health specialist into the multidisciplinary team.

The clinical cases supporting the data reviewed in the following sections have been compiled from hundreds of vertical band gastroplasty patients, thousands of Roux-en-Y gastric bypass cases, an ever growing number of adjustable gastric band patients, and a clinical trial of gastric stimulator cases. Considerations of the psychological sequelae of depression, anxiety, and addictions are discussed with specific reference to the impact of psychosocial stress, coping skills, and specific behaviors common to the severe/super obese archetype.

In furtherance of the learning goals outlined above, the literature review and psychological impressions presented are gathered heuristically from direct practice and are clinical in nature rather than anecdotal. As consideration is given to the often underserved and misconceived needs of this patient population, it is anticipated that a comprehensive multidisciplinary program that incorporates psychological service will be seen, not only of critical benefit in enhancing patient compliance, but also in securing patients' dramatic improvement in longer-term quality of life. A standardized psychological care model is outlined for a bariatric surgery program and thoughts offered regarding future research possibilities will conclude the discussion section of the chapter.

WHO

While the psychologist is well-suited for the advanced specialty training and delivery of services to the bariatric surgery patient population, psychiatry, psychiatric nursing, and social workers have also proved to be invaluable in meeting the needs of a comprehensive program. Key ingredients to consider in determining the efficacy of mental health specialists include empathy, authenticity, passion, and willingness to learn and better understand the maturational needs of the severely/super obese patient and their loved ones. It is also of the utmost importance for professionals to maintain an ability to be self-reflective in examining their own personal prejudices regarding the insidious nature of the disease.

WHY

Much of current literature reflects clinical appreciation for the fact that there is not a distinct *obese personality*. It is very important not to pathologize our brave and courageous patients, many of whom have demonstrated the lifelong determination and willpower to endure such humiliating treatments as jaw wiring and self-imposed starvation diets in an effort to control their disease. Clinical interviews routinely find that many patients have attempted and failed in excess of 20 diet programs before seeking bariatric surgery. Furthermore, it is important to note that only a very small percentage of people who need surgery actually present for surgery. In these special individuals, the spirit of hope is ignited. The power within this commonality can be tapped to help the patient take the needed steps beyond surgery and after weight loss to safely face the fact that they still have the disease of morbid obesity. (The healthy defense mechanism of denial, as it continues after surgery, can remain a contributing factor to the disease.) Despite the range of their commonalities, we must not labor under the misconception that bariatric surgery patients are all the same because, in practice, each of our patients presents with his or her own unique story. We must similarly not lose sight of the fact that the psychological dynamics of the morbid/super obese patients does differ from those who are less obese or their nonobese counterparts.

Clinical experience often coincides with research findings. Both perspectives reflect that, while the bariatric surgery patient does not suffer any greater psychiatric ailments or mental illness such as bipolar disorder or schizophrenia than the population at large, affective disorders (or simply put, emotional disorders such as depression, anxiety, symptoms of somatization, defense mechanism of denial, qualities like suspiciousness, and sense of loneliness) do occur with greater frequency. In fact, respectable reports identify that up to 95% of bariatric surgery patients acknowledge depressive symptoms, as identified in the Diagnostic and Statistical manual copyrighted by the American Psychiatric Association. Patients' self-defense mechanism of denial very often prevents them from recognizing these reported symptoms as signs of depression. There are various reasons for these affective disorders.

While researching and developing the Ardelt–Moorehead Addiction Scale, two potent factors impacting the behaviors of the morbidly/super obese individuals seeking surgical treatment were examined. These two factors have been identified as *craving* and an *inability to control*. Examining these two factors against the well-known *Three Factor Eating Inventory* developed by American psychologists Stunkard and Messick, two of their factors, i.e., *hunger* and *disinhibition*, were found to significantly correlate with the craving and the inability to control factors of the Ardelt–Moorehead (Addiction Scale). These findings indicate that high craving and high inability to control scores are related to our patients' feelings regarding hunger and a perceived inability to resist tempting smells or sight of food. This interpretation made sense to investigators and was not surprising; however, what was surprising and possibly ground breaking at that time was the finding that there was absolutely no correlation found between the craving and inability to control factors when compared to Stunkard and Messick's third factor, *cognitive restraint*. What this finding indicates is that for the morbidly/super obese patient seeking surgery, experiencing craving and inability to control their consumption of food represented a reaction to their affect, feelings, and emotions. It did not involve rational thoughts or the cognitive process. These findings offer an explanation for why the attempt to control eating behavior through behavioral modification alone is simply not successful long-term. It is felt that imparting this information to the patient may help them avoid experiencing shame for their inability to control their obesity by means other than surgery.

Removal of shame is an extremely relevant goal when working with the severely/super obese. To this end, it is important to understand the maturation and developmental needs of these patients to best appreciate how their ingrained thoughts trigger the affective system/emotional portion of the brain. We know through research that more than 75% of bariatric surgery patients have been obese since childhood. We also know that obese children receive less love, attention, and care from their caregivers and teachers than do their lean siblings. All too often obese children have learned to hate themselves because of the cultural prejudice and discrimination linked to severe obesity. Albert Stunkard and Thomas Wadden conducted research underscoring these points in a project where children under the age of six were showed silhouettes of an obese child. The children described the obese child as "lazy, dirty, stupid, ugly, cheat, and liar." As part of the project, drawings of children were shown of various weights and disfigurements to a variety of audiences, both adult and children. The audience, including the obese, rated the drawing of the obese child as least likable.

It has also been demonstrated that there is a progression in the severity of depression that correlates to the age of onset of obesity. The highest depression scores on paper-and-pencil psychological testing are found in adults who have been obese since early childhood, followed in severity by those who became obese during middle childhood and as adolescents with the least depression among individuals who had become obese as adults. Similar associations exist between age of obesity onset and the severity of *food addiction* and *inability to control* assessed by the Ardelt–Moorehead Addiction Scale, i.e., the more severe these conditions, the earlier the age of obesity onset. Many patients (2/3 of our population), in addition, have suffered early childhood abuse and more than 30% of patients report having grown up or currently live in an alcoholic household. It is apparent from such findings that surgery alone will not be sufficient to resolve these issues that, if left unattended, may interfere with weight-loss success.

Many preoperative bariatric patients report eating for reasons beyond physical hunger or need of physical satiety. These patients must come to terms with the fact that weight loss and, more importantly, weight-loss maintenance, even when achieved through bariatric surgery, requires a lifetime commitment of adhering to program guidelines. For a significant number of postoperative patients, this effort requires becoming aware of and taking responsibility for their decisions, choices, lifestyle behaviors, and learning to satisfy the need for emotional and psychological fulfillment and satiety by means other than eating. Thus, the successful bariatric patient may develop the motto of "I eat to live verses I live to eat." When both the bariatric team and patient population recognize the above realities, it becomes much easier to understand the essential importance of the Mental Health Specialist's involvement in a bariatric program beyond *patient screening*.

The Bariatric team must come to terms with the reality that, often following the weight loss or *Honeymoon* period, i.e., within the first 18 months following surgery, a patient who has not learned alternative coping skills and stress management techniques in managing both feelings and relationships may return to a preoperative, regressive style of eating. This behavior can return despite the fact that their new bodies tell them that they are physically full or even in the face of negative consequences that may occur due to noncompliant eating behaviors. The "diet of thoughts" beginning in early childhood, namely "I'm not good enough, not lovable enough, not deserving enough attention to meet my needs," can leave any heart starving. Helping the patient acquire the taste for a healthier diet of thoughts (e.g., through positive affirmations and progressive relaxation) can alter the negative self-fulfilling prophecy. Psychological satiety is needed to maintain weight loss following surgery once appetite returns. Therefore, it is important to address the reasons why people continue to eat when no longer feeling physically hungry and after reaching physical satiety.

The literature points out that proactive transformational coping skill, i.e., activities that help overcome destructive impulses, must be learned as a replacement for more regressive styles that rely on eating to manage chronic or acute stress. In addition to learning coping skills it is extremely valuable for bariatric surgery patients to own their legitimate rights in life and return to the absolute truth of deserving all the best that life has to offer.

WHAT, WHERE, AND WHEN

Overall, a psychodynamically structured environment founded on empathy, relationship, and rapport is a useful treatment milieu when treating bariatric surgery patients and their loved ones. In consideration of the cultural stigmatization, personal history, and often-neglected consequent maturational needs, the morbidly/super obese are well served by purposefully using empathy and warmth in the doctor–patient exchange. This requires the conscious implementation of a planned *good parent* treatment environment. Responding in an analytic or good parent manner rather than taking an authoritative *mean parent* stance, along with strong structural consistency in the multidisciplinary treatment settings, will help even the challenging suspicious patient have a positive emotional healing. Many patients attempt to recreate or recapitulate the dynamics involved in their family of origin while participating in a bariatric program. Remember Freud's discussion on repetition compulsion? The purpose of this repetition is an attempt at correcting and healing the early harmful experience.

Specifically, the range of mental health services offered to bariatric surgery patients may include the following: (1) An initial psychological or mental health evaluation with specialized assessment tools, (2) in-hospital psychological support, (3) ongoing brief support sessions when the patient is in the surgeon's office for follow-up care, (4) facilitation of the Bariatric Surgery Support Group meeting, and (5) when appropriate, referral to individual, group, or family psychotherapy.

Applied to this clinical patient group are both presurgical screening and clinical services for perioperative psychological planning purposes as well as the development of adequate postoperative psychosocial therapeutic support services. The former services document the patient's *psychological informed consent* and the latter create a climate of emotional healing throughout the first postoperative year. To this end, the best postoperative care begins with preoperative care. (In an effort to accomplish this, a useful audio CD, *The Gift and The Tool*,* may be offered to your patients). The principal goal

---

The Gift and The Tool: A Personal Guide for a Lifelong Journey. (©) The Gift and the Tool Enterprise) This is a 2-CD audio set for those living with the disease of severe/super obesity. Dramatically presented, it is a complete emotional guide for the bariatric surgery patient and their loved ones. CD 1 is an inspirational presentation helping to promote psychological informed consent. CD 2 contains a combination of relaxation techniques and positive affirmations to help prepare patients for surgery—the surgery itself—and for facing life and its challenges after surgery. Also included are five Quality of Life Questionnaires that will help measure progress—from presurgery to recovery to maintenance. Melodie K. Moorehead, PhD, the author of this chapter can be reached at the website (Drmoorehead.com).

of treatment services is to facilitate patient cooperation and adjustment in order to enhance long-lasting quality-of-life modifications in the face of patients' characteristics, emotional vulnerability, and any social withdrawal tendencies. Presurgery, patients are highly motivated. Seeking to set in place proactive habit formation, therefore, is wise at that time. Through active involvement in a comprehensive bariatric surgery program, the patient can develop skills that can help alter the diet of their thoughts while rediscovering their body. In order to secure these behavioral and attitudinal changes, in light of chronic psychological comorbidity, patients should be approached with comprehensive and pragmatic psychological programs of care.

It is valuable for each member of the multidisciplinary team to understand that the patient's decision to have bariatric surgery represents a transformational decision. This decision is typically arrived at following much deliberation and review of one's life and loss. It is important for the team to be aware of the value and power of the decision when referring the patient for the mental health evaluation. For most patients, their mental health evaluation, in fact, proves to be the first time they have had the ability to tell *their story*. Communicating the broad range of challenges and losses endured as a result of weight-related issues can prove to be a source of strength for the action that follows and that is required. Detailing one's history in a safe, empathic environment with the support of an understanding specialist can be a key step in the process of healing. The patients begin to let go of a lifelong history of personal shame and self-blame. Therefore, the evaluation is formulated on a broad psychoeducational model rather than as a narrower and more traditional clinical psychological evaluation. In this context, the evaluation provides important patient education while serving as a consultation to the bariatric surgeon, without the evaluation being reduced to a RED or GREEN LIGHT on the road to surgery. The psychological/mental health evaluation performed in this spirit can be used to help even psychologically challenged people face the emotional and behavior demands of bariatric surgery safely.

The evaluation report is designed, among other things, to advise the bariatric multidisciplinary team regarding the individual patient's needs and vulnerabilities, as well as any recommendations offered. The team together can then assist the patient to put in place any needed recommendations. This approach creates a safety net that addresses and helps cushion any anticipated potential postoperative adjustment difficulties. The successful multidisciplinary team uses the evaluation report to better understand their patient within providers' specific subspecialty. Some of the signs and symptoms of concern that may stand in the way of a person's ability to comply with needed protocols and postoperative adjustment may include

- chaotic/unstable lifestyle
- bulimia nervosa (active)
- dangerous noncompliance in psychiatric or medical treatment

- active substance abuse
- untreated psychiatric symptoms or symptoms not stabilized on medications
- suicide attempts or psychiatric hospitalizations within the last 12 months prior to assessment.

As these problem areas are identified, the mental health specialist's consulting relationship with the multidisciplinary team can prove critical in monitoring and directing the patient to those services necessary for adequate stabilization of problematic symptoms. At every step, it is essential for the mental health consultant to understand the surgeon's philosophy and expectations. While the above specific conditions may pose either significant or irreconcilable psychological barriers to patients' adaptation of program protocol, symptoms of severe (nonpsychotic) depressions, anxiety, posttraumatic shock, distorted body image/eating disorders, commonly applicable to our presenting surgical candidates, most often do not prelude bariatric surgery success.

The concept of the morbid/super obesity archetype, when well understood from a psychodynamic perspective, can be augmented from its iatrogenic nature for both provider and patient, to encompass an enhanced bridge of empathy, with targeted clinical pathways for specialized service delivery. It is also at this juncture that the team's mental health professional provides consultation to the other members in order that each provider may heighten their purposeful utilization of services to meet the needs of this deserving patient. The psychological understanding of the morbidly obese bariatric surgery patient affords each subspecialty enriched opportunities for quality care.

A comprehensive paper is available from the ASBS, *Suggestions for the Pre-Surgical Assessment of Bariatric Surgery Candidates*. For those most interested in this section, referring to the ASBS paper will further expound on the various aspects of a presurgery mental health evaluation as well as offer considerations regarding the choice and use of psychological instruments.

The evaluation includes a comprehensive, structured psychoeducationally oriented clinical interview. This interview focuses on obtaining a thorough psychosocial history of the individual and the individual's perception of family life. The weight history, with specific emphasis on the patient's relationship psychologically to food, dieting, and frustration tolerance, is of primary concern. Part of the weight history assessment includes an evaluation of the family weight and food use patterns. The clinical evaluation measures the level and depth of psychological functioning for each surgical candidate's emotional stamina, ego strength, defense and personality structure, coping strategies, characteristic cognitive and behavioral patterns, reasoning styles/problem-solving methods, and body image and self-esteem profiles. Of further interest is a conceptualization of existing social supports for each patient. Medical and psychological cofactors, including psychiatric history, are all pertinent. Of unique consideration is the patient's detailed understanding of the surgery, the after-care regimen, and longer term issues regarding compliance to program guidelines. Assessments of the patient's ad hoc problem-solving skills, a thorough mental status exam, and an evaluation of the patient's typical pain management threshold are additional factors of diagnostic relevance.

Psychological informed consent accomplishes two goals: (1) Helping prevent the patient from feeling overwhelmed and neglected, as has often been the perceived pattern of much of their lives and (2) reducing the program's litigation vulnerability. The clinical interview when structured as a psychoeducational model will afford the patient education regarding the possibilities of dramatic changes in many areas, such as important relationships, spiking in preoperative depression or anxiety, and transfer of addiction from food to other substances or activities. (It is often said by the bariatric surgery candidate, "I am a food addict.") Psychological informed consent is valuable and needed presurgically to help the patient who is vulnerable to experiencing one or more of these natural consequences.

For the purpose of this chapter, when evaluating any potential candidate for weight loss surgery, it is very important to maintain awareness that the disease of morbid or severe obesity kills and/or substantially reduces the quality of life of a person, while impacting the lives of family members. As life and death are often in balance, it is important for the evaluator to see their professional role within the context of the decision-making process of the larger team of whom the surgeon bears responsibility for determining the patients ultimate suitability for surgery. The evaluator's role, in the context of decision making is one of psychological consultation. This consultation provides an understanding of the patient's strengths and challenges rather than being a red flag to surgical candidacy. In this latter regard, it may be helpful to consider the mental health specialist in the bariatric arena being likened to the child custody evaluator in the legal arena during a contested marital divorce proceeding. While the judge or the attorneys may wish the psychologist to determine which parent might afford the preferred placement for the child, many commentators, relying on interpretation of American Psychological Association Guidelines, suggest that making such an ultimate determination involves a legal conclusion which, in fact, is outside the psychologist's expertise and training. It is suggested that just as in the legal arena, the preferred role of the psychologist is to limit his or her role to that of educating the courts as to the strengths and challenges of the particular parent, and thereby allowing the court to make a more informed legal decision as to the best placement for the child. So too, in the *surgical arena*, a well-prepared, in-depth evaluation report can similarly help the surgeon in better appreciating patient psychosocial dynamics, and thereby assist the surgeon in making a more informed medical/surgical determination as to the appropriateness of a particular patient. The surgeon, like the judge, has the responsibility for making ultimate decisions regarding patient care.

Clinicians and researchers specializing in the bariatric surgery field agree that people struggling with the disease of morbid/super obesity experience prototypic psychological distress. Certainly, following surgery coupled with existing pretreatment psychological stressors, it becomes clearer that the required, monumental postsurgical attitudinal and behavioral modifications needed can exacerbate the recovering patient's often fragile ego status, serving as precipitants to a period of more pronounced psychological vulnerability. The comorbidity of depression, following surgery, can support a profile of those patients with truncated cognitive perspectives, impaired self-esteem, and low frustration tolerance. In this prototypic, regressed psychological state, there is definitive indication for hand-in-hand psychological care of the population concurrent to the surgical intervention. While special attention may be needed for this portion of the population, all bariatric surgery patients can benefit by a program of psychological support. Including all patients in such a program negates further stigmatization of an already stigmatized group.

As the actual surgery is the central element of the entire change process, some have questioned whether there is a meaningful role of psychology during the hospital stay and subsequent outpatient medical follow-up visits. Psychological support at every stage can be invaluable in assisting the patient. One aspect of ongoing, supportive service is a focus on helping each person to manage the emotional stress, behavioral transitions, and demands that often occur during the course of hospitalization and the early adjustment period following discharge from hospital. Another aspect of service centers on working as part of a multidisciplinary outpatient team. In the surgeon's office, psychoeducational support offers an opportunity to the patients as they acquire the requisite new transformational coping skills as well as necessary personal comfort for successfully adapting to the lifestyle changes. Affording these services helps implement the positive changes necessary for patients to achieve their goals lifelong. It is one thing for the patient to plan and arrange for surgery; however, it is quite another dimension to actually enter the hospital, prepare for and recover from surgery, face the unknown, and cope with the uncertainties of the behavioral and lifestyle changes. One must also work through the sense of loss which can occur as the patient adjusts not only to what they have given up, i.e., the ability to turn to food for comfort, but also acknowledge, take ownership of, and to appreciate the positive changes that ensue. These changes must include the belief, "I am good enough, I am loveable, and I do deserve the attention I need." At every step along the way it is the goal of the mental health specialist to assist the patient in making the smoothest transition possible to their *new life and new beginning.*

In addition to the above range of psychological and mental health services, another significant aspect of the psychological and emotional journey for the bariatric surgery patient or prospective patient is the Bariatric Support Group. For many, these meetings are their first opportunities to free themselves from a profound social and emotional isolation and to encounter and become a part of a community of hope. It is quite common for our patients to feel misunderstood even *blamed* for seeking bariatric surgery, which is at times mistakenly viewed as the *easy way out*. The Support Group proves a venue to dispel this myth and educate the patient as to the credit they deserve as they embrace the range of challenges and demands that are a part of the bariatric program.

With the patient's commonly experienced history of despair, discrimination, hopelessness, depression, and anxiety, the overarching theme of the Support Group becomes one of personal transformation, new life, and a pride in accomplishment. Repeatedly, bariatric surgery patients will attest that through the surgery and the attendant improvements in health status and quality of life, they now have *two birthdays*, the day of their actual birth and the day of their surgery. What is it about the concept of *new birth* that makes it such a common theme? The answer becomes self-evident as the stories are shared: Abusive relationships end as patients no longer accept victimization; diabetes, chronic debilitating pain, and other life-threatening conditions resolve; parents become more actively engaged in their children's development; infertile couples give birth to long dreamed of children; and even less profound activities such as public seating, walking through a store, and participating in a range of leisure activities become an accepted part of life; job prospects, social and economic possibilities unfold. Is it any wonder that exhilarated patients proclaim that they are so pleased with their success that they would have the surgery again?" Even most of those unfortunates who experience significant complications reply "In a heart beat." Preoperatively, support groups give the patient scheduled for surgery a valuable opportunity to interact with people who have had the procedure. The preoperative patient is also able to meet people at all the different stages of recovery. This becomes an effective tool for managing patient expectations and reducing anxiety. It is also an effective way to help achieve and document informed consent.

Support group meetings can also be very useful to the postoperative patient. It can serve as a format for *giving back* to their program something of value. By sharing their personal stories, triumphs, trials, and tribulations, self-esteem is increased. By trusting and sharing one's experience in a group, people can learn that *slips* or even *lapses* in following program protocols do not have to end in *relapses* or *failure*.

The meetings can provide opportunities to learn how to handle feelings in new ways rather than turning to food. They can help individuals understand that while it is natural to fear the regain of weight, the power to sustain weight loss following surgery is always within their grasp.

DISCUSSION

Bariatric surgery is on the rise worldwide. One thing we can all agree on is that there is still so much to be learned about the disease of obesity. Some surgeons have asked psychology

specialists to help them better identify which surgical procedure is best suited for which patient. To this end, research is very much needed.

Using Bariatric Analysis and Reporting Outcome System (BAROS), a standardized reporting outcome system to quantify and define success and failure following bariatric surgery could help compare the effects of medical/surgical intervention across many different techniques and procedures in the following domains: (1) Percentage of excess weight loss, (2) resolution of comorbidities, and (3) quality of life. The information provided along with other psychology instruments may help the field to one day have the needed knowledge to identify patient characteristics that would be best suited to one surgery-type over another. Further, implementing BAROS clinically helps patients remain accountable. Documenting *success* versus *failure* with a broad range of scoring possibilities, including *excellent, very good, good, fair,* and *failure,* can help even patients with significant weight regain not score as *failure*. BAROS weighs all three domains (weight loss, resolution of comorbidities, quality of life) equally, so even when points are lost in the percentage of excess-weight-loss field, resolution of comorbidities and quality of life scores often maintain high value and when calculated in the standardized scoring system of BAROS an outcome of *good or fair* as opposed to *failure* can result.

Stratifying the range of success versus failure with standardized values can serve to reassure patients, hence lower anxiety for people returning to their surgeon with weight regain issues. The shame of weight regain, coupled with the history of multiple weight loss failures, leads a patient to think, "I have once again failed." Objectified reassurance is valuable to an anxious and shamed patient given that we know chronic anxiety plays a contributing role in the disease process of obesity.

Research is sorely warranted because it will scientifically determine the benefit that specialized bariatric mental health services offer, i.e., how building transformational coping skills (affirmations, changing the diet of thoughts, coupled with progressive relaxation) not only transforms regressive styles but also protects against transferring addiction qualities and behavior to another, leaving bariatric surgery patients vulnerable.

Further areas of interest might be: what addiction factors the morbidly obese share with their nonobese counterparts, the association between food addiction and body mass index, and the impact that different bariatric surgical procedures have on addiction factors.

Finally, the development of a superstructure for cost-effective psychological practice standards, responding specifically to the needs of bariatric surgery patients, is another worthy area of research. Such inquiry must lead to the development of sound clinical pathways aimed to increase patient cooperation and maximize successful weight reduction, resolving comorbidities and increasing the quality of life while minimizing the litigious impact often seen in bariatric surgery.

ACKNOWLEDGMENTS

Great appreciation is offered to my professional partner Michael S. Parish, JD LCSW, Psy, D. Thank you Michael for supporting the writing of this chapter, and particularly for permitting me to incorporate segments of your writing found in one of our office documents, *Why Are Psychological Support Services an Important Part of Your Bariatric Surgery Program?* Several of your thoughts and ideas are found in this chapter. While originally this office document was written to help our patients understand the value of psychology in bariatric surgery, your sensitivity and knowledge will now also help our professional community. Thank you Joan M. DiGregorio, PhD, my first professional partner; your original interest in the field of bariatric surgery psychology introduced me to bariatric surgery. To that end, I owe endless gratitude and recognition to Norman Samuels, MD, an early pioneer in bariatric surgery and the individual who is responsible for launching me into this third decade of service. The collegial resource and genuine friendship of Elisabeth Ardelt-Gattinger, PhD, and Cynthia Buffington, PhD, is more important than simple words can say. I offer lifelong appreciation for Emanuel Hell, MD; he is responsible for the international awareness regarding specialized psychology in bariatric surgery. Horacio Oria, MD, is needed to continue parenting BAROS throughout adoption into our bariatric community. Thanks to all the individuals involved in the writing of this book. The willingness to share our talents and experiences with one another are demonstrations of the passion inherent in this field. Recognition is given to all the early surgeons and allied health professionals of the ASBS and IFSO for helping our field continue to address the following: Bariatric surgery presents the greatest medical hope for lasting quality of life correction. When treating the disease, one cannot separate the emotional and psychological factors from the physical and biological. For that reason, every bariatric surgery patient is best served within a multidisciplinary team that includes a bariatric mental health specialist.

Suggested Readings

1. DiGregorio JM, Moorehead MK: The psychology of the bariatric surgery patients: A clinical report. *Obes Surg* 4:361–369, 1994.
2. Kleiner KD, Gold MS, Frost-Pineda K, Lenz-Brunsman B, Perri MG, Jacobs WS: Body mass index and alcohol use. *J Addict Dis* 23:105–118, 2004.
3. Kolotkin RL, Crosby RD, Pendelton R, Strong M, Gress RE, Adams T: Health-related quality of life in patients seeking gastric bypass surgery vs. non-treatment-seeking controls. *Obes Surg* 13:371–377, 2003.
4. Maddi SR, Fox SR, Khoshaba DM, Harvey RH, Lu JL, Persico M: Reduction psychopathology following bariatric surgery for morbid obesity. *Obes Surg* 11:680–685, 2001.
5. Maddi SR, Khoshaba DM, Persico, M, Bleeker, F, VanArsdall, G. Psychosocial correlates of psychopathology in a national sample of the morbidly obese. *Obes Surg* 7:397–404, 1997.
6. Mahoney Michael J: *Constructive Psychotherapy: A Practical Guide.* New York, Guilford Press, 2003.
7. Moorehead MK, Ardelt-Gattinger E, Lechner H, Oria HE: The validation of the Moorehead-Ardelt quality of life questionnaire II. *Obes Surg* 13: 684–692, 2003.
8. Sogg S, Mori D: The Boston interview for gastric bypass: Determining the psychological suitability of surgical candidates. *Obes Surg* 14, 370–380, 2004.
9. Stunkard Albert J, Wadden Thomas A: Psychological aspects of human obesity. *Human Obesity: General Aspects.* 1992; p. 352–358.
10. Allied Health Science Section Ad Hoc Behavioral Health Committee (Co-Chaired: Melodie K. Moorehead, Ph.D. and Cathy S. Reto, Ph.D., et al.): Suggestions for the pre-surgical psychological assessment of bariatric surgery candidates. American Society for Bariatric Surgery. 2004.
11. Oria HE, Moorehead MK: Bariatric analysis and reporting outcome system (BAROS). *Obes Surg*: 487–499, 1998.
12. Wadden TA, Sarwer DB, Arnold ME, Gruen D, O'Neil PM: Psychosocial status of severely obese patients before and after bariatric surgery. *Problems General Surg* 17:13–22, 2000.
13. Wadden TA, Stunkard AJ (eds.): *Handbook of Obesity Treatment.* New York, Guilford Press, 2002.
14. Wang GJ, Volkow ND, Thanos PK, Fowler JS: Similarity between obesity and drug addiction as assessed by neurofunctional imaging: A concept review. *J Addict Dis* 23:39–53, 2004.
15. Wolf AM, Falcone AR, Kortner B, Kuhlmann HW: BAROS: An effective system to evaluate the results of patients after bariatric surgery. *Obes Surg* 10:445–450, 2000.

10

Anesthetic Concerns

Jay B. Brodsky, MD • Luiz C. Lerner, MD

INTRODUCTION

Today more than 30% of adults in the United States are obese, and it is estimated that by the year 2025 that number will exceed 40%. Obesity is not confined to industrialized, developed nations like the United States, but has become a worldwide problem of epidemic proportions. There is no precise definition of when obesity actually begins. A patient is considered obese when the amount of body fat increases beyond the point where health deteriorates and life expectancy is shortened. The precursors of obesity include gender, genetic and environmental effects, ethnicity, education, and socioeconomic status. In industrialized countries obesity is more common in the lower socioeconomic groups, while in developing countries it is often associated with affluence.

Obesity affects every organ system and is the cause of many chronic medical problems. Obese patients have more annual admissions to the hospital, more outpatient visits, and higher prescription drug costs than nonobese adults. Obese patients also have "quality of life" issues than can include depression and a feeling of social incompetence. In 1991 the United States' National Institutes of Health Consensus Development Conference Panel recommended weight reduction surgery as the best alternative for extreme obesity for patients unable to lose weight by diet and exercise. Most of the medical conditions associated with extreme obesity are reversible following sustained surgical weight loss.

The number of bariatric surgical procedures performed in the United States in 2005 is estimated to have exceeded 150,000. Laparoscopy is now the preferred surgical approach since it is minimally invasive and allows high-risk morbidly obese patients to recover more rapidly with fewer complications than following open procedures.

This chapter will discuss anesthetic considerations for the obese patients undergoing bariatric surgery.

DEFINITIONS

Body mass index (BMI), an indirect measure of obesity, is calculated by dividing patient weight (kilograms, kg) by the square of their height (meters, m). BMI = kg/m^2. An individual with a BMI $\geq$ 30 kg/m^2 is said to be *obese*. "Morbid" obesity describes obesity that, if untreated, will significantly shorten life expectancy. A variety of definitions exist, but any patient with a BMI $\geq$ 40 kg/m^2 is considered to be "morbidly" obese. A patient with a BMI > 35 kg/m^2 who has serious medical comorbidities is also a candidate for weight loss surgery.

Since most anesthetic drugs are administered on the basis of either ideal body weight (IBW), lean body weight (LBW), or total body weight (TBW), the anesthesiologist must be familiar with these terms as they pertain to the obese patient.

IBW is a measure initially derived by life insurance companies to describe the weight statistically associated with maximum life expectancy. In the absence of weight tables, IBW can be easily estimated by the simple formula IBW = 22 × (h × 2), where 'h' is the patient's height.[1] Normal weight ranges between ±10% of IBW.

LBW is TBW minus the weight of body fat (FW). LBW includes muscles, bones, tendons, ligaments, and body water, while FW is adipose tissue. In normal patients, LBW should be about 80% TBW for males and 75% TBW for females. In nonobese patients, TBW approximates IBW. In morbid obesity, LBW is estimated by increasing IBW by 20%–30%.

PREOPERATIVE EVALUATION

Medical History

Obesity is associated with many chronic medical problems (Table 10–1). A patient who is moderately overweight probably carries no excess health risks, especially while still young. However, morbidity and mortality rise sharply with increasing age and BMI. Medical comorbidities must be recognized, and when possible optimized before elective bariatric surgery.

Table 10–1.

Medical Conditions Associated with Obesity

Organ System	Comorbidity
Respiratory	restrictive lung disease, asthma, obstructive sleep apnea (OSA) syndrome, obesity hypoventilation syndrome, Pickwickian syndrome
Cardiovascular	hypertension, cardiomegaly, congestive heart failure, coronary artery disease, peripheral vascular disease, pulmonary hypertension, thromboembolism, sudden death
Endocrine/ Metabolic	type 2 diabetes mellitus, Cushing's syndrome, hypothyroidism, hyperlipidemia, vitamin deficiency
Gastrointestinal	hiatal hernia, inguinal and ventral hernia, fatty liver (NASH), gallstones
Musculoskeletal	osteoarthritis on weight bearing joints, low back pain
Malignancy	breast, prostate, cervix, uterine, colorectal
Psychiatric	depression, low self-esteem

Any patient who has had previous bariatric surgery should be evaluated for metabolic changes that can include protein, vitamin, iron, and calcium deficiencies.

A list of all current medications must be available to the anesthesiologist, including nonprescription appetite suppressors and diet drugs. Many of these drugs can have important side effects. For example, the combination of phentermine and fenfluramine (phen–fen), which is no longer prescribed in the United States, is associated with serious heart and lung problems. Another weight loss medication, sibutramine, works in the brain by inhibiting the reuptake of norepinephrine, serotonin, and dopamine producing a feeling of "anorexia" which limits food intake. Sibutramine has been implicated as a cause of dysrhythmias and hypertension. Orlistat blocks digestion and absorption of dietary fat by binding lipases in the gastrointestinal tract and can cause deficiencies in fat-soluble vitamins (A, D, E, K). A reduction in vitamin K levels can increase the anticoagulation effects of coumadin.

Physical Examination

During the physical examination the anesthesiologist's attention is directed to the cardiac and pulmonary systems, and to head and neck anatomy in order to evaluate the airway for tracheal intubation.

Cardiovascular System

Cardiac output rises proportionally with increased weight. Stroke volume also increases since a greater total blood volume is needed to perfuse the added body fat. Increased cardiac output combined with normal peripheral vascular resistance leads to systemic hypertension. Mild to moderate hypertension is seen in most morbidly obese patients. The increased left ventricular wall stress caused by increased stroke volume and the resultant ventricular dilation leads to cardiac hypertrophy.[2]

Left ventricular dysfunction is often present in young, asymptomatic patients. Even normotensive patients have increased preload and after-load, increased mean pulmonary artery pressure (PAP), and elevated right and left ventricular stroke work. Since these patients are often not physically active, they may appear to be asymptomatic even in the presence of significant cardiovascular disease. Signs of pulmonary hypertension (exertional dyspnea, fatigue, syncope) should be sought and trans-esophageal echocardiography (TEE) obtained in symptomatic patients. Right heart failure is common in older patients. A medical consultation with a cardiologist may be indicated before bariatric surgery.

The ECG may show increased rate, changes in QRS voltage, left QRS axis shift, slowed conduction, and evidence of ischemia or previous myocardial infarction. The ECG even in normotensive morbidly obese patients may reveal left ventricular hypertrophy, cardiac chamber enlargement, ventricular ectopy, and other arrhythmias. Cardiac dysrhythmias are precipitated by chronic hypoxia (especially in patients with obstructive sleep apnea, OSA), hypercapnia, increased circulating levels of catecholamines, electrolyte disturbances caused by diuretic therapy, fatty infiltration of the conduction system, and ischemic heart disease.[3] Polycythemia suggests chronic hypoxemia.

Pulmonary System

Adipose tissue is metabolically active. Oxygen consumption and CO_2 production rise with increasing weight due to increased metabolic demands. The work of breathing is increased since more energy must be expended to carry the additional body mass, while respiratory muscle performance is impaired. The fatty chest and abdominal walls plus the increased pulmonary blood volume contribute to reduced pulmonary compliance. Mass loading of the thoracic and abdominal chest walls causes abnormalities in both lung volumes and gas exchange, especially when the patient is supine. The increased total respiratory resistance and decreased compliance associated with extreme obesity results in shallow, rapid breathing. Functional residual capacity (FRC) is significantly reduced due to a decrease in expiratory reserve volume, therefore total lung capacity is reduced. Airways close during normal ventilation. Continued perfusion of nonventilated alveoli will result in an oxygen tension (P_aO_2) that is lower than predicted for similar-aged nonobese patients. These changes increase in direct proportion with increasing BMI.[4] General anesthesia further reduces FRC.

Preoperative pulmonary function tests show a restrictive breathing pattern. For symptomatic patients, an arterial blood gas obtained while the patient breathes room air is useful to establish a baseline. Younger obese patients have an increased ventilatory response to hypoxia and a relatively decreased response to hypercapnia. Their arterial blood sample often demonstrates alveolar hyperventilation (P_aCO_2 30–35 mm Hg) and relative hypoxemia (P_aO_2 70–90 mm Hg) while breathing air.[5] With increasing age, sensitivity to CO_2 decreases so P_aCO_2 rises and P_aO_2 falls further.

A careful thorough preoperative assessment of patient's face, neck, and upper airway is always required since mask ventilation and tracheal intubation can be a challenge in some obese patients. A review of the patient's previous anesthetic records will reveal whether airway problems had been encountered during previous surgical procedures.

Obstructive Sleep Apnea Syndrome

Many obese patients maintain a normal P_aCO_2 during the day but have CO_2 retention, sleep disturbances, intermittent airway obstruction with hypoxemia, pulmonary hypertension, and cardiac arrhythmias at night. OSA syndrome is characterized by frequent episodes of apnea (>10-s cessation of airflow despite continuous respiratory effort against a closed airway) and hypopnea (50% reduction in airflow or reduction associated with a decrease of $S_pO_2 > 4\%$). OSA is frequently undiagnosed in patients scheduled for bariatric surgery.

Obesity is an important risk factor for OSA, but not every obese patient suffers from OSA.[6] OSA occurs more often in patients with large fat necks and high Mallampati (III and IV) scores. The patients may not be aware of symptoms, so it is important to interview their spouse. If OSA is present, they will describe loud snoring followed by silence as airflow ceases with obstruction, then gasping or choking as the patient awakes and airflow restarts. A definitive diagnosis of OSA can only be confirmed by polysomnography in a sleep laboratory. Because of fragmented sleep patterns, OSA patients may complain of daytime sleepiness and headaches. Chronic sleep apnea leads to secondary polycythemia, hypoxemia, and hypercapnia, all of which increase the risk of cardiac and cerebral vascular disease.

Patients with a history of snoring or a definitive diagnosis of OSA are often difficult to ventilate by mask, and their tracheas may be more difficult to intubate than similar weight patients without OSA. And OSA patients who use nasal continuous positive airway pressure (CPAP) devices at home should be instructed to bring them to the hospital to use following surgery.

If the patient is known or even suspected of having OSA they should be continuously monitored by pulse oximetry in the postoperative period, even following a completely uneventful operation.

Obesity Hypoventilation Syndrome

A small number of patients have the "obesity hypoventilation syndrome" (OHS), which is characterized by somnolence, cardiac enlargement, polycythemia, hypoxemia, and hypercapnia. OHS patients tend to be older, super obese (BMI > $50\,kg/m^2$), and have more restricted pulmonary function than other patients with OSA.

Hypoventilation is central and independent of intrinsic lung disease, and is probably due to a progressive desensitization of the respiratory center to hypercapnia from nocturnal sleep disturbances. In its most severe form, the "Pickwickian Syndrome," there is hypersomnolence, hypoxia, hypercapnia, pulmonary hypertension, right ventricular enlargement, and hypervolemia. These patients rely on a hypoxic ventilatory drive and may hypoventilate or even become apneic following emergence from general anesthesia after being given 100% O_2 to breathe.

Gastrointestinal and Urinary Systems

It is widely believed that morbidly obese patients are at greater risk for acid aspiration during induction of general anesthesia. Risk factors include increased intra-abdominal pressure, high incidence of gastroesophageal reflux disease (GERD) and hiatus hernia, increased gastric volume (usually >25 mL), and decreased gastric fluid pH (usually <2.5).[7] Recently this belief has been challenged. One study reported that fasting obese patients actually had a lower incidence of high-volume, low-pH gastric fluid than lean patients,[8] while another found no differences in gastric volume or pH between lean and moderately obese surgical patients.[9] Obese patients without symptoms of GERD have relatively normal gastroesophageal sphincter tone. Obese patients at special risk for gastric acid aspiration may be those with diabetes and gastroparesis.

Nonalcoholic steatohepatitis (NASH, "fatty hepatitis"), with or without liver dysfunction, is extremely common. Histologic abnormalities are present in the livers of as many as 90% of morbidly obese patients.[10] Preoperative liver function tests should be obtained, but they often do not reflect the actual severity of liver dysfunction. Alanine aminotransferase is the most frequently elevated liver enzyme. Surprisingly, liver clearance of many anesthetic agents is usually not altered with NASH.

There is increased renal blood flow and an increased glomerular filtration rate (GFR) associated with obesity. Renal clearance of drugs may be greater compared to the normal-weight patient. The most common renal abnormality seen is proteinuria.

PERIOPERATIVE CONSIDERATIONS

Premedication

Sedatives should be avoided. For the very anxious patient small amounts of midazolam (1–2 mg, iv) can be given. If a fiberoptic airway intubation is planned, atropine or glycopyrrolate will decrease oral secretions. Most medications for chronic hypertension are continued before surgery. An exception is the angiotensin-converting enzyme inhibitors, which should be stopped preoperatively since they can cause profound hypotension following induction of anesthesia. Diabetic medications (insulin, oral hypoglycemics) are usually withheld on the morning of surgery, but blood sugar levels must be closely monitored in the perioperative period. Antibiotics prophylaxis for wound infection, and heparin as prophylaxis against deep venous thrombosis are usually administered prior to surgery at the surgeon's request.

For protection against acid aspiration, an H_2-receptor antagonist can be given the night before and again on the morning of surgery along with 30 mL of nonparticulate antacid to increase gastric fluid pH and decrease gastric fluid volume.[11]

Patient Position

It is our practice to have the unpremedicated patient climb off the gurney and position him or herself on the operating room table. All pressure points must be carefully padded to avoid pressure sores, neurologic injury, and rhabdomyolysis. Special operating tables are available for patients weighing as much as 500 kg, and occasionally two conventional operating room tables must be placed together to accommodate even larger patients.

Laparoscopic bariatric operations are performed with the patient in the supine or reverse Trendelenburg position (RTP). In the supine position, FRC is markedly reduced causing V/Q mismatch and significant increases in O_2 consumption, cardiac output, and PAP.[12] A left lateral tilt will prevent inferior vena cava compression in the supine patient. The Trendelenburg (TP) and lithotomy positions further decrease lung volumes. If possible, the patient should always be in the RTP during surgery since in this position the diaphragm is "unloaded" and FRC is maximized.

Monitoring

Standard monitors (ECG, blood pressure cuff, pulse oximetry, end-tidal capnography, and temperature probe) are applied. Noninvasive cuff pressure may be inaccurate when the wrong size cuff is used or if the anatomy of the upper arm does not allow a proper fit. Cuff pressures can be obtained from the wrist or ankle. An arterial line is usually not needed, but is helpful for continuous blood pressure monitoring and arterial blood gas sampling in high-risk patients.

It is important to monitor urine output intraoperatively with an indwelling catheter. There is normally a transient decrease in urine output during laparoscopy, with return of normal kidney function following the release of the pneumoperitoneum.[13] A nerve stimulator is used to assess neuromuscular blockade, but excess fat may make surface electrodes inaccurate so needle electrodes are recommended. A depth of anesthesia monitor such as the BIS monitor can also be useful.

Central Venous Pressure (CVP) or Pulmonary Artery (PA) lines are usually not needed for routine procedures. Since venous access is often limited, a central line can be helpful for postoperative needs. It is important to recognize that the length of a standard intravenous catheter placed percutaneously in the neck of a very large patient may not be long enough to reach an intrathoracic location.

To date, there have been no published studies of TEE monitoring during bariatric surgery, so its utility in this patient population is still to be determined. However, if a TEE monitor is used, the probe must be withdrawn from the esophagus during critical parts of the procedure.

Pharmacologic Considerations

The physiologic changes in obesity affect the distribution, binding, and elimination of the various agents administered during general anesthesia. In routine, anesthetic practice drugs are usually administered on the basis of dose per unit body weight. This assumes that clearances and distribution volumes are proportional to weight—assumptions that may not be valid in extreme obesity.

Obese patients have a smaller than normal fraction of total body water, increased blood volume and cardiac output, greater than normal adipose content, increased total LBW, changed tissue protein binding from increased concentrations of free fatty acids, triglycerides, lipoproteins, cholesterol, and other serum constituents (Table 10–2). In addition, renal blood flow and GFR are increased and cardiopulmonary function may not be optimal. Hepatic clearance is usually normal or even increased in obese patients despite the presence of NASH. Drug dosing by monitoring clinical endpoints

Table 10–2.
Pharmacologic Considerations for the Obese Patient
Greater Than Normal Amount Adipose Tissue
Increased lean body weight
Increased blood volume
Smaller than normal fraction total body water
Increased cardiac output
Decreased pulmonary function
Increased protein and free fatty acids
Increased renal blood flow
Increased glomerular filtration rate
Abnormal liver function

(heart rate, arterial pressure, degree of sedation) may be more important than empirical dosing based on patient weight formulae.[14]

Highly lipophilic drugs have a significant increase in volume of distribution compared to nonobese patients and their loading dose is usually increased. Since their elimination half-lives are longer, maintenance dosing should be decreased to reflect IBW.[15] Non- or weakly lipophilic drugs are given based on LBW.[16] Systemic absorption of oral medications is not significantly affected by obesity.

Inhalational Agents

Desflurane with its low lipid solubility has been recommended based on the belief that a slow release of more lipid-soluble anesthetics from excess adipose tissue could prolong emergence from anesthesia.[17] Lower blood flow to adipose tissue may limit the initial delivery of volatile agent to the fat and liver and inhalational anesthetics are stored in the fat long after completion of surgery, but the concentration in the well-perfused brain and lungs of all volatile anesthetics rapidly decrease once that anesthetic is discontinued.[18] Therefore, all inhalational anesthetics, including isoflurane, are rapidly eliminated. With appropriate timing, there are no clinical differences in the recovery time after general anesthesia with any inhalational anesthetic agent.[19]

Induction Agents

Larger than normal doses of highly lipophilic drugs like propofol or thiopental are needed due to increased blood volume, cardiac output, and adipose. For anesthetic maintenance, the intravenous dosing regimen for propofol in theory should be based on TBW as in normal-weight patients. However, the cardiovascular effects of very large doses limit the amount that can be given to obese patients. Although patients require more induction agent, they are also more sensitive to these agents and maintenance dosage is based on LBW.

Muscle Relaxants

Pseudocholinesterase levels and extracellular fluid space are both increased in obesity. Relatively high doses of succinylcholine (1.0 mg/kg TBW) are needed for a rapid sequence anesthetic induction.[20]

Complete paralysis is especially important during laparoscopy to facilitate ventilation and to provide adequate space for visualization and maneuvering of the surgical equipment. Loss of pneumoperitoneum may indicate incomplete paralysis. Since non-depolarizing muscle relaxants are hydrophilic, there is limited distribution to adipose tissue and no clinical advantage between any of the commonly used agents. Neuromuscular recovery time is similar in obese and nonobese patients with atracurium, vecuronium, or rocuronium.[21] Relaxants should be administered in incremental doses based on IBW, and neuromuscular blockade must be completely reversed before extubation of the trachea.

Opioids

Opioids are highly lipophilic, and in theory, loading doses should be based on TBW. There is no evidence that lipophilic opioids last longer in morbidly obese patients and generous use of opioids must be discouraged to avoid respiratory depression. Small doses of fentanyl combined with a continuous infusion of a short-acting opioid like remifentanil is preferred for laparoscopy. The volume of distribution of remifentanil in obese patients is less than expected, probably because of hydrolysis by blood and tissue esterases. Remifentanil dosing is based on IBW.

Intravenous Fluids

Intraoperative fluid requirements are usually greater than would be anticipated in a normal-weight patient. Several liters of crystalloid should be given during a laparoscopic bariatric operation. Obese patients receiving 40 mL/kg of intravenous crystalloid had a faster recovery and fewer complications after cholecystectomy than patients receiving 15 mL/kg.[22] These results can only be extrapolated to morbidly obese patients since no investigation of fluid requirements for laparoscopic bariatric surgery has been performed. It is essential that adequate amounts of intravenous fluid be given to reduce postoperative renal failure, and to avoid other rare but serious complications such as rhabdomyolysis.[23]

GENERAL ANESTHESIA

Preoxygenation

Despite conflicting evidence that morbidly obese patients are at greater risk for acid aspiration, it remains prudent to establish a secure airway as quickly and as safely as possible. Patients cannot tolerate the supine position and should be preoxygenated in the RTP until S_pO_2 is 100% for several minutes.[24] The hemoglobin of an apneic obese patient will desaturate very quickly since FRC is reduced and O_2 reserves are limited.[25] Preoxygenation in the RTP can increase O_2 reserves, but may cause pooling of blood and hypotension.[26]

Tracheal Intubation

All patients undergoing bariatric surgery must have their tracheas intubated to allow controlled ventilation and to protect their airway from acid aspiration. Potential airway management problems (fat face and cheeks; limited range of motion of the head, neck, and jaw; small mouth and large tongue; excessive palatal and pharyngeal tissue; short/large neck; high Mallampati (III or IV) score) should all be evaluated during the preoperative visit. High Mallampati score and large neck circumference are the most reliable predictors of potential intubation difficulties.[27–29] If a problem is anticipated preoperatively, an "awake intubation" with a fiberoptic bronchoscope is recommended. Appropriate nerve blocks and topical anesthesia to the airway are applied, and sedative drugs are

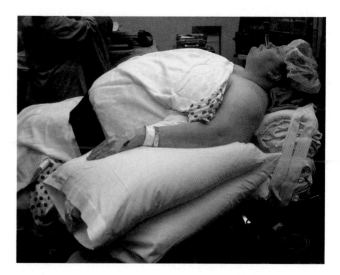

Figure 10–1. The proper position for a morbidly obese patient during preoxygenation, induction of general anesthesia, and tracheal intubation is shown. The head and upper body are ramped up in the "head elevated laryngoscopy position" in which an imaginary horizontal line connects the sternum with the ear. In this position the endoscopist's view of the vocal cords during direct laryngoscopy is significantly improved. The head of the bed is also in the reverse Trendelenburg position (RTP). The RTP maximizes lung volumes and delays hemoglobin desaturation during the intubation sequence.

kept to a minimum. It is important that the patient breathes supplemental O_2 during the intubation procedure.

Increasing weight or BMI are not risk factors for difficult laryngoscopy.[30] The most important strategy for insuring successful direct laryngoscopy is proper patient position. The patient must be placed with their head, upper body, and shoulders significantly elevated (stacked or ramped) so that their ear is level with the sternum (head elevated laryngoscopy position) (Figure 10–1). When a morbidly obese patient is in this position the endoscopist's view during direct laryngoscopy is significantly improved.[31]

For most patients a rapid intravenous induction with propofol and succinylcholine, combined with cricoid pressure, is the best means for securing the airway. A rapid sequence technique is important since bag and mask ventilation is often difficult due to upper airway obstruction, and reduced pulmonary compliance and gastric insufflation during ineffective mask ventilation will further increase the risk of regurgitation and acid aspiration. A second person experienced with airway management, preferably another anesthesiologist, must always be present to assist when difficulty is encountered.

Aids for difficult intubation, including a short laryngoscope handle, a variety of laryngoscope blades, special laryngoscopy equipment (Bullard laryngoscope, Wu laryngoscope) a gum elastic bougie, a light-wand, and equipment for crico-thyroidotomy and trans-tracheal jet ventilation, should also be available. A proseal laryngeal mask airway (LMA) or intubating LMA can serve as a *bridge* until an endotracheal tube is placed when difficulty is encountered.[32,33]

Mechanical Ventilation

Ventilation should be mechanically controlled during surgery. Morbidly obese patients breathing without assistance under general anesthesia are likely to hypoventilate. Patients should be ventilated with an F_iO_2 of 0.5–1.0 and a tidal volume 12–15 mL/kg IBW, preferably in the RTP. Larger tidal volumes will only marginally improve oxygenation while producing hypocapnia and potentially causing lung trauma.[34]

Peak ventilatory pressures and end-tidal CO_2 levels increase during laparoscopy.[35] If one wishes to limit these changes, minute ventilation can be adjusted by decreasing tidal volume and increasing respiratory rate. Pulmonary End Expiratory Pressure (PEEP) superimposed upon a large tidal volume can actually worsen hypoxemia by depressing cardiac output, which in turn will reduce O_2 delivery. Placement of subdiaphragmatic packs or retractors or changing to lithotomy or Trendelenburg positions will also impair ventilation.

The physiologic effects of the CO_2 pneumoperitoneum are usually well tolerated by the patient and require no intervention.[13] These effects include an elevation in peak inspiratory pressure combined with a decrease in tidal volume, a rise in end-tidal CO_2 and P_aCO_2, and a decrease in pH, and a rise in heart rate and mean arterial blood pressure. Maintaining the patient in the RTP minimizes the restriction of respiratory mechanics from the CO_2 insufflation.[36] All changes return to normal once the pneumoperitoneum is relieved.

As with any laparoscopic procedure, catastrophic complications such as massive gas embolism, pneumothorax, and pneumomediastinum can occur. The anesthesiologist must always be vigilant and recognize and treat these complications immediately.

The pneumoperitoneum can displace the diaphragm cephalad causing the position of the endotracheal tube to change. Occasionally, the endotracheal tube's tip can enter a bronchus, therefore tube displacement should always be considered in the differential diagnosis of hypoxemia during laparoscopy.[28,29]

Hemodynamic Changes

Pulmonary capillary wedge and PAP pressures may be elevated secondary to increased pulmonary blood volume and chronic hypoxemia. The surgical pneumoperitoneum can compress the inferior vena cava and femoral veins resulting in decreased blood return to the heart. During surgery there is usually an increase in heart rate, mean arterial pressure, and systemic vascular resistance, and a decrease in stroke volume, but the net result is cardiac output remaining unchanged or becoming only slightly decreased.[13]

ANESTHETIC TECHNIQUE

Our general anesthetic technique consists of an intravenous infusion of a short-acting opioid (remifentanil) supplemented with small amounts of fentanyl and/or dexmedetomidine. The patient is ventilated with an inhalational anesthetic (isoflurane, sevoflurane, or desflurane) with a F_iO_2 of 50%–100% O_2. Nitrous oxide can be used since it does not dilate the bowel during laparoscopic bariatric surgery, but its role is limited due to the high oxygen demand of many patients.[37]

Since the surgeon infiltrates the trocar sites with local anesthetics, deep levels of anesthesia are not required during wound closure. The inhalation agent is discontinued several minutes before surgery is completed but the remifentanil infusion is continued until the very end of the procedure. Once the remifentanil is stopped the patient is awake and their trachea can be extubated within 3 minutes.[38]

During laparoscopic bariatric procedures, the anesthesiologist is usually responsible for proper placement of the gastric tube to decompress the stomach and to help size the gastric pouch. They may be asked to help perform leak tests for anastomotic integrity, either by insufflation of the gastric tube or placement of saline or dye down the tube. It is extremely important that the gastric tube and anything else in the esophagus (such as a temperature probe or TEE probe) be completely withdrawn before the gastric pouch is stapled.

TEMPERATURE MAINTENANCE

Even though adipose tissue is a thermal isolator, patients become poikilothermic during general anesthesia. Heat loss may be exaggerated by the CO_2 pneumoperitoneum and when cold irrigating fluids are used. Warming blankets and other devices should be employed intraoperatively, and warmed intravenous and irrigating fluid are occasionally needed if there is a significant drop in temperature. Attempts to minimize heat loss with heated and humidified gas for the surgical pneumoperitoneum have been unsuccessful.[39]

POSTOPERATIVE CONSIDERATIONS

Position and Oxygenation

The semirecumbent and RTP positions maximize oxygenation by allowing the diaphragm to fall and FRC to increase. If hemodynamically stable, patients should have their airway extubated with their upper body elevated 30°–45°, and then be transferred from the operating room in that position.

Postoperative admission to an intensive care unit and/or mechanical ventilation is rarely needed. Factors that may necessitate ventilatory support include extremes of age, super obesity, coexisting cardiac disease or pulmonary disease and CO_2 retention, fever or infection, and an uncooperative or extremely anxious patient. The need for postoperative admission to an intensive care unit is relatively common after open bariatric procedures,[40] but rare after laparoscopic surgery.[41]

General anesthesia in morbidly obese patients results in a significant incidence of postoperative atelectasis.[42] Patients can become hypoxemic if supplemental O_2 is withheld in the immediate recovery period. Restoration of normal pulmonary function after open abdominal surgery may take several days.

OSA patients using nasal CPAP or bi-level positive airway pressure (BiPAP) at home should be instructed to bring their equipment to the hospital to use in the recovery room. These devices allow alveolar recruitment during inspiration and prevent alveolar collapse during expiration. In theory, CPAP could distend the gastric pouch, but its use following bariatric surgery has not been associated with anastomotic leaks.[43]

Antithrombosis

Thromboembolism is a major cause of postoperative mortality. Prolonged immobilization can lead to phlebothrombosis. The risk of thrombosis is further increased because of greater blood volume and relative polycythemia common in obese patients. Other risk factors include high fatty acid levels, hypercholesterolemia, and diabetes. In addition, morbidly obese patients demonstrate accelerated fibrin formation, fibrinogen-platelet interaction, and platelet function compared with controls. Anticoagulation or other prophylaxis measures should always be considered in the postoperative period, even for patients with epidural catheters.[44] A vena cava umbrella is occasionally placed preoperatively in older and high-risk patients, and sequential compression boots are often used during surgery. Early ambulation must be encouraged. Many patients can be ready for hospital discharge on the first or second postoperative day following laparoscopy.[41]

Postoperative Nausea and Vomiting

Obesity, per se, is not a risk factor for postoperative nausea and vomiting (PONV).[45] However, many patients undergoing bariatric procedures are at high risk (e.g., females, those receiving opioids, those undergoing emetogenic surgery) for PONV. Multimodal intraoperative prophylaxis with several antiemetic agents will reduce, but not eliminate, PONV. Dexamethasone (4–8 mg) should be a part of the therapeutic regimen.

Analgesia

Local anesthetic is infiltrated into the trocar sites during the procedure, so incisional pain in the immediate recovery period is much less than after a laparotomy.[46] Intravenous opioid patient-controlled analgesia (PCA) with drug dose based on IBW is usually satisfactory. Large amounts of opioids, especially longer acting opioids (morphine, demerol, hydromorphone), which can depress ventilation, should be avoided.

The use of non-opioid analgesic adjuncts should be instituted early. Dexmedetomidine, which has no respiratory depressant effects, is a useful alternative or supplement to opioids.[41] Nonsteroidal anti-inflammatory drugs are helpful initially, but should be discontinued within a day or two to avoid the potential complication of gastric ulceration.

References

1. Alpert MA, Hashimi MN: Obesity and the heart. *Am J Med Sci* 306:117–123, 1993.
2. Altermatt FR, Munoz HR, Delfino AE, Cortinez LI: Pre-oxygenation in the obese patient: Effects of position on tolerance to apnoea. *Br J Anaesth* 95:706–709, 2005.
3. Arain SR, Barth CD, Shankar H, Ebert TJ: Choice of volatile anesthetic for the morbidly obese patient: Sevoflurane or desflurane. *J Clin Anesth* 17:413–419, 2005.
4. Bardoczky GI, Yernault JC, Houben JJ, d'Hollander AA: Large tidal volume ventilation does not improve oxygenation in morbidly obese patients during anesthesia. *Anesth Analg* 81:385–388, 1995.
5. Bharati S and Lev M: Cardiac conduction system involvement in sudden death of obese young people. *Am Heart J* 129:273–281, 1995.
6. Brodsky JB: Positioning the morbidly obese patient for anesthesia. *Obes Surg* 12:751–758, 2002.
7. Brodsky JB, Lemmens HJ, Brock-Utne JG, Vierra M, Saidman LJ: Morbid obesity and tracheal intubation. *Anesth Analg* 94:732–736, 2003.
8. Brodsky JB, Lemmens HJM, Collins JS, Morton JM, Curet MJ, Brock-Utne JG: Nitrous oxide and laparoscopic bariatric surgery. *Obes Surg* 15:494–496, 2005.
9. Collins JS, Lemmens HJM, Brodsky JB, Brock-Utne JG, Levitan RM: Laryngoscopy and morbid obesity: A comparison of the "sniff" and "ramped" positions. *Obes Surg* 14:1171–1175, 2004.
10. Davila-Cervantes A, Dominguez-Cherit G, Borunda D, et al.: Impact of surgically-induced weight loss on respiratory function: A prospective analysis. *Obes Surg* 14:1389–1392, 2004.
11. de Menezes Ettinger JE, dos Santos Filho PV, Azaro E, Melo CA, Fahel E, Batista PB: Prevention of rhabdomyolysis in bariatric surgery. *Obes Surg* 15:874–879, 2005.
12. Dumont L, Mattys M, Mardirosoff C, Vervloesem N, Alle JL, Massaut J: Changes in pulmonary mechanics during laparoscopic gastroplasty in morbidly obese patients. *Acta Anaesthesiol Scand* 41:408–413, 1997.
13. Eichenberger A, Proietti S, Wicky S, et al.: Morbid obesity and postoperative pulmonary atelectasis: An underestimated problem. *Anesth Analg* 95:1788–1792, 2002.
14. Eriksson S, Backman L, Ljungstrom KG: The incidence of clinical postoperative thrombosis after gastric surgery for obesity during 16 years. *Obes Surg* 7:332–335, 1997.
15. Ezri T, Hazin V, Warters D, Szmuk P, Weinbroum AA: The endotracheal tube moves more often in obese patients undergoing laparoscopy compared with open abdominal surgery. *Anesth Analg* 96:278–282, 2003.
16. Ezri T, Medalion B, Weisenberg M, Szmuk P, Warters RD, Charuzi I: Increased body mass index per se is not a predictor of difficult laryngoscopy. *Can J Anesth* 50:179–183, 2003.
17. Farley DR, Greenlee SM, Larson DR, Harrington JR: Double-blind, prospective, randomized study of warmed humidified carbon dioxide insufflation vs standard carbon dioxide for patients undergoing laparoscopic cholecystectomy. *Arch Surg* 139:739–743, 2004.
18. Frappier J, Guenoun T, Journois D, et al.: Airway management using the intubating laryngeal mask airway for the morbidly obese patient. *Anesth Analg* 96:1510–1515, 2003.
19. Gaszynski TM, Strzelczyk JM, Gaszynski WP: Post-anesthesia recovery after infusion of propofol with remifentanil or alfentanil or fentanyl in morbidly obese patients. *Obes Surg* 14:1–7, 2004
20. Harter RL, Kelly WB, Kramer MG, Perez CE, Dzwonczyk RR: A comparison of the volume and pH of gastric contents of obese and lean surgical patients. *Anesth Analg* 86:147–152, 1998.
21. Helling TS, Willoughby TL, Maxfield DM, Ryan P: Determinants of the need for intensive care and prolonged mechanical ventilation in patients undergoing bariatric surgery. *Obes Surg* 14:1036–1041, 2004.
22. Holte K, Klarskov B, Christensen DS, et al.: Liberal versus restrictive fluid administration to improve recovery after laparoscopic

cholecystectomy. A randomize, double-blind study. *Ann Surg* 240:892–899, 2004.

23. Huerta S, DeShields S, Shpiner R, et al.: Safety and efficacy of postoperative continuous positive airway pressure to prevent pulmonary complications after Roux-en-Y gastric bypass. *J Gastrointest Surg* 6:354–358, 2002.

24. Jense HG, Dubin SA, Silverstein PI, O'Leary-Escolas U: Effect of obesity on safe duration of apnea in anesthetized humans. *Anesth Analg* 72:89–93, 1991.

25. Juvin P, Lavaut E, Dupont H, et al.: Difficult tracheal intubation is more common in obese than lean patients. *Anesth Analg* 97:595–600, 2003.

26. Juvin P, Vadam C, Malek L, Dupont H, Marmuse JP, Desmonts JM: Postoperative recovery after desflurane, propofol, or isoflurane anesthesia among morbidly obese patients: A prospective, randomized study. *Anesth Analg* 91:714–719, 2000.

27. Keller C, Brimacombe J, Kleinsasser A, Brimacombe L: The Laryngeal Mask Airway ProSeal$^{(TM)}$ as a temporary ventilatory device in grossly and morbidly obese patients before laryngoscope-guided tracheal intubation. *Anesth Analg* 94:737–740, 2002.

28. Kranke P, Apefel CC, Papenfuss T, et al.: An increased body mass index is no risk factor for postoperative nausea and vomiting. *Acta Anaesthesiol Scand* 45:160–166, 2001.

29. Lam AM, Grace DM, Manninen PH, Diamond C: The effects of cimetidine and ranitidine with and without metoclopramide on gastric volume and pH in morbidly obese patients. *Can Anaesth Soc J* 33:773–779, 1986.

30. Lemmens HJM, Brodsky JB: The dose of succinylcholine in morbid obesity. *Anesth Analg* 102(2): 438–42, 2006.

31. Lemmens HJM, Brodsky JB, Bernstein DP: Estimating ideal body weight—a new formula. *Obes Surg* 15:1082–1083, 2005.

32. Maltby JR, Pytka S, Watson NC, Cowan RA, Fick GH: Drinking 300 mL of clear fluid two hours before surgery has no effect on gastric fluid volume and pH in fasting and non-fasting obese patients. *Can J Anaesth* 51:111–115, 2004.

33. Marik P, Varon J: The obese patient in the ICU. *Chest* 113:492–498, 1998.

34. McCarty TM, Arnold DT, Lamont JP, Fisher TL, Kuhn JA: Optimizing outcomes in bariatric surgery. Outpatient laparoscopic gastric bypass. *Ann Surg* 242:494–501, 2005.

35. Moretto M, Kupski C, Mottin CC, et al.: Hepatic steatosis in patients undergoing bariatric surgery and its relationship to body mass index and comorbidities. *Obes Surg* 13:622–624, 2003.

36. Mortimore IL, Marshall I, Wraith PK: Neck and total body fat deposition in nonobese and obese patients with sleep apnea compared with that in control subjects. *Am J Resp Crit Care Med* 157:280–283, 1998.

37. Nguyen NT, Lee SL, Goldman C, et al.: Comparison of pulmonary function and postoperative pain after laparoscopic versus open gastric bypass: A randomized trial. *J Am Coll Surg* 192:469–477, 2001.

38. Nguyen NT, Wolfe BM: The physiologic effects of pneumoperitoneum in the morbidly obese. *Ann Surg* 241, 219–226, 2005.

39. Ogunnaike BO, Jones SB, Jones DB, Provost D, Whitten CW: Anesthetic considerations for bariatric surgery. *Anesth Analg* 95:1793–1805, 2004.

40. Pelosi P, Croci M, Ravagnan I, et al.: The effects of body mass on lung volumes, respiratory mechanics, and gas exchange during general anesthesia. *Anesth Analg* 87:654–660, 1998.

41. Perilli V, Sollazzi L, Bozza P, et al.: The effects of the reverse Trendelenburg position on respiratory mechanics and blood gases in morbidly obese patients during bariatric surgery. *Anesth Analg* 91:1520–1525, 2000.

42. Perilli V, Sollazzi L, Modesti C, et al.: Comparison of positive end-expiratory pressure with reverse Trendelenburg position in morbidly obese patients undergoing bariatric surgery: Effects on hemodynamics and pulmonary gas exchange. *Obes Surg* 13:605–609, 2003.

43. Servin F, Farinotti R, Haberer JP, Desmonts JM: Propofol infusion for the maintenance of anesthesia in morbidly obese patients receiving nitrous oxide. *Anesthesiology* 78:657–665, 1993.

44. Torri G, Casati A, Albertin A, et al.: Randomized comparison of isoflurane and sevoflurane for laparoscopic gastric banding in morbidly obese patients. *J Clin Anesth* 13:565–570, 2001.

45. Varin F, Ducharme J, Theoret Y, Besner JG, Bevan DR, Donati F: Influence of extreme obesity on the body disposition and neuromuscular blocking effect of atracurium. *Clin Pharmacol Ther* 48:18–25, 1990.

46. Vaughan RW, Bauer S, Wise L: Volume and ph of gastric juice in obese patients. *Anesthesiology* 43:686–689, 1975.

Physiology of Bariatric Operations

Restrictive Surgery

Edward E. Mason, MD, PhD, FACS

Gastroplasty was designed to restrict food intake without introducing bypass complications. It began in 1971 with horizontal gastroplasty and was changed to vertical in 1980, independently by many surgeons. The history helps explain what can cause success or failure. Small changes in design and technique too often lead to failure. Patients need to understand how to take care of their diminutive pouch in order to succeed. Overflow is a normal consequence of improper eating, but uncontrolled vomiting is abnormal and must be corrected before thiamine deficiency causes permanent injury or death (Wernicke–Korsakoff syndrome). Restriction operations are as effective as bypass operations in keeping patients alive for at least the first 8.3 years studied. Lifelong data may be needed to determine the best match of patients to operation type. Vertical pouches preserve the normal anatomy, which is important for preventing esophageal reflux. The ≤20 mL pouch size for gastroplasty is too small for an operation that bypasses

most of the small bowel. The pouch outlet for restriction operations is also too small for adding extensive small-bowel bypass in order to increase weight loss. Attempts to increase weight control by decreasing the pouch outlet below that recommended will lead to complications. Revision of vertical pouches that were too large initially and have enlarged to cause progressive increase in vomiting and weight gain should be revised to ≤20 mL, which will correct both complaints. Conversion to a bypass operation is not indicated for these complaints. Operative technique is important in determining whether the pouch is antireflux or causes reflux.

HISTORY

Dietary restriction of intake is the oldest and the least effective treatment for obesity. Surgery for obesity uses

(1) restriction, (2) malabsorption, and (3) manipulation of neurohumoral mechanisms for weight control. Gastric bypass for obesity was introduced in 1967 to restrict intake while avoiding the complications of intestinal bypass.[1] In 1971 horizontal gastroplasty was introduced as a means of eliminating the complications of gastric bypass, while maintaining the intake deficiency created by a small stomach pouch.[2] This was unsatisfactory because pouches were not measured and outlets were not stabilized. In addition, mobilization of the greater curvature brought the stomach into view for horizontal stapling, but when the fundus returned to its original position, the staple-line was slanted upward and emptying was like a cascade. This predisposed to obstruction, especially if the outlet was stabilized with a band that became adherent to adjacent tissues. Obstruction required endoscopy, which was difficult with the outlet high on the greater curvature. We needed a straight shot, which meant an outlet on the lesser curvature.

Beginning in 1980–81 pouches were changed from horizontal to vertical and moved to the lesser curvature to facilitate endoscopy. Michael Long described moving the pouch outlet to the lesser curvature and then, in successive patients, changing the slope of the staple-line from horizontal until it was vertical.[3] At the University of Iowa, a stapled circular window was made near the lesser curvature in order to facilitate vertical stapling and to allow placement of a Marlex mesh collar around the outlet without sewing or stapling it to the stomach wall. The volume of these vertical banded gastroplasty (VBG) pouches was measured and detailed descriptions of the operative technique were published and provided at surgical meetings.[4] Since restriction of intake was the only apparent mechanism for causing weight loss and maintaining a lower weight, a small measured pouch and a controlled outlet were crucial to success.

Failure occurred when pouches were too large. Surgeons, who attempted to increase weight loss by decreasing outlet size, soon abandoned the operation, blaming failure on the name of the operation instead of deviations from recommended technique.[5] As a result of the obesity epidemic that began in 1980, patients presenting were heavier each year. Surgeons and patients wanted more weight loss than a restriction operation could produce, which led to increased use of bypass operations. Training programs in laparoscopic surgery focused upon RYGB and adjustable gastric banding, which further decreased the use of any form of vertical gastroplasty. In 2005, in the United States, most of the operations were LRYGB. Concern remains about the late-in-life complications of bypass of the upper digestive tract, which was the reason for developing VBG in 1980.

REQUIREMENTS FOR SUCCESS OF RESTRICTION SURGERY

Both obesity and the surgical operations are life long and the operations are adjunctive. This means that success should be defined in terms of the effects of both the obesity and the operation over each patient's remaining life. Our medical care system is poorly designed for the lifelong monitoring, treatment, and documentation needed to determine success. To study the effect of an operation requires that the technique and patient care be standardized before lifelong study can begin. Our society worships what is new(s). What follows will be some observations about the changing practice of operations based upon the thesis that restriction of intake is the simplest and safest way to surgically control excessive body weight. The best restriction operation for the future has not been studied but can be hypothesized based upon a century of accumulated experience of many surgeons.

Patient Education

Success not only depends upon providing an optimum pouch, but also on a compliant patient who will chew well, eat small portions, and stop before vomiting (overflow/regurgitation). Control of intake is especially important with an operation, which is totally dependent upon restriction. These patients have not been able to reduce their meal size or change their eating habits before being provided a meal-sizing pouch of less than 20 mL compared with their total stomach capacity averaging 1700 mL. In addition, the outlet is stabilized to preserve a diameter of 11 mm so that the pouch will retain enough food to provide some sense of fullness. Both surgeons and patients must learn the anatomic requirements and limitations of the restriction pouch in order to make it work. Patients should be able to recognize a drawing of their operation and should know the measurements of pouch and outlet. They should practice eating out of a medicine glass before and early after the operation. If there is vomiting after the operation, more time should be spent in patient training as well as in review of the operative technique. Overflow is normal when patients overload the pouch but they should be able to prevent this by changes in eating habits. If a patient has uncontrollable vomiting, the reason must be found and corrected before depletion of thiamine results in nystagmus, loss of deep tendon reflexes, confusion, and rapid progression to coma and death, the Wernicke–Korsakoff syndrome.[6]

LONGEVITY AND FOLLOW-UP

We used the National Death Index (NDI) to provide what we believe to be a nearly complete follow-up for the length of life.[7] At an average postoperative time of 8.3 years for the first 654 deaths in a comparison of 7,185 patients after simple restriction operations with 11,787 patients after bypass operations, neither operative type has shown any advantage in keeping patients alive. Age, operative body mass index (BMI), gender, diabetes, hypertension, and smoking were predictive of longevity. It is important to extend the follow-up for mortality in these patients for sufficient years to detect any difference in the effect of operation type as early as it appears and to study the causes of death in the two groups of patients. This should provide help in advising patients regarding their choice of simple versus complex operations. It should also guide surgeons in recommending the type of operation for patients with type 2 diabetes. Unless simple restrictive operations are available, the information obtained from this study may be purely academic. The choice will then remain between bypass and gastric banding, or the surgeon's favorite operation and no operation.

DESIGN AND OPERATIVE TECHNIQUE

Pouch Configuration

Vertical banded gastroplasty was designed with the antireflux Collis gastroplasty in mind.[8] There are muscle fibers called the sling of Helvitius that encircle the junction of esophagus and stomach, cross at the angle of His, and descend along the lesser curvature of the stomach. This anatomy is important in preventing reflux and is preserved in the design of VBG. VBG, when properly performed, exaggerates the angle of His. Deitel et al. demonstrated that VBG is an antireflux operation.[10] Horizontal gastroplasty by contrast cuts across this complex musculature. One of the original requirements of any operation for obesity was reversibility. The stomach has long been known as a long tube (Magenstrasse) with a distensible attachment (sleeve). Vertical pouches make use of the upper end of the Magenstrasse, which preserves normal anatomy.

Placing a band around the upper stomach to create a small meal-limiting pouch has the advantages of no cutting or stapling but the resulting pouch is more like the one in horizontal gastroplasty rather than the vertical, lesser curvature pouch that replaced it. There tends also to be slippage between the band and the stomach wall, with enlargement of the pouch and tilting of the band, leading to obstruction of the pouch. Positioning of the band outside of the peritoneum posterior, and imbrication of the stomach anterior, has reduced the slippage. The importance of adjustment of the band has not been established. Comparisons made in the Swedish Obesity Subjects Study indicate that the weight loss and weight control are less after the adjustable band gastroplasty than after VBG, and much less than after RYGB.[11] A comparison by Suter et al. between results obtained with the Swedish Band and Lap Band showed no difference, with 50%–60% of patients obtaining satisfactory weight loss, but at least 10% developing severe long-term complications.[12]

The design and operative technique of gastroplasty should eliminate capacity for a large meal without creating acid reflux. The resulting pouch must have a stable configuration, volume, and outlet diameter. Foreign material used to stabilize the outlet should be kept at a minimum and protected from contamination since infection leads to migration into the lumen. The ideal gastroplasty pouch is too small for the short common channel of biliopancreatic diversion.

Decreasing the pouch outlet cannot increase weight loss and improve weight maintenance without increasing the risk of obstruction, staple-line disruption, migration of the foreign material into the lumen, and an unacceptable rate of re-operation. Failure to adhere to recommended technique has led to unsatisfactory results and abandonment of gastroplasty. When more is known about the lifelong effects of available operations, the need for a restriction operation may become evident for at least those patients whose obesity is less severe. Whether adjustable banding can substitute for vertical gastroplasty is yet to be proven. Operations are like dwellings—their protection and benefit depends upon the way they are constructed and the way they are used. The lifelong effects increase in importance over time for those operations that pass the earlier tests and remain in place. Experience from 100 years of digestive tract surgery serves as a guide for predicting the future of bypass operations but is of less help with restriction operations, which came with the newly recognized disease of severe obesity.

Pouch Volume

An advantage of the open technique is the ease of measuring the pouch volume under 70 cm of water pressure and then changing the placement of the stapler if the pouch is not the desired volume. The recording (documentation) of pouch measurements led to the use of smaller and smaller pouches over many years of experience with returning patients whose pouches had dilated to unacceptable size. Prevention of pouch dilatation depends upon decreasing the tension on the pouch wall from excessive pouch volume as dictated by the law of LaPlace ($T = Pr$) where T is the tension stretching the pouch wall, P is the difference in pressure across the wall, and r the radius of a cylindrical pouch. The pressure is dependent upon patient compliance in eating small amounts and chewing well so that the pouch is not over distended. The importance of LaPlace's law is that the larger the pouch the more it will distend. It is also evident that if the pouch is long it must be uniform in radius. If the upper end of the pouch is larger due to the staple-line reaching out on the fundus rather than at the angle of His, this area will distend and assume the shape of a sphere. The consequence may be sufficient tension at the cardia to cause reflux. Thus the operative technique determines whether the operation is antireflux or causes reflux. The pouch must be 20 mL or less in measured volume in order that over time the law of LaPlace will not result in excessive enlargement. A pouch that is too large at the outset may enlarge to a degree that the walls will overhang the outlet. If this is concentric enlargement, the pouch outlet sits in the middle with the shape of a volcano (Jamieson's description).[13] More often an enlarged pouch is asymmetric and the overhang is on one side. This may tilt the ring or collar and cause obstruction. This complication is analogous to the development of a Zenker's diverticulum, with the overhanging pouch assuming alignment with the vertical pouch and esophagus. The outlet into the main stomach may be displaced to the side and compressed by the tilted collar, silastic ring, or stabilizing sutures.

Outlet Length

Michael Long introduced a vertical gastroplasty that is similar to the silastic ring gastroplasty and VBG except for the outlet. Jamieson worked with Michael Long when this operation was introduced in 1980 and continued the study of the operation. He used three number-1 Ethibond sutures through the vertical staple-line starting at 4 cm below the angle of His and extending to 5.2 cm. These were tied around the lesser curvature over an indwelling 38–40 French bougie to provide a 12-mm outlet length. This compares with the 15-mm width of Marlex mesh used in VBG and 3 mm for silastic ring gastroplasty. In 1984, Jamieson used a 6-mm outlet length with two sutures (as used by Long) in 206 patients and compared the results with his preferred 12 mm with three sutures, used during 1983 and 1985. Percent excess weight loss at 5 years was 61% and 69% with the 12-mm and 52% with the 6-mm length of outlet. The revision rates were 3.5% and 3.7% for the 12 mm and 8.7% for the 6 mm length of outlet. These are the only data available comparing the effect of length of the outlet upon weight loss and revision rate for vertical gastroplasty. The distribution of operative weights for Jamieson's 512 patients was low with the most frequent BMI (kg/m^2) 35 and the range 25 to >60. These were open operations. The Michael Long gastroplasty would need to be adapted to the laparoscopic approach if it were to be competitive in today's market. Stapling in continuity from the angle of His, parallel to the lesser curvature, may be more difficult than stapling from a window to the angle as is performed laparoscopically in VBG.[14]

Outlet Size

When VBG was introduced, the Marlex mesh circumference used to stabilize the outlet was 5.0 cm. A few patients returned early following operation because of vomiting. Our response was to increase the circumference of the encircling mesh to 5.5 cm and to teach patients to drink and eat from a medicine glass during the early postoperative period. Patients were told to not swallow anything that was not converted to liquid by chewing. Fibrous foods that did not liquefy were to be spit out and then avoided. It was soon possible to resume the use of the 5.0-cm band with infrequent need for admission because of vomiting. Patients who were 225% of normal weight were provided 4.5-cm-circumference bands until it became evident that this was increasing the need for repair of disrupted staple-lines. Following this early experience, 5-cm bands were used in all patients regardless of weight.

In 1980, at the University of Iowa, we introduced the stapled window near the lesser curvature to facilitate vertical stapling to the angle of His and also allow placement of the Marlex mesh band around the pouch outlet and have

it remain in place without suturing the mesh to the stomach wall. The outlet required stabilization with an 11–12 mm diameter lumen, which was provided with an external 5.0-cm-circumference band. The goal was stabilization without obstruction. With small measured pouches it should not be necessary to divide the pouch from the rest of the stomach. Division does in theory increase the risk of contamination and infection, when there is foreign material, which increases the risk of migration into the lumen. The rapid infiltration of a mesh with a connective tissue should protect from contamination. Marlex mesh is relatively nonreactive but it is possible that low-grade irritation could combine with carcinogens in food and from the environment to cause cancer.

Four cancers have been reported, two after Marlex mesh,[15,16] one after a silastic ring,[17] and one after Gore-Tex.[18] Two additional patients with cancer after VBG have been operated upon at the University of Iowa, both following Marlex mesh. No cancers were found in the 7,185 patients with restriction operations in the IBSR search for deaths, which is another reason for continuing the NDI searches in this group of patients. There could be an effect of restriction in causing chronic irritation to the stomach lining. The thickness of stomach wall in the area of the outlet should be sufficient to fill the circle of Marlex mesh or other material used to stabilize the outlet. When the pouch was made long, stomach was pulled tightly through the stapler around the indwelling bougie in order to provide a small pouch. With the later use of shorter pouches, such tension was less necessary and the amount of stomach wall was increased, including that area where the outlet was created.

There are two major ways of calibrating the outlet of a restrictive pouch, which can be conveniently labeled external and internal. External calibration is with measurement of the Marlex mesh or silastic tube before it is applied. The internal diameter of the outlet should be functionally 11 mm if the sewn-in-place, circumferential, stabilizing material is 5 cm in length. This works fine with the mesh, measured without tension and marked before placement. The silastic ring may be secured with too much tension on the tie that is threaded through the lumen so that the outlet is too narrow. This is easy to correct if detected. The silastic ring can be replaced with less tension during the tie. A 32 French bougie must pass easily to avoid the need for a second operation. This is a test of lumen adequacy and not the calibration bougie. Jamieson uses three number-1 Ethibond sutures, stitched through the vertical staple-line over a length of pouch located 4–5.2 cm below the angle of His and tied around an indwelling 38–40 French bougie. The large bougie is used for calibration so that when the bougie is removed, and the stomach wall expands from the compression of the ties, the lumen will easily accept a 32 French bougie.

Reoperations

Some patients do not lose enough weight with a restriction operation. If the pouch is not large, conversion to RYGB may be justified. If however the history is one of satisfactory weight control for many years and a more recent failure of weight control, then restoration of a pouch ≤20 mL would seem the better operation. In a patient with a large pouch and a satisfactory result followed by a history of progressive vomiting, reflux, heartburn, and weight gain, the combination of weight gain and vomiting occurs because of the patient's inability to recognize when the large obstructed pouch is full. Reduction of a large pouch to 20 mL volume will relieve the vomiting and restore weight control in such a patient.

If a patient develops diabetes or has resumed treatment for diabetes with weight gain following a restriction operation then conversion to RYGB may be a better choice than revision of the restriction operation. Bypass of the pyloric muscle results in hypertonic gastric contents emptying directly into the small bowel, which stimulates peristalsis and this in turn causes food to reach the distal ileum where it stimulates the secretion of GLP-1, which is deficient in T2DM in the severely obese. GLP-1 increases insulin secretion and insulin receptor function.[19] It should be possible to treat recurrent type 2 diabetes with GLP-1 mimetics although there is as yet no experience with these new medications in patients who have had restriction operations. An advantage of the medication over bypass would be the ease of stopping the stimulation of islet tissue by stopping the medication. Bypass operations have caused nesidioblastosis, requiring pancreatic resection to control hypoglycemia from excessive insulin secretion.[20] This adds to the list of reasons for avoiding bypass operations if restriction will suffice.

When there is a need to reduce the size of the pouch of a VBG or other vertical gastroplasty, either a silastic ring gastroplasty or the Michael Long gastroplasty should be considered. At one time we were performing a complete new VBG within the old VBG and called this a Faberge. There may not be room for a second window without obstructing the emptying of the space between the old and new staple-lines. The use of a new vertical staple-line from the angle of His, parallel to the lesser curvature, and then stabilization with the three Ethibond sutures used by Jamieson does not require as much room for the new outlet and decreases the risk of contamination of Marlex mesh in an area that has more dissection and the associated serum and capillary bleeding, which can create an excellent culture medium. As with primary operations, it is important to make sure that the outlet is adequate before closing the operation by passing a 32 French bougie through the new outlet (and the old outlet if it is still present). The bougie should pass easily and if it does not, immediate replacement with less constricting ties will avoid prolonged inability to eat solid foods and another operation.

One of the concerns about converting a restriction operation to a bypass operation relates to pouch size. The more severe is the malabsorption the more is the need for eating larger meals, meats, and other foods. If the old pouch has remained small, it may not allow the overeating and eating of meat and other proteins that are needed to prevent protein malnutrition.

CONCLUSIONS

Restriction operations remain attractive for patients and surgeons who are concerned about the lifelong complications of bypass operations. The laparoscopic approach does not change the risks of bypass of the upper digestive tract, which led to the abandonment of Billroth II gastrectomy in midtwentieth century and the effort to replace gastric bypass with gastroplasty beginning in 1971.[21] This chapter provides some principles that should be considered in the evaluation and use of restriction operations.

References

1. Mason EE, Ito C: Gastric bypass. *Surg Clin N Am* 47:1345–1351, 1967.
2. Printon KJ, Mason EE: Gastric surgery for relief of morbid obesity. *Arch Surg* 106:428–431, 1973.
3. Long M, Collins JP: The technique and early results of high gastric reduction for obesity. *Aust N Z J Surg* 50:146–149, 1980.
4. Mason EE, Doherty C: Vertical banded gastroplasty for morbid obesity. *Dig Surg* 14:355–360, 1997.
5. Mason EE: Development and future of gastroplasties for morbid obesity. *Arch Surg* 138:361–366, 2003.
6. Mason EE: Starvation injury after gastric reduction for obesity. *World J Surg* 22:1002–1007, 1998.
7. Zhang W, Mason EE, Renquist KE, Zimmerman MB, IBSR Contributors: Factors influencing survival following surgical treatment of obesity. *Obes Surg* 15:43–50, 2005.
8. Mason EE: Vertical banded gastroplasty for obesity. *Arch Surg* 117:701–706, 1982.
9. Jackson AJ: The spiral constrictor of the gastroesophageal junction. *Am J Anat* 151:265–275, 1978.
10. Deitel M, Khanna RK, Hagen J, Ilves R: Vertical banded gastroplasty as an anti-reflux procedure. *Am J Surg* 155:512–516, 1988.
11. Sjöström L: Surgical intervention as a strategy for treatment of obesity. *Endocrine* 13:213–230, 2000.
12. Suter M, Giusti V, Worreth M, Heraief E, Calmes J-M: Laparoscopic gastric banding: A prospective, randomized, study comparing the Lapband and the SAGB: Early results. *Ann Surg* 241:55–62, 2005.
13. Jamieson AC: Determinants of weight loss after gastroplasty. *Prob Gen Surg* 9:290–297, 1992.
14. Lee W-J, Lai J-R, Huang M-T, Wu CC, Wei PL: Laparoscopic versus open vertical banded gastroplasty for the treatment of morbid obesity. *Surg Laparosc Endosc Percutan Tech* 11:9–13, 2001.
15. Sweet WA: Linitis plastica presenting as pouch outlet stenosis 13 years after vertical banded gastroplasty. *Obes Surg* 6:66–70, 1996.
16. Papakonstantinou A, Moustafellos P, Terzis I, Stratopoulos C, Hadjiyannakis E: Gastric cancer occurring after vertical banded gastroplasty. *Obes Surg* 12:118–120, 2002.
17. Zirak C, Lemaitre J, Lebrun E, Journe S, Carlier P: Adenocarcinoma of the pouch after silastic ring vertical gastroplasty. *Obes Surg* 12:693–694, 2002.
18. Jain PK, Ray B, Royston CM: Carcinoma in the gastric pouch after vertical banded gastroplasty. *Obes Surg* 13:136–137, 2003.
19. Mason EE: Ileal transposition and enteroglucagon/GLP-1 in obesity and (diabetic?) surgery. *Obes Surg* 9:223–228, 1999.
20. Service GJ, Thompson GB, Service FJ, Andrews JC, Collazo-Clavell ML, Lloyd RV: Hyperinsulinemic hypoglycemia with nesidioblastosis after gastric-bypass surgery. *N Engl J Med* 353:249–254, 2005.
21. Mason EE: History of obesity surgery. *Surg Obes Relat Dis* 1:123–125, 2005.

12

Physiology and Metabolism in Obesity Surgery: Roux-en-Y Gastric Bypass

Carolina G. Goncalves • Francesco Rubino • Stacy A. Brethauer • Philip R. Schauer, MD

INTRODUCTION

Surgical intervention has proven to be the most effective method for achieving persistent weight loss and reversing obesity-related metabolic abnormalities. The outcome of surgical treatment for morbid obesity varies according to their weight loss mechanisms.

Although Roux-en-Y gastric bypass (RYGB) is generally considered a mixed, restrictive–malabsorptive procedure, the mechanisms underlying the effects of this operation are incompletely understood. Growing evidence now suggests that diverse physiological changes also contribute to the impact of RYGB on body weight and amelioration of obesity-related comorbidities.[1,2]

Elucidating the actual mechanism of action of RYGB has become a priority because such knowledge may help devise new surgical procedures as well as identify targets for novel antiobesity and antidiabetic medications. This chapter reviews available data and the hypothesized mechanisms mediating the effects of RYGB.

ANATOMICAL CHANGES AFTER RYGB

There are several variations in the technique for the RYGB operation (antegastric, antecolic Roux-limb vs retrogastric, retrocolic; one layer vs two layers anastomosis; stapled vs hand-sewn-please see section IV); however, the commonly performed steps involve the creation of a 15–30 mL divided gastric pouch, a jejunojejunostomy with a 75–150 cm Roux limb, and an end-to-side gastrojejunostomy. The RYGB reduces gastric capacity by 90%–95%. The biliopancreatic limb includes the excluded stomach, duodenum, and proximal jejunum and drains bile, digestive enzymes, and gastric secretions. The mid-jejunum is anastomosed to the gastric pouch (Roux or alimentary limb) and carries ingested food. Food and digestive enzymes mix at the level of the jejunojejunostomy, and absorption takes place in this common channel that may vary in length depending on the patient's BMI.[3,4] Our current technique includes four main steps: (1) division of the jejunum 30–50 cm from the ligament of Treitz and measurement of a 75- or 150-cm (for patient with BMI > 50) Roux limb, (2) side-to-side stapled jejunojejunostomy between the Roux and biliopancreatic limb with closure of the mesenteric defect, (3) creation of a 15-mL divided gastric pouch, and (4) creation of a linear stapled end-to-side gastrojejunostomy with hand-sewn closure of the common opening over an endoscope.

The 75–100 cm Roux limb constitutes a short bypass; therefore the technique most commonly used for RYBG is not primarily a malabsorptive procedure. In an attempt to provide a more powerful malabsorptive element to the operation, the long limb or "distal gastric bypass" has been developed. The "distal" RYGB usually consists of an extended Roux limb (150–200 cm) and a 75–150-cm common channel.[5,6] Studies have shown that increasing the Roux limb in RYGB effectively increases the excess weight loss in super obese patients (BMI > 50 kg/m^2).[5,7–9] This increase in weight loss is attributed to the lengthened bypass of the foregut and induction of a state of increase malabsorption. However, a randomized prospective trial demonstrated that lengthening of the Roux limb did not increase weight loss for patients with a BMI lower than 50 kg/m^2.[10]

PHYSIOLOGICAL CHANGES AFTER RYGB

RYGB includes creation of a small gastric pouch and rearrangement of the gastrointestinal (GI) tract. This implies that there are several potential mechanisms that could influence energy homeostasis as a result of this operation:

- Gastric restriction, which could limit oral intake.
- Bypass of the duodenum and proximal small bowel (jejunum), which by diverting the bile and pancreatic enzymes may decrease the amount of bowel available for absorption as well as induce changes in proximal gut hormone secretion.
- Rapid delivery of food to ileum and colon, which could enhance the release of gut hormones produced by the intestinal L cells of the hindgut.[2]
- Gut hormonal changes. This anatomical rearrangement of the small bowel has the potential to change the hormonal milieu of the foregut and hindgut and ultimately contribute to the physiological changes and the sustained weight loss observed after the RYGB operation.

Restriction/Dumping

Gastric restriction is widely considered the primary mediator of weight loss after RYGB. In fact, the small residual gastric volume and the narrow outlet of the pouch both could reasonably reduce food intake. However, some evidences suggest that physiology of weight loss after RYGB is not so straightforward.

Indeed, unlike for purely restrictive procedures such as LAGB and VBG, the effect of RYGB on food intake behavior is not limited to early satiety during a meal and smaller meal sizes. Typically, in patients who have undergone RYGB, the feeling of satiety extends well beyond the immediate postprandial period, despite a lack of change in the perception of sweets or in the overall enjoyment of food.[11,12]

Furthermore, if gastric restriction was the only mechanism by which RYGB influences food intake, the energy homeostasis system would drive patients to compensate with increased meal frequency and calorie-dense foods in response to massive weight loss. Instead, patients who have undergone RYGB typically eat fewer meals and snacks per day and restrict consumption of calorie-dense foods.[13,14] In contrast, after purely restrictive procedures, patients can fail to lose weight if they consume highly caloric liquids that can pass easily through a small pouch and outlet.

The presence of the dumping symptoms after ingesting high-calorie drinks and sweets may cause some RYGB patients to develop an aversion to these foods. The dumping syndrome, a well-known complication of gastric resection for ulcer disease and of gastric bypass, may also be regarded as a potential beneficial side effect of the procedure. Early dumping symptoms occur within minutes of eating refined sugars and can include rapid heart beat, nausea, tremor, and faint feeling, sometimes followed by diarrhea. The small gastric reservoir and the increased gastric emptying after RYGB lead to rapid filling of the small bowel with hyperosmolar chyme, causing an osmotic overload and a shift of extracellular fluid into the bowel to restore isotonicity. This increase of fluid in the small bowel causes intestinal distension, cramping, vomiting, and diarrhea. Bowel distention stimulates the release of gut hormones including vasoactive intestinal peptide,[15] neurotensin,[16] serotonin,[17] and GLP-1,[18] and these hormones are related to diaphoresis, dizziness, and palpitations.

The late dumping syndrome occurs 1–4 hours after eating and is characterized by reactive hypoglycemia and sweating, dizziness, and fatigue. GLP-1 is suggested to be one of the modulators of the hypoglycemic response[19,20] because this hormone promotes nutrient assimilation via the stimulation of glucose-dependent insulin release and the inhibition of glucagons secretion.[21]

The association of dumping subsequent to sweet ingestion has been used to select bariatric surgical procedures based on patients' reported preoperative sweet intake.[22,23] Dumping symptoms, however, correlate poorly with the efficacy of RYGB as they occur only in some patients and after high-carbohydrate meals, and their intensity usually declines with time.[24] No difference in weight loss was found between RYGB classified as nondumpers versus dumpers, or between RYGB patients classified as sweet eaters versus nonsweet eaters.[25,26]

Malabsorption

The different techniques of RYGB operation can encompass different degrees of malabsorption. As described above, the usual length of the Roux limb is 75–100 cm, which promotes a small, and probably transient, degree of malabsorption. In the "distal" RYGB, however, the usual limb length varies from 150–200 cm. This operation maintains the same length of foregut bypass but is likely to result in greater nutrients malabsorption.

The majority of the ingested protein is absorbed in the duodenum. After RYGB, protein intake is limited due to restriction, and absorption occurs in the distal jejunum and ileum. Although protein malnutrition is very common after truly malabsorptive surgical procedures, it is rare after RYGB. It can occur, though, especially after long-limb or distal RYGB, and continuous monitoring of the patient's caloric and protein intake is mandatory (please see Chapter 39).[27]

Malabsorption of fat is also associated with RYGB procedure.[28,29] The causes include the exclusion of the duodenum from the regular intestinal transit that eliminates the physiological release of cholecystokinin (CCK), bile, and lipolytic enzymes.[30] Therefore, the delayed breakdown of dietary fats and delayed formation of micelles will limit the fat available for absorption. These changes are more pronounced in the "distal" RYGB. Undigested fat will eventually produce malabsorption and steatorrhea.

Gastric bypass may additionally alter carbohydrate digestion and absorption through several mechanisms. Reduced contact with mucosa and pancreatic enzymes and shortened transit time are the major contributors to carbohydrate malabsorption.[31] After RYGB, ingested carbohydrates pass through the Roux limb as intact polysaccharides and their digestion will not start until they pass the jejunojejunostomy. In jejunojejunostomy, they will interact with a small amount of basal amylase secreted from the pancreas through the biliopancreatic limb and will be hydrolyzed and absorbed in the remaining small instestine.[32] Carbohydrates are the sole energy source for the brain and red blood cells. If sufficient carbohydrate substrate is lacking, fat and protein are broken down through gluconeogenesis into carbohydrates to supply the nutritional substrate for the brain and red blood cells. Therefore, the deficiency of carbohydrates can secondarily lead to a deficiency in protein and reduction of fat stores.[32]

Vitamins and mineral deficiencies are a major concern after RYGB operations. The main micronutrients affected by bariatric surgery are vitamin B_{12} and folate, iron, and calcium.[33] After gastric bypass, vitamin B_{12} deficiency is due to malabsorption of dietary vitamin B_{12}. The absence of hydrochloric acid and pepsin restricts the cleavage of food-bound vitamin B_{12} from its protein carrier. Furthermore, the excluded stomach and bypassed duodenum prohibit binding of free B_{12} to intrinsic factor, preventing the absorption of crystalline vitamin B_{12} in the distal ileum. In spite of the substantial body storage of vitamin B_{12}, the estimated prevalence of vitamin B_{12} deficiency after RYGB range from 12% to 33%.[34]

Folate deficiency after RYGB range from 0% to 38%[26,34] and usually occurs secondary to decreased dietary intake. Although folate absorption occurs preferentially in the upper third of the small bowel, there is evidence that absorption can take place in the middle and distal small bowel with adaptation after surgery. Folate deficiency is preventable and corrected with multivitamin supplementation (1 mg/day).

The incidence of iron deficiency after RYGB ranges from 33% to 50% with a greater incidence in menstruating woman.[35–37] Iron deficiency is common secondary to decreased intake of heme iron and the decreased production of hydrochloric acid in the pouch. This relative achlorhydria does not permit the conversion of ferrous iron to the more absorbable ferric iron. Furthermore, the absorption of iron normally occurs in the duodenum, which is bypassed after the RYGB operation.

Calcium and thiamine (vitamin B_1) are also primarily absorbed in the duodenum. After RYGB these nutrients never enter the duodenum; therefore their absorption is significantly decreased. Calcium deficiency is common after RYGB, and many patients experience progressive bone loss over time to maintain normal serum calcium.[38,39] Consequently, metabolic bone disease represents a long-term potential risk associated with this operation. Thiamine deficiency occurs through the combination of a reduction in acid production by the gastric pouch, decreased food intake, and can be worsened by frequent episodes of vomiting. Due to the involvement of thiamine in carbohydrate metabolism, administration of glucose in the presence of thiamine deficiency can precipitate Wernicke's encephalopathy.[40–42] Therefore, patients presenting with mental status changes after bariatric surgery should receive parenteral thiamine prior to receiving glucose-containing intravenous fluids.

All fat-soluble vitamins (A, D, E, and K) are poorly absorbed after RYGB. Deficiency is more prevalent after "distal" or "long limb" RYGB because of the greater degree of fat malabsorption. Although there are no reports regarding complications due to fat-soluble vitamin deficiency after RYGB, delayed mixing of fat with pancreatic enzymes and bile salts is a potential problem when there is a short common channel.[4]

NEUROHORMONAL CHANGES

Changes in the network of signals involved in energy balance could also contribute to the effects of RYGB on body weight and glucose metabolism (see Chapter 5). As mentioned before, whereas the RYGB leads to significant weight loss with associated changes in fuel homeostasis, this does not result in a compensatory increase in appetite that typically follows most forms of nonsurgical weight loss.[43]

Peptides released from the GI tract have been shown to play an important role in appetite and food intake regulation through their actions on the hypothalamic arcuate nucleus (ARC).[44] The restructuring of the GI tract typical of the RYGB could alter the normal (or abnormal) gut–brain axis in obese patients.

In fact, after the RYGB operation, ingested nutrients bypass the remnant stomach, the duodenum, and the proximal jejunum, thus potentially changing the usual neuronal and

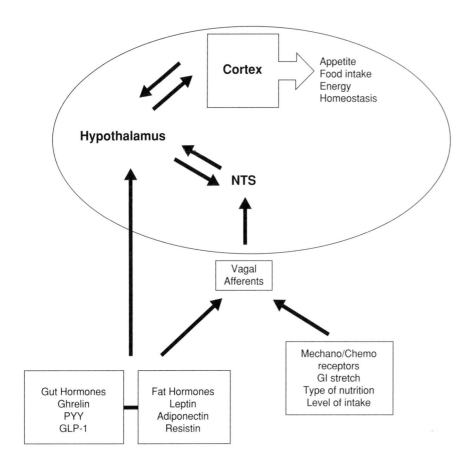

Figure 12–1. Gut–brain axis. Vagal sensory neurons convey information from gut hormones (ghrelin, PYY, and GLP-1), fat hormones (leptin, adiponectin, resistin), as well as mechano/chemoreceptor from the GI tract into the NTS. NTS transmit this information to the hypothalamus, which integrate neurohormonal signals and transmits it to the cortex that ultimately regulates appetite, food intake, and energy homeostasis. NTS has also connections with the cortex independently of the hypothalamus.

hormonal afferent gut signals to the nucleus tractus solitarius (NTS) and area postrema (AP).

Indeed, as illustrated in Figure 12–1, under normal physiologic conditions, vagal sensory neurons convey information from the GI tract (e.g., type of nutrition and level of intake, hormonal signals) into the NTS. From the NTS, these signals are transmitted to hypothalamic nuclei, which integrate neurohormonal signals from the gut and the adipose tissue and transmit the sum of hunger and satiety signals to the cortex that ultimately regulates appetite, food intake, and energy balance.[44−46] NTS, which is the viscerosensory nucleus of the dorsal vagus complex, can also induce satiety independently of the hypothalamus.[44−46] In summary, the CNS receives information from the periphery regarding the individual's energy balance through metabolic, neural, and endocrine signals, integrating and interpreting these signals to subsequently direct information to numerous organs to maintain energy homeostasis.[47] The fact that RYGB significantly alters the anatomy of the GI tract (where some of the components of this system are produced) means that the operation has the potential to influence energy homeostasis by more powerful ways than just mechanical restriction of food intake and nutrient malabsorption.

Gut Hormones

Several peptides released from the GI tract have been shown to regulate appetite and food intake, effecting orexigenic and anorexigenic outcomes.[47−50]

CCK is largely known as a short-term meal-related signal that is effective in maintaining appropriate meal size so that the daily regulation of energy intake is coordinated with energy usage and long-term body weight regulation. The role of CCK in inducing satiety after RYGB has not been established. CCK concentrations are expected to be lower after RYGB, because it is produced in intestinal I cells that are located primarily in the duodenum. Rubino et al. reported decreased levels of CCK after RYGB but the changes were not statistically significant.[51]

Ghrelin is another gut hormone that is strongly involved in the regulation of energy homeostasis.[52] Ghrelin is produced from the stomach in the preprandial state; it increases the expression of the orexigenic hypothalamic neuropeptide Y (NPY). In humans, plasma ghrelin concentration increases twofold before a meal and decreases within 1 hour after eating. In states of negative energy balance such as those caused by low-calorie diets, regular exercise, cancer anorexia, and anorexia nervosa, ghrelin concentrations are increased.[53]

Cummings and coworkers published a report suggesting that impairment in the secretion of ghrelin, an orexigenic hormone mainly produced in the stomach, might account for the loss of appetite and contribute to the weight loss effect of RYGB (see Chapter 15).[54] Other studies reporting ghrelin concentrations after RYGB have shown conflicting results (Table 12–1). The variations are possibly related to factors such as patient selection, size and orientation of gastric pouch, vagal denervation, and limb length between surgical anastomosis. Furthermore, acylated ghrelin stimulates food intake,

Table 12–1.

Changes in Ghrelin Concentrations After Gastric Bypass

Study	Change in Ghrelin Levels	Comments
Geloneze et al. 2003[55]	56% decrease in nondiabetics 59% decrease in diabetics	Ghrelin inversely related to changes in leptin
Fruhbeck et al. 2004[56]	Decreased ghrelin	Greater decrease after RYGB compared to AGB or BPD
Tritos et al. 2003[57]	45% reduction from preoperative 57% lower than lean controls	Low ghrelin response to OGTT
Cummings et al. 2002[54]	77% lower than normal weight controls 72% lower than matched obese controls	Meal fluctuation and diurnal rhythm of ghrelin were absent after gastric bypass
Leonetti et al. 2003[58]	Decreased ghrelin	Ghrelin after RYGB lower than after LASGB Lowest levels were in gastrectomy patients
Morinigo et al. 2004[1]	Decreased 6 weeks after surgery	Ghrelin changes correlated with insulin sensitivity and caloric intake
Stoeckli et al. 2004[59]	Ghrelin unchanged after surgery	Interpreted as impaired ghrelin response to weight loss
Faraj et al. 2003[60]	Increased during rapid weight-loss period Unchanged in weight-stable patients	Normal ghrelin secretion impaired in weight-stable patients
Holdstock et al. 2003[61]	62% increase at 12 months	Ghrelin and insulin inversely correlated

AGB, adjustable gastric banding; BPD, biliopancreatic diversion; OGTT, oral glucose tolerance testing; LASGB, laparoscopic adjustable silicone gastric banding.

while desacylated induces a negative energy balance by decreasing food intake and delaying gastric emptying. This difference may also confound ghrelin measurements and must be taken into consideration.[62]

Fasting plasma ghrelin concentrations have been reported to be decreased immediately,[63] 6 weeks,[1] 0.7 years,[64] and 1 year after the RYGB operation.[55] However, other studies have reported no change[59] or even an increase in fasting ghrelin concentrations after RYGB.[61]

In addition to changes in fasting plasma ghrelin concentrations, diurnal fluctuations on ghrelin have also been studied after gastric bypass. Gastric bypass promotes meal-related suppression,[1] premeal increases, and intermeal fluctuations in ghrelin levels.[54] Recent animal investigations also suggest that the exclusion of the intestinal foregut may per se be responsible for the restoration of physiologic patterns of ghrelin regulation in hyperphagic obese rats.[65]

Peptide YY (PYY) is a satiety hormone with highest tissue concentrations in distal segments of the GI tract (ileum and colon). This peptide is produced by intestinal L cells, is released into the circulation postprandially proportional to the food intake,[66] and acts within the ARC to inhibit the release of NPY.[67]

Glucagon-like peptide 1 (GLP-1) is an insulinotropic hormone secreted from the gut in response to luminal glucose.[68] GLP-1 acts mainly as an incretin, promoting postprandial insulin release, and improving pancreatic beta-cell function.[69] GLP-1 is suppressed in non-insulin-dependent diabetes mellitus (NIDDM). Administration of GLP-1 lowers blood glucose and reduces food intake in NIDDM patients.[70,71]

PYY and GLP-1 levels are expected to be higher after RYGB due to the greater nutrient flow to the ileum, where the majority of L cells are located. In fact, both GLP-1 and PYY levels are increased after surgical manipulations of the GI tract that accelerate nutrient delivery to the hindgut such as the jejuno–ileal bypass surgery in humans.[72] and ileal transposition in rodent models.[73,74]

Accordingly, Korner et al. showed an early-exaggerated rise in PYY after RYGB in humans.[75] These findings are consistent with experimental investigations using a RYGB rat model.[76] A recent prospective study showed a significant increase of both GLP-1 and PYY in response to a liquid meal 6 weeks after RYGB.[43]

Several studies have documented significant decrease in fasting and postprandial insulin levels, and reversal of insulin resistance has been observed as early as 1 week after

RYGB.[77] These observations are intriguing since insulin is a major player in the regulation of appetite as well as in glucose homeostasis.

Fat Hormones

Signals from body fat stores are related to the long-term regulation of energy homeostasis and maintenance of stable body weight. Leptin, adiponectin, and resistin are secreted by adipose tissue,[78] and these circulating bioactive peptides have emerged as factors that may modulate insulin resistance (see Chapter 5). The rapid improvement in insulin resistance following bariatric surgery is possibly mediated by changes in levels of incretin hormones, whereas the long-term changes may be modulated by adjustments in levels of circulating bioactive peptides generated by the decrease in fat mass.[79]

Leptin and insulin have critical roles in the regulation of food intake. Their receptors are richly expressed in the hypothalamic ARC. Leptin is secreted by adipose tissue in proportion to body fat mass.[78,80] Leptin acts on the CNS, particularly in the hypothalamus, suppressing food intake and stimulating energy expenditure.[81]

Obese individuals, however, often have increased leptin concentration. This is explained by a desensitization for the leptin signal by saturable transport of leptin across the blood–brain barrier and abnormalities in the extent of leptin receptor activation or signal transduction,[82] a phenomenon known as leptin resistance.[83] Leptin signaling is a decisive determinant of the ability of satiety signals to induce meal termination, and its action in the forebrain modulates both meal size and the hindbrain response to CCK.[84–86]

Leptin levels are decreased significantly after RYGB, with reports of reversal of the leptin-resistant state as early as 3 weeks postsurgery.[61,87] However, despite the significant decrease in leptin after RYGB, the relationship between changes in leptin concentrations and insulin resistance remain uncertain.

Adiponectin concentrations correlate inversely with total fat mass.[61,78] Adiponectin modulates insulin sensitivity, effectively enhancing glucose uptake while suppressing hepatic gluconeogensis.[88] Insulin resistance improves after weight loss and correlates with increased adiponectin concentrations.[60]

In rodents, adiponectin administration improves insulin sensitivity.[89] Adiponectin levels increase following RYGB.[60,90] Pories and colleagues reported an approximately 40% increase in adiponectin concentrations after RYGB.[91]

In a recent study, Vendrell et al. reported that preoperative resistin concentrations were a relevant predictor of weight loss 6 months after RYGB. However, there was no significant change in resistin levels following surgery (3.5–3.4 ng/mL).[90] The relationship between resistin and insulin resistance remains controversial and human studies have produced inconsistent results.[92–95] Further studies are necessary to establish whether an association exists between resistin, obesity, and insulin resistance.

Remarkably, both insulin and leptin levels decrease before substantial weight loss occurs following procedures that bypass the foregut (RYGB and BPD).[96,97] Therefore, it has been suggested that alteration of gut signaling secondary to the bypass of the small bowel may be responsible for these changes.[98]

MECHANISM OF DIABETES CONTROL AFTER RYGB

RYGB is not only effective in inducing weight loss but also results in a dramatic and rapid resolution of type 2 diabetes mellitus (T2DM).[77,98] More than 80% of patients with T2DM experience long-lasting remission of their disease and are able to discontinue all diabetic medications.[99]

This dramatic effect of surgery on T2DM cannot be accounted for by weight loss alone since most diabetic patients typically discontinue all of their medications at the time of discharge from the hospital, long before significant weight loss has occurred. These observations lead to speculations that alterations in gut-hormone release after RYGB may improve insulin secretion and/or action.[98]

Elucidating the mechanism of improvement of diabetes after RYGB would have crucial implications for both the management and understanding of this condition.

Rubino and Marescaux[100] have shown that Goto-Kakizki (GK) rats (a spontaneous nonobese model of T2DM) subjected to gastrojejunal bypass had improved glucose tolerance compared to sham-operated, food-restricted, and rosiglitazone-treated rats. This experiment suggests that the improvement of diabetes is a direct effect of the operation and not a secondary outcome of treating obesity or decreasing food intake and body weight.

In order to elucidate the molecular explanation of diabetes control after RYGB, it would be critical to understand which part of the typical anatomical rearrangement of RYGB is essential for the effect on diabetes.

Two hypotheses have been proposed. The "hindgut hypothesis" holds that diabetes control results from the expedited delivery of nutrient chime to the distal intestine, enhancing a physiologic signal that improves glucose metabolism.[101] A potential candidate mediator of this effect is GLP-1 or other distal gut peptides.

An alternative hypothesis is that the exclusion of the duodenum and proximal jejunum from the transit of nutrients may prevent secretion of a putative signal that promotes insulin resistance and type 2 diabetes ("foregut hypothesis").[98,102] Although no obvious candidate molecules can be identified with current knowledge, if proven true, this hypothesis might open new avenues in the search for the cause and cures of diabetes.

A recent study by Rubino and coworkers support the foregut hypothesis as a dominant mechanism in improving glucose homeostasis after RYGB.[103] In fact, this study shows that whereas DJB (gastrojejunostomy + duodenal exclusion as in RYGB) greatly improves diabetes in GK rats, performing an equivalent shortcut for ingested nutrients to the hindgut without excluding nutrient flow through the proximal intestine (via a simple gastrojejunostomy) does not improve diabetes in the same animal model. In addition, diabetic abnormalities of glucose tolerance return in DJB-treated animals when nutrient flow through the proximal intestine is surgically reestablished via the normal gastroduodenal route, despite preserving the gastrojejunostomy. Similarly, in animals that originally underwent a simple gastrojejunostomy without benefits, diabetes is greatly improved by a reoperation in which the proximal intestine is excluded from nutrient flow, but the gastrojejunostomy is left intact.

These findings demonstrate that isolating a segment of proximal intestine from nutrient flow is important in mediating the improvement of glucose tolerance in diabetic animals and suggest that a putative signal originating in the foregut might be involved in the pathophysiology of type 2 diabetes.

CONCLUSIONS AND FUTURE RESEARCH

Roux-en-Y gastric bypass is a powerful tool that results in massive weight loss and resolution of numerous obesity-related comorbidities. While the clinical success of this operation has been repeatedly demonstrated in large series, the underlying physiology that leads to this clinical success is not well understood. The complex interplay between adipose cells, the gut, the brain, and the immune system is dramatically altered by RYGB. The rapid induction of a negative energy balance after surgery, the limited foregut bypass, rapid nutrient delivery to the hindgut, and decreased adipocyte mass may all play important roles in durable weight loss, decreased satiety, improved insulin resistance, and resolution of the proinflammatory state associated with obesity. Further research is necessary to better define the exact physiologic changes that occur after RYGB and that mediate the effect of the operation. Improved understanding of this complex physiology will undoubtedly lead to important changes in the medical and surgical treatment of obesity and type 2 diabetes.

References

1. Moringo R, Moize V, Musri M, et al.: GLP-1, PYY, Hunger and satiety following gastric bypass surgery in morbidly obese subjects. *J Clin Endocrinol Metab* 91:1735–1740, 2006.
2. Cummings DE, Shannon MH, Foster-Schubert KE: Hormonal mechanisms of weight loss and diabetes resolution after bariatric surgery. *Surg Obes Related Dis* 1:358–368, 2005.
3. Schauer PR, Ikramuddin S, Hamad G, et al.: Laparoscopic gastric bypass surgery: Current technique. *J Laparoendosc Adv Surg Tech A* 13:229–239, 2003.
4. Alvarez-Leite JI: Nutrient deficiencies secondary to bariatric surgery. *Curr Opin Clin Nutr Metab Care* 7:569–575, 2004.
5. Brolin RE, LaMarca LB, Kenler HA, et al.: Malabsorptive gastric bypass in patients with superobesity. *J Gastrointest Surg* 6:195–203, 2002; discussion: 204–205.
6. Sugerman HJ, Kellum JM, DeMaria EJ: Conversion of proximal to distal gastric bypass for failed gastric bypass for superobesity. *J Gastrointest Surg* 1:517–525, 1997.
7. Freeman JB, Kotlarewsky M, Phoenix C: Weight loss after extended gastric bypass. *Obes Surg* 7:337–344, 1997.
8. Choban PS, Flancbaum L: The effect of Roux limb lengths on outcome after Roux-en-Y gastric bypass: A prospective, randomized clinical trial. *Obes Surg* 12:540–545, 2002.
9. MacLean LD, Rhode BM, Nohr CW: Long- or short-limb gastric bypass? *J Gastrointest Surg* 5:525–530, 2001.
10. Inabnet WB, Quinn T, Gagner M, et al.: Laparoscopic Roux-en-Y gastric bypass in patients with BMI <50: A prospective randomized trial comparing short and long limb lengths. *Obes Surg* 15:51–57, 2005.
11. Hafner RJ, Watts JM, Rogers J: Quality of life after gastric bypass for morbid obesity. *Int J Obes* 15:555–560, 1991.
12. Rand CS, Macgregor AM, Hankins GC: Eating behavior after gastric bypass surgery for obesity. *South Med J* 80:961–964, 1987.
13. Halmi KA, Mason E, Falk JR, et al.: Appetitive behavior after gastric bypass for obesity. *Int J Obes* 5:457–464, 1981.
14. Kenler HA, Brolin RE, Cody RP: Changes in eating behavior after horizontal gastroplasty and Roux-en-Y gastric bypass. *Am J Clin Nutr* 52:87–92, 1990.
15. Pan XR, Li GW, Hu YH, et al.: Effects of diet and exercise in preventing NIDDM in people with impaired glucose tolerance. The Da Qing IGT and diabetes study. *Diab Care* 20:537–544, 1997.
16. Blackburn AM, Christofides ND, Ghatei MA, et al.: Elevation of plasma neurotensin in the dumping syndrome. *Clin Sci (Lond)* 59:237–243, 1980.
17. Johnson LP, Sloop RD, Jesseph JE: Treatment of "dumping" with serotonin antagonists: Preliminary report. *Jama* 180:493–494, 1962.
18. Yamamoto H, Mori T, Tsuchihashi H, et al.: A possible role of GLP-1 in the pathophysiology of early dumping syndrome. *Dig Dis Sci* 50:2263–2267, 2005.
19. Gebhard B, Holst JJ, Biegelmayer C, et al.: Postprandial GLP-1, norepinephrine, and reactive hypoglycemia in dumping syndrome. *Dig Dis Sci* 46:1915–1923, 2001.
20. Toft-Nielsen M, Madsbad S, Holst JJ: Exaggerated secretion of glucagon-like peptide-1 (GLP-1) could cause reactive hypoglycaemia. *Diabetologia* 41:1180–1186, 1998.
21. Kreymann B, Williams G, Ghatei MA, et al.: Glucagon-like peptide-1 7-36: A physiological incretin in man. *Lancet* 2:1300–1334, 1987.
22. Sugerman HJ, Starkey JV, Birkenhauer R: A randomized prospective trial of gastric bypass versus vertical banded gastroplasty for morbid obesity and their effects on sweets versus non-sweets eaters. *Ann Surg* 205:613–624, 1987.
23. Sugerman HJ, Londrey GL, Kellum JM, et al.: Weight loss with vertical banded gastroplasty and Roux-Y gastric bypass for morbid obesity with selective versus random assignment. *Am J Surg* 157:93–102, 1989.
24. Cummings DE, Overduin J, Foster-Schubert KE: Gastric bypass for obesity: Mechanisms of weight loss and diabetes resolution. *J Clin Endocrinol Metab* 89:2608–2615, 2004.
25. Sugerman HJ, Kellum JM, Engle KM, et al.: Gastric bypass for treating severe obesity. *Am J Clin Nutr* 55:560S–566S, 1992.
26. Mallory GN, Macgregor AM, Rand CS: The influence of dumping on weight loss after gastric restrictive surgery for morbid obesity. *Obes Surg* 6:474–478, 1996.
27. Moize V, Geliebter A, Gluck ME, et al.: Obese patients have inadequate protein intake related to protein intolerance up to 1 year following Roux-en-Y gastric bypass. *Obes Surg* 13:23–28, 2003.
28. Pories WJ, Flickinger EG, Meelheim D, et al.: The effectiveness of gastric bypass over gastric partition in morbid obesity: consequence of distal gastric and duodenal exclusion. *Ann Surg* 196:389–399, 1982.
29. Leth RD, Abrahamsson H, Kilander A, et al.: Malabsorption of fat after partial gastric resection. A study of pathophysiologic mechanisms. *Eur J Surg* 157:205–208, 1991.
30. Tabrez S, Roberts IM: Malabsorption and malnutrition. *Prim Care* 28:505–522, 2001.

31. Kellum JM, Kuemmerle JF, O'Dorisio TM, et al.: Gastrointestinal hormone responses to meals before and after gastric bypass and vertical banded gastroplasty. *Ann Surg* 211:763–770, 1990; discussion: 770–771.

32. Ponsky TA, Brody F, Pucci E: Alterations in gastrointestinal physiology after Roux-en-Y gastric bypass. *J Am Coll Surg* 201:125–131, 2005.

33. Marcason W: What are the dietary guidelines following bariatric surgery? *J Am Diet Assoc* 104:487–488, 2004.

34. Brolin RE, Leung M: Survey of vitamin and mineral supplementation after gastric bypass and biliopancreatic diversion for morbid obesity. *Obes Surg* 9:150–154, 1999.

35. Amaral JF, Thompson WR, Caldwell MD, et al.: Prospective hematologic evaluation of gastric exclusion surgery for morbid obesity. *Ann Surg* 201:186–193, 1985.

36. Crowley LV, Seay J, Mullin G: Late effects of gastric bypass for obesity. *Am J Gastroenterol* 79:850–860, 1984.

37. Halverson JD: Micronutrient deficiencies after gastric bypass for morbid obesity. *Am Surg* 52:594–598, 1986.

38. von Mach MA, Stoeckli R, Bilz S, et al.: Changes in bone mineral content after surgical treatment of morbid obesity. *Metabolism* 53:918–921, 2004.

39. Coates PS, Fernstrom JD, Fernstrom MH, et al.: Gastric bypass surgery for morbid obesity leads to an increase in bone turnover and a decrease in bone mass. *J Clin Endocrinol Metab* 89:1061–1065, 2004.

40. Sola E, Morillas C, Garzon S, et al.: Rapid onset of Wernicke's encephalopathy following gastric restrictive surgery. *Obes Surg* 13:661–662, 2003.

41. Chaves LC, Faintuch J, Kahwage S, et al.: A cluster of polyneuropathy and Wernicke-Korsakoff syndrome in a bariatric unit. *Obes Surg* 12:328–334, 2002.

42. Loh Y, Watson WD, Verma A, et al.: Acute Wernicke's encephalopathy following bariatric surgery: clinical course and MRI correlation. *Obes Surg* 14:129–132, 2004.

43. le Roux CW, Aylwin SJ, Batterham RL, et al.: Gut hormone profiles following bariatric surgery favor an anorectic state, facilitate weight loss, and improve metabolic parameters. *Ann Surg* 243:108–114, 2006.

44. Berthoud HR: Mind versus metabolism in the control of food intake and energy balance. *Physiol Behav* 81:781–793, 2004.

45. Grill HJ, Kaplan JM: Interoceptive and integrative contributions of forebrain and brainstem to energy balance control. *Int J Obes Relat Metab Disord* 25(Suppl 5):S73–S77, 2001.

46. Grill HJ, Kaplan JM: The neuroanatomical axis for control of energy balance. *Front Neuroendocrinol* 23:2–40, 2002.

47. Strader AD, Woods SC: Gastrointestinal hormones and food intake. *Gastroenterology* 128:175–191, 2005.

48. Shepherd MF, Rosborough TK, Schwartz ML: Heparin thromboprophylaxis in gastric bypass surgery. *Obes Surg* 13:249–253, 2003.

49. Roth KA, Gordon JI: Spatial differentiation of the intestinal epithelium: Analysis of enteroendocrine cells containing immunoreactive serotonin, secretin, and substance P in normal and transgenic mice. *Proc Natl Acad Sci USA* 87:6408–6412, 1990.

50. Roth KA, Hertz JM, Gordon JI: Mapping enteroendocrine cell populations in transgenic mice reveals an unexpected degree of complexity in cellular differentiation within the gastrointestinal tract. *J Cell Biol* 110:1791–1801, 1990.

51. Rubino F, Gagner M, Gentileschi P, et al.: The early effect of the Roux-en-Y gastric bypass on hormones involved in body weight regulation and glucose metabolism. *Ann Surg* 240:236–242, 2004.

52. Gualillo O, Lago F, Gomez-Reino J, et al.: Ghrelin, a widespread hormone: insights into molecular and cellular regulation of its expression and mechanism of action. *FEBS Lett* 552:105–119, 2003.

53. Zigman JM, Elmquist JK: Minireview: From anorexia to obesity—the yin and yang of body weight control. *Endocrinology* 144:3749–3756, 2003.

54. Cummings DE, Weigle DS, Frayo RS, et al.: Plasma ghrelin levels after diet-induced weight loss or gastric bypass surgery. *N Engl J Med* 346:1623–1630, 2002.

55. Geloneze B, Tambascia MA, Pilla VF, et al.: Ghrelin: A gut-brain hormone: Effect of gastric bypass surgery. *Obes Surg* 13:17–22, 2003.

56. Fruhbeck G, Diez-Caballero A, Gil MJ, et al.: The decrease in plasma ghrelin concentrations following bariatric surgery depends on the functional integrity of the fundus. *Obes Surg* 14:606–612, 2004.

57. Tritos NA, Mun F, Bertkau A, et al.: Serum ghrelin levels in response to glucose load in obese subjects post-gastric bypass surgery. *Obes Res* 11:919–924, 2003.

58. Leonetti F, Silecchia G, Iacobellis G, et al.: Different plasma ghrelin levels after laparoscopic gastric bypass and adjustable gastric banding in morbid obese subjects. *J Clin Endocrinol Metab* 88:4227–4231, 2003.

59. Stoeckli R, Chanda R, Langer I, et al.: Changes of body weight and plasma ghrelin levels after gastric banding and gastric bypass. *Obes Res* 12:346–350, 2004.

60. Faraj M, Havel PJ, Phelis S, et al.: Plasma acylation-stimulating protein, adiponectin, leptin, and ghrelin before and after weight loss induced by gastric bypass surgery in morbidly obese subjects. *J Clin Endocrinol Metab* 88:1594–1602, 2003.

61. Holdstock C, Engstrom BE, Ohrvall M, et al.: Ghrelin and adipose tissue regulatory peptides: Effect of gastric bypass surgery in obese humans. *J Clin Endocrinol Metab* 88:3177–3183, 2003.

62. Asakawa A, Inui A, Fujimiya M, et al.: Stomach regulates energy balance via acylated ghrelin and desacyl ghrelin. *Gut* 54:18–24, 2005.

63. Lin E, Gletsu N, Fugate K, et al.: The effects of gastric surgery on systemic ghrelin levels in the morbidly obese. *Arch Surg* 139:780–784, 2004.

64. Chan JL, Mun EC, Stoyneva V, et al.: Peptide YY levels are elevated after gastric bypass surgery. *Obes Res* 14:194–198, 2006.

65. Rubino F, Zizzari P, Tomasetto C, et al.: The role of the small bowel in the regulation of circulating ghrelin levels and food intake in the obese Zucker rat. *Endocrinology* 146:1745–1751, 2005.

66. Adrian TE, Ferri GL, Bacarese-Hamilton AJ, et al.: Human distribution and release of a putative new gut hormone, peptide YY. *Gastroenterology* 89:1070–1077, 1985.

67. Batterham RL, Cowley MA, Small CJ, et al.: Gut hormone PYY(3-36) physiologically inhibits food intake. *Nature* 418: 650–654, 2002.

68. Orskov C, Wettergren A, Holst JJ: Secretion of the incretin hormones glucagon-like peptide-1 and gastric inhibitory polypeptide correlates with insulin secretion in normal man throughout the day. *Scand J Gastroenterol* 31:665–670, 1996.

69. Farilla L, Bulotta A, Hirshberg B, et al.: Glucagon-like peptide 1 inhibits cell apoptosis and improves glucose responsiveness of freshly isolated human islets. *Endocrinology* 144:5149–5158, 2003.

70. Vilsboll T, Krarup T, Sonne J, et al.: Incretin secretion in relation to meal size and body weight in healthy subjects and people with type 1 and type 2 diabetes mellitus. *J Clin Endocrinol Metab* 88:2706–2713, 2003.

71. Elahi D, McAloon-Dyke M, Fukagawa NK, et al.: The insulinotropic actions of glucose-dependent insulinotropic polypeptide (GIP) and glucagon-like peptide-1 (7-37) in normal and diabetic subjects. *Regul Pept* 51:63–74, 1994.

72. Narbro K, Agren G, Jonsson E, et al.: Pharmaceutical costs in obese individuals: Comparison with a randomly selected population sample and long-term changes after conventional and surgical treatment: The SOS intervention study. *Arch Intern Med* 162:2061–2069, 2002.

73. Rubino F, Gagner M, Marescaux J: Surgical treatment of type 2 diabetes mellitus. *Lancet* 358:668–669, 2001.

74. Strader AD, Vahl TP, Jandacek RJ, et al.: Weight loss through ileal transposition is accompanied by increased ileal hormone secretion

and synthesis in rats. *Am J Physiol Endocrinol Metab* 288:E 447–E453, 2005.

75. Korner J, Bessler M, Cirilo LJ, et al.: Effects of Roux-en-Y gastric bypass surgery on fasting and postprandial concentrations of plasma ghrelin, peptide YY, and insulin. *J Clin Endocrinol Metab* 90:359–365, 2005.

76. Suzuki S, Ramos EJ, Goncalves CG, et al.: Changes in GI hormones and their effect on gastric emptying and transit times after Roux-en-Y gastric bypass in rat model. *Surgery* 138:283–90, 2005.

77. Pories WJ, Swanson MS, MacDonald KG, et al.: Who would have thought it? An operation proves to be the most effective therapy for adult-onset diabetes mellitus. *Ann Surg* 222:339–350, 1995; discussion: 350–352.

78. Bartness TJ: Dual innervation of white adipose tissue: some evidence for parasympathetic nervous system involvement. *J Clin Invest* 110:1235–1237, 2002.

79. Ballantyne GH, Gumbs A, Modlin IM: Changes in insulin resistance following bariatric surgery and the adipoinsular axis: role of the adipocytokines, leptin, adiponectin and resistin. *Obes Surg* 15:692–699, 2005.

80. Mueller WM, Gregoire FM, Stanhope KL, et al.: Evidence that glucose metabolism regulates leptin secretion from cultured rat adipocytes. *Endocrinology* 139:551–558, 1998.

81. Webber J: Energy balance in obesity. *Proc Nutr Soc* 62:539–543, 2003.

82. El-Haschimi K, Pierroz DD, Hileman SM, et al.: Two defects contribute to hypothalamic leptin resistance in mice with diet-induced obesity. *J Clin Invest* 105:1827–1832, 2000.

83. Rosicka M, Krsek M, Matoulek M, et al.: Serum ghrelin levels in obese patients: The relationship to serum leptin levels and soluble leptin receptors levels. *Physiol Res* 52:61–66, 2003.

84. Peters JH, Ritter RC, Simasko SM: Leptin and CCK selectively activate vagal afferent neurons innervating the stomach and duodenum. *Am J Physiol Regul Integr Comp Physiol* 290:R1542–R1543, 2006.

85. Peters JH, Ritter RC, Simasko SM: Leptin and CCK modulate complementary background conductances to depolarize cultured nodose neurons. *Am J Physiol Cell Physiol* 290:C427–C432, 2006.

86. Kiely JM, Graewin SJ, Pitt HA, et al.: Leptin increases small intestinal response to cholecystokinin in leptin-deficient obese mice. *J Surg Res* 124:146–150, 2005.

87. Molina A, Vendrell J, Gutierrez C, et al.: Insulin resistance, leptin and TNF-alpha system in morbidly obese women after gastric bypass. *Obes Surg* 13:615–621, 2003.

88. Yamauchi T, Kamon J, Minokoshi Y, et al.: Adiponectin stimulates glucose utilization and fatty-acid oxidation by activating AMP-activated protein kinase. *Nat Med* 8:1288–1295, 2002.

89. Kubota N, Terauchi Y, Yamauchi T, et al.: Disruption of adiponectin causes insulin resistance and neointimal formation. *J Biol Chem* 277:25863–25866, 2002.

90. Vendrell J, Broch M, Vilarrasa N, et al.: Resistin, adiponectin, ghrelin, leptin, and proinflammatory cytokines: relationships in obesity. *Obes Res* 12:962–971, 2004.

91. Pender C, Goldfine ID, Tanner CJ, et al.: Muscle insulin receptor concentrations in obese patients post bariatric surgery: relationship to hyperinsulinemia. *Int J Obes Relat Metab Disord* 28:363–369, 2004.

92. Pfutzner A, Langenfeld M, Kunt T, et al.: Evaluation of human resistin assays with serum from patients with type 2 diabetes and different degrees of insulin resistance. *Clin Lab* 49:571–576, 2003.

93. Satoh H, Nguyen MT, Miles PD, et al.: Adenovirus-mediated chronic "hyper-resistinemia" leads to in vivo insulin resistance in normal rats. *J Clin Invest* 114:224–231, 2004.

94. Silha JV, Krsek M, Skrha JV, et al.: Plasma resistin, adiponectin and leptin levels in lean and obese subjects: Correlations with insulin resistance. *Eur J Endocrinol* 149:331–335, 2003.

95. Heilbronn LK, Rood J, Janderova L, et al.: Relationship between serum resistin concentrations and insulin resistance in nonobese, obese, and obese diabetic subjects. *J Clin Endocrinol Metab* 89:1844–1848, 2004.

96. Hickey MS, Pories WJ, MacDonald KG, Jr, et al.: A new paradigm for type 2 diabetes mellitus: Could it be a disease of the foregut? *Ann Surg* 227:637–643, 1998; discussion: 643–644.

97. De Marinis L, Bianchi A, Mancini A, et al.: Growth hormone secretion and leptin in morbid obesity before and after biliopancreatic diversion: relationships with insulin and body composition. *J Clin Endocrinol Metab* 89:174–180, 2004.

98. Rubino F, Gagner M: Potential of surgery for curing type 2 diabetes mellitus. *Ann Surg* 236:554–559, 2002.

99. Schauer PR, Burguera B, Ikramuddin S, et al.: Effect of laparoscopic Roux-en Y gastric bypass on type 2 diabetes mellitus. *Ann Surg* 238:467–484, 2003; discussion: 84–85.

100. Rubino F, Marescaux J: Effect of duodenal-jejunal exclusion in a non-obese animal model of type 2 diabetes: a new perspective for an old disease. *Ann Surg* 239:1–11, 2004.

101. Mason EE: Ileal [correction of ilial] transposition and enteroglucagon/GLP-1 in obesity (and diabetic?) surgery. *Obes Surg* 9:223–228, 1999.

102. Pories WJ, Albrecht RJ: Etiology of type II diabetes mellitus: role of the foregut. *World J Surg* 25:527–531, 2001.

103. Rubino F, Forgione A, Cummings DE, et al.: The mechanism of diabetes control after gastrointestinal bypass surgery reveals a role of the proximal small intestine in the pathophysiology of type 2 diabetes. *Ann Surg* 244:741–749, 2006.

13

Malabsorptive Procedures: Biliopancreatic Diversion—Scopinaro Procedure

Nicola Scopinaro, MD, FACS (Hons)

RATIONALE OF BILIOPANCREATIC DIVERSION

The main reason for failure of medical therapy of obesity in obtaining a stable body weight normalization is the reluctance of obese patients to permanently change their lifestyle and eating habits. These changes are temporarily easy to obtain by means of food-limitation surgical procedure, but when, in the long run, the patients are left with the original problem, the majority of them will not be able to maintain the changes indefinitely.

Forty years of worldwide experience with surgical treatment of obesity have demonstrated that the more the success of a procedure depends on patient's cooperation, the poorer the results are. This is the reason why malabsorptive methods, which require minimal patient's compliance, have always been the most effective obesity operations. The reduction of nutrient absorption was actually the first approach to surgical treatment of obesity. The fact that a new way had been opened and the early weight loss results with jejunoileal bypass (JIB) led to more than 100,000 of these operations performed in the United States through the years 1960s and

1970s. However, the analysis of late results and complications of JIB caused a drastic coolness of the initial enthusiasm. In addition to its complications, essentially due to indiscriminate malabsorption and the harmful effects of the long blind loop, the main problem with JIB is its narrow "therapeutic interval." In fact, the total length of the small bowel left in continuity is restrained within the range of 40–60 cm, a shorter or longer bypass resulting in life-threatening malabsorption or no weight reduction, respectively. On the other hand, the massive intestinal adaptation phenomena cause an increased absorptive surface leading out of the upper limits of the above range, with ensuing substantial recovery of energy absorption capacity.[1] This, in addition to the frequent need of restoration for major complications, ends in a high rate of failure with weight regain.[2,3] The high complication rate and the overall unsatisfactory weight loss results of JIB during the years around 1980 led to the general abandoning of malabsorption approach for obesity surgery, the gastric restriction procedures becoming those most frequently used.

Because of the absence of a blind loop and of the malabsorption essentially selective for fat and starch, biliopancreatic diversion (BPD) is free of the complications pertaining to JIB.[4,5] Moreover, BPD has a very wide "therapeutic interval" because by varying the length of the intestinal limbs, any degree of fat, starch, and protein malabsorption can be created, thereby adapting the procedure to the population's or even the patient's characteristics, to obtain the best possible weight loss results with the minimum of complications.[6] Finally, the selective energy malabsorption, in conjunction with this extreme flexibility, makes it easy to neutralize the consequences of intestinal adaptive phenomena, which, on the other hand, are little effective in BPD. In fact, since the absorption of protein and the other essential nutrients occurs in the alimentary limb (AL), the common limb can be created of any length at operation, including that which will result exactly in the desired fat absorption capacity after intestinal adaptation. The same applies to the length of the AL as far as starch absorption is concerned. The qualities of BPD have gradually led to reacceptance of malabsorption as a surgical approach to obesity therapy, the procedure in its many versions being increasingly performed worldwide.

Results and complications of BPD, after nearly 30 years of clinical use, are well known by all bariatric surgeons. Therefore, the main purpose of this chapter is to describe the physiology of the operation, the knowledge of which has increased considerably in the last years. A full understanding of the mechanisms of action of BPD is of paramount clinical importance, as it enables each surgeon to exploit the flexibility of the procedure to adapt it to its particular patients' population.[7]

CASE MATERIAL

Of the 2,900 patients operated on since May 1976, 1,993 (648 men and 1,345 women) underwent the "ad hoc stomach"

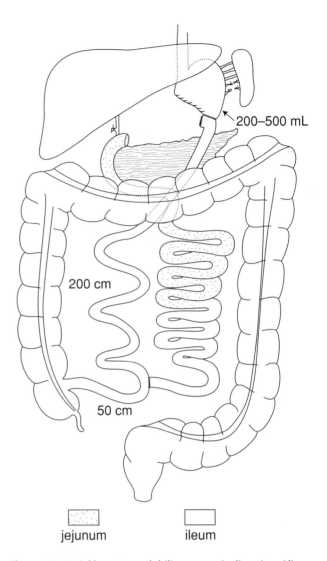

Figure 13–1. Ad hoc stomach biliopancreatic diversion. Alimentary limb, from gastroenterostomy to enteroenterostomy (EEA); biliopancreatic limb, from duodenum to EEA; and common limb, from EEA to ileocecal valve (ICV).

(AHS) type of BPD performed in open surgery by the same surgical team between June 1984 and Feb 2006. Mean age was 37 years (range, 11–70 years), mean weight was 128 kg (range, 73–236 kg), and mean excess weight was 69 kg (20–156), corresponding to 117% (41–311) and to a mean BMI of 47 kg/m^2 (29–87). Maximum follow-up was 21 years. The availability for follow-up evaluation was essentially total. The series of 143 patients submitted to laparoscopic BPD is described separately at the end of this chapter.

In the AHS BPD (Figure 13–1), the gastric volume, which is the main determinant of the initial weight loss (temporary food intake limitation due to decrease of appetite and occurrence of postcibal syndrome), and also influences the stabilization weight (see below), is adapted to the preoperative excess weight and other individual characteristics (sex, age, eating habits, socioeconomic status, and expected degree of compliance), with the aim of obtaining the best weight loss results with the minimum of nutritional complications.[8]

Intestinal lengths, which determine energy absorption and thus the weight of stabilization and its indefinite maintenance, were adapted to patient characteristics only in the last 14 years (as described below).

SURGICAL TECHNIQUE

Laparotomic

The operation consists of a distal gastrectomy with closure of the duodenal stump and a long Roux-en-Y reconstruction, where the enteroenterostomy (EEA) is placed on the distal ileum 50 cm proximal to the ileocecal valve (ICV), while the gastroenterostomy (GEA) is at 250 cm. Three intestinal limbs can then be recognized: the AL, from the GEA to the EEA (200 cm); the common limb (CL), from the EEA to the ICV (50 cm); and the biliopancreatic limb (BPL), from the ligament of Treitz to the EEA, which contains all the rest of the small bowel. A prophylactic cholecystectomy completes the operation.

After opening the abdomen through a midline xifoumbilical incision, the first intestinal step is the intestinal measurement. The small bowel is measured backward from the ICV to the ligament of Treitz and marking stitches are placed at 50 and 250 cm. It is very important that the small bowel is measured fully stretched, to make intestinal measurements reproducible in all hands. The ratio between the same small bowel fully loose and fully stretched is approximately half. The small bowel is then transected at the 250-cm level and the ileal mesentery is sectioned in depth. The EEA can be done with any technique, bringing the BPL to the left side of the AL.

The distal gastrectomy is done, the duodenal stump is closed, the gallbladder is removed, and a wedge liver biopsy is obtained. We are used to cutting the stomach on a TA 90 linear stapler placed as obliquously as possible, in order to compensate for the shortness of the ileal mesentery.

The gastric stump should be measured at all instances, which is very easy by filling with water (at the pressure of 35-cm H_2O) a condom which has been tied at the end of a nasogastric tube and pushed into the gastric stump. Gastric volume should be measured until the surgeon becomes able to evaluate it by sight.

The mesocolon is incised and the AL is brought into the supramesocolic space, checking for possible torsion. Any technique can be used for the GEA. We prefer to do it end-to-side, by cutting away the left corner of the gastric stump. The GEA is then anchored by two stitches to the mesocolic rent, to avoid intestinal kinkings and internal hernias. We always close the distal mesenteric defect and never the proximal. The last maneuver is the final intestinal check, starting from the ICV, with the surgeon following the AL and the first aid following the BPD.

Laparoscopic

The surgical technique entails the use of five trocars, placed in the positions illustrated in Figure 13–2. The gastrocolic

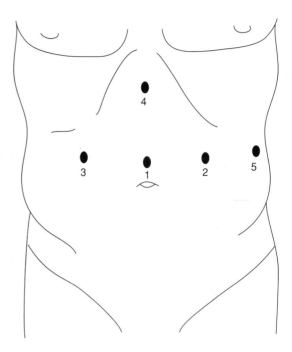

Figure 13–2. Trocar position in laparoscopic standard biliopancreatic diversion. 1: supraumbilical (10–12 mm), on the midline, 3–4 cm above the superior margin of the umbilicus; 2: left hypondriac (10–12 mm), along the left midclavicular line, about 6 cm below the costal margin; 3 right hypondriac (10–12 mm), along the right midclavicular line, about 6 cm below the costal margin; 4: xiphoid (10–12 mm), on the midline, 3 cm below the xiphoid; 5: left subcostal (5 mm), on the left costal margin, along the left middle axillary line.

ligament is incised at about its midpoint and the dissection, which is carried out with a harmonic scalpel, is performed until the traction of the large curve allows for the mobilization of the gastric fundus, which implies that the avascular area is always sectioned. The sectioning of the right gastroepiploic and the right gastric vessels completes the isolation of the duodenum, which is divided with single or double application of endoGIA 45. The small curve is then isolated cranially with the ultrasound scissors, stopping 1 or 2 cm before the trunk of the left gastric artery, and the gastric resection is carried out by repeated firing of endoGIA 45. The gastric volume is measured with the technique described above. A gastric sectioning from the greater curve, moderately stretched, at approximately 15 cm from the cardias to the lesser curve at 5 cm from the cardias corresponds to a gastric volume of about 300 mL. A distance of 20 cm along the greater curve corresponds to a volume of about 400 mL.

After the cholecystectomy has been carried out, the patient is placed in a slightly Trendelenburg position. The small bowel is measured backward from the cecum, fully stretched, using two forceps marked at 10 cm in alternating movements (Figure 13–3). A mark is left at 50 cm, the ileum is divided at 250 cm by using an endoGIA 45, and the mesentery is sectioned in depth with the ultrasonic scissors. The EEA is fashioned with a laterolateral technique, with an endoGIA 45 through two small enterotomies made by the harmonic

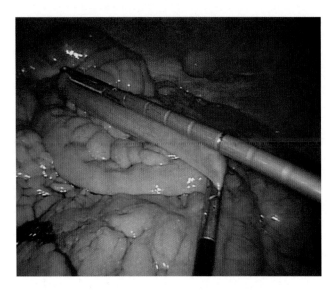

Figure 13–3. The small bowel is measured backward from the cecum, fully stretched, using two forceps marked at 10, 15, and 20 cm.

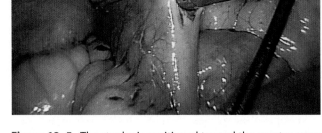

Figure 13–5. The stapler is positioned toward the greater curve in order to avoid the two suture lines being too close.

scalpel. The conjoined defect is closed with a manual running seromuscular suture.

The left angle of the gastric stump is then pulled into the submesocolic space through an incision performed in the transverse mesocolon over the ligament of Treitz (Figure 13–4). The distal intestinal stump is identified and perforated with the ultrasonic scissors at a distance from the suture line equal to the operative length of the endoGIA 45. The latter is used to perform a laterolateral isoperistaltic GEA on the posterior wall of the stomach, as close as possible to the distal angle and at midway between the suture line and the greater curve (Figure 13–5), with manual closure of the conjoined defect.

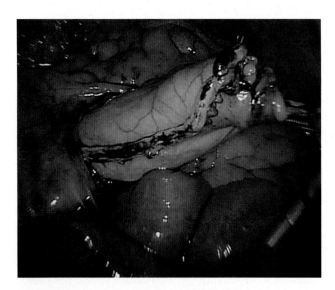

Figure 13–4. The left angle of the gastric stump is pulled into the submesocolic space through the mesocolic rent.

EATING HABITS

During the first postoperative months all patients undergoing BPD, due to the food stimulation of the ileum,[9] have reduced appetite, and they have early satiety, occasionally in association with epigastric pain and/or vomiting. These symptoms characterize the postcibal syndrome and are caused by rapid gastric emptying with subsequent distention of the postanastomotic loop. All these symptoms, which are more intense and last longer the smaller the gastric volume is, rapidly regress with time, most likely due to intestinal adaptation. One year after operation, the appetite and the eating capacity are fully restored and the patient's mean self-reported food intake is one and a half times as much as preoperatively, independently of gastric volume. Patients undergoing BPD must be aware that for the rest of their lives they will absorb minimal fat,[10,11] little starch, sufficient protein,[12,11] and nearly all mono- and disaccharides, short-chain triglycerides, and alcohol (i.e., the energy content of sugar, fruit, sweets, soft drinks, milk, and alcoholic beverages). They must also understand that when their body weight will have reached the level of stabilization the intake of these aliments may be varied as needed for individual weight adjustments.

Interestingly, the vasomotory phenomena characterizing the dumping syndrome are always absent after BPD, this indicating the lack of the specific receptors and/or the vasoactive gut hormones in the ileum that are thought to be implicated in the pathogenesis of dumping syndrome.

BOWEL HABITS

After full resumption of food intake, BPD subjects generally have two to four daily bowel movements of soft stools.

Most have foul-smelling stools and flatulence. These phenomena, which can be reduced by modifying eating habits or by neomycin or metronidazole or pancreatic enzyme administration, tend to decrease with time along with a reduction of bowel movement frequency and increased stool consistency. Diarrhea usually appears only in the context of postcibal syndrome, and then it rapidly disappears, being practically absent by the fourth month.[6] Sporadic acute gastroenterocolitis, generally lasting not more than a few days, may be observed, especially during the summer. Plasma prothrombin should be checked in these instances, as colonic bacterial flora are the main source of vitamin K in BPD subjects. Because the colon is also the main site of protein digestion/absorption after BPD, a longer period of diarrhea may result in lowering of serum protein concentration with spontaneous recovery after diarrhea has ceased.

The absence of diarrhea after BPD is easily explained considering that, unlike following JIB, the loss of bile salt into the colon was calibrated to about 750 mg/day by choosing the appropriate length for the common limb[11] and that, due to the lack of fat digestion, steatorrhea is essentially neutral, fecal pH being around 7. In fact, studies on intestinal transit time 1, 4, and 12 months after BPD showed, in comparison with preoperatively, a transport speed decreased by 50% in the small bowel but unchanged in the large bowel,[11,13] this being in keeping with the observed changes in gut hormones active on intestinal motility.[14]

WEIGHT LOSS

Weight reduction after AHS BPD in unrevised patients, when expressed as percent loss of the initial excess weight (IEW%L), was 71 ± 16 at 2 years (1,741 cases), 72 ± 16 at 4 years (1,555 cases), 73 ± 16 at 6 years (1,423 cases), 73 ± 15 at 8 years (1,347 cases), 74 ± 15 at 10 years (1,280 cases), 74 ± 15 at 12 years (1,120 cases), 75 ± 16 at 14 years (839 cases), 75 ± 16 at 16 years (417 cases), 76 ± 15 at 18 years (146 cases), and 77 ± 17 at 20 years (87 cases), with no differences between *morbidly obeses* and *super obeses* (IEW > 120%).[6] At 10 years, 90% of the operated patients had a reduction of the initial excess equal to or greater than 50%, the failure rate (loss of less than 25% of the excess) being 0.5%

As noted above, the initial weight loss is determined by the temporary forced food limitation that occurs immediately after operation. On the contrary, the weight of stabilization depends on the amount of daily energy absorption allowed by the BPD, as a consequence of a mechanism that acts permanently. As a rule, the operated patient fully recovers appetite and eating capacity before the stabilization weight is attained and therefore the final weight loss depends on the reduced energy intestinal absorption. The weight of stabilization is also influenced by the gastric volume, most likely because a smaller stomach, resulting in more rapid gastric emptying, accelerates intestinal transit, thereby reducing absorption.[15]

WEIGHT MAINTENANCE

The original philosophy for limitation of digestion in BPD was to delay the meeting between food and biliopancreatic juice in order to confine the pancreatic digestion to a short segment of small bowel. In the first experimental model of BPD, the length of BPL was only 30 cm and the one of the CL was equal to 1/7–1/10 of the small bowel total length, i.e., about 100 cm, so that the AL was about 7-m long. The analysis of changes in weight loss and in protein intestinal absorption in the BPD models that followed each other in the evolution of the operation[12,16–19] demonstrated that in the present model of BPD no pancreatic digestion occurs in the CL. Protein and starch digestion, which is only due to intestinal brush-border enzymes, occurs in the entire small bowel from the GEA to the ICV, while only fat absorption, which needs the presence of bile salts, is confined to the CL.

The extraordinarily good weight maintenance that occurs after BPD is exemplified by a group of 40 subjects who underwent the "half-half" (HH) type of operation, which differs from the AHS type only in that the stomach is larger and the AL is longer.[8] Comprehensibly, the weight reduction was smaller, but the weight attained was strictly maintained up to the twenty-fifth year of follow-up (Figure 13–6). Interestingly, these data are the only 25-year results ever reported in obesity therapy.

Some clinical-statistical observations on the modalities of this very long term weight maintenance indicate that body weight after BPD is essentially independent of individual and interindividual variations of food intake. This prompted us to investigate the relations between usual energy intake and energy intestinal absorption.

An absorption study was carried out,[20] the results of which are reported in Table 13–1, which demonstrated that the BPD digestive/absorptive apparatus has a maximum transport capacity for fat and starch, and thus energy. Consequently, all the energy intake that exceeds the maximum transport threshold is not absorbed; therefore, assuming that daily energy intake is largely higher than the aforementioned

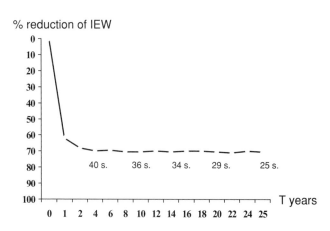

Figure 13–6. Changes in body weight after half-half biliopancreatic diversion.

Table 13–1.

Energy, Fat, Nitrogen, and Calcium Intestinal Apparent Absorption in 15 Subjects (3 Men) With Stable Body Weight 2–3 Years After BPD*

		Alimentary Intake	Fecal Loss	Apparent Absorption[†]	Apparent Absorption (%)
Energy (kcal/24 h)	mean	3070	1329	1741	58
	range	1840–4060	210–2590	1012–2827	32–71
Fat (g/24 h)	mean	130	89	39	28
	range	88–185	22–251	13–94	12–59
Nitrogen (g/24 h)	mean	27	12	15	57
	range	15–48	2.5–36	6.7–20	25–82
Calcium (mg/24 h)	mean	1994	1443	551	26
	range	1037–3979	−453–2565	−251–1414	−24–69

Fat and energy intake were not correlated with intestinal AA as absolute values, whereas a negative correlation was found between intake and intestinal AA as percent of the intake (Kendall rank test: fat $p < 0.05$, energy $p < 0.02$).

Nitrogen and calcium intake were correlated with intestinal AA as absolute values (Kendall rank test: nitrogen and calcium $p < 0.03$).

(Mean ± SD body weight: at the time of the operation 119 ± 24 kg; at the time of the study 75 ± 14 kg.)

[†]*Apparent absorption: Intake minus fecal loss.*

threshold, daily energy absorption is constant for each subject. In conclusion, the original intestinal lengths and gastric volume being equal, the interindividual variability of the weight of stabilization in BPD subjects is accounted for by interindividual differences of (1) original energy intestinal digestive-absorptive capacity per unit of surface; (2) intestinal adaptation phenomena; (3) intestinal transit time (which, in addition to gastric volume, can be influenced by the intake of fluids); (4) simple sugar intake; and (5) energy expenditure per unit of body mass. However, in each BPD individual, the weight of stabilization cannot be modified by any increase or decrease of fat–starch intake, provided the intake is greater than the maximum transport threshold. In reality, since the intestinal carrier becomes rapidly desaturated after the passage of food, an increased number of meals per day can also increase energy absorption, and this is confirmed by clinical experience.

The aforementioned results were confirmed by an overfeeding study, where 10 long-term BPD subjects kept a strictly stable body weight when fed their usual diet for 15 days and the same diet plus 2,000 fat–starch kcal/day (without increasing the number of meals per day) for 15 more days (Table 13–2).

When the food limitation effect has subsided and appetite and food intake are fully restored, the daily amount of energy absorption allowed by the BPD then remains the only determinant of body weight. Now, as it is known, in conditions of energy balance, energy expenditure must be equal to energy intake. If the latter changes and then remains constant, energy expenditure must also change until it equals the energy intake, and then remain constant. This change of energy expenditure can occur only as a consequence of change of body weight, and thus of the energy consumption that it produces.

Table 13–2.

Overfeeding Study in 10 Subjects 3–9 Years After BPD*

Subjects	Initial BW (kg)	BW on Usual Food Intake (kg)	BW After Overfeeding
1	77.7	78.0	78.0
2	90.0	90.5	89.2
3	97.0	96.5	95.7
4	73.0	72.7	73.4
5	89.1	88.8	90.3
6	68.5	68.0	68.5
7	102.8	103.5	103.0
8	87.0	87.0	86.5
9	66.5	66.0	66.0
10	70.5	70.0	71.0

Individual data of body weight at the beginning of the study, after a 15-day period on usual food intake (mean: ~3800 kcal/day) and after a 15-day period of overfeeding (usual food intake plus 2000 fat/starch kcal/day).

Table 13–3.

Body Weight, Body Mass Index, Fat Free Mass, and Resting Energy Expenditure in 53 Obese Subjects (11 Men) at Various Times Relative to BPD and in 30 Never-Obese Healthy Controls (Means ± SD)

	BW (kg)	BMI (kg/m^2)	FFM (kg)	REE (kcal/24 h)
Prior to BPD	127.6 ± 26.9	47.4 ± 9.5	64.3 ± 12.9	1591 ± 638
At one year	83.0 ± 15.4*	30.8 ± 5.6*	55.5 ± 8.3*	1578 ± 305
At two years	78.0 ± 12.6*	28.9 ± 4.4*	54.2 ± 8.6*	1600 ± 310
At three years	79.4 ± 13.8*	29.4 ± 4.8*	55.8 ± 8.6*	1580 ± 229
Controls	77.2 ± 11.0*	28.5 ± 4.3*	53.9 ± 7.1*	1317 ± 199

one-way ANOVA: *$p < 0.0001$ vs preop.

Since after BPD, the energy intake is represented by intestinal energy absorption, which is reduced in comparison with the preoperative energy intake/expenditure, body weight must decrease—as a consequence of the negative energy balance—until the consequent decrease of energy consumption leads to a total energy expenditure (TEE) equal to daily energy intestinal absorption. If we consider that in our patient population the mean preoperative TEE is about 2,100 kcal/day, the mean energy absorption is about 1,750 kcal/day, and the mean total energy consumption per kilogram of weight loss should not be less than 10 kcal/day,[20] it is evident that the difference between mean preoperative TEE and mean postoperative daily energy absorption cannot account for the mean weight lost at stabilization, corresponding to about 50 kg. Certainly, this phenomenon could also be explained by hypothesizing a reduced energy consumption of the kilograms of weight lost. Still, all of the many obese women with a preoperative TEE lower than 1,750 kcal/day lost weight after BPD. Therefore, an increase of energy expenditure per unit of body mass after BPD had to be hypothesized, already suggested by three previous studies,[21−23] demonstrating after BPD an energy expenditure greater than that theoretically expected after the observed weight reduction.

A longitudinal study on resting energy expenditure (REE) in 53 subjects with stable preoperative body weight prior to operation and at 1, 2, and 3 years after BPD was then carried out,[24] the results of which are reported in Table 13–3. Although the mean body weight was reduced by about 50 kg and the mean Fat Free Mass (FFM) by 8 kg, the mean REE at 1, 2, and 3 years was similar to the preoperative one.* This

means that, on an average, our subjects after BPD absorbed as much energy as they were eating before, which raises obvious questions about the reason for the weight loss.

The weight reduction in our sample can be explained considering the different energy expenditure of human body sectors. In fact, whereas adipose tissue consumes only about 5 kcal/kg/day,[25] the REE of muscle is about 18 kcal/kg/day and the energy consumption of internal organs is as high as about 360 kcal/kg/day.[26] Therefore, if the energy intake remains constant, a relatively small variation in internal organ mass must be balanced by a relatively large variation of the less-consuming body sectors, namely adipose tissue and muscles, so that the overall energy expenditure, which must equal the energy intake, remains unchanged.

Although plasma levels of the gut hormones that stimulate intestinal adaptation changes were found to be greatly increased after both JIB and BPD,[14] after the latter, differently from what happens following JIB, the entire bowel receives an intraluminal stimulus to adaptation,[27] which causes an increase in the size (Figure 13–7) and functional activity of the whole intestinal tract.[28,29] This obviously results in increased energy consumption, and thus, because the daily energy absorption cannot be modified, a negative energy balance causing a loss in the other body sectors such as to produce an identical decrease in energy consumption so that the eventual overall energy expenditure equals the energy intestinal absorption. Actually, the increase of energy expenditure attributable to the augmented bowel size–function fully accounts for the corresponding decrease owing to the loss of adipose tissue, muscle mass, and non-bowel visceral mass in our sample of operated patients, the net increase of visceral mass corresponding to about 1 kg or 360 kcal/day.[30] Therefore, in our 53 BPD subjects, on an average the weight loss can be entirely explained by the changes of body composition that follow the operation. Anyway, the presence of a great interindividual variability suggests that very different situations may exist. On one extreme, to a large increase of bowel mass with a low energy transport threshold should correspond the

---

*The difference existing between the mean postoperative TEE in this group calculated from REE with the 1.3 coefficient and the mean measured energy absorption (which corresponds to the mean TEE) in the absorption study group can be explained considering the intergroup variability (mean REE was 1424 kcal/day in the absorption study group and around 1600 in the energy expenditure study group) and a possible underreport of simple sugar intake in the alimentary diary of the absorption study group.

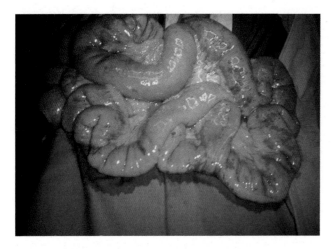

Figure 13–7. The small bowel 2 years after biliopancreatic diversion. Alimentary limb (Left). Biliopancreatic limb (Top right) and common limb (Bottom right).

threshold and partly on the changes of body composition consequent to the operation.

Another interesting consideration may be done concerning the differences existing in our population between men and women. In our sample, after weight stabilization, women weighed and consumed significantly less than men, and this means that they absorbed less than men per unit of intestinal surface. In fact, as said above, after BPD, energy expenditure is determined by intestinal energy absorption, so that a smaller energy expenditure must correspond to a smaller energy absorption. Therefore, intestinal lengths being equal, as is the case of our operated subjects, a smaller energy absorption can be explained only by a smaller absorption capacity per unit of intestinal length, and thus, since no significant differences were found in small bowel diameter and thickness between men and women in our population, a smaller absorption capacity per unit of intestinal surface. The same applies to height, i.e., taller individuals absorb more per unit of intestinal surface.

Finally, the existence of a positive correlation between the small bowel total length and the weight of stabilization demonstrates unequivocally that the absorption capacity per unit of intestinal surface, and thus length, is higher in longer small bowels. The existence of the above-mentioned natural differences between men and women and taller and shorter people, together with the correlations showing that the small bowel is longer in males and in taller people, makes it not necessary to create limb lengths inversely proportional to the small bowel total length to compensate this phenomenon. However, the surgeons who make the intestinal limbs directly proportional to the bowel length go into the opposite wrong direction.

After BPD, each operated subject has a fixed intestinal absorption capacity for fat and starch, which, in our study population, corresponds to about 40 g/day for fat and about 225 g/day for starch. Protein absorption varies, representing

maximum weight loss, the minimum corresponding to the opposite case, with all the possible intermediate situations where the weight loss is mainly due either to the decreased energy absorption or to the increased energy expenditure. For example, if in our sample men and women are considered separately (Table 13–4), the striking fall of REE after BPD in men suggests that weight loss is mainly due to decreased energy intestinal absorption. In contrast, the significant increase of REE observed in women, despite a 43-kg reduction of body weight, clearly indicates that in most cases the weight loss is entirely accounted for by the changes of LBM composition, with the consequent increase of energy expenditure per unit of body mass.

In conclusion, after BPD the weight maintenance is ensured by the existence of an intestinal energy transport threshold. The weight of stabilization depends partly on that

Table 13–4.

Body Weight, Body Mass Index, Fat Free Mass, and Resting Energy Expenditure in Obese Subjects Prior to and 1 Year, 2 Years, and 3 Years After BPD (Mean ± SD)

	BW (kg)	BMI (kg/m²)	FFM (kg)	REE (kcal/24 h)
Men (11)				
Prior to BPD	147.8 ± 32.9	49.3 ± 11.5	76.9 ± 18.6	2128 ± 979
At one year	91.5 ± 17.1*	30.4 ± 6.7*	62.6 ± 11.6†	1787 ± 346§
At two years	83.4 ± 13.0*	27.5 ± 4.0*	62.0 ± 12.6†	1752 ± 365§
At three years	85.0 ± 13.2*	28.0 ± 4.0*	63.7 ± 9.9†	1720 ± 251§
Women (42)				
Prior to BPD	120.5 ± 20.7	46.5 ± 8.8	60.1 ± 6.2	1425 ± 336
At one year	80.0 ± 13.7*	30.8 ± 5.3*	53.1 ± 5.0*	1508 ± 254
At two years	76.2 ± 11.9*	29.2 ± 4.5*	52.5 ± 4.3*	1546 ± 270†
At three years	77.6 ± 13.6*	29.8 ± 5.0*	53.3 ± 6.3*	1533 ± 200§

one-way ANOVA: §$p < 0.05$ *vs preop;* †$p < 0.02$ *vs preop;* *$p < 0.0001$ *vs preop.*

about 70% of the intake,[20] but it would be difficult to produce substantial changes in energy absorption by varying protein intake. Now, even considering the correlations with sex and height, the interindividual differences in energy absorption capacity per unit of intestinal length, producing different energy absorptions and thus energy expenditures with equal limb lengths, and the interindividual differences in body composition, producing different body weights with equal energy expenditures, could result, the limb lengths being equal, in very different stabilization weights. Therefore, the existence of highly caloric aliments (simple sugars, short-chain triglycerides, and alcohol), the absorption of which is unaffected by BPD, is of paramount importance for preventing excessive weight loss. Actually, many of our operated subjects (more frequently men) maintain their desired weight eating considerable amounts of the above aliments, in absence of which the use of BPD would be very difficult. The reverse is obviously represented by those operated subjects (more frequently women) who need to reduce to a minimum, or even to abolish at all the intake of simple sugars in order to attain and maintain the desired weight. Hopefully, routine preoperative measurements of REE and body composition will allow us to adapt limb lengths, and thus energy absorption, to these variables.

OTHER BENEFICIAL EFFECTS

The other benefits obtained after BPD are listed in Table 13–5. The percents of changes observed after the operation were calculated for each complication in patients with a minimum follow-up corresponding to the postoperative time after which there was generally no further substantial modification. Recovery and improvement were considered only when favorable changes were essentially maintained at all subsequent reexaminations. The observed beneficial effects are obviously not attributable to the BPD itself, but to the weight loss and/or the reduced nutrient absorption, the only two exceptions being the effects on glucose and cholesterol metabolism.[31,32]

In fact, out of the 2,410 (total series) AHS BPD patients with a minimum follow-up of 1 year, not only the 338 (14%) with preoperative simple hyperglycemia, or only the 150 (6.2%) with type 2 diabetes mellitus manageable with oral hypoglycemics, but also the 42 (1.7%) patients with preoperative type 2 diabetes mellitus requiring insulin therapy, 1 year after BPD and permanently thereafter, had normal serum glucose level without medication and on totally free diet. Comprehensibly, this is accompanied by serum insulin levels normalization, as demonstrated by us in cross-sectional[33] and longitudinal [serum insulin (mcU/mL) in 53 AHS BPD subjects: preop. 18 ± 10 mcU/mL; at 1 year, 5.2 ± 2.3; at 2 years, 4.6 ± 2.0; at 3 years, 6.0 ± 3.1; controls, 6.9 ± 2.6; ANOVA: each group vs preop. < 0.0001] studies, as well as normalization of insulin sensitivity (Table 13–6). Considering that about 20% of type 2 diabetes mellitus patients are not obese, and about 20% of formerly obese patients with type 2 diabetes mellitus still require insulin therapy after weight normalization by dieting, it must be concluded that simple weight loss

Table 13–5.

Other Beneficial Effects of AHS BPD

	Minimum Follow-Up (mo)	Disappeared (%)	Improved (%)	Unchanged (%)	Impaired (%)
Pickwickian syndrome* (2%)	1	100	—	—	—
Somnolence† (7%)	1	100	—	—	—
Hypertension‡ (42%)	12	80	14	6	—
Fatty liver§ (52%)	24	87	9	4	—
Leg stasis• (32%)	12	44	40	16	—
Hypercholesterolemia¶ (54%)	1	100	—	—	—
Hypertriglyceridemia (35%)	12	94	6	—	—
Hyperglycemia (14%)	4	100	—	—	—
Diabetes mellitus (6%)	4	100	—	—	—
Diabetes mellitus requiring insulin (2%)	12	100	—	—	—
Hyperuricemia (17%)	4	94	—	4	2
Gout (2%)	4	100#	—	—	—

(%) percent of patients with condition.
* Somnolence with cyanosis, polycythemia, and hypercapnia.
† In absence of one or more characteristics of pickwickian syndrome.
‡ Systolic $\geq$ 155, diastolic $\geq$ 95 mm Hg, or both.
§ More than 10%.
• Moderate or severe.
¶ More than 200 mg/mL (21% more than 240 mg/mL).
# Serum uric acid normalized, no more clinical symptoms.

Table 13–6.

Serum Glucose and Insulin Concentrations and Insulin Sensitivity (Euglycemic Hyperinsulinemic Clamp) in Obese Patients, in Subjects 2–4 years After BPD and in Lean Controls

		Obese Subjects	BPD Subjects	Lean Controls
No.		9	6	6
Glycemia (mg/dL)	Mean	99.1*	74.6	86.6*
	Range	63–116	69–81	83–92
Insulinemia (mcU/mL)	Mean	21.7	4.4§	10.3§
	Range	11–41	1–13	9–12
Glucose uptake (mg/kg/min)	Mean	2.9	9.3†	10.5†
	Range	1.7–7.2	6.8–11	8.5–12

Mann Whitney U test: $^*p < 0.01$ *vs BPD subjects;* $^§p < 0.03$ *vs obese patients;* $^†p < 0.001$ *vs obese patients.*

cannot account for the observed 100% recovery from type 2 diabetes mellitus after BPD.

The *primum movens* in the onset of type 2 mellitus in obesity could be, according to Randle,[34,35] an increased Free Fatty Acid (FFA) oxidation, which in turn inhibits glucose oxidation thus causing insulin resistance. More recently, it was suggested that insulin resistance could be caused by hyperinsulinemia due to decreased hepatic clearance of insulin secondary to increased FFA concentration in the portal blood.[36,37] In either case, the normalization of insulin sensitivity after BPD could be due to decreased lipid absorption and/or to reduction of intra-abdominal adipose tissue. Therefore, it would not be a specific action of BPD and it would also not explain the serum glucose normalization in the 20% of obese patients with type 2 diabetes mellitus who still require insulin therapy after weight normalization by dieting. Moreover, after BPD, serum glucose in previously diabetic patients is on the average already normalized 1 month after operation, when overweight is still greater than 80%, and this also suggests a specific action of BPD on glucose metabolism.

Now, if we consider that, independently of the *primum movens*, type 2 diabetes mellitus is characterized by a vicious circle where the high serum insulin level increases insulin resistance and vice versa, it is easily understood that any factor resulting in reduction of insulin production would beneficially affect that vicious circle. An interruption of the enteroinsular axis would be such a factor and this is what the specific action of BPD could be identified with. Indeed, the serum GIP concentration after BPD shows a substantially flat curve in response to the test meal, along with normalization of basal and meal-stimulated serum insulin levels.[13]

If this hypothesis is correct, BPD, reducing the insulin production, should result in impairment of type 1 diabetes mellitus, and this was the case for two young women in our series who, after BPD, in spite of the very good weight reduc-

tion, had to increase their insulin therapy by about 10 units per day.

Finally, though reduction of fat intake, and thus absorption, is common to any weight reduction method, the extreme and selective limitation of fat absorption consequent to BPD is not obtainable by any other means. Therefore, this should also be considered a specific action of the operation, with the consequent enhanced insulin sensitivity and reduced fat beta-toxicity.

There were four cases of late relapse of hyperglycemia in the 192 patients with preoperative type 2 diabetes mellitus, one at 3 years, and three at 5 years. None of them needed any therapy, as none ever had serum glucose values higher than 150 mg/dL. Two patients with severe preoperative diabetes never reached serum glucose normalization, but kept values below 150 mg/dL for more than 10 years on totally free diet and without any therapy.

Two specific actions of BPD account for the permanent serum cholesterol normalization in 100% of operated patients: the first is the calibrated interruption of the enterohepatic bile salt circulation (bile acids are electively absorbed by the distal ileum) that causes enhanced synthesis of bile acids at the expense of the cholesterol pool; the second specific action is the strongly reduced absorption of endogenous cholesterol consequent to the limitation of fat absorption.

The serum cholesterol level shows a stable mean reduction of approximately 30% in patients with normal preoperative values and 45% in patients who were hypercholesterolemic before the operation.[38] High-density lipoprotein (HDL) cholesterol remains unchanged, the reduction being entirely at the expense of low-density lipoprotein (LDL) and very low density lipoprotein (VLDL) cholesterol.[39] These results were maintained at long term, the HDL cholesterol showing a significant increase, in 51 BPD subjects at 6 years (total serum cholesterol: preop. 210 ± 46 mg/dL, postop.

Table 13–7.

Serum Cholesterol in 10 Subjects Before and 15–20 Years After HH BPD

Subjects	Preoperative Total Serum Cholesterol (mg/dL)	Serum Cholesterol 15-20 Years After HH BPD (mg/dL)	
		Total	HDL
1	205	116	47
2	140	125	38
3	150	140	52
4	210	158	65
5	280	158	73
6	230	127	61
7	180	118	35
8	285	120	36
9	189	130	59
10	260	171	33
Mean	213	136*	50

*Wilcoxon test: *p < 0.002 vs preop.*

124 ± 25 mg/dL, Student's *t* test, $p < 0.0001$; HDL cholesterol: preop. 44 ± 12 mg/dL, postop. 50 ± 15 mg/dL, Student's *t* test, $p < 0.03$) and at very long term in the 10 HH BPD subjects whose values were available 15–20 years after operation (Table 13–7). With the National Institutes of Health criterion of 200 mg/dL as the upper recommended limit for serum cholesterol, of the 2,888 (total series) obese patients submitted to BPD with a minimum follow-up of 1 month, 1,542 had hypercholesterolemia (612 had values higher than 240 mg/dL and 110 had values higher than 300 mg/dL). All of these patients had serum cholesterol values lower than 200 mg/dL 1 month after operation, and the values remained below that level at all subsequent examinations.

A very recent analysis of changes in glucose, triglyceride, cholesterol serum levels, and arterial blood pressure observed in all diabetic (fasting serum glucose > 125) AHS BPD patients in our series with a minimum follow-up of 10 years confirmed the excellent very long term effects of the operation on the major components of the metabolic syndrome.[40]

Gasbarrini et al.[41] submitted to HH BPD a lean young woman with familial chylomicronemia (serum triglycerides: 4,500 mg/dL; serum cholesterol: 502 mg/dL) and secondary type 2 diabetes mellitus (insulin 150 U/day to maintain serum glucose around 250 mg/dL). One year after operation she had gained 2 kg in weight; blood glucose, serum insulin, and insulin sensitivity were normal; serum triglycerides were 380 mg/dL; and serum cholesterol was 137 mg/dL, on totally free diet and without any medication. One year later, her younger sister with the same condition underwent the same operation with similar results.[42]

It is concluded that BPD may be effectively and safely used for the treatment of metabolic syndrome also in lean subjects.

NUTRITION

The easiest way to appraise nutritional status is to observe and talk to the subject. A person who looks well and exhibits complete well-being and ability to work, generally, has a good nutritional status. This has been the case for nearly all the AHS BPD patients once the early postoperative period has passed. Our studies on particular aspects of nutritional status showed normal immunological status,[43] physiological composition of the weight lost with attainment of a stable healthy body composition,[44] and capacity of getting pregnant, carrying out a normal pregnancy, and delivering healthy babies.[45]

NONSPECIFIC COMPLICATIONS

Increasing practice and experience led us out of the learning curve with BPD as far as immediate complications are concerned. When the first 738 subjects, the subsequent 500 subjects, and the last 755 subjects undergoing AHS BPD are evaluated separately, a stable reduction of operative mortality to less than 0.5% and the near disappearance of general and intra-abdominal complications are seen. Similarly, the incidence of wound complications appears to be steadily reduced to approximately 1% (Table 13–8).

In contrast, the incidence of nonspecific late complications, around 15% for incisional hernia ($\geq$3 cm)[46] and 1% for intestinal obstruction has not substantially changed throughout the years. Of note is the potential seriousness of biliopancreatic limb obstruction, which, because of its particular anatomo-functional situation, does not cause any specific clinical or radiological signs. However, it may lead to acute pancreatitis, which is more probable and more rapid in onset when the obstruction is more proximal. Any acute abdominal pain that raises suspicion of this complication should lead to an immediate search for duodenal and proximal jejunal distention (by ultrasound scan) and testing for abnormally high levels of serum amylase and bilirubin. If one or more of these signs are present, immediate laparotomy is mandatory.[47]

SPECIFIC LATE COMPLICATIONS

Anemia

The exclusion of the primary site for iron absorption in the alimentary tract causes this unavoidable complication. More

Table 13–8.

Immediate Complications Following AHS Biliopancreatic Diversion

	First 738 Subjects (June 1984–December 1990)	Subsequent 500 Subjects (December 1990–October 1999)	Last 755 Subjects (October 1999–Feb 2006)
Operative mortality	1.1% 3 heart arrest 3 pulmonary embolism 1 malignant hyperthermia 1 wound infection	0.4% 1 pulmonary embolism 1 GEA bleeding	0.3% 1 heart arrest 1 GEA leak and MOF
General complications	1.2% 5 pulmonary embolism 1 pneumonia 3 deep thrombophlebitis	0.2% 1 pulmonary embolism	0.4% 1 pulmonary embolism 3 deep thrombophlebitis
Surgical complications	2.7% 2 GEA leak 1 gastric perforation 2 intraperitoneal bleeding 6 wound dehiscence 9 wound infection	1.2% 3 wound infection 2 wound dehiscence 1 intraperitoneal bleeding	1.3% 2 intraperitoneal bleeding 3 wound dehiscence 5 wound infection

rarely, the anemia is due to folate deficiency and, exceptionally, to vitamin B_{12} deficiency (Schilling test gives normal results short term after BPD[11,48]). Anemia appears only in BPD patients with chronic physiologic (menstruation) or pathologic (hemorrhoids, stomal ulcer) bleeding. Reflecting the cause of the anemia, most cases are microcytic, fewer are normocytic, and a few are macrocytic. The general incidence of anemia after BPD in our population would probably be around 40%, but supplementation with periodic iron, folate, or both can reduce its occurrence to less than 5%. Over time, less supplementation is required.

Stomal Ulcer

BPD is a potentially ulcerogenic procedure.[49] Since the beginning of experimental work in dogs,[4] distal gastrectomy was preferred to gastric bypass[50] because it was thought to be more effective in preventing stomal ulcer[51] and because of the concern for the fate of the bypassed stomach.[52]

The incidence of stomal ulcer was initially rather high (12.5% with the HH BPD) because of the large residual parietal cell mass. Considering only the ulcers diagnosed in the first two postoperative years in order to allow comparisons among groups, the incidence was successively reduced to 9.1% in the first 132 consecutive patients submitted to AHS BPD, simply due to the reduced stomach size.[53] Some changes of surgical technique, namely preserving as much as possible of the gastrolienal ligament with its sympathetic nerve fibers[11] and shifting from end-to-end to end-to-side GEA, the latter being better vascularized and less prone to stenosis,[54] led to further progressive reduction (5.8% in the subsequent

650 cases). In the following group of 640 AHS patients operated on from January 1991 to March 1999 with a minimum follow-up of 2 years, thanks to H_2-blockers' oral prophylaxis[55] during the first postoperative year in patients at risk (see below), started at the beginning of 1991, the incidence of stomal ulcer in the first 2 years was further reduced to 3.3%.

If the totality of stomal ulcers in the first two groups are considered, they were significantly more frequent in men (14.4%) than in women (5.2%). Differently than what was reported in previous articles,[6,7,52] the incidence of stomal ulcer appeared unaffected by alcohol consumption, increased in men (though not significantly) by cigarette smoking, and significantly increased, more in women than in men, by the association of alcohol and smoke. Stomal ulcers responded well to medical treatment (100% healing with H_2-blocker therapy) and they showed no tendency to recur, provided the patient refrained from smoking. Endoscopic evidence of stomal ulcer was obtained in 52% of cases within the first postoperative year, in 26% of cases within the second year, and in 22% of cases, with progressively decreasing frequency, between the third and the tenth year. However, it must be considered that (1) most patients diagnosed in the second and the third year were symptomatic already in the first one; (2) most patients diagnosed at a greater distance from the operation had been treated (one or more times) previously because of specific symptoms; (3) many patients once or repeatedly treated because of specific symptoms had refused endoscopy at all instances; (4) in some cases operated patients with no endoscopic diagnosis had received H_2-blocker therapy from their family doctors; and (5) with the exception of one man, all patients with specific symptoms appearing after the second postoperative year were smokers, or smokers and drinkers. The consideration of all the above facts leads to the conclusions that (1) for BPD patients, not smokers or smokers/drinkers, the risk of developing a peptic ulcer is essentially confined to the first postoperative year and (b) the real incidence of stomal ulcer after BPD is certainly higher than that reported above.

Oral prophylaxis with H_2-blockers was started in 1991 because about one-fifth of ulcer healings in patients in the first two groups had occurred with GEA stenosis, requiring endoscopic dilatation or surgical revision with higher gastrectomy. Ranitidine was chosen because its intestinal absorption had proved to be normal.[54] Since in previous analyses[6,53] cigarette consumption appeared to increase the incidence of stomal ulcer in women more than in men, though not significantly, oral prophylaxis was given to all men and smoking women for the entire first postoperative year and to non-smoking women only for the first 2 months. The result of the prophylaxis was a reduction of stomal ulcer incidence in all the subgroups (men and women with or without alcohol and/or smoke), which was statistically significant only for the nonsmoking men, where no ulcer appeared in first 56 operated subjects during an overall 8-year follow-up period, while the incidence in nonsmoking women was unchanged. The differences present in the first two groups (men vs women and smokers/drinkers vs double abstinents) were still significant in the prophylaxis group, while the difference between smoking and nonsmoking men became significant, evidently due to the disappearance of ulcer in the second subgroup. The obvious conclusion was that oral H_2-blocker (more recently PPI) prophylaxis should be given to all BPD subjects for the entire first postoperative year. In fact, only one ulcer appeared in the 191 nonsmoking women operated on from March 1999, when all operated patients started receiving prophylaxis for the entire first postoperative year, with a minimum follow-up of 2 years. The difference with the incidence in the former group, receiving prophylaxis only for the first 2 months (7/186 or 3.8%), was not yet significant.

Bone Demineralization

The duodenum and proximal jejunum are selective sites for calcium absorption. However, our study on calcium intestinal absorption showed a more than sufficient mean apparent absorption in the 15 subjects on a free diet (Table 13–1). Moreover, intestinal absorption as an absolute value was positively correlated with the intake (Kendall rank test: $p < 0.03$), which means that, unlike fat and energy and similarly to protein, an increase of calcium intake results in increased absorption. Therefore, all of our patients are encouraged to maintain an oral calcium intake of 2 g/day (with tablets supplementation, if needed), while the daily requirement of vitamin D, as well as of all other vitamins and trace elements, is contained in a multi-integrator that all patients are recommended to take for all life, though both in old[56,57] and recent (unpublished data) studies serum levels of vitamin D_2 and D_3 were found to be normal in nearly all our BPD subjects.

When natural history of bone disease was investigated by us in obese patients and operated subjects not taking any supplementations 1–10 years after BPD, histomorphologic signs of mild to severe bone demineralization (cross-sectional study on 252 transiliac bone biopsies after double-labeling with tetracycline, 58 of which preoperatively) were present in 28% of the obese patients and 62% of the operated subjects. Slightly low levels of serum calcium and high levels of alkaline phosphatase were found in about 20% of the subjects in that study, with no significant differences between obese patients and operated subjects or between operated subjects with and without bone alterations. Serum magnesium, phosphorus, and 25-hydroxyvitamin D levels were essentially normal both prior to and after operation. The prevalence and severity of metabolic bone disease (MBD) increased after BPD until the fourth year [prevalence: preop. 16/58, at 4 year 15/21, chi-square test $p < 0.001$; severity (subjects with moderate or severe MBD): preop. 7/58, at 4 year 8/21; chi-square test $p < 0.01$], at which point they tended to regress. Long-term (6–10 year) mineralization status was not significantly worse than that observed before operation. Patients with the most severe preoperative alterations, i.e., the older and the heavier patients, showed a sharp improvement in bone mineralization status compared to their preoperative status (prevalence of moderate or severe MBD in patients over 45-year-old: preop. 25%, at 1–2 year 29%, at 3–5 year 33%, and at 6–10 year 11%; in patients with an IEW greater than 120% these values were, respectively, 24%, 28%, 53%, and 14%).[11,56–58]

The histomorphology data were in total agreement with the clinical findings. Bone pain attributable to demineralization (with prompt regression after calcium, vitamin D only when needed, and diphosphonate therapy) was observed in 6% of patients, generally between the second and fifth postoperative years (maximum prevalence: 2.4% during the fourth year) and more rarely on long term (10–20 years). Four cases of rib fractures and one case of vertebral crash were reported so far in patients undergoing AHS BPD.

The pathogenesis of bone demineralization in obese patients is unclear. The bone problems caused by BPD do not seem to differ substantially from those reported in 25%–35% of postgastrectomy subjects with duodenal exclusion for peptic ulcer[59–61] and in one-third of patients with gastric bypass for obesity.[62] The mechanism is very likely a decreased calcium absorption causing an augmented parathyroid hormone (PTH) release which is generally sufficient to normalize serum calcium level at the expense of bone calcium content. During the first postoperative years, the adverse effect of reduced calcium absorption seems to prevail over the beneficial one of the weight loss, whereas the opposite happens at long term, this being more evident in the subjects with the most severe preoperative alterations.

Recently, it has been suggested that low albumin level is also implicated in the pathogenesis of MBD after BPD.[63]

In our experience, oral calcium supplementation seems to be able both to prevent and to cure bone alterations caused by BPD, monitored by computerized bone mineralometry.

Still, the observations that, on one hand, most of our operated patients do not take the recommended calcium supplementations while very few develop serious MBD, and, on the other hand, the bone problems caused by BPD seem to be more severe in the United States,[64,65] suggest that great differences in calcium requirement and metabolism exist among populations and individuals in the same population. Vitamin D synthesis in the skin at different latitudes probably also plays a major role. It is important to remember that parenteral vitamin D supplementation should not be used in the treatment of MBD unless low serum levels have been documented. In fact, an excess of vitamin D can cause bone damage similar to that caused by its deficiency.

Neurological Complications

Peripheral neuropathy and Wernicke encephalopathy, early complications caused by excessive food limitation,[66] have now totally disappeared (none in the last consecutive 1,969 operated subjects of the total series with a minimum follow-up of 1 year) because of prompt administration of large doses of thiamin to patients at risk, i.e., those reporting a very small food intake during the early postoperative weeks.

Protein Malnutrition

Characterized by hypoalbuminemia, anemia, edema, asthenia, and alopecia, protein malnutrition (PM) represents the most serious late specific complication of BPD, and its correction generally requires 2–3 weeks of parenteral feeding.

Our understanding of the pathogenesis of PM following BPD has considerably improved during the last years. Protein intestinal absorption (measured by means of I-125 albumin) was investigated at the beginning of the clinical experimentation[12] and the study was repeated after completion of the developmental phase,[17] and later again,[18] with similar results. Still, the observed, about 30%, protein malabsorption did not seem to explain the occurrence of PM. A determinant contribution came from the more recent and complete study on intestinal absorption mentioned above. In fact, the comparison between alimentary protein intestinal absorption (73%) and nitrogen apparent absorption (Table 13–1) revealed a mean loss of endogenous nitrogen of about 5 g/day, corresponding to protein about 30 g/day, i.e., approximately fivefold the normal value. The extra nitrogen lost, which, due to the length of the BPL, should not contain un-reabsorbed pancreatic enzymes, could be represented by increased cell desquamation and, hypothetically, by active albumin secretion, both caused by the chronic irritation due to malabsorption. Assuming that 40 g/day protein requirement with a loss of about 6 g/day is normal, all calculations made, the average post-BPD protein requirement should be about 90 g/day, which is quite reasonable considering that the 15 long-term subjects in our study had an average intake of about 170 g/day.

The increased loss of endogenous nitrogen, if confirmed at short term, would result of much greater importance in the first months following BPD, when the forced food limitation causes a negative balance both for energy and nitrogen, thus creating a condition of protein-energy malnutrition (PEM). For the latter, as is known, two subtypes can be identified: the marasmic form (MF) and the hypoalbuminemic form (HAF). In MF PEM, which represents effective metabolic adaptation to starvation, both energy and nitrogen deficits are present. The ensuing hypoinsulinemia allows lipolysis and proteolysis from skeletal muscles, which supply aminoacids for visceral pool preservation and hepatic synthesis of glucose, which in turn is necessary for brain, heart, and kidney metabolism as well as for the oxidation of fatty acids. This, in association with protein sparing due to negative energy balance, ensures both energy and protein homeostasis. The result is a loss of weight due to reduction of adipose tissue and muscle mass in a state of complete well-being. In contrast, in HAF PEM the nitrogen deficit is associated with a normal or near-normal energy (carbohydrate) supply. This causes hyperinsulinemia, which inhibits both lipolysis and skeletal muscle proteolysis. Not being able to draw on its protein stores, and in the absence of protein sparing, the organism reduces visceral protein synthesis, with consequent hypoalbuminemia, anemia, and immunodepression. The result is a severely ill person with body weight unchanged or increased, maintained adipose tissue size, and lean body composition pathologically altered with decreased visceral cell mass and increased extracellular water.

During the early post-BPD period, preservation of protein homeostasis, already threatened by the negative energy–protein balance due to the food limitation, would be made more difficult by the presence of an increased endogenous nitrogen loss which should be counterbalanced. If operated patients devote the reduced eating capacity mainly to protein-rich food, they compensate for the loss and, like starving individuals, develop MF PEM, which is the goal of the procedure. If, on the contrary, they eat mainly carbohydrates, the nitrogen loss would make the HAF PEM even more severe than kwashiorkor. Paradoxically, starving patients are in a better metabolic situation, because they can draw on their protein store to try to satisfy the requirement and compensate for the loss. Therefore, HAF PEM is milder in patients who take protein-rich food compared to carbohydrate-eaters. Between the two extremes, HAF PEM of varying severity can take place in patients with mixed intake, depending on (1) how much smaller the protein intake is than the protein loss and (2) how much the relatively excessive energy intake prevents skeletal muscle proteolysis and protein sparing.

The presence of increased endogenous nitrogen loss also explains late sporadic PM, which, even if rarely, may occur at any length of time from the BPD in case of reduced food intake for any reason, or in case of prolonged diarrhea due to nonspecific enterocolitis. PM is usually more severe in the latter situation because, the colon being an important site of protein digestion/absorption after BPD,[17] protein absorption may be more affected than carbohydrate absorption.

The goal of treatment of early PM, when significant excess weight is still present, is to change the PEM from HAF into MF, providing the patient the possibility of exploiting their energy and protein stores. This state is easily obtained by annulling alimentary carbohydrate intake and, taking into account the protein intake, administering intravenously only amino acids in amounts sufficient to compensate for the endogenous protein loss. In contrast, therapy for late PM, when body weight is normal or near-normal, must be aimed at eliminating PEM and restoring normal nutritional status, with parenteral feeding that includes both the nitrogen and the energy necessary to restore the amino acid pool, reestablish the anabolic condition, and resynthesize deficient visceral protein.

The pathogenesis of PM after BPD is then multifactorial, depending on some operation-related (biological) variables (gastric volume, intestinal limb lengths, individual capacity of intestinal absorption and adaptation, amount of endogenous nitrogen loss) and some patient-related (psychological and environmental) variables (customary eating habits, ability to adapt them to the requirements, socioeconomic status). In most cases, PM is limited to a single episode that occurs during the first or the second year, the patient-related factors being preeminent. Delayed appearance of sporadic PM (see above) is increasingly less frequent as time passes.[67] The operation-related factors are of greater importance in the recurrent form of PM, usually caused by excessive malabsorption and requiring elongation of the common limb; rarely, it is due to excessive duration of the food limitation mechanism (permanent decrease of appetite and occurrence of the postcibal syndrome), generally in conjunction with poor protein intake, which may require restoration of intestinal continuity.[6,68]

In addition to the increased endogenous nitrogen loss, with its impact on daily protein requirement, another important phenomenon acting in the same direction is the overgrowth of colonic bacterial flora. The latter would not affect protein requirement if protein were not absorbed by the colonic mucosa. In reality, we demonstrated that, both in BPD and in intact subjects, colon has the capacity of absorbing about 50% of a load of 10-g albumin directly instilled into the cecum.[17] This absorption capacity is considerable and it is fully exploited in BPD, otherwise there would be no protein malabsorption. If we consider that in the experiment mentioned above albumin was given as a bolus, whereas in our absorption study the fraction of the 60-g protein meal not absorbed in the small bowel reached the cecum diluted by the intestinal transit, we must conclude that the colon is a very important site for protein absorption in BPD. Therefore, overgrown bacterial flora, the synthesis of which partly or totally occurs at the expense of alimentary protein escaped to absorption in the small bowel, reduces protein absorption by the colonic mucosa, thus increasing protein malabsorption and protein requirement.

It is interesting to note that in BPD there is a sort of counterbalance mechanism between increased endogenous nitrogen loss and bacterial overgrowth on one side, both caused by malabsorption and both increasing protein requirement, and food intake on the other side, which exerts a protective action against PM. Actually, the BPD subjects who eat more, having a greater malabsorption, are likely to have a greater endogenous nitrogen loss and a greater colonic bacterial overgrowth, but this is compensated by the greater protein intake. On the contrary, the BPD subjects who eat less are also likely to have a smaller occurrence of these two factors of increased protein requirement. Clearly, this phenomenon does not favor the subjects with great intake of protein-poor food. The absorption study mentioned above was carried out in conditions of free diet, and thus in the presence of considerable malabsorption. A new study is being planned aimed at determining endogenous nitrogen loss in a group of long-term BPD subjects kept at a balanced diet containing 1,000 cal/day. Theoretically, these subjects should not have fat and starch malabsorption, and thus they should have little, if any, increase of endogenous nitrogen loss. Moreover, having little or no colonic bacterial overgrowth, they could exploit colonic protein absorption capacity to complete alimentary protein absorption. In other words, our hypothesis is that in conditions of energy intake lower than energy absorption threshold, BPD has little effect on energy and protein absorption and requirement. The observation that the two subjects with familial chylomicronemia submitted to BPD did not lose weight, and that many of our long-term BPD subjects who, especially with aging, spontaneously reduce their food intake, probably in many cases below the energy absorption threshold, lose weight without becoming malnourished, would support this hypothesis. If it were confirmed by the planned study, this would explain why the incidence of PM is so little both in the early postoperative period and in the late sporadic form.

At a remote phase of BPD development, in an attempt to accelerate and increase the weight loss, we drastically reduced mean gastric volume to about 150 mL, obtaining, in addition to excellent weight reduction (near 90% of the IEW at 2 years), a catastrophic approximate 30% incidence of PM with 10% recurrence rate. With the aim of decreasing the PM incidence without losing the benefit of the small stomach, the gastric volume was adapted to the patient's initial EW (ad AHS BPD, June 1984). In fact, the original philosophy of the AHS was to confine the risk of PM to patients who required greater weight loss. It resulted in a 17.1% incidence of PM with 8.3% recurrence, and the mean weight reduction remained at a very satisfactory 77% of the IEW (initial 192 AHS BPD patients with a minimum follow-up of 2 years), the higher weight of stabilization being evidently due to the larger mean stomach volume (about 350 mL) with the consequent slower intestinal transit and greater energy absorption. Indeed, BPD patients with a more than 300-mL gastric remnant lost significantly less than those with a smaller stomach. Subsequently, sex, age, and the other patient-related variables were also taken into account in the choice of gastric volume, with the new rationale of allowing only patients with the best individual characteristics to take advantage of the risk/benefit of a smaller stomach. This new policy, entailing an increase of mean gastric volume to about 400 mL, led to a further reduction of PM incidence, which progressed with the progressive increase in number and improvement in use of the criteria for adapting the stomach volume to the patient's character-istics. In fact, among the subsequent 859 AHS BPD patients, the first 430 had a PM incidence of 13.5% with 6.0% recurrence, the IEW loss decreasing to 75%, whereas the second 429 had a PM incidence of 8.2% with 3.5% recurrence, at the price of only 2% mean reduction of the IEW loss (decreased to 73%). At that point, the disappearance of any significant negative correlation between gastric volume and occurrence of PM meant that stomach size had no more influence on PM incidence. In order to further reduce the incidence of this complication while preserving the best possible weight loss, we decided to increase intestinal absorption in the patients at risk. Most of those, in our series, are in the southern Italian population, where the main energy source is carbohydrates, the compliance is smaller, and the financial status is lower. In the first subgroup noted above, the incidence of PM was 8.7% with 4.3% recurrence in the 230 patients from northern Italy, whereas it was 19.0% with 8.0% recurrence in the 200 patients from southern Italy; in the second subgroup the corresponding values were 4.5% with 1.8% in 221 northern Italian patients and 11.9% with 5.3% in 208 southern Italian patients.

Starting from September 1992, our policy was to create a 200-cm AL in all patients from North, unless their individual characteristics were strongly negative, and a 300-cm AL in the patients from South, unless their individual characteristics were strongly positive; some patients in each group had an intermediate length of 250 cm. Among the 146 patients from North who had reached a minimum follow-up of 2 years in 1999 (10 with a >200-cm AL) only two subjects with a 200-cm AL had early episodic PM (1.4%). Among the 147 from the South (125 with a >200-cm AL) PM occurred in the early episodic form in two cases with a >200-cm AL and one case with a 200-cm AL (2.0%), and in the recurrent form in two cases of the first group and one of the second (2.0%). The overall incidence in the whole population of 293 operated patients was 2.7%, with 1.0% recurrence. This excellent result was obtained, as expected, at the expense of mean reduction of IEW, which dropped to 71% (73% in the 158 patients with 200-cm AL and 68% in the 135 with >200-cm AL); the patients from North lost 73% and those from South lost 69%.

Interestingly, a longer AL should reduce the risk of PM with a double mechanism of action. On one hand, it increases protein absorption in the small bowel. On the other hand, by also increasing starch absorption, it reduces energy malabsorption and then the loss of endogenous nitrogen and the colonic bacterial overgrowth, which results in an increased protein absorption also in the colon and in a decreased protein requirement.

On the basis of this experience, starting from March 1999, we are now adapting gastric volume and intestinal lengths (200–250 cm) to each patient according to all his/her individual characteristics, independently of his/her origin, this new policy being called "ad hoc stomach–ad hoc alimentary limb (AHS–AHAL)" BPD (Figure 13–8).

Out of the 392 patients operated on from March 1999 to February 2004 (min. follow-up 2 years), 282 had a 200-cm AL and 110 had a 250-cm AL. One psychotic patient had

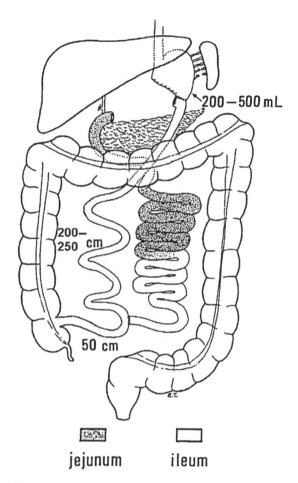

Figure 13–8. Ad hoc stomach–ad hoc alimentary limb biliopancreatic diversion, with the alimentary limb varying from 200 to 250 cm.

a 300-cm AL. Four cases of early PM (1.4%) and one case of recurrent PM (0.4%) were observed in the first group, while one early (0.9%) and one recurrent PM occurred in the second group. Therefore, the overall incidence of PM in the 392 operated patients was 1.8%, with 0.5% recurrence rate. Both patients with recurrent PM underwent elongation, while another patient in the first group was elongated because of chronic diarrhea without PM. Mean excess weight reduction was 70% (71% in the first group and 66% in the second).

The updated figure of recurrent PM in the above-mentioned group of 293 patients who have now reached a minimum follow-up of more than 8 years (max. 13 years) is 2.0% (4 patients with 200-cm AL and 2 with a >200-cm AL). Three of these patients underwent elongation of the CL, and 2 restoration. Late sporadic PM occurred in 4 patients (1.4%) in the same group. These figures make BPD, in our hands, not only the most effective but also the safest (lowest revision rate) of all the existing bariatric procedures.

MINOR OR RARE LATE COMPLICATIONS

Among the 1,804 AHS BPD patients with a minimum follow-up of 2 years, the following minor or rare complications were observed or reported: 80 (4.4%) cases of impairment or appearance of hemorrhoids, 29 (1.6%) cases of anal rhagades, 9 (0.5%) cases of perianal abscess, 58 (3.2%) cases of acne, 12 (0.7%) cases of inguino-perineal furuncolosis, 46 (2.5%) cases of night blindness, 4 cases of lipothymias from hypoglycemia, 2 cases of transient dumping syndrome, 1 case of bypass arthritis, and 1 case of gallstone ileus. These complications showed a decreasing incidence in our population of operated patients. Anyway, they occur more rarely as time passes and tend to disappear in the long term.

Halitosis after BPD could be due either to food stagnation in a virtually achloridric stomach, which can be avoided by correct execution of the GEA, or to pulmonary expiration of ill-smelling substances resulting from malabsorption, the oral administration of pancreatic enzymes being of use in these cases. This unpleasant side effect has also become less common in our series, currently affecting less than 5% of the operated patients.

BPD causes oxalate hyperabsorption, but not hyperoxaluria, though oxalate urinary excretion in the operated patients is significantly higher than in controls.[69] The procedure can then be considered a remote cause of kidney stone formation, keeping in mind that not even hyperoxaluria can cause this complication in the absence of cofactors, the first of which is decreased urinary volume from dehydration. The incidence of kidney stones in our series (5/1,804 or 0.3%) does not differ from that of the general population. Thirty-two needle kidney biopsies obtained at long-term relaparotomy in BPD patients failed to demonstrate any microscopic or ultrastructural alterations (unpublished data: study in cooperation with Dr. Thomas Stanley, VA Hospital, Los Angeles, CA, 1984).

LATE MORTALITY

Specific late mortality consisted of eight cases of PM (inadequately treated elsewhere) and one case of Wernicke's encephalopathy. Semispecific mortality (i.e., the operation being a remote cause of death) included eight cases of alcoholic cirrhosis (the pharmacological effect of alcohol is enhanced by the distal gastrectomy due to more rapid intestinal absorption) and four cases of obstruction of the biliopancreatic limb (late or no diagnosis elsewhere).

LAPAROSCOPIC BILIOPANCREATIC DIVERSION

One hundred and forty-three subjects underwent laparoscopic BPD between March 2000 and May 2003.[70] The surgical technique was the one described above, with the exception of the first six cases, who had a GEA performed according to the technique described by Gagner[71] using a 25-mm circular stapler. This technique was abandoned due to the difficulty with introducing the 25-mm stapler into the distal ileum. Moreover, we detected a high incidence of

stenosis of the gastroileal anastomosis. Conversion to open surgery was necessary for 7 cases (3 of whom were treated with Gagner's technique) in the first 24 (9%) patients and for no case in the last consecutive 119 operated patients.

There were 25 males and 118 females. Mean age at operation was 34 years (18–57), mean weight was 120 kg (range 80–192), mean excess weight was 106% (64–186%), and mean BMI was 44 (range 35–61). Mean follow-up was 36 months (max. 74). Early complications were three wound infections (all after conversion) and four stomal ulcers. Late complications were three GEA stenosis (two with Gagner's technique); six stomal ulcers; one PM, seven incisional hernias; two intestinal obstructions (one due to internal hernia). Mean loss of the preoperative excess weight was 62% in the 119 subjects at 1 year, 71% in the 99 at 2 years, 68% in the 71 at 3 years, 70% in the 45 at 4 years, and 73% in the 23 subjects at 5 years. The other beneficial effects (specific and nonspecific) were the same as in the open series.

The similarity of these results to the ones obtained in the open series allows us to believe that the long-term outcome of laparoscopic BPD will be the same as that of the laparotomic. An exception is represented by the strikingly higher incidence of stomal ulcer, with 2.8% appearance as an early complication, which is an exceptional event in the open series. This could be interpreted as a negative effect of the learning curve, with too high dissection of the greater curve (see above).[11]

BAROS EVALUATION

In order to assess BPD outcome according to the BAROS criteria,[72] on December 2000, we sent out a questionnaire to the first consecutive 1,800 AHS BPD subjects with a minimum follow-up of 2 years (max. 14 years). The response rate was 51%. The mean total score was 5.1 ± 2.2, which represents a very good result according the outcome group scoring key. In details, 3% of patients were classified as *failures*, while results were *fair* in 11%, *good* in 23%, *very good* in 40%, and *excellent* in 23% of cases.

When the AHS group was compared with the AHS–AHAL group, the results were: failure 6%, fair 11%, good 24%, very good 36%, and excellent 23% in the first group; failure 2%, fair 6%, good 20%, very good 47%, and excellent 25% in the second group. Mean reduction of the IEW at the maximum follow-up for each subject (2–14 years) was 71% in the first group and 65% in the second group, with a revision rate of 9% in the first group and 1% in the second. Particularly, the increase in the "quality of life" score (0.8 in the first group and 1.3 in the second, $p < .001$) shows greater patients' satisfaction, despite lower weight loss, in the AHS–AHAL BPD patients.

A random sample of 100 nonresponder patients were reached by phone and asked about their satisfaction with the operation. Eighty-seven of the interviewees, independently of the different reasons why the questionnaire had not been sent back, declared to be pleased with their BPD, thus proving the reliability of the examined sample.

CONCLUSIONS

The studies carried out during the last years have greatly enlarged our knowledge of the physiology of BPD. Such knowledge has enabled us to make better use of the procedure, thereby improving its cost/benefit ratio considerably.

Biliopancreatic diversion is unanimously considered the most effective procedure for the surgical treatment of obesity. Like any other powerful weapon, it can be dangerous if used improperly. Twenty-seven years of careful investigation and clinical experience made it, in our hands, also a very safe remedy. It was a very a long "learning curve," consisting essentially of increasingly adapting the operation to the patient's individual characteristics, so the best weight loss results be reserved to the subjects at low risk of nutritional complications, accepting less weight reduction in the less compliant patients to minimize potential nutritional problems.

Our criteria of assessment are based on our personal experience with our cohort of patients, and therefore they are largely subjective; on the other hand, to try to standardize them would be of little use when dealing with a different population. All surgeons willing to obtain the best results with BPD should follow our example, finding the criteria to be used to adapt the operation to the patients in their population according to their individual characteristics. The flexibility of the procedure is such that, theoretically, the best combination of stomach volume and intestinal lengths could be identified for each patient. Obviously, the adaptation must be based on a profound knowledge of all the mechanisms of action of BPD, which are sufficiently understood today to allow any good-will surgeon to obtain the best results at the lowest price in all patients.

References

1. Scopinaro N: Intervento in Tavola rotonda su: Trattamento medico-chirurgico della obesità grave. *Accad Med* 88–89:215–234, 1974.
2. Halverson JD, Scheff RJ, Gentry K, et al.: Jeunoileal bypass. Late metabolic sequelae and weight gain. *Am J Surg* 140:347–350, 1980.
3. MacLean LD, Rhode BM: Surgical treatment of obesity: metabolic implications. In: Griffen WO, Printen KJ (eds.): *Surgical Management of Morbid Obesity*. New York, Marcel Dekker, 1987; p. 205–233.
4. Scopinaro N, Gianetta E, Civalleri D, et al.: Bilio-pancreatic by-pass for obesity, I: An experimental study in dogs. *Br J Surg* 66:613–617, 1979.
5. Scopinaro N, Gianetta E, Civalleri D, et al.: Bilio-pancreatic by-pass for obesity, II: Initial experience in man. *Br J Surg* 66:619–620, 1979.
6. Scopinaro N, Gianetta E, Adami GF, et al.: Biliopancreatic diversion for obesity at eighteen years. *Surgery* 119:261–268, 1996.
7. Scopinaro N, Adami GF, Marinari GM, et al.: Biliopancreatic diversion. *World J Surg* 22:936–946, 1998.
8. Scopinaro N, Gianetta E, Friedman D, et al.: Evolution of biliopancreatic bypass. *Clin Nutr* 5(Suppl):137–146, 1986.
9. Koopmans HS, Sclafani A: Control of body weight by lower gut signals. *Int J Obes* 5:491–494, 1981.
10. Gianetta E, Civalleri D, Bonalumi U, et al.: Studio dell'assorbimento lipidico dopo bypass biliopancreatico per l'obesità. *Min Diet e Gastr* 27:65–70, 1981.
11. Scopinaro N, Gianetta E, Civalleri D, et al.: Biliopancreatic diversion. In: Griffen WO, Printen, KJ (eds.): *Surgical Management of Morbid Obesity*. New York, Marcel Dekker, 1987; p. 93–162.
12. Gianetta E, Civalleri D, Bonalumi U, et al.: Studio dell'assorbimento proteico dopo bypass bilio-pancreatico per l'obesità. *Min Diet e Gastr* 26:251–256, 1980.
13. Bonalumi U, Moresco L, Gianetta E, et al.: Il tempo di transito intestinale nel bypass biliopancreatico. *Min Chir* 35:993–996, 1980.
14. Sarson DL, Scopinaro N, Bloom SR: Gut hormone changes after jeunoileal or biliopancreatic bypass surgery for morbid obesity. *Int J Obes* 5:513–518, 1981.
15. Scopinaro N, Marinari GM, Adami GF, et al.: The influence of gastric volume on energy and protein absorption after BPD. *Obes Surg* 2:125–126, 1999.
16. Scopinaro N, Gianetta E, Civalleri D, et al.: Two years of clinical experience with biliopancreatic bypass for obesity. *Amer J Clin Nutr* 33:506–514, 1980.
17. Bonalumi U, Cafiero F, Caponnetto A, et al.: Protein absorption studies in biliopancreatic bypass patients. *Int J Obes* 5:543, 1981.
18. Friedman D, Caponnetto A, Gianetta E, et al.: Protein absorption (PA) and protein malnutrition (PM) after biliopancreatic diversion (BPD). In: *Proceedings of the Third International Symposium on Obesity Surgery*. Genoa, Italy, September 1987; p. 20–23.
19. Scopinaro N, Marinari GM, Gianetta E, et al.: The respective importance of the alimentary limb (AL) and the common limb (CL) in protein absorption (PA) after BPD. *Obes Surg* 7:108, 1997.
20. Scopinaro N, Marinari GM, Camerini G, et al: Energy and nitrogen absorption after biliopancreatic diversion. *Obes Surg* 10:436–441, 2000.
21. Adami GF, Campostano A, Bessarione D et al.: Resting energy expenditure in long-term postobese subjects after weight normalization by dieting or biliopancreatic diversion. *Obes Surg* 3:397–399, 1993.
22. Greco AV, Tatarranni PA, Tacchino RM, et al.: Daily energy expenditure in postobese patients. *Int J Obes* 17:27, 1993.
23. Marinari G, Simonelli A, Friedman D, et al.: Very long-term assessment of subjects with "half-half" biliopancreatic diversion. *Obes Surg* 5:124, 1995.
24. Adami GF, Campostano A, Gandolfo P, et al.: Body composition and energy expenditure in obese patients prior to and following biliopancreatic diversion for obesity. *Eur Surg Res* 28:295–298, 1996.
25. Nelson KM, Weinsier RL, Long CL, et al.: Prediction of resting energy expenditure from fat-free mass and fat mass. *Am J Clin Nutr* 56:848–856, 1992.
26. Holliday MA: Metabolic rate and organ size during growth from infancy to adolescence and during late gestation and early infancy. *Pediatrics* 47:101–117, 1971.
27. Dowling RH: Small bowel adaptation and its regulation. *Scand J Gastroenterol* 74(Suppl):53–75, 1982.
28. Stock-Damgé C, Aprahamian M, Raul F, et al.: Small intestinal and colonic changes after biliopancreatic bypass for morbid obesity. *Scand J Gastroenterol* 21:1115–1123, 1986.
29. Evrard S, Aprahamian M, Hoeltzel A, et al.: Trophic and enzymatic adaptation of the intestine to biliopancreatcic bypass in the rat. *Int J Obes* 17:541–547, 1993.
30. Scopinaro N, Gianetta E, Adami GF, et al.: Recenti acquisizioni fisiopatologiche e nuove strategie d'uso nella diversione biliopancreatica. In: *Proceedings of the "Novantottesimo Congresso della Società Italiana di Chirurgia.*, Rome, October 13–16, 1966; 2: p. 37–62.
31. Scopinaro N, Adami GF, Marinari G, et al.: The effect of biliopancreatic diversion on glucose metabolism. *Obes Surg* 7:296–297, 1997.
32. Marinari G, Adami GF, Camerini G, et al.: The effect of biliopancreatic diversion on serum cholesterol. *Obes Surg* 7:297, 1997.
33. Scopinaro N, Sarson DL, Civalleri D, et al.: Changes in plasma gut hormones after biliopancreatic bypass for obesity. A preliminary report. *Ital J Gastroenterol* 12:93–96, 1980.
34. Randle PJ, Newsholme EA, Garland PB: Regulation of glucose uptake by muscle. 8. Effects of fatty acids, ketone bodies and pyruvate, and of alloxan-diabetes and starvation, on the uptake and metabolic fate of glucose in rat heart and diaphragm muscles. *Biochem J* 93:652–665, 1964.

35. Randle PJ, Garland PB, Newsholme EA, et al.: The glucose fatty acid cycle in obesity and maturity onset diabetes mellitus. *Ann N Y Acad Sci* 131:324–333, 1965.

36. Stromblad G, Bjorntorp P: Reduced hepatic insulin clearance in rats with dietary-induced obesity. *Metabolism* 35:323–327, 1986.

37. Peiris AN, Mueller RA, Smith GA, et al.: Splanchnic insulin metabolism in obesity. Influence of body fat distribution. *J Clin Invest* 78:1648–1657, 1986.

38. Gianetta E, Friedman D, Adami GF, et al.: Effects of biliopancreatic bypass on hypercholesterolemia and hypertriglyceridemia. In: *Proceedings of the Second Annual Meeting of the American Society for Bariatric Surgery*, Iowa City, IA, June 13–14, 1985; p. 138–142.

39. Montagna G, Gianetta E, Elicio N, et al.: Plasma lipid and apoprotein pattern in patients with morbid obesity before and after biliopancreatic bypass. *Atheroscl Cardiovasc Dis* 3:1069–1074, 1987.

40. Scopinaro N, Marinari GM, Camerini GB, et al.: Specific effects of biliopancreatic diversion on the major components of metabolic syndrome. *Diab Care* 28:2406–2411, 2005.

41. Gasbarrini G, Mingrone G, Greco AV, et al.: An 18-year-old woman with familial chylomicronaemia who would not stick to a diet. *Lancet* 348:794, 1996.

42. Mingrone G, Henriksen FL, Greco AV, et al.: Triglyceride-induced diabetes associated with familial lipoprotein lipase deficiency. *Diabetes* 48:1258–1263, 1999.

43. Adami GF, Civalleri D, Gianetta E, et al.: In vivo evaluation of immunological status after biliopancreatic bypass for obesity. *Int J Obes* 9:171–175, 1985.

44. Adami GF, Barreca A, Gianetta E, et al.: Body composition in subjects with surgically obtained stable body weight normalization. *Int J Obes* 13:55–58, 1989.

45. Friedman D, Cuneo S, Valenzano M, et al.: Pregnancies in an 18-year follow-up after biliopancreatic diversion. *Obes Surg* 5:308–313, 1995.

46. Friedman D, Traverso E, Adami G, et al.: Incisional hernias following biliopancreatic diversion (BPD). *Obes Surg* 6:304, 1996.

47. Gianetta E, Friedman D, Traverso E, et al.: Small bowel obstruction after biliopancreatic diversion. *Probl Gen Surg* 9:386–389, 1992.

48. Civalleri D, Scopinaro G, Gianetta E, et al.: Assorbimento della vitamina B_{12} dopo bypass biliopancreatico per l'obesità. *Min Diet Gastroenterol* 28:181–188, 1982.

49. Mann FC, Williamson CS: The experimental production of peptic ulcer. *Ann Surg* 77:409–422, 1923.

50. Mason EE, Ito C: Gastric bypass in obesity. *Surg Clin North Am* 47:1345–1352, 1967.

51. Storer EH, Woodward ER, Dragstedt LR: The effect of vagotomy and antrum resection on the Mann-Williamson ulcer. *Surgery* 27:526–530, 1950.

52. Scopinaro N, Gianetta E, Friedman D, et al.: Biliopancreatic diversion for obesity. *Probl Gen Surg* 9:362–379, 1992.

53. Civalleri D, Gianetta E, Friedman D, et al.: Changes of gastric acid secretion after partial biliopancreatic bypass. *Clin Nutr* 5(Suppl):215–220, 1986.

54. Gianetta E, Friedman D, Adami GF, et al.: Present status of biliopancreatic diversion (BPD). In: *Proceedings of the Third International Symposium on Obesity Surgery.* Genoa, Italy, September, 20–23, 1987; p. 11–13.

55. Adami GF, Gandolfo P, Esposito M, et al.: Orally-administered serum ranitidine concentration after biliopancreatic diversion. *Obes Surg* 1:293–294, 1991.

56. Compston JE, Vedi S, Gianetta E, et al.: Bone histomorphometry and vitamin D status after biliopancreatic bypass for obesity. *Gastroenterology* 87:350–356, 1984.

57. Compston JE, Vedi S, Watson GJ, et al.: Metabolic bone disease in patients with biliopancreatic bypass. *Clin Nutr* 5(Suppl): 221–224, 1986.

58. Adami GF, Compston JE, Gianetta E, et al.: Changes in bone histomorphometry following biliopancreatic diversion. In: *Proceedings of the III International Symposium on Obesity Surgery*, Genoa, Italy, September, 20–23, 1987; p. 46–47.

59. Williams JA: Effects of upper gastro-intestinal surgery on blood formation and bone metabolism. *Br J Surg* 51:125–134, 1964.

60. Eddy RL: Metabolic bone disease after gastrectomy. *Am J Med* 8:293–302, 1984.

61. Fisher AB: Twenty-five years after Billroth II gastrectomy for duodenal ulcer. *World J Surg* 8:293–302, 1984.

62. Crowley LV, Seay J, Mullin GT Jr, et al.: Long term hematopoietic and skeletal effects of gastric bypass. *Clin Nutr* 5(Suppl):185–187, 1986.

63. Marceau P, Biron S, Lebel S, et al.: Does bone change after biliopancreatic diversion? *J Gastrointest Surg* 6:690–698, 2002.

64. Fox SR: The use of biliopancreatic diversion as a treatment for failed gastric partitioning in the morbidly obese. *Obes Surg* 1:89–93, 1991.

65. Chapin BL, LeMar, HJ, Jr, Knodel DH, et al.: Secondary hyperparathyroidism following biliopancreatic diversion. *Arch Surg* 131:1048–1053.

66. Primavera A, Schenone A, Simonetti S, et al.: Neurological disorders following biliopancreatic diversion. In: *Proceedings of the Third International Symposium on Obesity Surgery*, Genoa, Italy, September, 20–23, 1987; p. 48–49.

67. Gianetta E, Friedman D, Adami GF, et al.: Etiological factors of protein malnutrition after biliopancreatic diversion. *Gastroenterol Clin North Am* 16:503–504, 1987.

68. Scopinaro N, Gianetta E, Friedman D, et al.: Surgical revision of biliopancreatic bypass. *Gastroenterol Clin North Am* 16:529–531, 1987.

69. Hofmann AF, Schnuck G, Scopinaro N, et al.: Hyperoxaluria associated with intestinal bypass surgery for morbid obesity: Occurrence, pathogenesis and approaches to treatment. *Int J Obes* 5:513–518, 1981.

70. Scopinaro N, Marinari GM, Camerini G: Laparoscopic standard biliopancreatic diversion: Technique and preliminary results. *Obes Surg* 12:362–365, 2002.

71. Ren GJ, Patterson E, Gagner M: Early results of laparoscopic biliopancreatic diversion with duodenal switch: A case series of 40 consecutive patients. *Obes Surg* 10:514–523, 2000.

72. Oria HE, Moorehead MK: Bariatric analysis and reporting outcome system (BAROS). *Obes Surg* 8:487–499, 1998.

14

Malabsorptive Procedures: Duodenal Switch

Picard Marceau, MD, PhD • Simon Biron, MD, MSc • Frédéric-Simon Hould, MD •
Stéfane Lebel, MD • Simon Marceau, MD • Odette Lescelleur, MD •
Christine Simard, MD • Serge Simard, MSc

Our understanding of the physiological basis underlying biliopancreatic diversion (BPD) has evolved during the last two decades. Initially, 25 years ago, when presented by Scopinaro and his colleagues, the procedure was seen as a simple technique to decrease caloric absorption particularly by decreasing fat absorption. Shortening the gut and controlling the action of bile were the two fundamental mechanisms on which the procedure was based. The reversibility of the procedure and the fact that normal eating habits were preserved made the procedure very appealing. Later, another major mechanism was discovered. Absence of food in the first part of the gut decreases levels of hormones (known to be involved in the development of obesity and diabetes) secreted by this part of the gut. At the same time, food diverted directly into the last part of the gut increases levels of hormones (known to decrease insulin secretion and to help prevent obesity) secreted by this segment. These hormonal

changes, which directly affect the cause of obesity, are an additional reason to prefer this approach.[1]

Convinced from our clinical experience that morbid obesity is a metabolic disease, rather than due to abnormal eating habits, BPD became our procedure of choice and helped demonstrate that obesity is indeed a disease of the gut. BPD is a procedure intended to change the pathology underlying morbid obesity.

Removing bile from the outlet of the stomach is an ulcerogenic procedure.[2] To prevent ulcers, it was initially suggested that BPD be accompanied by a partial gastrectomy, which was the classic ulcer preventing procedure at the time, in similar circumstances. Later it was shown that replacing distal gastrectomy by a sleeve gastrectomy (SG) and a duodenal switch better preserved normal gastric physiology, without interfering with the basic function of the procedure. The changes meant same weight loss without compromising the

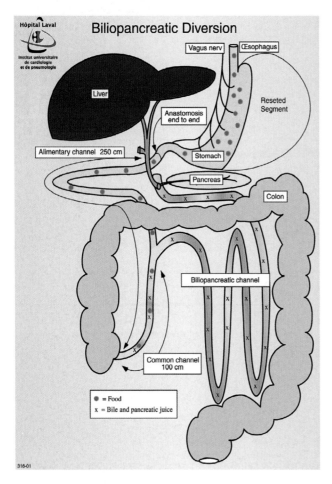

Figure 14–1. Duodenal switch.

and lesser protein deficiency compared to a 50-cm channel, and it has also been shown that the SG causes less side effects, such as dumping, than does the distal gastrectomy. We consider these two matters as settled not only from the available data but also because these changes are so physiologically sound that until new challenging data are presented there is no interest in debating the question.

On the other hand, there are no data comparing different lengths of the "alimentary channel." For convenience, we have used the 250-cm channel as suggested by Scopinaro.[6] However, we are conscious that in the future, for better results, it may become apparent that other factors should be considered in setting the length of the "alimentary channel."

Many other questions remain unanswered about duodenal switch (DS), for example: Is there a need for individualization of intestinal length? Is gastric resection always necessary? How much stomach should be resected? In the long term, is food ingestion decreased after gastric resection? Until better data are available our best source of information remains our clinical experience. In the absence of a prospective study, we are limited to retrospective studies and search for data that could help understand the physiology involved. In this chapter, we report four clinical situations that provide valuable information on how DS works:

1. The first situation was the failure of stapled duodenum; this revealed the predominant role of the bypass itself in producing both the early loss and its maintenance.
2. The second source of information was the retrospective study of revisions for either excessive or insufficient weight loss. It showed that precision in the measurement of intestinal lengths is unrealistic and unnecessary.
3. A third source of information was from the study of a gastric specimen removed during surgery. We can demonstrate that the extent of the resection did not influence long-term results.
4. Finally, other information came from our experience with simple gastrectomy versus intestinal bypass (IB) for the first stage of a two-stage duodenal switch.

Each of these clinical experiences has contributed to our comprehension of DS physiology.

FAILURE OF A STAPLED DUODENUM

In 1990, while very pleased with our 6 years of experience with Scopinaro's BPD, we felt that avoiding distal gastrectomy and its side effects would improve the procedure. We decided to preserve the pylorus and do a SG and a duodenal switch as proposed by Demeester for alkaline gastritis.[7] Since it was an innovative procedure, in the context of bariatric surgery, for greater safety and reversibility, we did not section the duodenum but only obstructed the normal duodenal pathway with a stapling device. And just proximal to the obstructed duodenum a new food passage was constructed by an end-to-side ileo duodenal anastomosis (Figure 14–2). Unfortunately, over a period of time, the normal duodenal

basic function of the procedure and produced fewer side effects. The procedure was called "duodenal switch" and represents a variant of the conventional BPD (Figure 14–1). It has the same fundamental physiologic mechanism with fewer side effects.[3–5]

BPD has three components, and all three have both positive and negative effects. The components are as follows: (1) the length of gut left in contact with food: the "alimentary channel"; (2) the length of intestine where bile is allowed to be involved in the digestive process: the "common channel"; (3) the size of the remaining stomach: the "gastric remnant." All three factors individually and concomitantly influence weight loss, side effects, as well as complications.

The ideal construction of a BPD is not yet established. It is not known whether it would be preferable to individualize the construction, according to certain patient characteristics such as age, sex, height, BMI, etc. There are no data relating any of the three components of the BPD with long-term results. Evaluation is difficult since one must balance maintained weight loss against subjective and objective side effects and short- and long-term complications. Even if good randomized long-term series existed, the subjective aspect related to "quality of life" remains unevaluated.

It has already been shown[3,4] that a 100-cm common channel produces the same weight loss with lesser diarrhea

Parietal Gastrectomy & Duodenal Switch

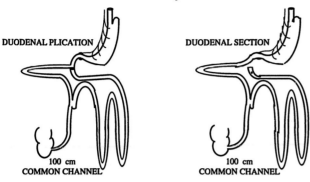

Figure 14–2. Duodenal switch with stapled or sectioned duodenum.

pathway reopened (partially or totally) in some patients, letting food and bile pass through and thus making the bypass nonfunctional. The reopening was a slow process whose major impact became evident only after 2 years. Many patients did not obtain adequate weight loss while others started regaining weight.[8,9] In subsequent operations, the duodenum was sectioned instead of being clamped. There were 216 patients who had the DS done with the clamping method.

Patients were appropriately informed and together we decided to let nature take its course and not do systematic search. When it was evident that recanalization had occurred, the patients were reoperated to section the duodenum exactly where it had been clamped initially. In most cases, the reopening process was asymptomatic but manifested by inadequate weight loss.

Out of the 216 patients, 158 (73%) required duodenum closure. In 63 patients (29%), the expected initial weight loss did not occur. In 95 patients (44%), weight regain occurred after the expected weight loss. In 58 patients (27%), secondary closure was not necessary since the weight loss was maintained or there was no endoscopic and radiologic evidence of dehiscence. After the secondary duodenal closure, patients' weight loss resumed but did not reach the loss obtained after primary duodenal closure. The reason for this is not clear (Table 14–1).

This experience showed that the IB itself contributes not only to the maintenance of weight but is also responsible for the "initial weight loss." It is evident that in a DS, we create a short gut syndrome. Leaving only 250 cm of intestine in contact with food creates a temporary insufficient absorption causing weight loss until natural mechanisms succeed in improving absorption and stop the weight loss. This is the basis of this procedure. The gastric resection increases early weight loss but does little to maintain the loss.

EXPERIENCE WITH REVISIONS

Our experience with revisions done to increase or decrease the effect of duodenal switch provided another source of information. Out of 1,171 patients, after 8 years of follow-up, it was found that 21 patients (1.8%) have been reoperated for insufficient weight loss and 7 (0.6%) for malabsorption. When revision was done to increase weight loss in the 21 patients, the alimentary channel was found to be much longer than expected. In 19 patients, the length of both the alimentary and the common channels were found to be more than 40% longer than the expected 250/100 cm. On the other hand, in 7 patients when revisions were done to decrease malabsorption, all measurements of both channels were found to be within 15%, the expected 250/100 cm representing the normal variation of different measuring techniques. In cases of excessive weight regain, we interpret these findings to mean that the lengthening of the channels was not due to different measuring techniques but was due to a compensatory mechanism. On the contrary, in the cases of excessive malabsorption, there was no compensatory lengthening. Initial faulty measurement remains a possible explanation, but in our opinion very unlikely.

When revision was done to increase weight loss, three different approaches were used. In 12 patients, channels were shortened to the conventional 250/100. This caused an

Table 14–1.

Failure of Stapled Duodenum*

	n	Weight Loss (kg)	% Weight Loss	Follow Up (mo)
Pts with clamped duodenum	216	37.0 ± 18.4	29.7 ± 12.0	160.7
Pts with second closure	158	35.4 ± 17.8	28.6 ± 12.0	161.5
Pts without second closure	58	41.3 ± 19.2	32.7 ± 11.6	161.0
Pts with primary closure	229	45.2 ± 22.0	34.3 ± 10.9	133.5

*In some patients submitted to a duodenal switch, the duodenum was obstructed by staple line instead of being sectioned. With time the duodenum reopened, weight loss stopped, and patients regained weight. Once the duodenum was closed again, weight loss resumed, without reaching the level of loss obtained after primary duodenal closure. The reason for that is not clear.

additional loss of 13 ± 8 kg. In 5 patients, in addition to shortening the channels to 250/100, an additional piece of stomach was removed along the greater curvature. This caused an additional loss of 12.8 ± 7.4 kg. Finally in 4 patients, instead of shortening the gut only an additional SG was done. This caused an additional weight loss of 10.5 ± 6.8 kg. There was no relation between the changes in intestinal length and the subsequent weight loss.

When revision was done to improve absorption in 7 patients, both channels were lengthened. The common channel was doubled to a mean of 212 cm (range 150–325 cm) and the alimentary channel lengthened by a third to a mean of 334 cm (range 250–460 cm). These changes corrected the malabsorption but produced only a small weight gain of 6.7 ± 9 kg. Here again, there was no relation between the amount of intestine lengthened and the subsequent weight gain.

We found two important sources of information in this clinical experience. One was the great variation in the individual capacity to recover from a "too short" intestine. Most patients will increase absorption to meet their needs and a few will not or will remain borderline; while others will over compensate the shortening. The second point was that precise measurements of limbs are not necessary. Within certain limits, individual capacity to recover from intestinal shortening makes variations in measuring techniques less important.

Of the two channels, the common and the alimentary, greater attention should be given to the common, which is responsible for the steatorrhea. Being shorter, its capacity to lengthen is more limited. The alimentary channel need only be short enough to decrease absorption but long enough to remain within the range of compensation. In our view, it is this individual compensatory mechanism, which makes using the same measurements appropriate for all patients.

EXTENT OF STOMACH REMOVED

More information came from studying the amount of stomach removed and its effect on weight loss and protein absorption. We do not routinely measure the size of the stomach left in place and it varies between surgeons. To see whether extended gastric resection contributed to long-term weight loss, we looked at the weight of the stomach removed (available on the pathology report) and the actual weight loss of these patients. We studied 504 consecutive "duodenal switches" performed more than 5 years earlier.

Since male stomachs are bigger, specimens from men were heavier (137 ± 36 g versus 106 ± 29 g, $p < 0.0001$). Specimens were also weakly related to patients' weight ($r = 0.34$, $p < 0.0001$), height ($r = 0.32$, $p < 0.0001$), and BMI ($r = 0.21$, $p < 0.0001$) in both men and women, accounting for about 10% in the variation. For all practical purposes, there was no relation between the amount of stomach removed and the long-term weight loss. After 8 years, the variation in the weight of the resected stomach explained less than 2% of the variation in the long-term weight loss.

On the other hand, considering the important role of the stomach in protein digestion [10,11] and the advantage in preserving it, we looked for a relationship between the extent of resection and the future risk of protein deficiency. Protein deficiency was defined as the risk of having had a serum albumin level below 32 gm/L anytime, during follow up. This has been seen in 22% of patients. The more the stomach removed, the greater the risk of protein deficiency. For each additional 25 gm of stomach removed, the risk was increased by 32% in men and by 66% in women ($p < 0.03$). In women the prevalence of incidental hypoalbuminemia increased from 16 to 28.6%, depending on whether the stomach removed was in the lower or the upper third.

This clinical observation speaks in favour of limiting the gastric resection, which does not contribute greatly to long-term weight loss but may compromise protein absorption. We need longer follow up to evaluate the indication to do re-resection in cases of revision as it has been proposed.[12]

EXPERIENCE WITH TWO-STAGE DUODENAL SWITCH

Another experience helped better understand the respective roles of the intestinal switch itself versus gastrectomy. In rare circumstances, to decrease the surgical risk of a complete procedure, it may be indicated to perform it in two stages. This raises a question: What should be done first? Among 892 consecutive DS, this situation was met on 20 occasions (2.2%). IB was done first on 16 occasions and SG alone on 4 occasions. Despite the limited number of cases and the complexity of each situation, a review of these patients helped better understand the respective role of the two components in a DS. The main reasons for choosing a two-stage procedure are given in Table 14–2. In 11 patients, the decision was made before

Table 14–2.

Reason for Choosing a Two-Stage Duodenal Switch

	Decision Before Surgery	Decision During Surgery
Intestinal bypass only ($n = 16$) (IB)	7 severe medical problem 2 strangulated inc hernia	3 technical difficulties 2 cirrhosis 2 carcinoid
Sleeve gastrectomy only ($n = 4$) (SG)	1 fecal incontinence 1 revision gastroplasty	1 carcinoid 1 cirrhosis

In 20 patients, it was decided to do a two-stage duodenal switch. The decision was made before surgery in 11 patients and at laparatomy in 9 patients. In most patients, the clinical situation was complex and many factors were involved.

Table 14–3.

Clinical Characteristics of Patients Submitted to Intestinal Bypass Alone Versus Gastrectomy Alone as the First Stage of a Two-Stage Duodenal Switch

	Intestinal Bypass (n = 16)	Sleeve Gastrectomy (n = 4)
Sex F/M	9/7	2/2
Age (mean, years)	56.8 ± 12.0	45.9 ± 12.3
>60 yrs	10	1
BMI (mean, kg/m²)	50.2 ± 7.1	47.6 ± 16.5
Diabetes	12	1
with insulin	9	0
HTA	15	2
Sleep apnea	11	2
Dyslipidemia	9	1
Cirrhosis	4	1
Follow up (mo, mean)	21.9 ± 15.4	30 ± 20.7

As the first stage of a two-stage duodenal switch, a group had the intestinal bypass (IB) without the gastrectomy and the other group, only the sleeve gastrectomy (SG) without the intestinal bypass. The characteristics of each group are presented. IB group was heavier, sicker, and older.

surgery and in 9 patients the decision was made after laparotomy findings. In most patients, the situation was complex with more than one reason for choosing the two-stage approach. Age was often a deciding factor.

Clinical characteristics of the two groups are presented in Table 14–3. The IB group was heavier, older, and sicker with more comorbidities. IB alone rather than gastrectomy alone gave better results both in terms of weight loss and improvement in comorbidities. For IB patients, the second stage has not been necessary even after 5 years.

For both IB and SG groups, early weight loss (within the first 6 months) was about the same, between 20–35 kg. But after a year, 3 of the 4 SG patients started to regain weight: during the second year they gained 14, 23, and 26 kg, respectively. Only 1 of the 2 SG patients, with a follow up greater than 2 years, has maintained a weight loss (26.6 kg). All 6 IB patients, with a follow up greater than 2 years, have maintained their loss, which averages 39.9 kg; 4 have been followed for more than 3 years.

The effect on comorbidities was also much greater in the IB group. Dyslipidemia present in 9 IB patients resolved in all cases but not in the one with dylipidemia in the SG group. Sleep apnea in all 16 IB patients was cured or improved. It

was improved in only 1 out of 2 in SG patients. Non-insulin-dependant diabetes was similarly cured or partly improved in both groups. All 9 IB patients who had been taking insulin were able to discontinue it. Hypertension was only partly improved in both groups.

Patients in IB groups required appropriate follow up. Diarrhea (not requiring treatment) was present in 1 patient. Ulcer-preventing medication and supplements (vitamins, calcium, and iron) were supervised. None of the patients complained of hyperacidity symptoms, and for them to take antiulcer medication requires insistence. It has been reported that DS alone without gastrectomy is followed by as much as 30% incidence of peptic ulcer.[13] We have no explanation for this major difference. Our experience with SG alone was limited to only 4 cases. Our "early" results were similar to those reported by others.[14–16] It is with longer follow up that the procedure failed. We do not think this to be a matter of technique.

The concordance between these four clinical experiences demonstrates that in a DS, the basic mechanism resides in the intestinal switch itself. The role of the gastrectomy is marginal. Shortening the intestine, decreasing the role of bile, and letting food enter directly into the distal intestine form the basis of this procedure. The gastrectomy increases early weight loss but only slightly influences the long-term weight maintenance. We consider using IB alone more often in older and sicker patients when the operative risk is high since gastric secretion decreases with age [17] and the danger of peptic ulcer is decreased.

CONCLUSION

These four observations emphasize the predominant role of the intestinal switch over the gastrectomy in the process of weight loss. This procedure is not based on food restriction. Its basic mechanisms are as follows: (1) the entrance of food directly into the distal gut, bypassing the proximal gut; (2) the decreased role of bile; (3) the creation of a short gut situation. This changes intestinal hormone secretion, decreases fat absorption, and forces nature itself to improve absorption until a new equilibrium is established. The capacity to improve absorption varies with individuals but it is usually within reach when about half the intestine remains.

Spontaneous reopening of the stapled duodenum stopped weight loss and caused weight regain despite the presence of a smaller stomach. A BPD without gastrectomy is as efficient in improving comorbidities even if weight loss is not as important (not shown here). The gastrectomy itself contributes little to the long-term weight maintenance. Increased gastric resection does not increase long-term weight loss but does increase the risk of protein deficiency.

In our opinion precise technique in measuring the alimentary channel (250 cm) is not very important. The capacity of each individual to compensate surpasses the variation in measuring technique. The 40% lengthening in the situations of insufficient weight loss and the absence of lengthening in the situations of malabsorption cannot be simply explained by inaccurate measurement. This conclusion is supported by the absence of correlation between change in length and the resulting weight loss after revisions. It is remarkable that a simple reversible switch of intestine is so efficient in correcting the disorder of morbid obesity. It represents a major contribution to the understanding of this disease and it demonstrates that morbid obesity is a disease of the gut.

References

1. Marceau P: Contribution of bariatric surgery to the comprehension of morbid obesity. *Obes Surg* 15:3–10, 2005.
2. Mann FC, Williamson CS: The experimental production of peptic ulcer. *Ann Surg* 77:409–422, 1923.
3. Marceau P, Hould FS, Simard S, et al.: Biliopancreatic diversion with duodenal switch. *World J. Surg* 22:947–954, 1998.
4. Marceau P, Hould FS, Lebel S, Marceau S, Biron S: Malabsorptive obesity surgery. *Surg Clin North Am* 81:1113–1127, 2001.
5. Marceau P, Biron S, Hould FS, Lebel S, Marceau S: Malabsorption procedure in surgical treatment of morbid obesity. In: *Problems in General Surgery.* Philadelphia, PA, Lipponcott Williams & Wilkins, 2000; 17: p. 29–39.
6. Scopinaro N, Gianetta E, Friedman D, Adami GF, Traverso E, Bachi V: Evolution of biliopancreatic bypass. *Clin Nutr* 5:137–146, 1986.
7. Demeester TR, Fuchs KH, Ball CS, Albertucci M, Smyrk TC, Marcus JN: Experimental and clinical results with proximal end-to-end duodeno jejunostomy for pathologic duodenogastric reflux. *Ann Surg* 206:414–426, 1987.
8. Marceau P, Biron S, Bourque RA, Potvin M, Hould FS, Simard S: Biliopancreatic diversion with a new type of gastrectomy. *Obes surg* 3:29–35, 1993.
9. Lagacé M, Marceau P, Marceau S, et al.: Biliopancreatic diversion with a new type of gastrectomy: Some previous conclusions revisited. *Obes Surg* 5:411–118, 1995.
10. Gianetta E, Friedman D, Adami GF, et al.: Etiologic factors of protein malnutrition after BPD. *Gastrpenterol Clin NA* 16:503–504, 1987.
11. Scopinaro N, Marinari GM, Adami GF, et al.: The influence of gastric volume on energy and protein absorption after BPD. *Obes Surg* 2:125–126, 1999.
12. Gagner M, Rogula T: Laparoscopic reoperative sleeve gastrectomy for poor weight loss after biliopancreatic diversion with duodenal switch. *Obes Surg* 13:649–654, 2003.
13. Cossu ML, Noya G, Tonolo GC, et al.: Duodenal switch without gastric resection: Results and observations after 6 years. *Obes Surg* 14:1354–1359, 2004.
14. Baltasar A, Serra C, Perez N, Bon R, Bengochea M, Ferri L: Laparoscopic sleeve gastrectomy: A multi-purpose bariatric operation. *Obes Surg* 15:1124–1128, 2005.
15. Almogy G, Crookes PF, Anthone GJ: Longitudinal gastrectomy as a treatment for the high-risk super-obese patient. *Obes surg* 14:492–497, 2004
16. Moonhan S, Kim WW, Oh JH: Results of laparoscopic sleeve gastrectomy at 1 year in morbidly obese Korean patients. *Obes Surg* 14:492–497, 2004.
17. Grossman MI, Kirsner JB, Gillespie IE: Basal and histalog-stimulated gastric secretion in control subjects and in patient with peptic ulcer or gastric cancer. *Gastroenterology* 45:14, 1963.

Possible Hormonal Mechanisms Mediating the Effects of Bariatric Surgery

David E. Cummings, MD • Karen E. Foster-Schubert, MD • Molly J. Carlson, MD •
Michael H. Shannon, MD • Joost Overduin, PhD

INTRODUCTION

The ever-worsening problem of obesity has become so prevalent and is so strongly associated with medical comorbidities and mortality that it has begun to overtake infectious diseases as the most significant contributor to ill health worldwide.[1–7] Despite the obvious public health benefits (and financial rewards) that would accrue from the development of truly effective pharmacotherapy for obesity, medical and behavioral approaches remain limited in their efficacy, facilitating no more than a 5–10% loss of body weight, and recidivism after even this modest weight loss is nearly universal.[8–11] A principal reason for this is that body weight is regulated by a powerful homeostatic system that, in response to weight loss, triggers compensatory changes in appetite and energy expenditure to promote weight regain.[12] Importantly, even minor weight loss confers disproportionate health benefits, in terms of ameliorating obesity-related comorbidities.[7] Thus, obese individuals benefit greatly from the mild weight loss that can often be achieved with medical/behavioral approaches; however, more substantial and durable weight reduction would clearly be of even greater value. Fortunately, body-weight regulation researchers have made stunning recent advances,[13] and it is widely hoped that these insights into the physiology of energy homeostasis will yield far more effective antiobesity pharmaceuticals in the future.

At present, however, bariatric surgery is the only method that dependably produces major, long-lasting weight loss.[14,15] In contrast to the transient 5–10% weight reduction typical of nonsurgical methods, modern bariatric operations can facilitate 35–40% loss of body weight, and most of this is maintained for at least 15 years.[14–19] Not surprisingly, such massive weight loss is accompanied by improvements in virtually every obesity-related complication yet studied.[10,15–18,20] This includes an almost miraculous resolution after certain procedures of diabetes mellitus (DM), which is traditionally considered a relentless, progressive disease. Selected operations completely reverse DM in over 80% of cases,[16–18,21–24] by mechanisms that very likely extend beyond the effects of weight reduction alone.[20,25]

The energy homeostasis system that normally constrains weight loss is evidently either overcome or circumvented by bariatric surgery, which improves body weight and glucose tolerance by mechanisms that are incompletely understood. Elucidating these mechanisms is a high priority, and as such knowledge should lead not only to the greater refinement of bariatric procedures but also, hopefully, to the ultimate harnessing of some of these capabilities into novel pharmaceuticals. Moreover, it is important to improve our understanding of bariatric surgery because the number of operations performed is increasing dramatically, e.g., in the United States the number increased from an estimated 29,000 in 1999 to over 100,000 in 2003.[26] In this chapter, we review the known and hypothesized mechanisms that mediate some of the impressive effects of bariatric surgery on body weight and diabetes, focusing particularly on the Roux-en-Y gastric bypass (RYGB), which, in the United States, is considered to be the gold-standard operation.[27]

TYPES OF BARIATRIC SURGERY

Intestinal malabsorption and gastric restriction are the two most obvious mechanisms to explain weight loss after bariatric surgery, and the types of operations are traditionally categorized based upon which of these changes they primarily induce. Malabsorptive procedures, including the former jejunoileal bypass (JIB)[28] and more modern biliopancreatic diversion (BPD) and duodenal switch duodenal switch, reconstruct the small intestine to reduce the area of mucosa available for nutrient absorption. BPD and duodenal switch causes at least as much long-term weight loss as does any bariatric operation,[14] but their complications are also greater than those following most other procedures.[15]

Purely restrictive bariatric operations promote weight loss by limiting gastric capacity and constricting the flow of ingested food. Gastroplasty is the classic example,[29] modified by Edward Mason and colleagues from the original horizontal-banded version to the improved vertical-banded gastroplasty (VBG).[30] Although VBG effectively limits the amount of food that can be consumed at one sitting and causes 30–50% reduction of excess body weight within the first 1–2 years, long-term results are often disappointing.[15]

Patients can accommodate to gastric restriction by eating frequent, small meals and calorie-dense foods, such as milkshakes.[14] A nearly 80% failure rate has been reported after 10 years,[31] and randomized, prospective trials as well as sequential, comparative studies consistently show that VBG is less effective than RYGB at inducing and maintaining weight loss.[17,18,32–36] Consequently, VBG has fallen out of favor[14,19] and has been replaced by another purely restrictive operation, adjustable gastric banding (AGB).[37,38] Approved for use in the United States in 2001, this operation is rapidly becoming more prevalent there, and it is the most common bariatric procedure in many other parts of the world. Essentially an adjustable variant of VBG, this approach offers the advantages of a gastric constriction that can be noninvasively titrated according to needs, a lack of anastomoses, and ease of laparoscopic placement. Weight loss after AGB is usually less impressive than that following RYGB, but short- and long-term complications are also less common.[14,17,18]

The modern RYGB resulted from several improvements upon a gastric bypass operation developed in 1969 by Mason and Ito,[39] who observed that postgastrectomy patients with a small residual gastric remnant experienced substantial weight loss. Results from RYBG are genuinely impressive. Patients typically lose 35–40% of total body weight, and most of this effect persists for at least 15 years.[14–19] As expected, such massive weight loss ameliorates almost all obesity-related morbidities, most notably DM.[16] Although RYGB creates significant gastric restriction, and malabsorption can also occur with long-limb variants, the precise mechanisms mediating the effects of this procedure on body weight and glucose homeostasis are not fully understood. (These will be discussed in detail later in this chapter.) The 1991 NIH Consensus Development Panel endorsed only VBG, gastric banding, and RYGB,[27] and the last of these has emerged as the most widely used bariatric operation in the United States.[40]

MECHANISMS CAUSING WEIGHT LOSS AFTER RYGB

Traditional Mechanisms: Gastric Restriction, Malabsorption, and Dumping

Although the mechanisms causing weight loss after purely malabsorptive or restrictive bariatric operations are readily apparent, less obvious physiologic changes may also contribute to the profound impact of RYGB on body weight and glucose homeostasis. Unquestionably, gastric restriction plays a role. Because of the reduced functional gastric capacity, post-RYGB patients experience early satiety, and consequently, they eat smaller meals.[41,42] If this were the only mechanism at work, however, the energy homeostasis system would drive patients to compensate with increased meal frequency and to favor calorie-dense foods, in response to massive weight loss. Instead, people who have undergone gastric bypass paradoxically eat fewer meals and snacks per day.[42,43] Similarly, in a rat model of RYGB, postsurgical animals lose weight by consuming not only smaller meals but also fewer of them.[44] Equally counter-intuitively, post-RYGB patients voluntarily restrict consumption of calorie-dense foods, such as fats, concentrated carbohydrates, ice cream, and sweetened beverages.[42,43] Presumably because of these changes in eating behavior, RYGB is more effective than VBG, even though the degree of gastric restriction (i.e., proximal pouch volume and stomal aperture) is at least as great or greater after VBG as after RYGB.[45] Randomized, prospective trials consistently demonstrate that RYGB causes 50–80% loss of excess body weight as opposed to only 30–50% loss after the equally restrictive VBG, and the former operation is also more effective at reducing appetite.[17,18,20,32–36] Moreover, weight loss resulting from RYGB is considerably more durable than that following VBG. Similarly, gastric bypass is usually more effective than AGB,[17,18,46] even though the degree of gastric restriction in the latter procedure can be increased essentially infinitely.

It is often hypothesized that RYGB produces more weight loss than does VBG because of malabsorption and/or dumping syndrome, which can result only from the former operation. Although some malabsorption does transiently occur even after a standard proximal RYGB, the portion of the small intestine still in digestive continuity (representing a majority of intestinal length) subsequently adapts with villous hypertrophy to increase absorption.[47–49] Consequently, clinically significant malabsorption—judged by indices such as levels of albumin, prealbumin, and fecal fat—is not observed after proximal RYGB.[14,47,50–53] Moreover, randomized, prospective trials show that the weight loss from RYGB is comparable to that following the radical, malabsorptive JIB,[54,55] even though only ~3 feet of small intestine is bypassed with RYGB compared to 12–18 feet with JIB.[45]

Dumping symptoms (nausea, bloating, colic, diarrhea, lightheadedness, diaphoresis, and palpitations) occur in some patients who have undergone RYGB, typically after high-carbohydrate meals. Although these symptoms can promote a negative conditioning response to sweets, the severity of dumping does not correlate with the efficacy of weight loss after RYGB,[56] and it is unlikely that dumping plays a major role in weight loss overall.

A key reason explaining why RYGB is more effective than VBG is because of the profound loss of appetite that typically results from RYGB but is less consistent after VBG.[14] The decrease in hunger after RYGB is not explained by early satiety from gastric restriction alone because it extends well beyond the immediate postprandial period. Moreover, it occurs despite a lack of change in the perception of sweets as being delicious or in the overall enjoyment of food.[42,57,58] Levels of the two most well-established anorexigenic adiposity hormones, leptin and insulin,[12] decrease appropriately after RYGB,[59,60] as expected with weight loss. Thus, these hormones do not account for the reduction in hunger and the postoperative regulation of body weight at a new, reduced level. Alterations in gut hormones have long been hypothesized to mediate these effects, but those initially examined—cholecystokinin, serotonin, and vasoactive intestinal peptide—are unaffected by gastric bypass.[61,62]

Effects of RYGB on Levels of the Orexigenic Hormone Ghrelin

Several years ago, we hypothesized that impairment of ghrelin secretion might account, in part, for the loss of hunger that accompanies RYGB, potentially contributing to weight reduction.[63] Ghrelin is a gastrointestinal peptide hormone that is the only known circulating orexigen (appetite stimulant).[64–67] Endogenous levels increase markedly before meals and decrease after food intake in humans as well as other species—both among individuals fed on fixed schedules and in those initiating meals voluntarily in the absence of cues related to time or food.[36,68,69] These and other findings support the hypothesis that ghrelin stimulates mealtime hunger and contributes to meal initiation.

Additional data also implicate ghrelin in long-term body weight regulation—a potential unique orexigenic counterpart to leptin in this process.[36] Several lines of evidence support this assertion.[70] Ghrelin regulates neuronal activity in classical body-weight regulatory centers in the brain, including the hypothalamus, caudal brainstem, and midbrain reward centers. Chronic ghrelin administration increases body weight, through anabolic effects on food intake, energy expenditure, and fuel utilization. Conversely, chronic blockade of ghrelin signaling in adult animals decreases body weight, and genetic ablation of the gene for either ghrelin or its receptor yields mice that are resistant to diet-induced obesity.[71,72] Lastly, circulating ghrelin levels correlate inversely with measures of adiposity, and ghrelin secretion responds to alterations in energy stores with compensatory adaptations.[73] For example, ghrelin levels increase with weight loss resulting from numerous causes, including caloric restriction, cancer anorexia, eating disorders, Huntington's disease, chronic exercise, and end-stage failure of the heart, lungs, liver, or kidneys.[36,63,70] Conversely, weight gain resulting from diverse interventions reduces ghrelin levels, indicating bidirectional adaptive regulation. The implication of these observations is that an increase in ghrelin levels may constitute one of the adaptive responses to weight loss, which characterizes long-term energy homeostasis and promotes weight regain after volitional weight reduction.

Ghrelin is produced primarily by the stomach and, to a lesser extent, the duodenum, i.e., the exact organs most affected by RYGB.[74] Because ingested nutrients are dominant regulators of ghrelin production and because the majority of ghrelin-producing tissue is permanently excluded from contact with enteral nutrients after RYGB, we hypothesized that RYGB disrupts ghrelin regulation. In a study examining 24-h ghrelin profiles, we found that among people who had undergone RYGB 1.4 ± 0.4 years earlier, integrated area-under-curve daily ghrelin values were 77% lower than those of lean controls and 72% lower than those of matched-obese controls.[63] These low-ghrelin levels were especially remarkable in view of the 36% weight loss that had been experienced by the RYGB group—a change that would stimulate ghrelin secretion if achieved by other means. Moreover, the 24-h profiles of post-RYGB individuals were completely flat, displaying neither the prandial oscillations nor diurnal rhythm characteristic of normal ghrelin profiles.[68]

Numerous other groups have subsequently examined the effects on ghrelin of RYGB as performed at their centers, and there are now at least 17 reports from human studies on this topic. Six prospective investigations found that ghrelin levels decreased after RYGB, despite massive weight loss.[75–80] Five others, including our own, reported abnormally low levels of ghrelin in post-RYGB patients, compared with those in matched-obese or lean controls.[63,81–84] Four additional prospective studies observed no change in ghrelin levels after RYGB, despite massive weight loss—an observation generally interpreted as reflecting an impairment of the normal response of ghrelin to weight loss.[60,85–87] Finally, two groups found that ghrelin levels increased after RYGB, as expected with other modes of weight loss.[88,89] Although these two reports are outliers, they are solid studies with relatively large numbers of subjects and prospective designs. One implication of this heterogeneity is that there may be subtle differences in surgical technique, which lead to suppression or at least constraint of ghrelin levels after RYGB in many, but not all, surgeons' hands. A significant longitudinal decrease in ghrelin levels, despite major weight loss, was also observed in two recently developed rat models of RYGB.[90,91] In one of these, the magnitude of the fall in ghrelin concentrations was the best predictor of the amount of weight lost, a finding that provides more direct evidence favoring a causal role for impaired ghrelin secretion in RYGB-induced weight reduction.[90] If it is ultimately proven that impairment of the ghrelin response to weight loss contributes to the long-lasting efficacy of RYGB, it will be important to elucidate the mechanisms by which this occurs so that the effect can be sought expressly.

Our initial hypothesis was that RYGB suppresses ghrelin secretion through a process known as "override inhibition."[63] This is a phenomenon in which hormones that are normally secreted in response to an episodic stimulus are paradoxically inhibited when that stimulus occurs continuously. By this mechanism, gonadotropins and GH are paradoxically suppressed by continuous delivery of their normally pulsatile secretagogues, GnRH and GHRH, respectively.[92,93] In the case of ghrelin, the normal stimulus would be an empty stomach and duodenum—a condition that is rendered permanent by RYGB. The possibility that ghrelin-producing cells in the gut are subject to override inhibition is suggested by several lines of evidence that we have summarized elsewhere.[36] The override inhibition hypothesis predicts that bariatric procedures that do not exclude the majority of ghrelin-producing tissue (i.e., the gastric fundus) from contact with enteral nutrients would not impair ghrelin secretion. Consistent with this prediction, weight loss achieved by VBG, AGB, or BPD is associated with either unchanged or, more commonly, increased ghrelin levels in longitudinal studies (Cummings, D.E. and

Clement, K. unpublished observations; see also Refs. 60, 76, 77, 80, and 94–106.)

The override inhibition hypothesis, if valid, has clinical implications for surgical design.[107] According to this model, the position of the staple line partitioning the stomach in RYGB could be a critical determinant of weight loss. Placing this partition even slightly too far to the left would include part of the fundus—the richest source of ghrelin—in the upper gastric pouch, thus failing to exclude it from contact with food and undermining override inhibition. It is conceivable that this physiology contributes to the lesser efficacy of horizontal-compared to vertical-banded gastric bypasses.[15] Similarly, a short biliopancreatic limb (between the distal gastric remnant and the jejunojejunal anastomosis) could allow reflux of ingested nutrients from the Roux anastomosis into the ghrelin-rich stomach and duodenum. Interestingly, in one of the two studies of RYGB that reported a normal increase of ghrelin levels in response to weight loss,[88] patients had among the shortest biliopancreatic limbs and the widest upper gastric pouches of RYGB patients examined in ghrelin investigations to date.[107] The study also reported more modest weight loss (29.7%) than is typically seen after RYGB (35–40%), and less than was reported in most other studies of RYGB and ghrelin.[107]

The override inhibition hypothesis is called into question, however, by our rat experiments designed to locate the putative sensor that detects ingested nutrients and suppresses ghrelin levels in response to them. Unexpectedly, we found that nutrients infused into the stomach and constrained there with a reversible pyloric cuff did not affect ghrelin levels, which were significantly suppressed by nutrients infused when the cuff was opened.[108] Complimentary results have subsequently been reported in humans.[109] Moreover, we found that in rats nutrients delivered into the proximal jejunum suppressed ghrelin entirely as well as did nutrients injected into either the stomach or proximal duodenum.[110] In other words, prandial ghrelin regulation does not require the presence of nutrients in either the stomach or duodenum, i.e., the principal sites of ghrelin production. Thus, it seems less likely that exclusion of ingested nutrients from these areas after RYGB would disrupt ghrelin regulation.

An alternate hypothesis is that ghrelin regulation is perturbed after RYGB because of denervation of autonomic input to ghrelin-producing tissue in the foregut. We found that in rats vagotomy eliminates the increase of ghrelin levels that normally accompanies weight loss, as is often observed after RYGB.[111] Severing of vagal input to the foregut is accomplished variably by different surgeons performing RYGB and so this hypothesis could explain some of the heterogeneity in data pertaining to the effect of this operation on ghrelin levels.[107] A neural mechanism might also explain the very rapid decline in ghrelin levels, which is observed within 24 h after the operation, before suppression via override inhibition from an empty stomach and duodenum would be predicted to occur.[76,77] Interestingly, vertical-banded gastroplasty promotes greater weight loss if accompanied by a full truncal vagotomy.[112]

Effects of Gastric Bypass Surgery on Hindgut Satiety Peptides: PYY, GLP-1, and Oxyntomodulin

In addition to altering circulating ghrelin levels, certain kinds of bariatric surgery, including RYGB, may promote weight loss, in part, by expediting delivery of ingested nutrients to the distal intestine, thereby reducing food intake by accentuating the complex mechanisms underlying the "ileal brake." In this long-observed phenomenon, the presence of nutrients in the ileum suppresses gastrointestinal motility, gastric emptying, small intestinal transit, and ultimately, food intake. Neural mechanisms are implicated in this response, as well as hormones such as neurotensin and several products of proglucagon secreted from intestinal L-cells, including glucagon-like peptide-1 (GLP-1), peptide YY (PYY), oxyntomodulin, and enteroglucagon.[113,114] All of these peptides are produced primarily by the ileum and colon.

Beyond inhibiting gastrointestinal motility, some of these hindgut hormones function as satiety factors by modulating neuronal activity in the afferent vagus nerve, by acting directly on the brain, or both. A processed form of PYY called PYY_{3-36} decreases appetite and food intake when injected at physiologic levels in humans, and chronic administration can reduce body weight in rodents.[115,116] Similarly, exogenous administration of either GLP-1 or oxyntomodulin decreases food intake in humans as well as in experimental animals.[114,117-119] All of these hindgut peptides are released postprandially into the circulation in proportion to the caloric content of ingested food, consistent with their proposed roles as satiety hormones.[117,120]

Because PYY, GLP-1, and oxyntomodulin are secreted from the distal intestine in response to enteral nutrient exposure, bariatric procedures that expedite delivery of ingested nutrients to the hindgut should increase postprandial and possibly basal levels of these peptides. Operations predicted to exert such an effect include JIB, BPD, and RYGB because all of these procedures remove the pylorus and some portion of the small intestine from the pathway taken by ingested food. As predicted, PYY, GLP-1, neurotensin, and enteroglucagon are all increased in response to meals and/or at baseline following JIB.[61,103,121-125] Although this operation is no longer performed, it represents a useful and very longstanding model of markedly enhanced nutrient delivery to the distal intestine. Early studies indicated that JIB stimulated humoral levels of one or more nonaversive, appetite-suppressing factors, because nonoperated rats ate substantially less after receiving injections of post-JIB donor blood than after receiving control blood, without manifesting any signs of illness or discomfort.[126] Although the identity of this circulating anorexic factor was unknown at that time, subsequent studies have shown that basal and postprandial levels of PYY, GLP-1, and neurotensin are elevated for as many as 20 years after JIB in humans.[123] Similarly, fasting and postprandial PYY levels increase after nonbariatric surgeries that expedite nutrient delivery to the hindgut, such as extensive small-bowel resection.[127,128] In a rat model of JIB, postoperative PYY levels

are also increased, and pharmacologic antagonism of PYY signaling increases food intake in these animals.[103] This finding provides direct evidence for a causal role of increased PYY levels in reducing food intake after bariatric surgery.

The meal-related rise of PYY levels is also markedly enhanced after RYGB.[84,87,103,129,130] Following ingestion of a small meal, people who have undergone this operation display an early and exaggerated PYY response, with as much as a 10-fold postprandial increase in plasma levels, compared with only a minimal prandial response among lean or BMI-matched, nonsurgical controls.[84,103,129,130] Peak PYY levels, as well as area–under–curve values, are markedly higher in post-RYGB patients than in controls.[84,103,129,130] Elevated PYY concentrations are also observed in a recently developed rat model of RYGB.[91] These findings are in marked contrast to the blunted prandial PYY response normally observed in nonoperated obese, compared to lean, individuals.[84,103,116,129] Moreover, the degree of postprandial satiety reported by patients with RYBG has been found in some studies to correlate with the magnitude of the meal-related PYY surge.[84,87]

Like PYY, other products of distal intestinal L-cells, including GLP-1, also display markedly increased circulating levels following bariatric operations that significantly expedite nutrient delivery to the hindgut. Several studies of JIB, which greatly enhances hindgut nutrient exposure, show increased GLP-1 levels after surgery, both within the first year and as late as 20 years postoperatively.[103,121-123] Similarly, the major intestinal bypass created with BPD causes clear increases of GLP-1 levels, especially in response to meals.[131,132] The impact of the much shorter intestinal bypass rendered by RYGB is less obvious, and some studies in humans and rodents have shown only equivocal changes in GLP-1 or none at all.[91,133] However, enteroglucagon, a marker of L-cell secretion, is increased after RYGB as it is after BPD,[87,125,134] and several very recent studies have, indeed, reported exaggerated GLP-1 responses to meals following RYGB in humans.[87,103,130]

The effects of bariatric surgery on oxyntomodulin levels have not been reported. However, since this satiety peptide is released from distal intestinal L-cells in response to enteral nutrient exposure, the impact of bariatric operations on oxyntomodulin levels should mirror the effects described above for PYY, GLP-1, and enteroglucagon.

MECHANISMS OF DIABETES RESOLUTION AFTER BARIATRIC SURGERY

Type 2 DM is the obesity-related comorbidity that is most dramatically ameliorated by RYGB. In five large studies, examining a total of 3,568 people undergoing RYGB, diabetic patients enjoyed complete remission of their disease at rates ranging from 82% to 98%, with most studies showing resolution in ~83% of cases.[16,21-24] Similarly, a systematic meta-analysis of 136 studies, involving a total of 22,094 patients, reported that gastric bypass completely resolved DM in 84% of cases.[18] In these studies, the reversal of impaired glucose tolerance without DM was nearly universal. Patients whose DM remitted were able to discontinue all diabetic medications and manifest normal fasting glucose and glycosylated hemoglobin levels. In a longitudinal examination of obese people with impaired glucose tolerance followed for ~5.5 years, bariatric surgery lowered the rate of progression from this condition to frank DM by more than 30-fold.[135] Thus, RYGB is a highly effective method to prevent and reverse DM, which is traditionally regarded as a progressive, incurable disease.

The most obvious mechanism to explain this effect is the beneficial impact of weight loss on insulin sensitivity. Indeed, patients who have lost substantial weight following RYGB display increased levels of adiponectin (which enhances insulin sensitivity) and muscle insulin receptor concentration, as well as reductions in intramuscular lipids and fatty acyl-CoA molecules (moieties that cause insulin resistance).[136–138] As predicted from these changes, glucose transport in incubated muscle fibers is greatly enhanced after RYGB, and whole-body glucose disposal during a euglycemic clamp has been reported to increase from 27% to 78% of that observed in normal-weight controls.[139] Similarly, insulin sensitivity as measured by minimal modeling increases approximately 4–5-fold after RYGB-induced weight loss.[136,138] Importantly, all these changes have been observed a year or more after surgery and could thus result from major weight loss, rather than from RYGB *per se*.

The beneficial effects of RYGB on DM, however, cannot be accounted for by weight loss alone. Perhaps the most impressive observation supporting this assertion is that previously diabetic patients can very often discontinue all of their diabetes medications by the time of discharge from the hospital after RYGB (~1 week or less post-operatively), which is long before major weight loss has occurred.[21,25]

What mechanisms could explain this dramatic, rapid reversal of DM? The most pedestrian (although quite possibly valid) is that patients consume no food in the immediate postoperative period and so their pancreatic β-cells are not challenged. Starvation-induced alleviation of DM is well known. A few days later, patients gradually escalate their oral intake; but by the time they begin to eat reasonably normally at home, they are losing weight and in a state of negative energy balance—a condition that improves glucose tolerance. Eventually, amelioration of DM can be accounted for by the well-known effects of weight loss to increase insulin sensitivity, thereby decreasing glucotoxicity and lipotoxicity, to improve β-cell function.

Although these mechanisms undoubtedly help improve glucose tolerance after RYGB, they are unlikely to explain the entire phenomenon. Patients who undergo purely restrictive bariatric operations, such as gastroplasty or gastric banding, also experience a period of postoperative food deprivation followed by major weight loss. Yet DM resolves in only approximately half of cases following these procedures, compared with 84% of cases after gastric bypass.[18] More importantly, DM resolves over months to years after restrictive procedures, consistent with mechanisms resulting secondarily from weight loss. In contrast, resolution of DM

occurs within days to weeks following RYGB, long before major weight loss has occurred,[21] suggesting that additional mechanisms related to the operation itself are also at work.

Diabetes Resolution Following Bariatric Surgery: Role of Ghrelin

To explain RYGB-induced DM resolution, a more interesting possibility (which may act in concert with the above mechanisms) is that favorable alterations in gut hormones improve insulin secretion and/or action. Ghrelin, which typically decreases after this operation, exerts several diabetogenic effects.[36] Exogenous ghrelin delivery increases levels of GH, cortisol, and epinephrine—three of the four classical counterregulatory hormones—in addition to decreasing secretion of the insulin-sensitizing hormone, adiponectin.[70] Beyond these hormonally mediated mechanisms that oppose insulin action, ghrelin directly antagonizes insulin-mediated intracellular signaling events pertaining to glucose metabolism in cultured hepatocytes.[140] Lastly, ghrelin administration suppresses insulin secretion, even in the face of ghrelin-induced hyperglycemia.[141] Thus, at least at pharmacologic doses, ghrelin hinders insulin secretion and action, and accordingly, chronic administration of ghrelin receptor agonists impairs glucose tolerance in humans.[142] If these effects are physiologic, and ghrelin acts as an "anti-incretin" to limit peripheral glucose utilization in the fasted and preprandial state, then suppression of ghrelin levels after RYGB could help improve glucose homeostasis.

Diabetes Resolution Following Bariatric Surgery: Role of Hindgut Hormones

An even more attractive putative mediator of the antidiabetic effects of RYGB is GLP-1. This hormone and glucose-dependent insulinotropic peptide (GIP) are the classical incretins that augment insulin secretion in response to ingested food. Furthermore, GLP-1 exerts proliferative and antiapoptotic effects on pancreatic β-cells.[143] It may also improve insulin sensitivity, at least indirectly,[144] while decreasing food intake and body weight. Consequently, methods to enhance GLP-1 signaling show great promise for the treatment of type 2 DM,[114] and the first of many new medications in this arena has recently been approved for clinical use. As detailed above, enhanced secretion of GLP-1 and other L-cell products occurs following bariatric operations that expedite delivery of nutrients to the hindgut, including RYGB, BPD, and JIB; and indeed, these are the bariatric procedures that most effectively and rapidly reverse DM.[18,125] Remarkably, BPD improves insulin sensitivity even more than does RYGB,[145] and nearly everyone with DM who undergoes BPD experiences complete remission of the disease.[18,21] Augmentation of GLP-1 levels could plausibly account for some of the impressive antidiabetic and weight-reducing effects of bariatric procedures that creates shortcuts for ingested nutrients to access the distal intestine.

In support of this hypothesis are intriguing rodent experiments in which a portion of the ileum is resected and inserted into the duodenum or proximal jejunum.[146] Without creating any restrictive or malabsorptive physiology, such ileal interpositions can cause significant reductions in food intake and body weight, with improved glucose homeostasis, presumably by placing the hormone-rich ileum in close contact with ingested nutrients, thus enhancing ileal brake physiology. Consistent with this mechanism, ileal interposition increases levels of PYY, GLP-1, and enteroglucagon, and it inhibits gastric motility and emptying.[113,146-149] Importantly, even in experiments in which no change in food intake or body weight was observed following ileal interposition, diabetic rats nevertheless displayed improved glucose tolerance and substantially elevated GLP-1 levels.[150] These findings are consistent with a role for GLP-1 in mediating the antidiabetic effects of bariatric operations that enhance ileal nutrient exposure, independent of, or in addition to, body weight alterations.

Recent independent publications have described a number of patients suffering pathologic overgrowth of pancreatic beta cells (nesidioblastosis) following RYGB, accompanied by life-threatening hyperinsulinemic hypoglycemia.[151,152] Although there are only a handful of such cases known to date, the vanishingly rare *de novo* development of nesidioblastosis in adulthood and the overrepresentation of this condition in post-RYGB patients make it likely that there is a causal link between that operation and occasional beta-cell overgrowth.[153] Since GLP-1 levels are increased after RYGB, and since GLP-1 can stimulate beta-cell neogenesis and proliferation while inhibiting apoptosis (at least in rodents),[143] it is conceivable that enhanced GLP-1 secretion could contribute to beta-cell overgrowth following RYGB. Indeed, some of the post-RYGB patients with nesidioblastosis had extraordinarily high GLP-1 levels.[152] However, GLP-1 receptor agonists have never been found to cause beta-cell overgrowth when used clinically, and even at doses that substantially exceed peak endogenous activity, such agents ameliorate diabetes far less impressively than does either RYGB or BPD. These operations improve glucose homeostasis through multiple mechanisms, among which increased GLP-1 secretion may act in concert with antidiabetic effects of weight loss, reduced caloric intake, decreased ghrelin levels, and perhaps changes in PYY, oxyntomodulin, or factors yet to be discovered.

Importantly, nesidioblastosis probably represents the pathologic extreme of a phenomenon that benefits the vast majority of patients with diabetes who undergo RYGB. Although rare nesidioblastosis should now technically be added to the list of bariatric surgical complications, the concept that RYGB might stimulate beta-cell re-growth is far more exciting than worrisome, as it offers prospects for a genuine cure of DM.[153]

Diabetes Resolution Following Bariatric Surgery: Role of the Intestinal Foregut

Although all bariatric operations promote weight loss and improve glucose homeostasis, RYGB and BPD are the fastest and most effective current procedures to achieve both endpoints.[18,21,154,155] These operations cause durable remissions of DM in >80% of cases, typically within days after surgery.[16,18,59,155,156] RYGB and BPD both exclude the intestinal foregut from digestive continuity, whereas purely restrictive operations, which exert less impact on DM, do not exclude this segment. Thus, it has been hypothesized that bypass of the hormonally active intestinal foregut is an important determinant of the antidiabetic effects of these procedures.[59,154] As articulated above, suppression or constraint of ghrelin secretion from the bypassed foregut is one candidate mechanism to explain some of the effects of RYGB on weight loss and glucose homeostasis, but it is very unlikely that ghrelin explains all of these actions.

A series of elegant studies by Rubino et al. provides support for the hypothesis that bypassing only the intestinal foregut exerts antidiabetic effects.[157] Using Goto-Kakizaki rats—a spontaneous, nonobese model of type 2 DM—these investigators evaluated the actions of RYGB that are specifically related to exclusion of the duodenum and proximal jejunum, independent of those resulting from gastric restriction and bypass. In a novel surgical procedure, the stomach was left unperturbed, but food was diverted from the stomach to the proximal jejunum with a gastrojejunal anastomosis. This "duodenal–jejunal bypass" (DJB) represents a stomach-sparing bypass of approximately the same amount of intestinal foregut as is excluded in RYGB. (The entire duodenum was bypassed. Of the jejunum, 12 cm was included in the alimentary limb and 8 cm in the biliopancreatic limb. Thus, 20 cm of jejunum was incapable of absorbing nutrients, i.e., ~20% of the ~100-cm-long rat small intestine.) Experimental animals displayed similar food intake and body weight as did sham-operated controls, indicating that foregut bypass alone is not sufficient to cause weight loss in these rats. This is not surprising, since the DJB creates no gastric restriction, bypasses too little intestine to cause malabsorption, and does not involve a vagotomy. The results support assertions made above that malabsorption following the degree of foregut bypass typical of proximal RYGB is unlikely to be a major contributor to weight loss.

The most interesting finding in this study was that DJB rats displayed significant improvements in glucose tolerance compared with sham-operated controls, despite equivalent body weights in the two groups. Compared with controls, bypassed animals had lower fasting glucose levels at all postoperative time points for 9 months, which is equivalent to decades of life in humans. They also had a lower glucose nadir after insulin injection and lower area–under–curve glucose values in response to oral glucose loads at 1, 2, and 32 weeks after surgery. The DJB resulted in better glycemic control than did either rosiglitazone therapy or substantial weight loss from food restriction.

The markedly improved glucose homeostasis of diabetic rats following DJB could result from one or both of the two main components of this operation: exclusion of the intestinal foregut from digestive continuity and/or expedited delivery of nutrients to the hindgut due to bypass of the pylorus and a short segment of upper intestine. The latter feature might, theoretically, increase GLP-1 levels, thereby improving glucose tolerance. To distinguish between these two possibilities, Rubino et al. modified the DJB in Goto-Kakizaki rats, allowing nutrients to exit the stomach into not only the proximal jejunum (via the gastrojejunostomy) but also through an intact pylorus into the beginning of the duodenum (via the normal route).[158] Without altering the degree of shortcut for ingested nutrients to reach the hindgut, this reestablishment of nutrient passage through the duodenum and proximal jejunum eliminated the antidiabetic effects of DJB. The authors went on to show that they could dynamically reverse or reestablish diabetes by excluding or restoring, respectively, nutrient passage through the intestinal foregut, independent of the gastrojejunal shortcut for nutrients to reach the hindgut. Finally, they showed that the normal DJB is not associated with elevated GLP-1 levels, presumably because this bypass is too short to enhance substantially the delivery of nutrients to the ileum and colon.

The important implication of these findings is that bypass of the intestinal foregut (e.g., as accomplished by RYGB and BPD) can ameliorate type 2 DM independently of changes in food intake and body weight, through mechanisms that remain unclear. Rubino et al. hypothesized alterations in gut hormones, to explain their results, and consistent with this, they subsequently showed that DJB lowers ghrelin levels in obese Zucker rats.[159] Because ghrelin exerts prodiabetic effects (*vide supra*), this reduction in the hormone could contribute to improved glucose homeostasis. Furthermore, unlike normal or Goto-Kakizaki rats, obese Zucker rats subjected to DJB ate less and lost weight compared with animals that underwent gastric banding or sham operations, an effect potentially related to the impact of DJB on ghrelin in Zucker rats. Other candidate foregut molecules to explain the effects of DJB are not obvious. The incretin hormone GIP, produced primarily by the foregut, is stimulated by ingested nutrients and promotes insulin secretion. Bypass of the foregut should, theoretically, decrease GIP levels, and there is little consensus on the actual effect of intestinal bypass operations on this hormone; various reports claim decreased, unchanged, or increased postoperative levels.

SUMMARY AND CONCLUSIONS

In summary, the mechanisms mediating weight loss and improved glucose tolerance after RYGB may include the following: (1) gastric restriction, leading to early satiety, small meal size, and negative conditioning; (2) bypass of the foregut, impairing ghrelin secretion via still-cryptic mechanisms, possibly affecting additional undiscovered intestinal foregut factors, and causing mild malabsorption in the case of long-limb variations only; (3) expedited delivery of nutrients to the hindgut, enhancing the ileal brake, and stimulating the release of PYY and GLP-1, which may decrease food intake and increase glucose tolerance. Dumping symptoms accompanying ingestion of concentrated carbohydrates may contribute in some people. These hypotheses and the others articulated herein are but a few of many possible explanations for the weight-reducing and antidiabetic effects of bariatric surgery, as numerous gut hormones have yet to be examined in this context. Clearly, this is an arena rich with opportunities for research that should ultimately elucidate all of the mechanisms underlying the dramatic actions of bariatric operations, hopefully allowing us to replicate some of these effects with new medications to treat obesity and diabetes.

References

1. Ogden CL, Carroll MD, Curtin LR, et al.: Prevalence of overweight and obesity in the United States, 1999–2004. *JAMA* 295:1549, 2006.
2. Mokdad AH, Ford ES, Bowman BA, et al.: Prevalence of obesity, diabetes, and obesity-related risk factors 2001. *JAMA* 289:76, 2003.
3. Deitel M: Overweight and obesity worldwide now estimated to involve 1.7 million people. *Obes Surg* 13:329, 2003.
4. Manson JE, Willett WC, Stampfer MJ, et al.: Body weight and mortality among women. *N Engl J Med* 333:677, 1995.
5. Calle E, Thun M, Petrelli J, et al.: Body-mass index and mortality in a prospective cohort of U.S. adults. *N Engl J Med* 341:1097, 1999.
6. Friedrich MJ: Epidemic of obesity expands its spread to developing countries. *JAMA* 287:1382, 2002.
7. Kopelman PG: Obesity as a medical problem. *Nature* 404:635, 2000.
8. Yanovski SZ, Yanovski JA: Obesity. *N Engl J Med* 346:591, 2002.
9. Bray GA, Tartaglia LA: Medicinal strategies in the treatment of obesity. *Nature* 404:672, 2000.
10. McTigue KM, Harris R, Hemphill B, et al.: Screening and interventions for obesity in adults: Summary of the evidence for the U.S. Prevention Services Task Force. *Ann Intern Med* 139:933, 2003.
11. Safer DJ: Diet, behavior modification, and exercise: A review of obesity treatments from a long-term perspective. *Southern Med J* 84:1470, 1991.
12. Cummings DE, Schwartz MW: Genetics and pathophysiology of human obesity. *Annu Rev Med* 54:453, 2003.
13. Schwartz MW, Woods SC, Porte D, et al.: Central nervous system control of food intake. *Nature* 404:661, 2000.
14. Brolin RE: Bariatric surgery and long-term control of morbid obesity. *JAMA* 288:2793, 2002.
15. Mun EC, Blackburn GL, Matthews JB: Current status of medical and surgical therapy for obesity. *Gastroenterology* 120:669, 2001.
16. Pories WJ, Swanson MS, MacDonald KG, et al.: Who would have thought it? An operation proves to be the most effective therapy for adult-onset diabetes mellitus. *Ann Surg* 222:339, 1995.
17. Sjostrom L, Lindroos AK, Peltonen M, et al.: Lifestyle, diabetes, and cardiovascular risk factors 10 years after bariatric surgery. *New Engl J Med* 351:2683, 2004.
18. Buchwald H, Avidor Y, Braunwald E, et al.: Bariatric surgery: A systematic review and meta-analysis. *JAMA* 292:1724, 2004.
19. Jones KB, Jr.: Experience with the Roux-en-Y gastric bypass, and commentary on current trends. *Obes Surg* 10:183, 2000.
20. Cummings DE, Overduin J, Foster-Schubert KE: Gastric bypass for obesity: Mechanisms of weight loss and diabetes resolution. *J Clin Endocrinol Metab* 89:2608, 2004.
21. Schauer PR, Burguera B, Ikramuddin S, et al.: Effect of laparoscopic Roux-en Y gastric bypass on type 2 diabetes mellitus. *Ann Surg* 238:467, 2003.
22. Sugerman HJ, Wolfe LG, Sica DA, et al.: Diabetes and hypertension in severe obesity and effects of gastric bypass-induced weight loss. *Ann Surg* 237:751, 2003.
23. Wittgrove AC, Clark GW: Laparoscopic gastric bypass, Roux-en-Y-500 patients: Technique and results, with 3–60 month follow-up. *Obes Surg* 10:233, 2000.
24. Schauer PR, Ikramuddin S, Gourash W, et al.: Outcomes after laparoscopic Roux-en-Y gastric bypass for morbid obesity. *Ann Surg* 232:515, 2000.

25. Pories WJ: Diabetes: The evolution of a new paradigm. *Ann Surg* 239:12, 2004.

26. Steinbrook MD: Surgery for severe obesity. *New Engl J Med* 350:1075, 2004.

27. NIH CDCP: Gastrointestinal surgery for severe obesity. *Ann Intern Med* 115:956, 1991.

28. Payne JH, DeWind LT: Surgical treatment of obesity. *Am J Surg* 118:141, 1969.

29. Pace WG, Martin EW, Tetrick T, et al.: Gastric partitioning for morbid obesity. *Ann Surg* 190:392, 1979.

30. Mason EE: Vertical banded gastroplasty for obesity. *Arch Surg* 117:701, 1982.

31. Balsiger BM, Poggio JL, Mai J, et al.: Ten and more years after vertical banded gastroplasty as primary operation for morbid obesity. *J Gastrointest Surg* 4:598, 2000.

32. Nightengale ML, Sarr MG, Kelly KA, et al.: Prospective evaluation of vertical banded gastroplasty as the primary operation for morbid obesity. *Mayo Clin Proc* 67:304, 1991.

33. Howard L, Malone M, Michalek A, et al.: Gastric bypass and vertical banded gastroplasty—A prospective randomized comparison and 5-year follow-up. *Obes Surg* 5:55, 1995.

34. Sugerman HJ, Starkey J, Birkenhauer R: A randomized prospective trial of gastric bypass versus vertical banded gastroplasty for morbid obesity and their effects on sweets versus non-sweets eaters. *Ann Surg* 205:613, 1987.

35. Naslund I: A prospective randomized comparison of gastric bypass and gastroplasty. *Acta Chir Scand* 152:681, 1986.

36. Cummings DE, Shannon MH: Roles for ghrelin in the regulation of appetite and body weight. *Arch Surg* 138:389, 2003.

37. Bo O, Modalsli O: Gastric banding, a surgical method of treating morbid obesity: Preliminary report. *Int J Obes* 7:493, 1983.

38. Kuzmak L: Stoma adjustable silicone gastric banding. *Prob Gen Surg* 9:298, 1992.

39. Mason EE: Gastric bypass. *Ann Surg* 170:329, 1969.

40. Must A, Spadano J, Coakley EH, et al.: The disease burden associated with overweight and obesity. *JAMA* 282:1523, 1999.

41. Trostler N, Mann A, Zilberbush N, et al.: Weight loss and food intake 18 months following vertical banded gastroplasty or gastric bypass for severe obesity. *Obes Surg* 5:39, 1995.

42. Halmi KA, Mason E, Falk JR, et al.: Appetitive behavior after gastric bypass for obesity. *Int J Obes* 5:457, 1981.

43. Kenler HA, Brolin RE, Cody RP: Changes in eating behavior after horizontal gastroplasty and Roux-en-Y gastric bypass. *Am J Clin Nutr* 52:87, 1990.

44. Xu Y, Ohinata K, Meguid MM, et al.: Gastric bypass model in the obese rat to study metabolic mechanisms of weight loss. *J Surg Res* 107:56, 2002.

45. Sugerman HJ: Morbid Obesity. In: Greenfield LJ (ed.): *Surgery: Scientific Principles and Practice*. Philadelphia, PA, J.B. Lippincott, 1993; p. 702.

46. Biertho L, Steffen R, Ricklin T, et al.: Laparoscopic gastric bypass versus laparoscopic adjustable gastric banding: A comparative study of 1200 cases. *J Am Coll Surg* 197:536, 2003.

47. Brolin RE, LaMarca LB, Kenler HA, et al.: Malabsorptive gastric bypass in patients with superobesity. *J Gastrointest Surg* 6:195, 2002.

48. le Roux CW, Bloom SR: Why do patients lose weight after Roux-en-Y gastric bypass? *J Clin Endocrinol Metab* 90:591, 2005.

49. Friedman HI, Chandler JG, Peck CC, et al.: Alterations in intestinal structure, fat absorption and body weight after intestinal bypass for morbid obesity. *Surg Gynecol Obstet* 146:757, 1978.

50. Faraj M, Jones P, Sniderman AD, et al.: Enhanced dietary fat clearance in postobese women. *J Lipid Res* 42:571, 2001.

51. MacLean LD, Rhode BM, Nohr CW: Long- or short-limb gastric bypass? *J Gastrointest Surg* 5:525, 2001.

52. Naslund I: Gastric bypass versus gastroplasty: A prospective study of differences in two surgical procedures for morbid obesity. *Acta Chir Scand Suppl* 536:44, 1987.

53. MacLean LD, Rhode BM, Nohr CW: Late outcome of isolated gastric bypass. *Ann Surg* 231:524, 2000.

54. Griffen WO, Young VL, Stevenson CC: A prospective comparison of gastric and jejunoileal bypass for morbid obesity. *Ann Surg* 186:500, 1977.

55. Mason EE, Printen KJ, Blommers TJ, et al.: Gastric bypass for obesity after ten years experience. *Int J Obes* 2:197, 1978.

56. Mallory GN, Macgregor AM, Rand CS: The Influence of dumping on weight loss after gastric restrictive surgery for morbid obesity. *Obes Surg* 6:474, 1996.

57. Rand CS, Macgregor AM, Hankins GC: Eating behavior after gastric bypass surgery for obesity. *South Med J* 80:961, 1987.

58. Hafner RJ, Watts JM, Rogers J: Quality of life after gastric bypass for morbid obesity. *Int J Obes* 15:555, 1991.

59. Hickey MS, Pories WJ, MacDonald KG, Jr, et al.: A new paradigm for type 2 diabetes mellitus: Could it be a disease of the foregut? *Ann Surg* 227:637, 1998.

60. Stoeckli R, Chanda R, Langer I, et al.: Changes of body weight and plasma ghrelin levels after gastric banding and gastric bypass. *Obes Res* 12:346, 2004.

61. Kellum JM, Kuemmerle JF, O'Dorisio TM, et al.: Gastrointestinal hormone responses to meals before and after gastric bypass and vertical banded gastroplasty. *Ann Surg* 211:763, 1990.

62. Pappas TN: Physiological satiety implications of gastrointestinal antiobesity surgery. *Am J Clin Nutr* 55:571S, 1992.

63. Cummings DE, Weigle DS, Frayo RS, et al.: Human plasma ghrelin levels after diet-induced weight loss and gastric bypass surgery. *New Engl J Med* 346:1623, 2002.

64. Kojima M, Hosoda H, Date Y, et al.: Ghrelin is a growth-hormone-releasing acylated peptide from stomach. *Nature* 402:656, 1999.

65. Tschop M, Smiley DL, Heiman ML: Ghrelin induces adiposity in rodents. *Nature* 407:908, 2000.

66. Nakazato M, Murakami N, Date Y, et al.: A role for ghrelin in the central regulation of feeding. *Nature* 409:194, 2001.

67. Wren AM, Small CJ, Ward HL, et al.: The novel hypothalamic peptide ghrelin stimulates food intake and growth hormone secretion. *Endocrinology* 141:4325, 2000.

68. Cummings DE, Purnell JQ, Frayo RS, et al.: A preprandial rise in plasma ghrelin levels suggests a role in meal initiation in humans. *Diabetes* 50:1714, 2001.

69. Cummings DE, Frayo RS, Marmonier C, et al.: Plasma ghrelin levels and hunger scores in humans initiating meals voluntarily without time- and food-related cues. *Am J Physiol Endocrinol Metab* 287:E297, 2004.

70. Cummings DE, Foster-Schubert KE, Overduin J: Ghrelin and energy balance: Focus on current controversies. *Curr Drug Targets* 6:153, 2005.

71. Wortley KE, del Rincon JP, Murray JD, et al.: Absence of ghrelin protects against early-onset obesity. *J Clin Invest* 115:3573, 2005.

72. Zigman JM, Nakano Y, Coppari R, et al.: Mice lacking ghrelin receptors resist the development of diet-induced obesity. *J Clin Invest* 115:3564, 2005.

73. McLaughlin T, Abbasi F, Lamendola C, et al.: Plasma ghrelin concentrations are decreased in insulin-resistant obese adults relative to equally obese insulin-sensitive controls. *J Clin Endocrinol Metab* 89:1630, 2004.

74. Ariyasu H, Takaya K, Tagami T, et al.: Stomach is a major source of circulating ghrelin, and feeding state determines plasma ghrelin-like immunoreactivity levels in humans. *J Clin Endocrinol Metab* 86:4753, 2001.

75. Geloneze B, Tambascia MA, Pilla VF, et al.: Ghrelin: A gut-brain hormone: Effect of gastric bypass surgery. *Obe Surg* 13:17, 2003.

76. Fruhbeck G, Caballero AD, Gil MJ: Fundus functionality and ghrelin concentrations after bariatric surgery. *New Engl J Med* 350:308, 2004.

77. Lin E, Gletsu N, Fugate K, et al.: The effects of gastric surgery on systemic ghrelin levels in the morbidly obese. *Arch Surg* 139:780, 2004.

78. Couce M, Cottam D, Esplen J, et al.: Central *vs.* peripheral ghrelin: Impact on human obesity. NAASO annual meeting. *Obes Res* 11(Suppl A):35, 2003.

79. Morinigo R, Casamitjana R, Moize V, et al.: Short-term effects of gastric bypass surgery on circulating ghrelin levels. *Obes Res* 12:1108, 2004.

80. Fruhbeck G, Rotellar F, Hernandez-Lizoain JL, et al.: Fasting plasma ghrelin concentrations 6 months after gastric bypass are not determined by weight loss or changes in insulinemia. *Obes Surg* 14:1208, 2004.

81. Tritos NA, Mun E, Bertkau A, et al.: Serum ghrelin levels in response to glucose load in obese subjects post-gastric bypass surgery. *Obes Res* 11:919, 2003.

82. Leonetti F, Silecchia G, Iacobellis G, et al.: Different plasma ghrelin levels after laparoscopic gastric bypass and adjustable gastric banding in morbid obese subjects. *J Clin Endocrinol Metab* 88:4227, 2003.

83. Fruhbeck G, Diez-Caballero A, Gil MJ, et al.: The decrease in plasma ghrelin concentrations following bariatric surgery depends on the functional integrity of the fundus. *Obes Surg* 14:606, 2004.

84. Korner J, Bessler M, Cirilo LJ, et al.: Effects of Roux-en-Y gastric bypass surgery on fasting and postprandial concentrations of plasma ghrelin, peptide YY, and insulin. *J Clin Endocrinol Metab* 90:359, 2005.

85. Faraj M, Havel PJ, Phelis S, et al.: Plasma acylation-stimulating protein, adiponectin, leptin, and ghrelin before and after weight loss induced by gastric bypass surgery in morbidly obese subjects. *J Clin Endocrinol Metab* 88:1594, 2003.

86. Copeland P, Davis P, Kaplan L: Weight loss after gastric bypass is associated with decreased plasma gastric inhibitory polypeptide without a significant change in circulating ghrelin. NAASO annual meeting. *Obes Res* 11(Suppl A):17, 2003.

87. Borg CM, le Roux CW, Ghatei MA, et al.: Progressive rise in gut hormone levels after Roux-en-Y gastric bypass suggests gut adaptation and explains altered satiety. *Br J Surg* 93:210, 2006.

88. Holdstock C, Engstrom BE, Obrvall M, et al.: Ghrelin and adipose tissue regulatory peptides: Effect of gastric bypass surgery in obese humans. *J Clin Endocrinol Metab* 88:3177, 2003.

89. Vendrell J, Broch M, Vilarrasa N, et al.: Resistin, adiponectin, ghrelin, leptin, and proinflammatory cytokines: Relationships in obesity. *Obes Res* 12:962, 2004.

90. Stylopoulos N, Davis P, Pettit JD, et al.: Changes in serum ghrelin predict weight loss after Roux-en-Y gastric bypass in rats. *Surg Endosc* 19:942, 2005.

91. Suzuki S, Ramos EJ, Goncalves CG, et al.: Changes in GI hormones and their effect on gastric emptying and transit times after Roux-en-Y gastric bypass in rat model. *Surgery* 138:283, 2005.

92. Belchetz PE, Plant TM, Nakai Y, et al.: Hypophysial responses to continuous and intermittent delivery of hypothalamic gonadotropin-releasing hormone. *Science* 202:631, 1978.

93. Rittmaster RS, Loriaux DL, Merriam GR: Effect of continuous somatostatin and growth hormone-releasing hormone (GHRH) infusions on the subsequent growth hormone (GH) response to GHRH: Evidence for somatotroph desensitization independent of GH pool depletion. *Neuroendocrinology* 45:118, 1987.

94. Foschi D, Corsi F, Rizzi A, et al.: Vertical banded gastroplasty modifies plasma ghrelin secretion in obese patients. *Obes Surg* 15:1129, 2005.

95. Hanusch-Enserer U, Brabant G, Roden M: Ghrelin concentrations in morbidly obese patients after adjustable gastric banding. *New Engl J Med* 348:2159, 2003.

96. Nijhuis J, van Dielen FM, Buurman WA, et al.: Ghrelin, leptin and insulin levels after restrictive surgery: A 2-year follow-up study. *Obes Surg* 14:783, 2004.

97. Schindler K, Prager G, Ballaban T, et al.: Impact of laparoscopic adjustable gastric banding on plasma ghrelin, eating behaviour and body weight. *Eur J Clin Invest* 34:549, 2004.

98. Dixon AF, Dixon JB, O'Brien P E: Laparoscopic adjustable gastric banding induces prolonged satiety: A randomised blind crossover study. *J Clin Endocrinol Metab* 90:813, 2005.

99. Ram E, Vishne T, Diker D, et al.: Impact of gastric banding on plasma ghrelin, growth hormone, cortisol, DHEA and DHEA-S levels. *Obes Surg* 15:1118, 2005.

100. Hanusch-Enserer U, Cauza E, Brabant G, et al.: Plasma ghrelin in obesity before and after weight loss after laparoscopical adjustable gastric banding. *J Clin Endocrinol Metab* 89:3352, 2004.

101. Langer FB, Reza Hoda MA, Bohdjalian A, et al.: Sleeve gastrectomy and gastric banding: Effects on plasma ghrelin levels. *Obes Surg* 15:1024, 2005.

102. Mariani LM, Fusco A, Turriziani M, et al.: Transient increase of plasma ghrelin after laparoscopic adjustable gastric banding in morbid obesity. *Horm Metab Res* 37:242, 2005.

103. le Roux CW, Aylwin SJ, Batterham RL, et al.: Gut hormone profiles following bariatric surgery favor an anorectic state, facilitate weight loss, and improve metabolic parameters. *Ann Surg* 243:108, 2006.

104. Adami GF, Cordera R, Marinari G, et al.: Plasma ghrelin concentration in the short-term following biliopancreatic diversion. *Obes Surg* 13:889, 2003.

105. Garcia-Unzueta MT, Fernandez-Santiago R, Dominguez-Diez A, et al.: Fasting plasma ghrelin levels increase progressively after biliopancreatic diversion: One-year follow-up. *Obes Surg* 15:187, 2005.

106. Adami GF, Cordera R, Andraghetti G, et al.: Changes in serum ghrelin concentration following biliopancreatic diversion for obesity. *Obes Res* 12:684, 2004.

107. Cummings DE, Shannon MH: Ghrelin and gastric bypass: Is there a hormonal contribution to surgical weight loss? *J Clin Endocrinol Metab* 88:2999, 2003.

108. Williams DL, Cummings DE, Grill HJ, et al.: Meal-related ghrelin suppression requires postgastric feedback. *Endocrinology* 144:2765, 2003.

109. Parker BA, Doran S, Wishart J, et al.: Effects of small intestinal and gastric glucose administration on the suppression of plasma ghrelin concentrations in healthy older men and women. *Clin Endocrinol (Oxf)* 62:539, 2005.

110. Overduin J, Frayo RS, Cummings DE: Role of the duodenum and macronutrient type in prandial suppression of ghrelin. NAASO annual meeting. *Obes Res* 11(suppl A):21, 2003.

111. Williams DL, Grill HJ, Cummings DE, et al.: Vagotomy dissociates short- and long-term controls of circulating ghrelin. *Endocrinology* 144:5184, 2003.

112. Kral JG, Gortz L, Hermansson G, et al.: Gastroplasty for obesity: Long-term weight loss improved by vagotomy. *World J Surg* 17:75, 1993.

113. Strader AD, Vahl TP, Jandacek RJ, et al.: Weight loss through ileal transposition is accompanied by increased ileal hormone secretion and synthesis in rats. *Am J Physiol Endocrinol Metab* 288:E447, 2005.

114. Drucker DJ: Enhancing incretin action for the treatment of type 2 diabetes. *Diabetes Care* 26:2929, 2003.

115. Batterham RL, Cowley MA, Small CJ, et al.: Gut hormone PYY (3-36) physiologically inhibits food intake. *Nature* 418:650, 2002.

116. Batterham RL, Cohen MA, Ellis SM, et al.: Inhibition of food intake in obese subjects by peptide YY3-36. *N Engl J Med* 349:941, 2003.

117. Deacon CF: Therapeutic strategies based on glucagon-like peptide 1. *Diabetes* 53:2181, 2004.

118. Cohen MA, Ellis SM, Le Roux CW, et al.: Oxyntomodulin suppresses appetite and reduces food intake in humans. *J Clin Endocrinol Metab* 88:4696, 2003.

119. Gutzwiller JP, Goke B, Drewe J, et al.: Glucagon-like peptide-1: A potent regulator of food intake in humans. *Gut* 44:81, 1999.

120. Adrian TE, Ferri GL, Bacarese-Hamilton AJ, et al.: Human distribution and release of a putative new gut hormone, peptide YY. *Gastroenterology* 89:1070, 1985.

121. Naslund E, Backman L, Holst JJ, et al.: Importance of small bowel peptides for the improved glucose metabolism 20 years after jejunoileal bypass for obesity. *Obes Surg* 8:253, 1998.

122. Naslund E, Gryback P, Backman L, et al.: Distal small bowel hormones: Correlation with fasting antroduodenal motility and gastric emptying. *Dig Dis Sci* 43:945, 1998.

123. Naslund E, Gryback P, Hellstrom PM, et al.: Gastrointestinal hormones and gastric emptying 20 years after jejunoileal bypass for massive obesity. *Int J Obes Relat Metab Disord* 21:387, 1997.

124. Sorensen TI, Lauritsen KB, Holst JJ, et al.: Gut and pancreatic hormones after jejunoileal bypass with 3:1 or 1:3 jejunoileal ratio. *Digestion* 26:137, 1983.

125. Sarson DL, Scopinaro N, Bloom SR: Gut hormone changes after jejunoileal (JIB) or biliopancreatic (BPB) bypass surgery for morbid obesity. *Int J Obes* 5:471, 1981.

126. Atkinson RL, Brent EL: Appetite suppressant activity in plasma of rats after intestinal bypass surgery. *Am J Physiol* 243:R60, 1982.

127. Andrews NJ, Irving MH: Human gut hormone profiles in patients with short bowel syndrome. *Dig Dis Sci* 37:729, 1992.

128. Adrian TE, Savage AP, Fuessl HS, et al.: Release of peptide YY (PYY) after resection of small bowel, colon, or pancreas in man. *Surgery* 101:715, 1987.

129. Chan JL, Mun EC, Stoyneva V, et al.: Peptide YY levels are elevated after gastric bypass surgery. *Obesity* 14:194, 2006.

130. Morinigo R, Moize V, Musri M, et al.: GLP-1, PYY, hunger, and satiety following gastric bypass surgery in morbidly obese subjects. *J Clin Endo Metab* 91:1735, 2006.

131. Lugari R, Dei Cas A, Ugolotti D, et al.: GLP-1 secretion and plasma dipeptidyl peptidase IV activity in morbidly obese patients undergoing biliopancreatic diversion. *Horm Metab Res* 36:111, 2004.

132. Valverde I, Puente J, Martin-Duce A, et al.: Changes in GLP-1 secretion after biliopancreatic diversion or vertical banded gastroplasty in obese subjects. *Obes Surg* 15:387, 2005.

133. Clements RH, Gonzalez QH, Long CI, et al.: Hormonal changes after Roux-en Y gastric bypass for morbid obesity and the control of type-II diabetes mellitus. *Am Surg* 70:1, 2004.

134. Meryn S, Stein D, Straus EW: Pancreatic polypeptide, pancreatic glucagon, and enteroglucagon in morbid obesity and following gastric bypass operation. *Int J Obes* 10:37, 1986.

135. Long SD, O'Brien K, MacDonald KG Jr, et al.: Weight loss in severely obese subjects prevents the progression of impaired glucose tolerance to type II diabetes. A longitudinal interventional study. *Diabetes Care* 17:372, 1994.

136. Pender C, Goldfine ID, Tanner CJ, et al.: Muscle insulin receptor concentrations in obese patients post bariatric surgery: Relationship to hyperinsulinemia. *Int J Obes Relat Metab Disord* 28:363, 2004.

137. Gray RE, Tanner CJ, Pories WJ, et al.: Effect of weight loss on muscle lipid content in morbidly obese subjects. *Am J Physiol Endocrinol Metab* 284:E726, 2003.

138. Houmard JA, Tanner CJ, Yu C, et al.: Effect of weight loss on insulin sensitivity and intramuscular long-chain fatty acyl-CoAs in morbidly obese subjects. *Diabetes* 51:2959, 2002.

139. Friedman JE, Dohm GL, Leggett-Frazier N, et al.: Restoration of insulin responsiveness in skeletal muscle of morbidly obese patients after weight loss. Effect on muscle glucose transport and glucose transporter GLUT4. *J Clin Invest* 89:701, 1992.

140. Murata M, Okimura Y, Iida K, et al.: Ghrelin modulates the downstream molecules of insulin signaling in hepatoma cells. *J Biol Chem* 277:5667, 2002.

141. Broglio F, Arvat E, Benso A, et al.: Ghrelin, a natural GH secretagogue produced by the stomach, induces hyperglycemia and reduces insulin secretion in humans. *J Clin Endocrinol Metab* 86:5083, 2001.

142. Svensson J, Lonn L, Jansson JO, et al.: Two-month treatment of obese subjects with the oral growth hormone (GH) secretagogue MK-677 increases GH secretion, fat-free mass, and energy expenditure. *J Clin Endocrinol Metab* 83:362, 1998.

143. Drucker DJ: Glucagon-like peptide-1 and the islet beta-cell: Augmentation of cell proliferation and inhibition of apoptosis. *Endocrinology* 144:5145, 2003.

144. Zander M, Madsbad S, Madsen JL, et al.: Effect of 6-week course of glucagon-like peptide 1 on glycaemic control, insulin sensitivity, and beta-cell function in type 2 diabetes: A parallel-group study. *Lancet* 359:824, 2002.

145. Muscelli E, Mingrone G, Camastra S, et al.: Differential effect of weight loss on insulin resistance in surgically treated obese patients. *Amer J Med* 118:51, 2005.

146. Koopmans HS, Ferri GL, Sarson DL, et al.: The effects of ileal transposition and jejunoileal bypass on food intake and GI hormone levels in rats. *Physiol Behav* 33:601, 1984.

147. Ueno T, Shibata C, Naito H, et al.: Ileojejunal transposition delays gastric emptying and decreases fecal water content in dogs with total colectomy. *Dis Colon Rectum* 45:109, 2002.

148. Ohtani N, Sasaki I, Naito H, et al.: Effect of ileojejunal transposition of gastrointestinal motility, gastric emptying, and small intestinal transit in dogs. *J Gastrointest Surg* 3:516, 1999.

149. Mason EE: Ileal [correction of ilial] transposition and enteroglucagon/GLP-1 in obesity (and diabetic?) surgery. *Obes Surg* 9:223, 1999.

150. Patriti A, Facchiano E, Annetti C, et al.: Early improvement of glucose tolerance after ileal transposititon in a non-obese type 2 diabetes rat model. *Obes Surg* 15:1258, 2005.

151. Service GJ, Thompson GB, Service FJ, et al.: Hyperinsulinemic hypoglycemia with nesidioblastosis after gastric bypass surgery. *New Engl J Med* 353:249, 2005.

152. Patti ME, McMahon G, Mun EC, et al.: Severe hypoglycemia post-gastric bypass requiring parital pancreatectomy: Evidence for inappropriate insulin secretion and pancreatic islet hyperplasia. *Diabetologia* 48:2236, 2005.

153. Cummings DE: Gastric bypass and nesidioblastosis—Too much of a good thing for islets? *N Engl J Med* 353:300, 2005.

154. Greenway SE, Greenway FL, Klein S: Effects of obesity surgery on non-insulin-dependent diabetes mellitus. *Arch Surg* 137:1109, 2002.

155. Rubino F, Gagner M: Potential of surgery for curing type 2 diabetes mellitus. *Ann Surg* 236:554, 2002.

156. Scopinaro N, Adami GF, Marinari GM, et al.: Biliopancreatic diversion. *World J Surg* 22:936, 1998.

157. Rubino F, Marescaux J: Effect of duodenal-jejunal exclusion in a non-obese animal model of type 2 diabetes: A new perspective for an old disease. *Ann Surg* 239:1, 2004.

158. Rubino F, Forgione A, Cummings DE, et al.: The mechanism of diabetes control after gastrointestinal surgery reveals a role of the proximal small intestine in the pathophysiology of type 2 diabetes. *Ann Surg* 244:741, 2006.

159. Rubino F, Zizzari P, Tomasetto C, et al.: The role of the small bowel in the regulation of circulating ghrelin levels and food intake in the obese Zucker rat. *Endocrinology* 146:1745, 2005.

16

Metabolic Syndrome: Diagnosis, Clinical Presentations, and Surgical Treatment

Bruno Geloneze, MD, PhD

INTRODUCTION

Over the last 60 years, there has been an impressive change in the human environment, behaviors, and lifestyle. These changes have resulted in an increase in both type 2 diabetes and macrovascular disease (myocardial infarction and cerebral ischemic disease). These rises must be attributed to the greater prevalence of obesity and consequent pathophysiologic condition, the so-called metabolic syndrome.[1] It has been estimated that 190 million people worldwide have diabetes and it is likely that this will increase to 324 million by 2025.[2] This epidemic is taking place both in developed and developing countries and the combination of obesity, diabetes, and metabolic syndrome is now recognized as one of the major threats to human health in the twenty-first century.

Considering the obesity epidemic as the major cause of increasing prevalence of metabolic syndrome, we assumed that obesity-related insulin resistance is the major cause of the metabolic derangement in this population. Insulin resistance is defined clinically as a state in which a given increase in plasma insulin in an individual causes less of an effect in lowering the plasma glucose than it does in a normal population.

METABOLIC SYNDROME—HISTORICAL NOTES

The first description corresponding to the metabolic syndrome comes from a paper of Kylin, a Swedish physician who, in 1923, pointed out a clustering of hypertension, hyperglycemia, and gout.[3] In 1947, Vague reported that obesity phenotype, android or male-type obesity, was associated with the metabolic abnormalities often seen with diabetes and with cardiovascular disease.[4] The clinical importance of the syndrome was highlighted some years later by Reaven, who described the existence of a cluster of metabolic abnormalities, with insulin resistance as a central pathophysiological feature, and named it "Syndrome X."[5] The metabolic syndrome has several synonymous syndromes including the deadly quartet,[6] insulin resistance syndrome,[7] and dysmetabolic syndrome.[8] More important than giving a name is providing a definition for the syndrome.

DEFINITION OF THE METABOLIC SYNDROME

The first attempt at a global definition of the metabolic syndrome was in 1999 by the World Health Organization (WHO)

Consultative Group[9] (Table 16–1). Critics of the WHO definition identified several limitations, of which the most important related to the use of the euglycemic clamp to measure insulin sensitivity, making the definition virtually impossible to use either in clinical practice or epidemiological studies. Later, a new version of WHO definition had considered the fasting levels of insulin instead of the euglycemic clamp to measure insulin resistance.[10] This definition also introduced waist circumference (94 cm for men and 80 cm for women) as the measure of centripetal adiposity and included modified cut points for other components.

The National Cholesterol Education Program of the United Sates introduced the ATP III definition 2 years later[11] (Table16–1). This definition did not have a specific measure of insulin resistance and adopted a less glucose-centric approach by treating all components with equal importance. Waist circumference was maintained as the measure of obesity using higher cut points (102 cm for men and 88 cm for women). The ATP definition has been popular because of its simplicity in that its components are easily and routinely measured in most clinical and research settings, also in severe obese subjects.

A modification of the ATPIII definition was also developed by the American Association of Clinical Endocrinologists (AACE) based on the belief that insulin resistance was the core feature.[12] The AACE listed four factors identifying abnormalities of the metabolic syndrome: elevated triglycerides, reduced HDL-cholesterol (HDL-C), elevated blood pressure, and elevated fasting and post-load glucose. Obesity, diagnosis

Table 16–1.

Current Definitions of the Metabolic Syndrome

WHO (1999)	EGIR (1999)	ATP III (2001)
Diabetes or impaired glucose tolerance or insulin resistance* plus two or more of the following: 1. Obesity: BMI >30 kg/m^2 or WHR >0.9 (M), >0.85 (F) 2. Dyslipidemia: Triglycerides ≥150 mg/dL or HDL-C <35 mg/dL (M), <39 (F) 3. Hypertension: Blood pressure ≥140/90 mm Hg or medication 4. Microalbuminuria: Albumin excretion ≥20 μg/min or Alb/Creatinine >30 mg/g	Insulin resistance*or hyperinsulinemia (for nondiabetics) plus two or more of the following: 1. Central obesity: Waist circumference ≥94 cm (M), ≥80 cm (F) 2. Dyslipidemia: Triglycerides ≥177 mg/dL or HDL-C <39 mg/dL 3. Hypertension: Blood pressure ≥140/90 mm Hg or medication 4. Fasting plasma glucose: ≥110 mg/dL (6.1 mmol/L)	Three or more of the following: 1. Central obesity: Waist circumference ≥ 102 cm (M), ≥88 cm (F) 2. Dyslipidemia: Triglycerides ≥150 mg/dL 3. Low HDL-C: <40 mg/dL (M), <50 (F) 4. Hypertension: Blood pressure ≥135/85 mm Hg or medication 5. Fasting plasma glucose: ≥110 mg/dL (6.1 mmol/L)

Defined as the top quartile of fasting insulin in the nondiabetic population.
WHR, waist hip ratio; HDL, high-density lipoprotein.

of hypertension, non-European ancestry, or age greater than 40 years and a sedentary lifestyle were listed as factors that increase the likelihood of the syndrome, rather than as key identifying abnormalities. The omission of abdominal obesity as a component in the AACE definition has evoked much criticism, considering the growing evidence that it is a major risk factor for type 2 diabetes and cardiovascular disease.[13]

A review on the prevalence of the syndrome, using different criteria, has been published.[14] However, comparisons of prevalence for different populations are difficult considering the utilization of several definitions of metabolic syndrome. According to the studies that include subjects 20–25 years and older, the prevalence varies in urban population from 8% (India) to 24% (United States) in men and from 7% (France) to 46% (Iran) in women. In an interesting demonstration of the effect of ethnicity on the metabolic syndrome, Ford et al. studied the prevalence of the syndrome among US adults and found that non-Hispanic whites had lower rates compared to Mexican Americans, and African American men had lower rates compared to non-Hispanic white and Mexican American men.[15]

The prevalence of metabolic syndrome in the morbid obese population has not been described. There are also some opened questions: (1) What is the best definition of metabolic syndrome to use in a given morbid obese population or individual? (2) Having a definition, is it necessary to apply it in order to identify high risk individuals for type 2 diabetes or cardiovascular disease? In fact, the prevalence of these conditions in massive obese subjects is high and the morbid obesity per se would be enough to identify high-risk individuals.

During the last 7 years we have been conducting an epidemiological study named BRAMS (Brazilian Metabolic Syndrome Study) in regard to study clinical presentations of the metabolic syndrome and its underlying physiopathological mechanisms in about 2,000 patients.[16] In this cohort, there are 480 individuals with BMI above 40. Considering the NCEP/ATP III criteria, the prevalence of metabolic syndrome in this group is 89%. The remaining eumetabolic group is younger than the whole group (35 vs 39 years) and has a lower BMI (40.6 ± 2 vs 50.3 ± 2 kg/m2; $p < .001$). We can speculate that a significant part of this group will be dysmetabolic and classified as having metabolic syndrome if they gain some additional weight or when they became older.

New Definition for Metabolic Syndrome

In light to overcome controversies on the limitations in the current definitions, the International Diabetes Federation (IDF) has proposed a new, more practical definition which would be applicable globally for the identification of people at high risk of cardiovascular disease and diabetes[17] (Table 16–2). The IDF Group recognized that central obesity was an important determinant of the metabolic syndrome (Table 16–2). In fact, visceral fat accumulation determined by CT scan or ultrasound has been demonstrated to have a strong correlation with the development of metabolic and cardiovascular disease.[18,19] The consensus group placed particular empha-

Table 16–2.

New Definition for Metabolic Syndrome (International Diabetes Federation)

Central Obesity
Waist circumference * (ethnicity specific)
    Euripides: male ≥94 cm, female ≥80 cm
    South Asians: male ≥90 cm, female ≥80 cm
    Chinese: male ≥90 cm, female ≥80 cm
    Japanese: male ≥85 cm, female ≥90 cm
    Ethnic South and Central America = male ≥90 cm, female ≥80 cm
    Sub Saharan Africans, Eastern Mediterranean, Arabians = use European data **

Plus any two of the following
    Raised triglycerides: ≥150 mg/dL
    Reduced HDL-C: <40 mg/dL (males), <50 mg/dL (females)
    Raised blood pressure: ≥130 (systolic) or ≥85 mm HGg (diastolic)
    Raised fasting plasma glucose ***
        Fasting plasma glucose ≥100 mg/dL
        or previously diagnosed type 2 diabetes

*If BMI > 30 kg/m^2 then central obesity can be assumed and waist circumference does not need to be measured.
** In the United States the ATP III values (102 cm for male and 88 cm for female) are likely to continue to be used for clinical purpose.
*** In clinical practice, impaired glucose tolerance is also acceptable.

sis on developing criteria for central obesity, which would be appropriate for a wide variation of populations. However, no mention was placed in regard to the use of this new definition in a special and also prevalent population, the morbidly obese subjects.

In recent times, the metabolic syndrome has been the subject of vigorous debate. Some authors questioned whether this condition can in fact be labeled a syndrome, as the cause is not fully recognized, and whether it serves any purpose other than labeling and medicalizing people.[20,21] There are even some suggestions that the concept of metabolic syndrome has been driven by the pharmaceutical industry to create new markets.[22]

Despite these concerns, the necessity in identifying people with increasing risk for diabetes and cardiovascular diseases exists. Furthermore, it is reasonable to accept the causal association between obesity, insulin resistance, and increasing risk for these conditions. Then, we believe that metabolic syndrome was not created for commercial purposes, since the syndrome would not be incidentally created 80 years ago for future exploratory purposes.

It is reasonable to assume that in people with severe obesity, the presence or not of metabolic syndrome could influence metabolic and cardiovascular outcomes. The Scandinavian Obesity Survey will answer these questions following severe obese subjects submitted or not to a bariatric procedure. As expected, the great majority of this cohort of severe obese subjects has metabolic syndrome.

METHODS FOR ASSESSING INSULIN RESISTANCE

Insulin resistance can be assessed by several methods, all of which estimate the relationship between plasma glucose and plasma insulin. The gold standard for assessing insulin resistance is the euglycemic clamp.[23] This difficult, time-consuming research technique measures the effect of a constant infusion of insulin on glucose utilization under conditions in which plasma glucose level is kept constant by administering intravenous glucose. A somewhat easier research technique that can be applied to larger numbers of subjects and to repeated measurements in the frequently sampled intravenous glucose tolerance test has been analyzed by the Minimal Model of Bergman.[24] This involves administering an intravenous bolus of glucose and measuring plasma glucose and insulin frequently over 2 hours. Despite the intrinsic difficulty of complex methods, our group has applied clamp studies for severe subjects showing significant improvement in insulin sensitivity along with weight loss.[25,26]

Another short-term and suitable test is the insulin tolerance test (ITT).[27] The ITT consists of a bolus of 0.1 U/insulin and collections of plasma glucose frequently from 0 to 15 minutes. Plasma glucose $t^{1/2}$ is calculated from the slope of least square analysis of plasma glucose concentrations from 3 to 15 minutes after insulin injection. Using this technique we demonstrate a clear correlation between improvement in insulin sensitivity and amelioration in glucose and lipid homeostasis after bariatric surgery, reinforcing the importance of insulin resistance in the physiopathological basis of metabolic profile in severe obese subjects.[28]

Currently, the most commonly used method in clinical practice and in studies of bariatric surgery follow-ups, because of its simplicity, is the homeostasis model assessment (HOMA) model, which requires only the measurements of the fasting plasma insulin and fasting plasma glucose.[29] The model is derived from a computer program that assesses the relationship between fasting plasma insulin and plasma glucose levels, in a large population of normally glucose-tolerant individuals. From the data, a simple formula for the calculation of HOMA index for insulin resistance (HOMA-IR) can be used:

HOMA-IR = (fasting plasma insulin [uU/ml])
    × fasting plasma glucose [mmol/l]/22.5

or

HOMA-IR = (fasting plasma insulin [uU/ml])
    × fasting plasma glucose [mg/l]/405

The HOMA model has been used in several epidemiological studies.[16,30–32] In the BRAMS study, normal subjects showed a HOMA-IR of 1.66 ± 0.79 (1.65 ± 0.81 in women and

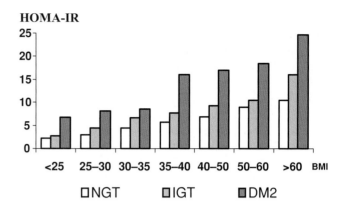

Figure 16–1. Insulin resistance measured by HOMA model across a range of glucose tolerance and adiposity: From normal glucose tolerance to diabetes and from normal weight to super super obesity. NGT, normal glucose tolerant; IGT, impaired glucose tolerant; DM2, type 2 diabetes. *Data from BRAMS (Brazilian Metabolic Syndrome Study).*

1.69 ± 0.72 in men). Considering the patients whose HOMA-IR is above the ninetieth percentile as insulin resistant subjects, we found a threshold value for insulin resistance of 2.71. This threshold is comparable to that in Bonora's study (i.e., 2.77),[27] but it is fairly low compared with the recently published study of Stern et al. (i.e., 4.65 for BMI > 28.9 kg/m^2 and 3.60 for BMI > 27.5 kg/m^2).[33] Therefore, we calculated the HOMA-IR threshold in those subjects who fulfilled the criteria of normal subjects. There is a marked rise in HOMA-IR in high degrees of adiposity. HOMA-IR is also influenced by the glucose tolerance status (Figure 16–1).

ETIOLOGY OF METABOLIC SYNDROME

Insulin resistance, as noted previously, can be caused by many different factors. In the severe obese group of patients, the major cause of insulin resistance is the obesity per se.[34] However, even severe obese subjects may have other underlying causes for the presence and intensity of metabolic derangement. Most individuals have insulin resistance for the following reasons: a genetic abnormality involving one or more steps of the insulin action cascade,[35] an increase in the secretion of counter-regulatory hormones (e.g., glucocorticoids, catecholamines, glucagons, or growth hormone), the use of pharmacological agents that can generate insulin resistance (e.g., glucocorticoids), fetal malnutrion predisposing to the development of insulin resistance in postnatal life, and obesity and decreased physical activity.[36] The factors leading to the development of insulin resistance are not mutually exclusive, and frequently interrelated. Insulin resistance causes physiologic alterations that bring out specific metabolic diseases in individuals who have the susceptible genetic background. In fact, after similar surgical-induced weight loss, patients have different metabolic impact probably related by the maintenance of other pathophysiological mechanisms beyond obesity, i.e., unknown genetic factors.

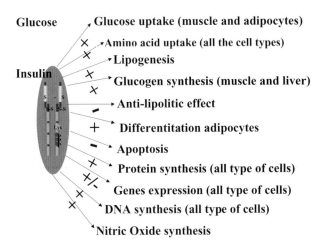

Symbols: (+) = positive effect; (-) = negative effect

Figure 16–2. Diverse biological effects of insulin. When insulin binds its receptor, resultant activation of the insulin signaling cascade leads to multiple effects on several biological processes, including glucose and lipid uptake/metabolism, gene expression/protein synthesis, and cell growth, division, and survival.

In human beings and various other vertebrates, the main anabolic and anticatabolic hormone is insulin. This hormone stimulates glucose, protein, and lipid metabolism, as well as RNA and DNA synthesis, by modifying the activity of a variety of enzymes and transport processes within the cell (Figure 16–2). The knowledge of the molecular pathways of insulin action is crucial to unravel the pathogenesis of type 2 diabetes mellitus and metabolic syndrome, and other insulin-resistant states such as obesity, an insulin resistance state per se.[34] Insulin is the most potent anabolic hormone known and is essential for appropriate tissue development,

growth, and maintenance of whole-body glucose homeostasis (Figure 16–3). This hormone is secreted by the beta cells of the pancreatic islets of Langerhans in response to increased circulating levels of glucose and amino acids after a meal, with a response modulated by gastrointestinal hormones named incretins.[37] Insulin regulates glucose homeostasis at many sites, by reducing hepatic glucose output (via deceased gluconeogenesis and glucogenolysis) and increasing the rate of glucose uptake, mainly into skeletal muscle, heart, and adipose tissue. In muscle and fat cells, the clearance of circulating glucose depends on the insulin-stimulated translocation of GLUT-4 glucose transporters to the cell surface. In addition, insulin stimulates the synthesis in liver and muscle by activation of glycogen synthase and inhibition of glycogen phosphorylase. Insulin also affects lipid metabolism by increasing fatty acid and triglyceride synthesis in liver and fat cells, also by inhibiting lipolysis and fatty acid release from triglyceride synthesis in liver and fat, and by inhibiting ketogenesis in liver. Regarding the metabolism of proteins, insulin stimulates the uptake of amino acids by hepatocytes and muscle cells and, in parallel, enhances protein synthesis in muscle cells, liver, and adipose tissue. In addition, this hormone inhibits protein degradation in skeletal muscle. As a result of the action of insulin, hepatocytes accumulate glycogen, triglycerides, and protein and inhibit glucose release, while in skeletal muscle, this hormone favors glucose uptake, glycogen synthesis, and protein accretion. In adipose tissue, insulin enhances glucose uptake, lipogenesis, and esterification of fatty acids, while it inhibits the release of fatty acids; all these effects lead to enhanced accumulation of triglycerides in adipose cells.[38] In a given patient, as he/she eats large amounts of food, an increased production of insulin will act as an anabolic hormone, accumulating energy in the main tissue for storage, the adipose tissue.

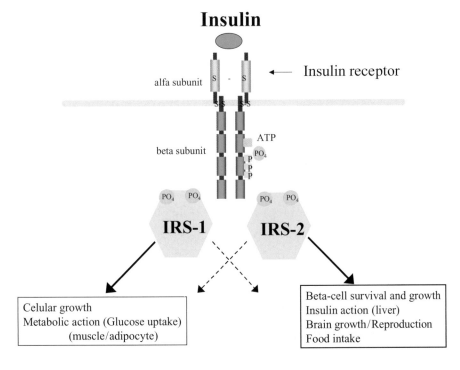

Figure 16–3. Interaction between insulin and the insulin receptor substrate (IRS) proteins. Insulin activates the insulin signaling cascade largely through its interaction with the IRS proteins. Phosphorylation of IRSs proteins results in a number of downstream effects. IRS-1 and IRS-2 have different but overlapping functions. While IRS-1 has a predominant role in cell growth and insulin metabolic action in muscle and adipose tissue, the effects of IRS-2 are better defined in the beta cell and liver, in addition to its role in brain growth, reproduction, and food intake.

MOLECULAR MECHANISMS OF INSULIN RESISTANCE

Insulin resistance means an impaired biological response by target organs to insulin.[39] Impaired signaling at the receptor level results in a cascade of events within the target tissue, which in turn results in impaired glucose transport and a compensatory insulin secretion to overcome the insulin resistance. There are several signaling pathway defects implicated in insulin resistance. The most studied pathway involves the phospatidylinositide 3-kinase (PI3-kinase) and protein kinase B (Akt) pathway. Both insulin and insulin growth factor have effects on the same receptor but have different intracellular signaling pathways[35] (Figure 16–4). Upon binding to their receptor, in the insulin sensitive state, there is autophosphorylation of the beta subunit, which mediates noncovalent but stable interaction between the receptor and cellular proteins. Several proteins are then rapidly phosphorylated on tyrosine residues by ligand-bound insulin receptors, including receptor substrate 1 (IRS-1). IRS docking proteins bind strongly to the enzyme PI3-kinase, a heterodimer consisting of a p85 regulatory subunit and a p110 catalytic subunit, via SH-2 domain interaction with the p85 subunit.[40] Insulin and insulin-like growth factor 1 stimulation increases the amount of PI3-kinase associated with IRSs, and the binding process is associated with increased activity of the enzyme. Activation of this enzyme is essential for transducing the actions of these peptides in insulin sensitive tissues. The interruption or the impairment of this signaling cascade results in a resistance to actions of insulin with resulting hyperinsulinemia.[41] Although hyperinsulinemia may compensate for resistance to some biological actions of insulin, it may result in overexpression of insulin action in tissues with normal or minimally impaired insulin sensitivity. One simple clinical signal of hyperinsulinism in obese subjects is the presence of acantose nigricans, a gray-brown velvety discoloration and increased thickness of the skin, usually at the neck, groin, axillae, and under the breasts.[42] Thus, accentuation to other actions gives rise to diverse clinical manifestations and sequelae of the insulin resistance syndrome. Hyperinsulinemia may continually stimulate the mitogenic insulin-signaling pathway, thus exerting its detrimental influence on cardiovascular disease.[43]

CLINICAL PRESENTATIONS OF METABOLIC SYNDROME IN THE OBESE PATIENT

Obese subjects develop insulin resistance, which usually compensates for the decreased effects on glucose metabolism by increasing insulin secretion to maintain a normal glucose metabolism.[44] This state of compensated hyperinsulinemia interacts with the underlying genetic constitution of the individual. This interaction determines the phenotypic response and the clinical effects of the insulin resistance and hyperinsulinemia. If insulin resistance develops in an individual who has pancreatic beta cells with limited functional capacity, then type 2 diabetes will develop. Polycystic ovary syndrome (PCOS) will develop if insulin resistance occurs in women who have ovarian enzymes that are abnormally regulated, promoting a state of hyperandrogenism.[45]

Insulin resistance also interacts with each individual's genetic background to determine which of the components of metabolic syndrome will be manifest. Besides, this interaction will determine how severe the metabolic syndrome will be and the extent to which they will accelerate atherosclerosis and cause macrovascular disease.

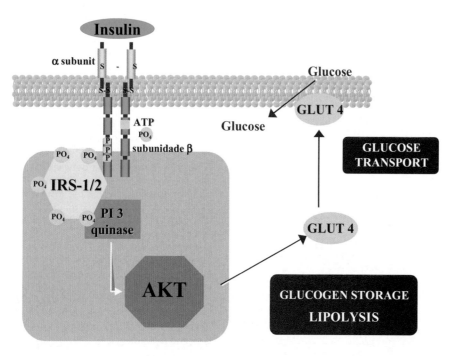

Figure 16–4. Molecular mechanism for insulin action. Binding of insulin to its receptors activates tyrosine kinase, resulting in autophosphorylation of tyrosine residues on the receptor β-subunit. This in turn leads to phosphorylation of several protein substrates (IRSs) activating the downstream cascade necessary for stimulation of glucose transport.

Type 2 Diabetes

The vast majority of population has beta cell function that is adequate to fulfill normal tissue insulin requirements. These individuals have beta cells that have considerable reserve function and could increase insulin secretion as much as necessary.[46] There is, however, a significant segment of every population whose beta cells have limited reserve function. In these individuals, the development of insulin resistance raises the tissue insulin requirements beyond insulin secretory capabilities of the beta cells, and hyperglycemia ensues.[47] The great increase in the prevalence of type 2 diabetes can be attributed to changing lifestyles that have created an enormous number of people with insulin resistance, and probably 25%–33% of these individuals will have beta cell abnormalities, which will lead to the development of type 2 diabetes.[48] In severely obese subjects, the degree of insulin resistance is so high that beta cell function could be exhausted after an intense exposure to constant and intense necessities of insulin production.

The key to understanding the natural history of type 2 diabetes in obese subjects is the knowledge of the evolution of beta cell function in individuals who have the genetic predisposition for, and go on to develop, type 2 diabetes.[49] If a given severe obese subject has a production of insulin that overcomes the prevailing insulin resistance, then type 2 diabetes will not develop. Otherwise, these patients would develop the insulin resistance syndrome with the intrinsic increasing risk of cardiovascular disease. The presence of diabetes in these patients raises the risk of cardiovascular diseases. The earliest clinically significant change in insulin secretion is a decrease in early meal-mediated insulin secretion. The consequence of this delay following a meal is an exaggerated rise in plasma glucose in the first hour (normal value <140 mg/dL) and a prolongation of the rise such that the 2-hour plasma glucose is elevated above normal levels (<120 mg/dL). As the beta cell abnormalities progress, the next defect to develop is a progressive loss in the quantity of insulin secreted in response to nutrients, such that the amount of insulin secreted is inadequate relative to the degree of insulin resistance.[50] At this stage, the 2-hour postprandial plasma glucose rises progressively with time from 140 mg/dL to finally exceed 200 mg/dL. From this point in time, there is a progressive loss of beta-cell insulin secretory function. At the time of clinical diagnosis of type 2 diabetes, beta cell function is approximately 50% of normal for the prevalent BMI, and this decreases, approximately, 50% each subsequent 6 years.[51] After 10–15 years, most patients are sufficiently beta cell deficient and they require some form of insulin in their treatment program.[52]

Accelerated Atherosclerosis and Macrovascular Disease

Many prospective studies in diverse ethnic populations have shown that hyperinsulinemia is a powerful predictor of the development of type 2 diabetes (relative risk five- to sixfold increased).[53–55] Similarly, other components of insulin resistance syndrome, such as central obesity, 2-hour postglu-cose challenge plasma glucose levels, blood pressure, plasma triglycerides, and low HDL-C have also been shown to be predictors of the development of type 2 diabetes. Appropriate models show that insulin resistance cluster has a relative risk for type 2 diabetes, which is increased by 13-fold.

Individuals with insulin resistance and hyperinsulinemia have other components of metabolic syndrome at the time when they are normoglycemic or have intolerance to glucose. This means that cardiovascular risks, and accelerated atherosclerosis, are occurring many years before the development of any of the clinical syndromes, such as type 2 diabetes or vascular disease. Insulin resistance is associated with other components of metabolic syndrome. A number of studies measuring intimal–medial thickness of the carotid artery by B-mode ultrasound have shown an increase in individuals with insulin resistance and obesity. It is presumed that this reflects changes in other arteries, such as the coronary arteries.[56]

The question whether insulin resistance is a significant risk factor for a cardiovascular disease is a difficult one. Scant data are available in severe obese subjects. The problem that is difficult to solve is the determination of cardiovascular risk of metabolic syndrome as a whole and how much each of the components of the syndrome independently, and selectively, contribute to the cardiovascular risk. Three questions are still open to discussion: (1) Are the cardiovascular risks of the components greater than the sum of the parts? (2) Are the cardiovascular risks of the components of the metabolic syndrome additive, or are a few more dominant? (3) Is there a stage in the development of cardiovascular disease where the disease process is no longer dependent on insulin-resistance-associated risk factors, and, in contrast, where the subclinical disease progresses with little or no dependence on risk factors? These questions are still a matter of discussion, but there is no doubt in regard to the potential beneficial metabolic effect of treating obesity. There are several bariatric series showing after surgery some improvement in insulin resistance, individual components of the metabolic syndrome, and the overall reversion of the syndrome.

IMPROVEMENT AND RESOLUTION OF CLINICAL CONDITIONS ASSOCIATED WITH METABOLIC SYNDROME AFTER BARIATRIC SURGERY

Type 2 Diabetes

The prevention, improvement, and reversion of type 2 diabetes are observed across all the bariatric surgical techniques (Table 16–3).

One of the first surgical series on diabetic subjects was the Greenville study in which 165 patients were operated by the gastric bypass and 83% of them had a remission of the diabetes along with a 14-year follow-up.[57] Other important study is the Swedish Obesity Subjects, in which 2,010 patients after different bariatric procedures were compared to 2,037

Table 16–3.

Reversion of Diabetes 2 Year After Bariatric Surgery

Surgical Procedure	Reversion of Type 2 Diabetes %	95% CI
Biliopancreatic diversion or Duodenal switch	98.9	96.8–100%
Gastric bypass	83.7	77.3–90.1%
Gastroplasty	71.6	55.1–88.2%
Gastric Banding	47.9	29.1–66.7%

Adapted, with permission, from Buchwald et al.: Bariatric Surgery. A systematic review and Meta-Analysis. JAMA 292: 1724–1737, 2004.

controls who underwent conventional clinical management. After 2 years, the prevalence was 8% in the control group and 1% in the operated group. After 10 years, the prevalence raised to 24% in the control group and to 7% in the operated group.[58] In a recent meta-analysis, Buchwald and coworkers reported a resolution of diabetes in 76.8% of 1,846 patients.[59] Otherwise, improvement of glucose homeostasis is usually observed in all patients, along with reducing requirements of antidiabetic drugs.[60] There was a difference in metabolic outcomes, according to the type of surgery, with better results reported in disabsorptive procedures (biliopancreatic diversion and duodenal switch) (Table 16–3). There is no specific data available in regard to micro- and macrovascular diabetic complications after surgical treatment of diabetes.

Dyslipidemia

The outcome of dyslipidemia was significantly improved across all surgical procedures. These results extend to hyperlipidemia, hypercholesterolemia, and hypertriglyceridemia. Surgical-induced weight loss leads to a decrease in plasma free fatty acids, lower triglycerides, raise in HDL-C, decrease in LDL-cholesterol (LDL-C), and shift in the LDL particle atherogenic pattern from a preponderance of the small dense particles to one of the large buoyant particles.[61] The best results are found in the disabsorptive techniques, showing improvement in 99.1% patients with biliopancreatic diversion and 96.9% patients with duodenal switch.[59] Scopinaro and coworkers have reported a reversion of dyslipidemia in near total of 2,241 operated subjects with a maximum follow-up of 21 years.[62] In the meta-analysis of Buchwald, considering the pooled data of all surgical procedures, there was an average reduction of 33.2 mg/dL in total cholesterol, 29.3 mg/dL in LDL-C, 79.6 mg/dL in trygliceries, and a raise in HDL-C of 5 mg/dL.

The underlying mechanisms for the antidyslipidemic effect of bariatric surgery are related with reduction in the total lipidic and caloric ingestion, improvement in insulin sensitivity, and lipid disabsorption in biliopancreatic diversion/duodenal switch.

Hypertension

The studies have shown an average reversion of hypertension in 61.7% (95% CI, 55.6%–67.8%).[59] The clinical outcome of hypertension, including reversion or improvement, was 78.5% (95% CI, 70.8%–86.1%). The underlying mechanisms for the antihypertensive surgical effect are related with reduction in hyperinsulinemia and insulin resistance,[28] reduction in sympathetic hyperactivation due to reduction in leptin levels,[63] and reduction in intra-abdominal hypertension.[64] This reduction in blood pressure seems to be independent of the surgical procedure performed.[59] One of the major complications of hypertension is the renal failure. Recent studies have shown stabilization or even better an improvement in renal function after massive weight loss.[65]

Infertility

Severe obesity is characterized by several sexual hormonal dysfunctions leading to some degree of infertility. In men, there is hypogonadotrophic hypogonadism due to an enhanced testosterone conversion to estrogen mediated by aromatase in the increased amount of adipose tissue.[66] In women, there is a massive conversion of estradiol in estrone by the same mechanism observed in severe obese men, a raised action of adipose aromatase. In a recent series was reported a prevalence of PCOS in 35% of morbid obese women that was resolved after bariatric surgery along with improvement in the hyperandrogenism.[67] The ultimate proof that insulin resistance through its compensatory hyperinsulinemia significantly contributes to the pathogenesis of PCOS has come from interventional studies with drugs that decrease insulin resistance. Metformin and glitazones, both insulin sensitizers, have been shown to decrease hyperinsulinemia and plasma androgen levels and correct menstrual irregularities through restoration of ovulation.[68] The amelioration of fertility in the PCOS group after surgery may be dependent on the improvement in the insulin sensitivity.

Procoagulant State

It has been shown for several decades that individuals with obesity are at increased risk of death from coronary artery disease. It is now suspected that this increase in macrovascular disease is, at least in part, the result of the presence of metabolic syndrome and insulin resistance. Detailed analysis of coagulation and fibrinolytic systems in individuals with severe obesity has shown that several factors, which influence thrombus development or dissolution, are altered and appear to be a part of metabolic syndrome.[69] These factors, which have a significant correlation with either insulin resistance or hyperinsulinemia, are elevated levels of plasminogen activator inhibitor-1 (PAI-1), von Willebrand factor, fibrinogen, and factor VII.[70] Some bariatric series have shown an overall improvement in these factors contributing for the reduction in the procoagulant state of the obesity-related metabolic syndrome.[71,72]

Endothelial Dysfunction

The endothelium lines the blood vessels and regulates blood flow and proliferation and migration of the adjacent vascular smooth muscle cells. Endothelial cells generate vasoconstrictor and vasodilator molecules to control vascular tone. They also produce growth factors (i.e., IGF-1), generate an inflammatory response, and modulate the thrombotic process.[73] Endothelial cells can be viewed as having two opposite functions: On the one hand these cells promote vasoconstriction, inflammation, proliferation, and thrombosis, which can ultimately lead to atherosclerosis. On the other hand, these cells promote vasodilatation and minimize inflammation, proliferation, and thrombosis, and are antiatherogenic.[74] Changes in insulin sensitivity and in adiposity after bariatric surgery are related to reduction in products of a dysfunctional endothelium as E-selectin, PAI-1, adhesion molecules, and oxidative stress biomarkers.[75]

BARIATRIC SURGERY AND NATURAL HISTORY OF METABOLIC SYNDROME

Prevention of Diabetes

The metabolic syndrome is a condition with increasing risk for the development of type 2 diabetes. An expected beneficial effect of bariatric surgery is to prevent type 2 diabetes in this population. Clinical interventional studies have demonstrated some beneficial effect of weight loss in preventing the evolution from prediabetic states (impaired fasting glucose or impaired glucose tolerance) to overt diabetes.[76] In bariatric surgical studies, the described impact is more pronounced. In fact, gastric bypass has been associated with diabetic prevention in high-risk individuals with pre-diabetes, in about 99%–100%.[77] The first work focusing the surgical diabetic prevention was published by Long and coworkers.[78] They found a relative risk for developing diabetes 30 times greater in obese patients who refused bariatric surgeries for several reasons in comparison to the operated subjects.

Cardiovascular Mortality

The reversion of metabolic syndrome could lead to a potential improvement in life expectancy. An extensive study with 43,457 women with a 12-year follow-up has shown that an intentional weight loss of at least 9 kg was associated with a 53% reduction in obesity-associated mortality.[79] Increasing evidences associate longevity with bariatric surgery. The Swedish Obese Subjects Study in diabetic patients has shown 9% mortality at 9 years in the operated group and

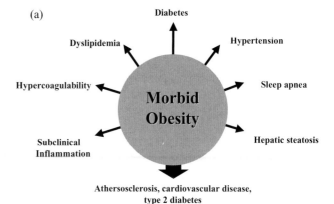

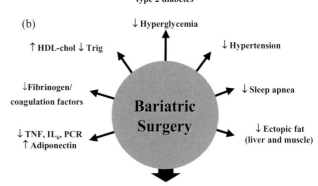

Figure 16–5. Clinical presentations of metabolic syndrome in morbid obesity and its potential reversion with bariatric surgical treatment.

28% mortality in the control group.[80] The major cause of deaths in this group is cardiovascular disease. Other groups studying 1,035 operated patients in comparison with 5,746 controls have demonstrated a 5-year follow-up reduction in the relative risk of death by 89% with an absolute significant mortality reduction of 5.49%.[81]

Considering the underlying physiopathological mechanisms linking cardiovascular events and features of the metabolic syndrome, we can assume that reduction in mortality rates in surgical-treated patients is, at least in part, mediated by the reversion or amelioration of the metabolic syndrome[82] (Figure 16–5(a) and (b)).

CONCLUSIONS

Bariatric surgery is an effective treatment for sustained weight loss in morbid obese subjects. A marked reduction in the insulin resistance is found after surgical-induced weight loss.[25,26,28,44] We have shown a sustained improvement in insulin sensitivity at 6 years after surgery.[83] This phenomenon affects directly the pathophysiologic basis of the metabolic syndrome. Considering the prevailing diagnostic criteria, there is a reversion or cure of the metabolic syndrome in the great majority of the patients after bariatric surgery (Figure 16–5(a) and (b)).

In 1995, a landmark article on bariatric surgery was published.[84] That paper had a provocative title, "Who would have thought it? An operation proves to be the most effective therapy for adult-onset diabetes mellitus." The authors pointed for the clinical findings, but they also recognized the limited knowledge about the reasons for such marked metabolic improvement. Few years later, the same group had asked a new question: "A new paradigm for type 2 diabetes mellitus: could it be a disease of the foregut?" reinforcing their perception for considering type 2 diabetes a surgical condition.[85]

In times of increasing rates of obesity, we propose another provocative question: Is metabolic syndrome a surgical condition in severe obese subjects? Considering the impressive data in regard to beneficial effects of bariatric surgery on major components of metabolic syndrome and also on the improvement in insulin resistance, the answer is yes.[86]

References

1. Zimmet P, Magliano D, Matsuzawa Y, Alberti G, Shaw J: The metabolic syndrome: A global health problem and a new definition. *J Atheroscler Thromb* 12:295–300, 2006.
2. Alberti G, Zimmet P, Shaw J, Bloomgarden Z, Kaufman F, Silink M: Type 2 diabetes in the young: The evolving epidemic. The international diabetes federation consensus workshop. *Diabetes Care* 27:1798–1811, 2004.
3. Kylin E. Studien ueber das Hypertonie-Hyperglyka "mie-Hyperurika" miesyndrome. *Zentralblatt fuer Innere Medicin* 44:105–127, 1923.
4. Vague J: La differentiation sexuelle. Facteur determinant dès formes de l'obesité. *Presse Méd* 30:339–340, 1947.
5. Reaven G: The role of insulin resistance in human disease. *Diabetes* 37:1595–1607, 1988.
6. Kaplan N: The deadly quartet: Upper-body obesity, glucose intolerance, hypertriglyceridemia, and hypertension. *Arch Intern Med* 149:1514–1520, 1989.
7. DeFronzo R, Ferrannini E: Insulin resistance. A multifaceted syndrome responsible for NIDDM, obesity, hypertension, dyslipidemia and atherosclerotic cardiovascular disease. *Diabetes Care* 14:173–194, 1991.
8. Groop L, Orho-Melander M: The dysmetaboli syndrome. *J Intern Med* 250:105–120, 2001.
9. Alberti K, Zimmet P: Definition, diagnosis and classification of diabetes mellitus. Part 1: Diagnosis and classification of diabetes mellitus. Report of WHO consultation. *Diabet Med* 15:539–553, 1998.
10. Balkau B, Charles MA: Comment on the provisional report from the WHO consultation. European group for the study of insulin resistance (EGIR). *Diabet Med* 16:442–443, 1999.
11. Executive summary of the third report of the National Cholesterol Education Program (NCEP): Expert panel on detection, evaluation, and treament of high blood cholesterol in adults (ATP III). *JAMA* 285:2486–2497, 2001.
12. American College of Endocrinology Task Force on the Insulin Resistance Syndrome: American College of Endocrinology Position Statement on the insulin resistance syndrome. *Endocr Pract* 9:236–252, 2003.
13. Zimmet P, Alberti KG, Shaw J: Global and societal implications of the diabetes epidemic. *Nature* 414:782–787, 2001.
14. Cameron AJ, Shaw JE, Zimmet P: The metabolic syndrome: Prevalence in worldwide populations. *Endocrinol Metab Clin North Am* 33:351–376, 2004.
15. Ford ES, Giles WH, Dietz WH: Prevalence of the metabolic syndrome among US adults: Findings from the third national health and nutrition examination survey. *JAMA* 287:356–359, 2002.
16. Geloneze B, Repetto EM, Geloneze SR, Tambascia MA, Ermetice MN: The threshold value for insulin resistance (HOMA-IR) in an admixtured population. IR in the Brazilian Metabolic Syndrome Study. *Diabetes Res Clin Pract* 72:219–220, 2006.
17. Alberti KG, Zimmet P, Shaw J., Metabolic syndrome—a new world definition. A consensus statement from the International Diabetes Federation. *Diabet Med* 23:469–480, 2006.
18. Ribeiro-Filho FF, Faria AN, Azjen S, Zanella MT, Ferreira SRG: Methods of estimation of visceral fat: Advantages of ultrasonography. *Obes Res* 11:1488–1494, 2003.
19. Ribeiro-Filho FF, Faria AN, Kohlmann O Jr, et al.: Ultrasonography for the evaluation of visceral fat and cardiovascular risk. *Hypertension* 38:713–717, 2001.
20. Kahn R, Buse J, Ferrannini E, Stern M: The metabolic syndrome: Time for a critical appraisal. Joint statement from the American Diabetes Association and the European Association for the study of diabetes. *Diabetes Care* 28:2289–2304, 2005.
21. Grundy SM: Metabolic syndrome: Connecting and reconciling cardiovascular and diabetes worlds. *J Am Coll Cardiol* 47:1093–1100, 2006.
22. Gale EA: The myth of the metabolic syndrome. *Diabetologia* 48:1679–1683, 2005.
23. DeFronzo R, Tobin J, Andres R. Glucose clamp technique: A method for quantifying insulin secretion and resistance. *Am J Physiol* 237:E214–E223, 1979.
24. Bergman RN: Lilly lecture. Toward physiological understanding of glucose tolerance. Minimal-model approach. *Diabetes* 38:1512–1527, 1989.
25. Pereira JA, Lazarin MA, Pareja JC, de Souza A, Muscelli E: Insulin resistance in nondiabetic morbidly obese patients: Effect of bariatric surgery. *Obes Res* 11:1495–1501, 2003.
26. Muscelli E, Mingrone G, Camastra S, et al.: Differential effect of weight loss on insulin resistance in surgically treated obese patients. *Am J Med* 118:51–57, 2005.
27. Bonora E, Moghetti P, Zancanaro C, et al.: Estimates of in vivo insulin action in man: Comparison of insulin tolerance tests with euglycemic and hyperglycemic glucose clamp studies. *J Clin Endocrinol Metab* 68:374–378, 1989.
28. Geloneze B, Tambascia MA, Pareja JC, Repetto EM, Magna LA: The insulin tolerance test in severely obese patients undergoing bariatric surgery. *Obes Res* 9:763–769, 2001.
29. Matthews D, Hosker JP, Rudenski AS, Naylor BA, Trecher DF, Turner RC: Homeostasis model assessment: Insulin resistance and β-cell function from fasting plasma glucose and insulin concentration in man. *Diabetologia* 28:412–419, 1985.
30. Bonora E, Targher G, Alberiche M, et al.: Homeostasis model assessment closely mirrors the glucose clamp technique in the assessment of insulin sensitivity. *Diabetes Care* 23:57–63, 2000.
31. Bonora E, Formentini G, Calcaterra F, et al.: HOMA-estimated insulin resistance is an independent predictor of cardiovascular disease in type 2 diabetic subjects: Prospective data from the Verona Diabetes Complications Study. *Diabetes Care* 25:1135–1141, 2002.
32. Haffner SM, Kennedy E, Gonzalez C, Stern MP, Miettinen H: A prospective analysis of the HOMA model. The Mexico City Diabetes Study. *Diabetes Care* 19:1138–1141, 1996.
33. Stern SE, Williams K, Ferrannini E, DeFronzo RA, Bogardus C, Stern MP: Identification of individuals with insulin resistance using routine clinical measurements. *Diabetes* 54:333–339, 2005.
34. Natali A, Ferrannini E: Hypertension, insulin resistance, and the metabolic syndrome. *Endocrinol Metab Clin North Am* 33:417–429, 2004.
35. Saad MJ, Araki E, Miralpeix M, Rothenberg PL, White MF, Kahn CR: Regulation of insulin receptor substrate-1 in liver and muscle of animal models of insulin resistance. *J Clin Invest* 90:1839–1849, 1992.

36. Kahn CR: Diabetes. Causes of insulin resistance. *Nature* 373:384–385, 1995.

37. Gautier JF, Fetita S, Sobngwi E, Salaun-Martin C: Biological actions of the incretins GIP and GLP-1 and therapeutic perspectives in patients with type 2 diabetes. *Diabetes Metab* 31:233–242, 2005.

38. Saltiel AR: New perspectives into molecular pathogenesis and treatment of type 2 diabetes. *Cell* 104:517–529, 2001.

39. Sowers JR, Sowers PS, Peuler JD: Role of insulin resistance and hyperinsulinemia in development of hypertension and atherosclerosis. *J Lab Clin Med* 123:647–652, 1994.

40. Rhodes CJ, White MF: Molecular insights into insulin action and secretion. *Eur J Clin Invest* 32(Suppl3):3–13, 2002.

41. Sowers JR: Insulin and insulin-like growth factor in normal and pathological cardiovascular physiology. *Hypertension* 29:691–699, 1997.

42. Dunaif A, Green G, Phelps R, et al.: Acanthosis nigricans, insulin action, and hyperandrogenism: Clinical, histological, and biochemical findings. *J Clin Endocrinol Metab* 73:590–595, 1991.

43. Wang CC, Goalstone ML, Draznin B: Molecular mechanisms of insulin resistance that impact cardiovascular biology. *Diabetes* 53:2735–2740, 2004.

44. Ferrannini E, Camastra S, Gastaldelli A, et al.: Beta-cell function in obesity: Effects of weight loss. *Diabetes* 53(Suppl 3):S26–S33, 2004.

45. Schroder AK, Tauchert S, Ortmann O, Diedrich K, Weiss JM: Insulin resistance in patients with polycystic ovary syndrome. *Ann Med* 36:426–439, 2004.

46. Gerich JE: The genetic basis of type 2 diabetes mellitus: Impaired insulin secretion versus impaired insulin sensitivity. *Endocr Rev* 19:491–503, 1998.

47. Kahn SE: The importance of beta-cell failure in the development and progression of type 2 diabetes. *J Clin Endocrinol Metab* 4:372–389, 2001.

48. Stumvoll M, Gerich J: Clinical features of insulin resistance and beta cell dysfunction and the relationship to type 2 diabetes. *Clin Lab Med* 21:31–51, 2001.

49. Scheen AJ: From obesity to diabetes: Why, when and who? *Acta Clin Belg* 55:9–15, 2000.

50. Pimenta W, Korytkowski M, Mitrakou A, et al.: Pancreatic beta-cell dysfunction as the primary genetic lesion in NIDDM. Evidence from studies in normal individuals with a first-degree NIDDM relative. *J Am Med Assoc* 273:1855–1861, 1995.

51. UK Prospective Diabetes Study (UKPDS) Group: UKPDS 16. Overview of 6 years' therapy of type II diabetes: A progressive disease. *Diabetes* 44:1249–1258, 1995.

52. Levy J, Atkinson AB, Bell PM, McCance DR, Hadden DR: Beta-cell deterioration determines the onset and rate of progression of secondary dietary failure in type 2 daibetes mellitus: The 10-year follow-up of the Belfast Diet Study. *Diabet Med* 15:290–296, 1998.

53. Festa A, D'Agostino R Jr, Howard G, et al.: Chronic subclinical inflammation as part of the insulin resistance syndrome: The Insulin Resistance Atherosclerosis Study (IRAS). *Circulation* 102:42–47, 2000.

54. Hanley AJG, Stern MP, Willians K, Haffner SM: Homeostasis model assessment of insulin resistance in relation to the incidence of cardiovascular disease. *Diabetes Care* 25:1177–1184, 2002.

55. Haffner SM: The metabolic syndrome: Inflammation, diabetes mellitus, and cardiovascular disease. *Am J Cardiol* 97:3A–11A, 2005.

56. Rohani M, Jogestrand T, Ekberg M, et al.: Interrelation between the extent of atherosclerosis in the thoracic aorta, carotid intima-media thickness and the extent of coronary artery disease. *Atherosclerosis* 179:311–316, 2005.

57. Sjostrom CD, Peltonen M, Wedel H, Sjostrom L: Differentiated long-term effects of intentional weight loss on diabetes and hypertension. *Hypertension* 36:20–25, 2000.

58. Sjostrom L, Lindroos AK, Peltonen M, et al.: Swedish obese subjects study scientific group. Lifestyle, diabetes, and cardiovascular risk factors 10 years after bariatric surgery. *N Engl J Med* 351:2283–2293, 2004.

59. Bushwald H, Avidor Y, Braunwad E, et al.: Bariatric surgery. A systematic review and meta-analysis. *JAMA* 292:1724–1737, 2004.

60. Cummings DE, Overduin J, Foster-Schubert KE: Gastric bypass for obesity: Mechanisms of weight loss and diabetes resolution. *J Clin Endocrinol Metab* 89:2608–2615, 2004.

61. Brizzi P, Angius MF, Carboni A, et al.: Plasma lipids and lipoprotein changes after biliopancreatic diversion for morbid obesity. *Dig Surg* 20:18–23, 2003.

62. Scopinaro N, Marinari GM, Camerini GD, Papadia FS, Adami GF: Specific effects of biliopancreatic diversion on the major components of metabolic syndrome: A long-term follow-up study. *Diabetes Care* 28:2406–2411, 2005.

63. Geloneze B, Tambascia MA, Pareja JC, Repetto EM, Magna LA, Pereira SG: Serum leptin levels after bariatric surgery across a range of glucose tolerance from normal to diabetes. *Obes Surg* 11:693–698, 2001.

64. Sugerman HJ: Effects of increased intra-abdominal pressure in severe obesity. *Surg Clin North Am* 81:1063–1075, 2001.

65. Agnani S, Vachharajani VT, Gupta R, Atray NK, Vachharajani TJ: Does treating obesity stabilize chronic kidney disease? *BMC Nephrol* 6:7 2005.

66. Karagiannis A, Harsoulis F: Gonadal dysfunction in systemic diseases. *Eur J Endocrinol* 152:501–513, 2005.

67. Escobar-Morreale HF, Botella-Carretero JI, Alvarez-Blanco F, Sancho J, Millan JL: The polycystic ovary syndrome associated with morbid obesity may resolve after weight loss induced by bariatric surgery. *J Clin Endocrinol Metab* 90:6364–6369, 2005.

68. Erhmann DA: Polycystic ovary syndrome. *N Engl J Med* 352:1223–1236, 2005.

69. Goichot B, Grunebaum L, Desprez D, et al.: Circulating procoagulant microparticles in obesity. *Diabetes Metab* 32:82–85, 2006.

70. Mertens I, Verrijken A, Michiels JJ, Van der Planken M, Ruige JB, Van Gaal LF: Among inflammation and coagulation markers, PAI-1 is a true component of the metabolic syndrome. *Int J Obes.* 30:1308–1314, 2006.

71. Uzun H, Zengin K, Taskin M, Aydin S, Simsek G, Dariyerli N: Changes in leptin, plasminogen activator factor and oxidative stress in morbidly obese patients following open and laparoscopic Swedish adjustable gastric banding. *Obes Surg* 14:659–665, 2004.

72. van Dielen FM, Buurman WA, Hadfoune M, Nijhuis J, Greve JW: Macrophage inhibitory factor, plasminogen activator inhibitor-1, other acute phase proteins, and inflammatory mediators normalize as a result of weight loss in morbidly obese subjects treated with gastric restrictive surgery. *J Clin Endocrinol Metab* 89:4062–4068, 2004.

73. Vita JA: Endothelial function and clinical outcome. *Heart* 91:1278–1279, 2005.

74. Landmesser U, Hornig B, Drexler H: Endothelial function: A critical determinant in atherosclerosis? *Circulation* 109(21 Suppl 1):II27–II33, 2004.

75. Willians IL, Chowienczyk PJ, Wheatcroft SB, et al.: Endothelial function and weight loss in obese humans. *Obes Surg* 15:1055–1060, 2005.

76. Inzucchi SE, Sherwin RS: The prevention of type 2 diabetes mellitus. *Endocrinol Metab Clin North Am* 34:199–219, 2005.

77. Eisenberg D, Bell RL: The impact of bariatric surgery on severely obese patients with diabetes. *Diabetes Spectr* 16:240–245, 2003.

78. Long SD, O'Brien K, MacDonald KG Jr, et al.: Weight loss in severely obese subjects prevents the progression of impaired glucose tolerance to type II diabetes. A longitudinal interventional study. *Diabetes Care* 17:372–375, 1994.

79. Williamson DF, Pamuk E, Thun M, Flanders D, Byers T, Heath C: National Prospective study of intentional weight loss and mortality

in overweight white men aged 40–64 years. *Am J Epidemiol* 149:491–503, 1999.

80. Sjostrom CD, Peltonen M, Sjostrom L: Blood pressure and pulse pressure during long-term weight loss in the obese: The Swedish Obese Subjects (SOS) Intervention Study. *Obes Res* 9:188–195, 2001.

81. Christou NV, Sampalis JS, Liberman M, et al.: Surgery decreases long-term mortality, morbidity, and health care use in morbidly obese patients. *Ann Surg* 240:416–423, 2004.

82. Geloneze B, Geloneze SR, Picolo M, Repetto EM, Murro AL, Tambascia MA: Metabolic syndrome as a surgical condition. *Obes Surg* 12:459, 2002.

83. Lima MMO, Pareja JC, Tambascia MA, Repetto EM, Thé C, Geloneze B: Insulin sensitivity after gastric bypass. A 6-year prospective study. *Diabetes* 54(Suppl 2):A203, 2005.

84. Pories WJ, Swanson MS, MacDonald KG, et al.: Who would have thought it? An operation proves to be the most effective therapy for adult-onset diabetes mellitus. *Ann Surg* 222:339–350, 1995.

85. Hickey MS, Pories WJ, MacDonald KG Jr, et al.: A new paradigm for type 2 diabetes mellitus: Could it be a disease of the foregut? *Ann Surg* 227:637–643, 1998.

86. Geloneze B, Pareja JC: Does bariatric surgery cure metabolic syndrome? *Arq Bras Endocrinol Metab* 50:400-407, 2006.

17

The Learning Curve

Michael L. Schwartz, MD, PhD • Raymond L. Drew, MD

I. METHODS

II. RESULTS

III. DISCUSSION

The learning curve in laparoscopic bariatric surgery has been described by experts in the field as

1. "daunting and far more demanding of the surgeon's patience and tenacity"[1];
2. "a long and arduous journey"[2];
3. "a technically challenging procedure with a steep learning curve"[3];
4. "a high degree of difficulty translates into a steep learning curve."[4]

These statements certainly cause anxiety in the surgeon who starts a program on laparoscopic bariatric surgery.

Every paper that has addressed the issue of the learning curve has noted that operative times decrease with experience. Operative time is really not an issue. The issue is whether the surgeon experiences a cluster of serious complications and deaths early in their experience. The length of this steep and treacherous learning curve is around 100 cases, as measured by various complications such as bowel obstruction,[5] leaks,[6] or all complications.[7–9] Flum[10] reported that this learning curve applies to open as well as laparoscopic bariatric operations. We, along with several other authors,

do not think that the learning curve need be dangerous for patients.[11–13]

METHODS

We have attempted to measure the slope of our learning curve by quantifying our errors. We conceptualized a program of laparoscopic Roux-en-Y gastric bypass (lap RYGBP) in August 1998 and performed our first laparoscopic operation in February 1999. Both authors were experienced in bariatric surgery, having performed approximately 1,500 open bariatric operations during their careers. Each surgeon attended a separate 2-day course in laparoscopic bariatric surgery. In addition, laparoscopic gastric bypasses were performed on seven experimental animals, with approval of the animal experimentation committee. Laparoscopic staplers were used on six open cases prior to our first clinical lap RYGBP.

Guidelines for patient selection for laparoscopic surgery were established prior to the series. Initially patients with a waist measurement less than 125 cm, BMI less than 50 kg/m², and no prior upper abdominal surgery were selected. Patients with central obesity, as determined by physical examination and waist/hip ratio, were avoided. These guidelines were later liberalized to include patients with a waist measurement of 150 cm. No revisions of any previous bariatric operation were attempted with the laparoscopic approach.

The laparoscopic operation attempted to duplicate our experience with open operations.[14] The laparoscopic operation created a 20 mL or less gastric pouch. A 12-mm banded gastroenterostomy was created with a linear stapler. The stapler defect was sutured to complete the anastomosis. The biliopancreatic limb was 15–30 cm in length and the Roux-en-Y limb was 75–150 cm depending on the patients' BMI.[15] The enteroenterostomy was created with two 45-mm or one 60-mm stapler. The stapler defect was closed with an additional 45-mm stapler or hand sutured. The Roux-en-Y limb was routed retrocolic and retrogastric. The mesenteric, transverse mesocolon and Petersen's defects were closed with permanent suture.

There were several differences between the laparoscopic and the open procedure (see Chapters 3 and 4). In the lap procedure the gastric pouch was lesser curvature based. In the open procedure, the gastric pouch was based on anterior-oblique pouch.[14,16] The open RYGBP band was created from the linea alba. The lap RYGBP band was created from cadaver or autogenous fascia lata. With both the lap and the open operation, the fascia band was marked for radiographic identification with 90-mm stapler and placed at the gastroenterostomy.

We analyzed our first 1,000 consecutive cases to estimate the difficulty of learning the laparoscopic gastric bypass. Preoperatively, waist, hips, height, and weight were measured. All patients conformed to NIH guidelines for bariatric surgery.[17]

Data was placed into a prospectively designed database (eMD Bariatrics, Exemplo Medical). Postoperatively, operative time was recorded. The frequency and seriousness of complications and the rate of conversion from laparoscopic to open bariatric surgery was used to estimate the difficulty of learning bariatric surgery. The patients were divided into consecutive groups of 100 patients each to analyze the data.

Complications included a leak from the GI tract, pulmonary embolus, small bowel obstruction/internal hernia, postoperative GI bleed causing a 5-gm/dL decrease in hemoglobin or requiring transfusion, stenosis of the GI tract requiring dilation or reoperation, intraoperative bleeding requiring transfusion or conversion to an open operation, and intra-abdominal infection or a wound problem that required return to the operating room.

Conversion from laparoscopic to open gastric bypass was performed whenever the operating surgeon thought a safe operation could not be conducted laparoscopically. The reason for the conversion was noted in the operative report and recorded in the database.

RESULTS

The average age of the patients was 41.9 years, average BMI was 47.1 kg/m², and 89.1% of the patients were female. Average waist measurement per patient group is shown in Figure 17–1. This trend was significant ($p < 0.001$) using a linear regression analysis. Operating time decreased during the series (Figure 17–1). This was also significant ($p < 0.001$) using a linear regression analysis.

Complications of lap RYGBP are listed in Table 17–1. The numbers for each individual complication were too small

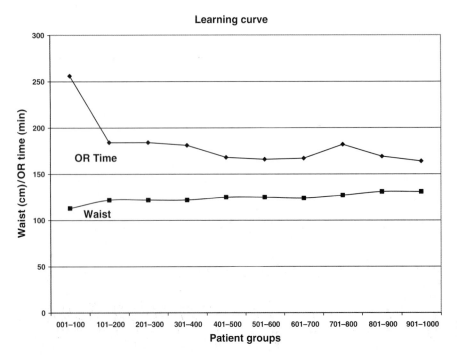

Figure 17–1. Average OR time (minutes) and average waist size (centimeters) in 1,000 laparoscopic gastric bypass patients grouped by 100s.

Table 17–1.

Major Complications in 1,000 Laparoscopic Gastric Bypass Patients Grouped by 100s

Patient Group	Stenosis	Leak	PE	SBO/Internal Hernia	Post-Op Bleed	Intra-OP Bleed	Abdominal Infection	Total
001–100	5	1	0	2	0	0	2	10
101–200	6	2	0	1	2	0	0	11
201–300	4	1	1	0	2	0	0	8
301–400	6	0	0	2	2	1	1	12
401–500	2	0	0	0	1	2	0	5
501–600	7	0	1	0	3	1	1	13
601–700	5	0	1	0	0	1	0	7
701–800	0	0	0	2	3	1	0	6
801–900	2	2	0	0	2	1	1	8
901–1000	5	0	0	0	0	0	0	5
Totals	42	6	3	7	15	7	5	85

to analyze separately therefore they were added together. Figure 17–2 shows the number of total serious complications graphed in sequential patient groups. The Cochrane-Armitage test showed that a significant trend ($p < 0.05$) occurred after 500 cases. Stenosis of the GI tract accounted for 42 of the 85 complications. Stenosis was analyzed separately (Figure 17–3). There were no trends in this data analyzed by the Cochrane-Armitage test. The frequency of conversion varied considerably from group to group (Figure 17–4), but there were no trends evident.

In 2002, a surgeon in our group decided to begin doing bariatric surgery. He had been trained in open bariatric surgery during his residency. He assisted on 14 open and 19 laparoscopic gastric bypasses performed by the authors. He

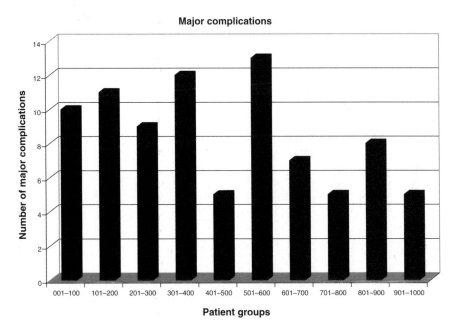

Figure 17–2. Major complications in 1,000 laparoscopic gastric bypass patients grouped by 100s.

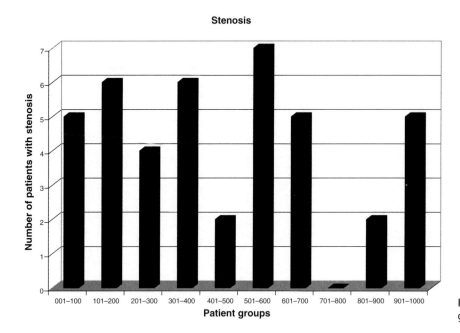

Figure 17–3. Stenosis in 1,000 laparoscopic gastric bypass patients grouped by 100s.

performed, as primary surgeon, 20 open and 21 laparoscopic bypasses with assistance of the authors. He then began his own series performing open and laparoscopic surgery with the assistance of a surgical technician who had assisted the authors with over 1,000 laparoscopic bariatric procedures. During his first 100 laparoscopic gastric bypasses, he had no deaths, no leaks, and no pulmonary emboli. Early complications consisted of one wound infection. Late complications were one stenosis at the gastroenterostomy, two incisional hernias, and one internal hernia.

DISCUSSION

Table 17–2 compares our complications to the series of Wittgrove,[20] Schauer,[4,19] and Higa.[18] Both our major and minor complications are included. Our data compare very favorably with these series. While we were learning laparoscopic bariatric, our patients were not experiencing unusually high complication rates.

The learning curve of bariatric laparoscopic surgery was difficult but it was not dangerous for our patients. The

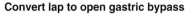

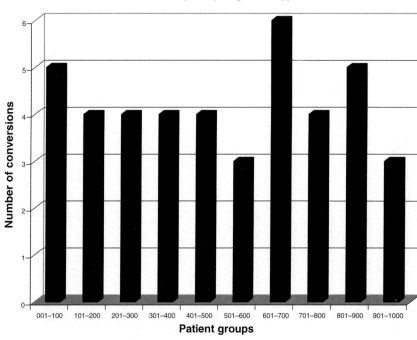

Figure 17–4. Conversion from laparoscopic to open gastric bypass in 1,000 patients grouped by 100s.

Table 17–2.

Literature Comparison of Complications After Laparoscopic Roux-En-Y Gastric Bypass

	Present Study	Higa[18]	Schauer[4,19]	Wittgrove[20]
Cases	1,000	1,040	275	1,000
Deaths	0.1%	0.1%	0.4%	0.0%
GI leaks	0.6%	0.0%	1.5%	2.8%
PE	0.3%	0.3%	0.8%	—
Hemorrhage	2.2%	0.6%	3.3%	1.2%
GI stenosis	4.2%	5.8%	4.7%	3.8%
Infection	1.5%	0.1%	—	8.0%
SBO	0.3%	—	1.5%	0.8%
Internal hernia	0.3%	2.5%	0.7%	—

operative time for our first 100 cases averaged 240 minutes compared to 156 minutes for our last 100 cases. We operated on progressively larger patients during our learning curve. The average waist measurement increased by 10 cm during the series. Therefore, we learned to operate on larger patients more efficiently.

The complication rate in this series was not different than the largest published series in the literature. There was no evidence of a cluster of complications near the initial part of this series. Our only death was near the end of the series. The most dreaded and lethal[21] complications, leak, and pulmonary emboli occurred at a rate similar to other large series.

There are actually three separate learning curves in laparoscopic bariatric surgery. The first is learning to do open bariatric surgery. The second is learning to care for bariatric patients. The third is learning to perform advanced laparoscopic surgery. Our preparation before beginning the series was directed at our deficiency, which was advanced laparoscopic surgery. We attempted to overcome this deficiency by extra preparation on an animal model and the use of laparoscopic staple devices on open cases. This strategy was successful.

The effect of fellowship training in eliminating the learning curve has been shown.[12,13] We have demonstrated that this learning curve can be eliminated by proctoring a surgeon. Kligman[11] has started a laparoscopic bariatric program without experiencing an initial cluster of complications. He was selective in choosing patients for the laparoscopic approach. Fernandez[22] reported that older patients, males,

and patients with multiple comorbidities are more likely to leak and/or expire after gastric bypass surgery. Perhaps, these patients should be avoided as well.

In conclusion, laparoscopic bariatric surgery can be learned without undue risk to the patient. Following are our recommendations for starting a laparoscopic program:

1. Training—obtain proper training by a proctor or fellowship.
2. Patient selection—Select patients with BMI <50 kg/m^2, waist <125 cm. Avoid central obesity and reoperative bariatric surgery.
3. Operating team—Assemble a reproducible operative team including anesthesia, surgical assistants, nurses, and scrub technicians.
4. Equipment—Obtain crystal-clear video equipment, surgical staplers, suturing devices, trocars, and laparoscopic instruments of high quality and train the operating team in their use.

References

1. Wittgrove AC, Clark G, Schubert KR: Laparoscopic gastric bypass, Roux-en-Y: Technique and results in 75 patients with 3-30 months follow-up. *Obes Surg* 6:500–504, 1996.
2. Higa KD, Boone KB, Ho T, et al.: Laparoscopic Roux-en-Y gastric bypass in morbid obesity: Technique and preliminary results of our first 400 patients. *Arch Surg* 135:1029–1033, 2000.
3. Papasavas PK, Caushaj PF, McCormick JT, et al.: Laparoscopic management of complications following laparoscopic Roux-en-Y gastric bypass for morbid obesity. *Surg Endosc* 17: 610–614, 2003.
4. Schauer PR, Ikramuddin S: Laparoscopic surgery for morbid obesity. *Surg Clin North Am* 81:1145–1179, 2001.
5. Nguyen NT, Huerta S, Gelfand D, et al.: Bowel obstruction after Roux-en-Y gastric bypass. *Obes Surg* 14:190–196, 2004.
6. DeMaria EJ, Sugerman, HJ, Kellum JM: Results of 281 consecutive total laparoscopic Roux-en-Y gastric bypasses. *Ann Surg* 235:640–647, 2002.
7. Gould JC, Garren MJ, Starling JR: Lessons learned from the first 100 cases in a new minimally invasive bariatric surgery program. *Obes Surg* 14:618–625, 2004.
8. Oliak D, Ballantyne GH, Weber P, et al.: Laparoscopic Roux-en-Y gastric bypass: Defining the learning curve. *Surg Endosc* 17:405–408, 2003.
9. Schauer P, Ikramuddin S, Hamad G, et al.: The learning curve for laparoscopic Roux-en-Y gastric bypass is 100 cases. *Surg Endosc* 17:212–215, 2003.
10. Flum DR, Dellinger EP: Impact of gastric bypass operation on survival: A population based analysis. *J Am Coll Surg* 199:543–551, 2004.
11. Kligman MD, Thomas C, Saxe J: Effect of the learning curve on early outcomes of laparoscopic Roux-en-Y gastric bypass. *Am Surg* 69:304–309, 2003.
12. Kothari SN, Boyd WC, Larson CA, et al.: Training of a minimally invasive bariatric surgeon: Are laparoscopic fellowships the answer? *Obes Surg* 15:323–329, 2005.
13. Oliak D, Owens M, Schmidt HJ: Impact of fellowship training on the learning curve for laparoscopic gastric bypass. *Obes Surg* 14:197–200, 2004.
14. Drew RL, Linner JH: Revisional surgery for severe obesity with fascia banded stoma Roux-en-Y gastric bypass. *Obes Surg* 2:249–354, 1992.
15. Brolin RE, Kenler HA, Gorman JY, et al.: Long-limb gastric bypass in the super obese. *Ann Surg* 215:387–395, 1992.

16. Linner JH: Gastric operations: Specific techniques. In: Linner JH (ed.): *Surgery for Morbid Obesity.* New York, Springer, 1984; pp. 65–93.

17. Gastrointestinal surgery for severe obesity. Consensus development conference panel, National Institutes of Health. *Ann Intern Med* 115:956–961, 1991.

18. Higa KD, Boone KB, Ho T: Complications of the laparoscopic Roux-en-Y gastric bypass: 1,040 patients—what have we learned? *Obes Surg* 10:509–513, 2000.

19. Schauer PR, Ikramuddin S, Gourash W, et al.: Outcomes after laparoscopic Roux-en-Y gastric bypass for morbid obesity. *Ann Surg* 232:515–529, 2000.

20. Wittgrove AC, Endres JE, Davis M, et al.: Perioperative complications in a single surgeons experience wit 1000 consecutive laparoscopic Roux-en-Y gastric bypass operations for morbid obesity. *Obes Surg* 12:457–458, 2002.

21. Melinek J, Livingston E, Cortina G, et al.: Autopsy findings following gastric bypass surgery for morbid obesity. *Arch Pathol Lab Med* 126:1091–1095, 2002.

22. Fernandez AZ Jr, DeMaria EJ, Tichansky DS, et al.: Experience with over 3000 open and laparoscopic bariatric procedures: Multivariate analysis of factors related to leak and resultant mortality. *Surg Endosc* 18:193–197, 2004.

Technical Procedures

18

Laparoscopic Restrictive Procedures: Adjustable Gastric Banding

Karl Miller, MD

Bariatric surgery offers a long-term solution for the problem of severe obesity. The major benefits of sustained weight loss include the reversal of numerous obesity-related illnesses, making bariatric surgery one of the most powerful therapies in current clinical practice. Laparoscopic adjustable gastric banding (LAGB) is proving to be an acceptable form of bariatric surgery because of its safety, effectiveness, long-term weight-loss maintenance, and reversibility. The success or failure of this type of operation depends more than almost any other on the patient's cooperation and compliance. The patient needs to be fully informed about obesity as a disorder, the operative procedure, possible complications, warning signs and symptoms, and the postoperative follow-up. In 2003, worldwide adjustable gastric banding was one of the three leading procedures, with 24% of all bariatric procedures.[1,2]

The adjustable gastric band is a 12 mm wide soft silicone band with an elastic balloon that can be inflated by injection, according to individual need. The band is fitted around the upper part of the stomach, dividing it into two sections: the smaller section is above the band and has a capacity of about 10–20 mL (pouch), and the larger section is below the band (Figure 18–1). This constriction is called stoma. Besides the obvious assets of laparoscopic surgery, the proposed advantages of gastric banding include reversibility and the possibility of adjusting the band's stoma size. It should be hoped and expected that the treatments for obesity available today will be superceded by better treatments in the next 20 years. It is an asset of the band that it can be removed easily and the stomach anatomy remains intact. Removing the band is a minor laparoscopic procedure that can be performed on an outpatient basis, but this results in weight regain. Adjustable gastric banding has become popular since 1985 as a means of achieving gastric restriction and treating morbid obesity. Adjustable silicone gastric banding as described by Kuzmak[3]

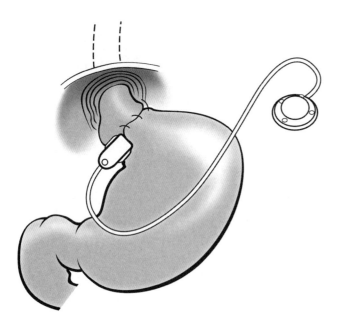

Figure 18–1. Adjustable gastric banding with gastropexy.

and the Swedish adjustable gastric banding proposed by Hallberg and Forsell[4] permit regulation of gastric restriction.

Early experience gained in Europe with the LAP-BAND System made by Bioenterics (Inamed Corp., USA) led to repeated modification of the technique and resulted in great improvements in the outcome.[5,6] As with the adjustable band, the so-called Swedish Adjustable Gastric Band (SAGB, Obtech AG, ETHICON), which makes a smaller pouch, significantly reduced the postoperative complication rate.[7,8] Meanwhile, an increasing number of different bands are now available (Table 18–1).

Public and professional concerns about the quality of care and surgical outcomes are associated with the explosive growth in bariatric surgery over the past decade. The use of standardized operations and clinical pathways to permit objective evaluation and interinstitutional comparisons of outcomes is one criterion of a program of Centers of Excellence (COE) in bariatric surgery.[9]

Regardless of the surgical technique, the allied health-supporting aspect of patient care requires a primary place in any bariatric program. As patients prepare for their surgery, education and guidance for nutrition, lifestyle changes, physiology, and psychosocial development should be clearly addressed. When proctoring new surgeons, it is important to advise utilization of the multidisciplinary model from a practical standpoint. A standardized pathway of the patient, accompanied by the multidisciplinary team, is mandatory in this field of surgery (Figure 18–2), and recommended by the National Institutes of Health, the multidisciplinary approach addresses the complexity of the disease being treated.[10]

PATIENT SELECTION

In the case of obesity surgery, it is quite difficult to ascertain the relative importance of patients' true expectations; often medical reasons are given, but the driving force is cosmetic or social. Denial of disease affects the patient's cooperation with monitoring and follow-up. Obesity is a "chronic disorder that requires a continuous care model of treatment."[11] Although there are only a few comparative studies on the frequency, intensity, or mode of follow-up, close regular follow-up visits have become routine in most centers.[12]

Table 18–1.

Different Brands and Features

Feature	SAGB and SAGB Quick Close	Inamed (LAP-BAND®)	Inamed (Vanguard®)	Heliogast®	AMI Band®	Mid-Band®	Minimizer®
Type of band system	high volume/ low pressure	low volume/ high pressure	high volume/ low pressure	low volume/ high pressure	low volume/ high pressure	high volume/ low pressure	low volume/ high pressure
Balloon configuration	large balloon, 9 mL inflates internally	small balloon, 4 mL inflates internally	large balloon, 10 mL inflates internally	balloon 5 mL inflates internally and lateral	5 mL inflates internally	9 mL inflates internally and externally	small balloon, 3 mL inflates internally
Clinical efficacy	multiple clinical papers	multiple clinical papers	no clinical papers	small number of clinical papers, limited long-term weight loss	no clinical papers	no clinical papers	no clinical papers

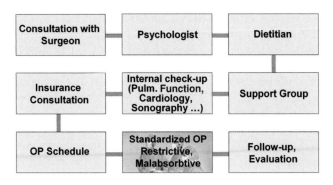

Figure 18–2. Clinical pathway.

Kral and Kissileff[13] list numerous preoperative parameters, the predictive powers of which have been investigated throughout the history of obesity surgery. Relatively few preoperative predictive parameters have been evaluated over long periods. Although it is possible to create a risk profile from several parameters, it is questionable whether such a profile has any use in determining candidacy for surgery, because there are no other effective treatment options for severe obesity; even relatively poor results after restrictive surgery are superior to the results of nonoperative modalities. The most important uses of predictors are for preoperative education and optimization and potentially for patient allocation to generically different operations according to the mode of action (restrictive vs diversionary). The majority of parameters are behavioral. This is logical, recognizing that antiobesity surgery is truly a behavioral surgery.[13]

SURGICAL TECHNIQUE

The main differences in technique for gastric banding are: By means of a calibration balloon positioned in the stomach, the site of incision is determined at the small curvature. Another so called "pars flaccida technique" starts at the medial edge of the right crus of the diaphragm after incision of the pars flaccida of the lesser omentum dissecting to the angle of HIS. Tunnelled suturing is obligatory to prevent band slippage and to ensure that the fundus does not slide under the band. We also recommend gastropexy in addition to the stomach wall suture (fundus sutured to the left side of the diaphragm) (Figure 18–1).

Perigastric Technique

Four to five trocars are introduced with the patient lying in half-sedentary position (Figure 18–3, A). With a calibration balloon positioned in the stomach, the site of the incision is determined at the small curvature. At this site, a 0.5–1-cm window is placed closed to the cardia. The fenestration is continued along the posterior wall of the gastroesophageal junction up to the angle of His. Thereafter, the endodissector (Inamed Corp., USA) is introduced and attached to the end of the catheter. The catheter end of the gastric band is

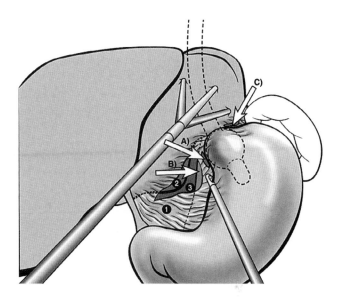

Figure 18–3. Surgical techniques. (A) Perigastric technique; (B) pars flaccida technique; (C) Angle of His. (1) Lesser omentum (pars flaccida); (2) caudate lobe of the liver; (3) right crus of the diaphragm.

placed around the cardia. For final positioning of the band, the calibration balloon in the cardia is filled up to 10–15 mL. Beneath this so-called pouch the band is closed with a special sealing device. Three to four seromuscular sutures are made in the large curvature to prevent the band from slipping. The catheter end of the band is brought outward via a 15-mm or 18-mm trocar and is connected here to the port, which is fixed below the anterior rectus sheet with four nonresorbable interrupted sutures.

"Pars Flaccida" Technique

After the pars flaccida is opened, the right crus is dissected (Figure 18–3, B). The procedure involves blunt dissection of the esophageal hiatus, with special care taken to preserve the hepatic branch of the vagus nerve. After the dissection of the left crus, the phrenogastric ligament at the angle of His is opened. The band is introduced through a 15-mm or 18-mm trocar. A blunt articulating dissector "Goldfinger" (Obtech, Ethicon) is passed under laparoscopic visualization through the retroesophagogastric opening. The band is placed, without entering the omental bursa on the posterior side of the stomach, in a dissected tunnel above the arteria gastica sinistra and the vagus branch. The fat and vagus nerve on the lesser curvature are included within the loop of the band. A small pouch (relaxed pouch of 10 mL) is created and secured with a row of tunnellating sutures. Three to four tunnellating sutures are placed on the ventral side, below and above the band, to ensure its stable anterior position. The sutured end flaps of the band are rotated all the way down at the lesser curvature. The port is placed on the anterior rectus sheath or on the lower part of the sternum with four nonresorbable interrupted sutures. A large loop of the tube is left inside the abdomen to prevent the tube from ripping off the port due to extensive movement of the patient.

Combination (Pars Flaccida–Perigastrica) Technique

The band is placed following the pars flaccida technique. The lesser curvature containing the nerve of Latarjet is dissected from the gastric wall in the direction of the right crus. The end of the tube is transported behind the esophagus from the left to the right side of the hiatus. The next step is to advance the tube along the gastric wall to the marked opening. After the removal of the articulating dissector, the band is pulled into position without force and the adherent tissue can be dissected under laparoscopic view. The closing procedure is not different from previous techniques. Stomach-to-pouch sutures are placed as close as possible to the greater curvature to prevent band migration.

POSTOPERATIVE FOLLOW-UP

By using gastrografin, a contrast medium-enhanced roentgenogram is made on the first postoperative day. If the findings are negative, the patient is permitted to take fluids, followed by a structured diet. The stoma is finally adjusted above the port after 4–6 weeks in the outpatient department. The bands are slowly filled by consecutive injections into the port of a radiology contrast medium (Iopamiro® isotonic 300 mg J/mL, Gerot Pharmazeutika Vienna, Austria). The band's stoma diameter is adjusted in all bands postoperatively after 5–6 weeks by qualified medical staff. The final total volume in the band averages between 6 and 8.5 mL in the SAGB and 3–5 mL in the LAP-BAND. Patients are always requested to drink some liquid after filling the band and are kept in hospital for a short while to make sure that they are comfortable with the new stoma diameter. The port area is disinfected with a swab imbibed in chlorhexidine spirit 5% for at least 3–5 minutes before the injection. Previous studies have pointed out the importance of disinfection to avoid port infection. Patient follow-up is performed every third month during the first year if requested by the patient and thereafter routinely once a year. Band adjustments and follow-up is routinely performed under fluoroscopy.

Low Pressure—High Pressure Bands

The bands function on two concepts: low pressure–high volume and high pressure–low volume. To fullfill the criteria of a low pressure–high volume system, the band must have a large overall balloon surface. Fried and Lechner[8] carried out a study to investigate the theoretical and clinical levels of adjustable band volume–pressure features and their possible influence on band-related complications.

When the low pressure–high volume system (SAGB) was filled with 5.2 mL of fluid, needed on an average to achieve a sufficient stoma diameter, a pressure of 40 mm Hg was created. By filling the high pressure–low volume system (LAP-BAND System) with 2.8 mL of fluid, needed to achieve a sufficient stoma diameter, a mean pressure of 120 mm Hg

was created. Intake of barium for the x-ray studies caused a rise of pressure to 82 mm Hg on an average in SAGB patients and a rise of pressure to 135 mm Hg on average in LAP-BAND patients. Some of these adverse effects could be related to the relatively high pressure exerted by the band on the esophageal and gastric wall. The SAGB (Obtech Medical, Baar, Switzerland) was engineered as a low-pressure device and has been introduced into clinical practice.[14–16]

The reason for band-related complications after adjustable banding is likely multifactorial. The restrictive function of the adjustable band is based on the physical principles of gastric narrowing over the stoma by pressure and force applied through the inner-band balloon and vice versa by food passage through the stoma toward the band. According to Fried et al.,[8] band slippage and erosions are significantly linked to a high pressure–low volume band system (Table 18–2).

Table 18–2.

Meta-Analysis of Band Slippage/Erosion Rates of High Pressure vs. Low Pressure Band Systems[8,17,18]

Band Slippage/ Erosion	SAGB® %	Lap-Band® %	Follow-up Months (max)
Miller and Hell[19] (n = 156)	1	2	28
Berrevoet et al.[20] (n = 91)	0	9	18
Frering[21] (n = 1418)	0	64	16
Nowara[22] (n = 108)	0	3	48
Fabre[23] (n = 229)	3	38	18
Ponson et al.[24] 2002 (n = 101)	3	3	9
Nocca et al.[25] (n = 214)	12	42	24
Suter et al.[17]* (n = 180)	8	11	36
Miller and Hell[18]* (n = 100)	2	8	88
Total (mean value, n = 2597)	3.2	20	31.4

Prospective randomized study.

WEIGHT LOSS AND COMORBIDITY

The most commonly reported measures were weight loss (WL), reduction of BMI, and percentage of excess weight lost (EWL), and these provide a broad perspective on the long-term weight reduction achieved by LAGB. All studies reported achieved weight loss in their overall patient populations with both the LAP-BAND and SAGB. Weight loss is given in the literature as BMI 43–46 kg/m^2 preop to BMI 28–32 kg/m^2 postop. A target of 50–60% reduction of excess weight is achievable.[26] Combined international data show that weight loss after gastric banding is characterized by steady progressive weight loss over a 2–3-year period, followed by stable weight up to 6 years. This pattern reflects the benefit of adjustability. For the international series, the %EWL at 2 years has been between 52% and 65%. Weiner et al.[27] reported that the mean BMI of all patients fell from 46.8 to 34.0 kg/m^2 within 1 year. After 3 years, BMI fell to 32 kg/m^2. The median BMI of the first 100 patients, with a band in place, was 32 kg/m^2 after 8 years. Distribution at 8 years showed that 19% of patients had an excess weight loss of 61–100%. Substantial weight reduction was observed in a study by Buchwald et al.,[1,2] which was conducted by both meta-analytic techniques and simple pooling across studies using weighted means. The mean (95% CI) percentage of excess weight loss by meta-analysis at the outcome time point for which comorbidities were assessed was 47.5% (40.7%–54.2%) for gastric banding.[1,2] Belachew et al.[28] have demonstrated that 80% of patients reduced their excess weight by 60%. O'Brien et al.[29] report excess weight loss of 51% in the first year, 58% in the second, 61% in the third, and 68% in the fourth year postop. Studies with a follow-up of over 5 years confirm that the weight loss is long term.[26] A prospective randomized study in our department, comparing two bands, documented a mean excessive weight loss of 64% and no difference in weight loss between LAP-BAND system® and SAGB® after 9-years follow-up.[18] Combined international data show that weight loss after LAGB placement is characterized by steady progressive weight loss over a 2–3-year period, followed by stable weight for 6 years. This pattern reflects the benefit of adjustability. Vella and Galloway[30] have that LAGB results in approximately 60% (43%–78%) excess weight loss at 3 years. A random effects model was used in the meta-analysis published by Buchwald et al.[1,2] The mean (95% CI) percentage of excess weight loss was 61.2% (58.1–64.4%) for all patients, 47.5% (40.7–54.2%) for patients who underwent gastric banding, 61.6% (56.7–66.5%) for those who underwent gastric bypass, 68.2% (61.5–74.8%) for those who underwent gastroplasty, and 70.1% (66.3–73.9%) for those who underwent biliopancreatic diversion or duodenal switch. Chapman et al.[26] reported, in a summary of comparative studies, comparable results of LAGB and Roux-en Y gastric bypass (RYGB). Up to 2 years, LAGB results in less weight loss compared to RYGB; from 2 to 4 years there is no significant difference in the weight loss between LAGB and RYGB, but the quality of data is only moderate.[26]

The Adelaide Study, found that medical comorbidities either improved (47%) or resolved (43%) in all but 9% of patients who had unsatisfactory weight loss.[31] They reported that 60% of the patients who initially had any obesity-related comorbidity, were free of medication for those comorbidities 3 years after surgery.[31] Buchwald et al.[1,2] reported that for all types of bariatric surgery, diabetes resolved completely in 77% of cases and improved or resolved in 86%, hypertension resolved completely in 62% and improved or resolved in 78%, hyperlipidemia improved in 70%, and obstructive sleep apnea resolved in 85%. The LAGB is proving to be extremely safe and is able to facilitate good weight loss as well as maintain weight loss over time.

QUALITY OF LIFE

Severe obesity has been associated with disordered eating, impaired quality of life (QoL), and decreased physical activity. QoL is significantly improved after obesity surgery, both in terms of life expectancy[32] and physical activity as well as satisfaction.[33] According to an analysis by Weiner et al.,[34–36] QoL improves significantly in 92% of patients. In one of our studies we have shown a direct correlation between QoL and BMI.[37] Moreover, statistically significant improvements in all areas of life (social contacts, physical activity, self-confidence, sexuality, and work and family life) were demonstrated after a BMI reduction of 5.7. The Moorehead-Ardelt Quality of Life Questionnaire was originally developed as a disease-specific instrument to measure postoperative outcomes of self-perceived QoL in obese patients.[38] Five key areas were examined: self-esteem, physical well-being, social relationships, work, and sexuality. Each of these questions offered five possible answers, which were given + or − points according to a scoring key. The Bariatric Analysis and Reporting Outcome System (BAROS), developed by Oria and Moorehead,[32] has now become the accepted assessment method for QoL and treatment outcome after bariatric surgery. The BAROS assessment score covers weight loss (−1 for weight increase to +3 for 75–100% excess weight loss), comorbidity (−1 for deterioration to +3 for completely resolved), and the QoL questionnaire (self-esteem, physical activity), social contacts, job satisfaction, and sexuality (−3 max. and +3 min.). Points are lost for complications (1 point) and reoperation (1 point). A score of 7–9 points is thus an excellent result, that of 4–6 points is good, and that of 1–3 points is a satisfactory score, with −3 to 0 points indicating a failed treatment. The health status and QoL assessment after surgery for obesity is summarized in Table 18–3. Favretti et al.[40] reports on 170 LAP-BAND system patients, with excellent and good results in 48%. The failure rate in this group is reported as 10%. A large number of case series reported postoperative increases in QoL or satisfaction with operative outcomes for LAGB.[17,34–36,40–42] The BAROS score revealed good, very good, and excellent results in 92% of patients.

Table 18–3.

Health Status and Quality of Life (QoL) After Surgical Treatment for Obesity According to Hell et al.[39]

	VBG	AGB	Y-RGB	*P*
Weight loss	1.6	1.5	2.7	*P* < 0.05
Comorbidity	2.57	2.48	1.9	n.s.
QoL	1.96	2.01	2.55	n.s.
BAROS	6.13	5.99	7.15	*P* < 0.05
Total score				
Failure %	3	3	0	n.s.
Fair %	3	7	7	n.s.
Good %	13	17	10	n.s.
Very good and excellent %	71	73	83	n.s

BAROS, bariatric analysis and reporting outcome system; VBG, vertical banded gastroplasty; AGB, adjustable gastric banding; Y-GBP, roux-en-Y gastric bypass.

EDUCATION AND FUTURE ASPECTS

Surgical treatment for obesity has proved that it is the best and the most effective means of preventing the life-threatening complications and serious degenerative problems associated with pathological obesity. It is indicated by the ineffectiveness of nonsurgical treatment methods and the high risk resulting from untreated obesity.[43,44] Safe, effective surgical treatment methods increase life expectancy and QoL for patients with extreme excess weight and is by the way health cost effective.[45]

Attention to technical details is of utmost importance for a safe, standardized, and effective operation. Most studies show the importance of complying both with the developed operating technique and the correct follow-up procedure to avoid complications. According to the available data, adjustable gastric banding operations meet the criteria of a low-risk laparoscopic alternative in the treatment of obesity. Notwithstanding its advantages, minimally invasive operative treatment of morbid obesity is associated with a certain degree of surgical risk, which is reported to be less than 1% in the literature.[46] Nevertheless, laparoscopic adjustable gastric banding appears to be the surgical method of choice in the future. The results reported in the literature as well as our own experience show that the method is difficult to learn but is associated with a markedly lower postoperative morbidity for the patient. Adjustable gastric banding is a surgical method that provides the patient a very early feeling of satiety and

increases the QoL in morbidly obese patients. It should be kept in mind that the operation marks the beginning of treatment. Control examinations at standardized close intervals, performed in cooperation with psychologists and dietitians, are essential to ensure the long-term success of this therapy. Without the patient's cooperation, no adiposity operation will be successful on a long-term basis.

References

1. Buchwald H, Williams SE: Bariatric surgery worldwide 2003 *Obes Surg* 14:1157–1164, 2004.
2. Buchwald H, Avidor Y, Braunwald E, et al.: Bariatric surgery. A systematic review and meta-analysis *JAMA* 292:1724–1737, 2004.
3. Kuzmak L: Silicone gastric banding: A simple and effective operation for morbid obesity. *Contemp Surg* 28:13–18, 1986.
4. Hallberg D, Forsell P: Ballongband vid behandling av massiv Gvervikt. *Svensk Kirwgi* 43:106, 1985.
5. Belachew M, Legrand M, Jaquet N: Laparoscopic placement of adjustable silicone gastric banding in the treatment of morbid obesity: An animal model experimental study. *Obes Surg* 3:140–141, 1993.
6. Favretti F, Cadiere GB, Segato G: Laparoscopic adjustable gastric banding (LAP-BAND®): How to avoid complications. *Obes Surg* 7:352–358, 1997.
7. Forsell P, Hellers G: The Swedish adjustable gastric banding for morbid obesity—Nine year experience and a four year follow-up of patients operated with a new adjustable band. *Obes Surg* 7:345–351, 1997.
8. Fried M, Lechner W, Kormanova K: Physical principles of available adjustable gastric bands: How they work. *Obes Surg* 14:1118–1122, 2004.
9. Champion JK, Pories WJ. 2004 ASBS Consensus Conference. Centers of Excellence for bariatric surgery. *Surg Obes Relat Dis* 1:148–151, 2005.
10. National Institutes of Health Consensus Development Conference: Gastrointestinal surgery for severe obesity. *Obes Surg* 1:257–266, 1991.
11. Goodrick GK, Poston WS, II Foreyt JP: Methods for voluntary weight loss and control: Update 1996. *Nutrition* 12:672–676, 1996.
12. Miller K, Hell E: Laparoscopic surgical concepts of morbid obesity. *Langenbecks Arch Surg* 388:375–384, 2003.
13. Kral JG, Kissileff HR: Surgical approaches to the treatment of obesity. *Ann Behav Med* 9:15–19, 1987.
14. Forsell P, Hallberg D, Hellers G: Gastric banding for morbid obesity: Initial experience with a new adjustable band. *Obes Surg* 3:369–374, 1993.
15. Wright TA, Kow L, Wilson T, et al.: Early results of laparoscopic Swedish adjustable gastric banding for morbid obesity. *Br J Surg* 87:362, 2000.
16. Hesse UJ, Berrevoet F, Ceelen W, et al.: Adjustable silicone gastric banding and the Swedish adjustable gastric banding in treatment of morbid obesity. *Chirurgie* 72:14–18, 2001.
17. Suter M, Giusti V, Worreth M, Heraief E, Calmes JM: Laparoscopic gastric banding: A prospective, randomized study comparing the Lapband and the SAGB: early results. *Ann Surg* 241(1):55–62, 2005.
18. Miller KA, Hell E: Adjustable silicone gastric band (Lap-Band) vs. Swedish adjustable gastric band (SAGB)—long-term results of a prospective randomized study. *Surg Obes Rel Dis* 1:(3):222, 2005.
19. Miller K, Hell E: Laparoscopic adjustable gastric banding: A prospective 4-year follow-up study. *Obes Surg* 9:183–187, 1999.
20. Berrevoet F, Pattyn P, Cardon A, et al.: Retrospective analysis of laparoscopic gastric banding technique: Short-term and mid-term follow-up. *Obes Surg* 9:272–275, 1999.
21. Frering V, Vicard P, Stagni R, et al.: Laparoscopic gastric banding: Incidence of complications according to type of gastric band. *Le Journ de Coeliochir* 35:21–24, 2000.

22. Nowara H: Egyptian experience in laparoscopic adjustable gastric banding. *Obes Surg* 11:70–75, 2001.

23. Fabre J, Nocca D, Lemoin C, et al.: Comparative study between Lap-Band® and Swedish adjustable gastric banding. *Obes Surg* 11:404, 2001 (Abstr 91).

24. Ponson A, Janssen I, Klinkenbijl J: Laparoscopic adjustable gastric banding: A prospective comparison of two commonly used bands. *Obes Surg* 12:579–582, 2002.

25. Nocca D, Fabre JM, Jacquet E, et al.: Perigastric versus pars flaccida technique in laparoscopic horizontal banded gastroplasty. *Le Journ de Coeliochir* 42:23–28, 2002.

26. Chapman AE, Kiroff G, Game P, et al.: Laparoscopic adjustable gastric banding in the treatment of obesity: A systematic literature review. *Surgery* 135:326–351, 2004.

27. Weiner R, Blanco-Engert R, Weiner S, Matkowitz R, Schaefer L, Pomhoff I: Outcome after laparoscopic adjustable gastric banding—8 years experience. *Obes Surg* 13(3):427–434, 2003.

28. Belachew M, Legrand M, Vincent V, et al.: Laparoscopic adjustable gastric banding. *World J Surg* 22:955–963, 1998.

29. O'Brien P, Brown W, Smith A, et al.: Prospective study of a laparoscopically placed, adjustable gastric band in the treatment of morbid obesity. *Br J Surg* 85:113–118, 1999.

30. Vella M, Galloway DJ: Laparoscopic adjustable gastric banding for severe obesity. *Obes Surg* 13(4):642–648, 2003.

31. National Institutes of Health, National Heart, Lung, and Blood Institute, in cooperation with the National Institute of Diabetes and Digestive and Kidney Diseases. Clinical guidelines on the identification evaluation, and treatment of overweight and obesity in adults: The evidence report. NHLBI report 98-4083, September 1998.

32. Oria HE, Moorehead MK: Bariatric analysis and reporting outcome system (BAROS). *Obes Surg* 8:487–499, 1998.

33. Miller K, Hell E, Schoen E, Ardelt E: Quality of life outcome of patients with the LAP BAND vs vertical banded gastroplasty: Results of a long-term follow-up study. *Obes Surg* 8:359, 1998.

34. Weiner R, Wagner D, Datz M, Bockhom H: Quality of life outcome after laparoscopic gastric banding. *Obes Surg* 9:336, 1999.

35. Weiner R, Datz M, Wagner D, et al.: Quality-of-life outcome after laparoscopic adjustable gastric banding for morbid obesity. *Obes Surg* 9:539–545, 1999.

36. Weiner R, Wagner D, Bockhorn H: Laparoscopic gastric banding for morbid obesity. *J Laparoendosc Adv Surg Tech A* 9:23–30, 1999.

37. Miller K, Mayer E, Pichler M, Hell E: Quality-of-life outcomes of patients with the LAP-BAND® versus nonoperative treatment of obesity. Preliminary results of an ongoing long-term follow-up study. *Obes Surg* 7:280, 1997.

38. Moorehead MK, Ardelt-Gattinger E, Lechner H, Oria HE: The validation of the Moorehead-Ardelt quality of life questionnaire II. *Obes Surg* 13(5):684–692, 2003.

39. Hell E, Miller K, Moorehead MK, Samuels N: Evaluation of health status and quality of life after bariatric surgery: Comparison of standard roux-en-Y gastric bypass, vertical banded gastroplasty and laparoscopic adjustable gastric banding. *Obes Surg* 10:214–219, 2000.

40. Favretti F, Cadiere GB, Segato G, et al.: Bariatric analysis and reporting outcome system (BAROS) applied to laparoscopic gastric banding patients. *Obes Surg* 8:500–504, 1998.

41. Schok M, Geenen R, van Antwerpen T, et al.: Quality of life after laparoscopic adjustable gastric banding for severe obesity: Postoperative and retrospective preoperative evaluations. *Obes Surg* 10:502–508, 2000.

42. Stieger R, Thurnheer M, Lange J: Morbid obesity: 130 consecutive patients with laparoscopic gastric banding. *Schweiz Med Wochenschr* 128:1239, 2000.

43. Drenick EJ, Bale GS, Seltzer F, Johnson DG: Excessive mortality and causes of death in morbidly obese men. *JAMA* 243:443–445, 1980.

44. Wadden TA: Treatment of obesity by moderate and severe caloric restriction. Results of clinical research trials. *Ann Intern Med* 119:688–693, 1993.

45. Sampalis JS, Liberman M, Auger S, Christou NV: The impact of weight reduction surgery on health-care costs in morbidly obese patients. *Obes Surg* 14:725–730, 2004.

46. De Jong JR, van Ramshorst B: Re-interventions after laparoscopic gastric banding. *Obes Surg* 8:386, 1998.

19

Laparoscopic Restrictive Procedures: Sleeve Gastrectomy

Camilo Boza, MD • Michel Gagner, MD, FRCSC, FACS

Laparoscopic sleeve gastrectomy (LSG) for treatment of morbid obesity was first described as a part of the more complex operation, biliopancreatic diversion with duodenal switch (BPD/DS). The LSG was developed as a first-stage procedure in high-risk patients with a body mass index (BMI) of more than 60 to obtain an initial weight loss with low morbidity and mortality.[1] Early series of laparoscopic BPD/DS reported a 38% rate of major complications, with 6% mortality rate in patients with BMI greater than 65. Our group described a two-stage laparoscopic BPD/DS on these patients. With this approach, the mortality rate dropped to 0% and morbidity rate to 6%. LSG has been described increasingly as a first-stage procedure of gastric bypass, and even more as an alternative to other restrictive procedures such as gastric banding in patients with lower BMI. Recent studies have shown encouraging results during the first year with low morbidity and good quality of life.[2]

The sleeve gastrectomy (not laparoscopic) was incorporated by Marceau and colleagues[3] as an improvement of the distal gastrectomy performed by Scopinaro in BPD.[4] This modification decreased the capacity of the gastric reservoir and lowered the parietal cell mass to minimize the ulcerogenicity. However, it maintained the antropyloric pump and avoided the dumping syndrome. Conceptually, a similar technique has been described with good results: The Magenstrasse and Mill procedure. The "street of stomach" (gastric tube) is created by dividing the gastric mill completely from a hole performed in the antrum with a circular stapler, and multiple firings on linear staplers toward the angle of His. In this procedure, the stomach is left in place.[5]

As a restrictive procedure, the LSG could have an advantage over the adjustable gastric banding and vertical banded gastroplasty, because of the hormonal effect of the procedure. Complete removal of the greater curvature and fundus produces lower levels of ghrelin, which enhances the results on the control of food intake.

OPERATIVE TECHNIQUE

Patients are positioned with the legs split in the reverse Trendelenburg position with assurance of proper support to the extremities. The surgeon stands between the legs with the assistants on both sides. Seven ports are inserted routinely. Pneumoperitoneum is established to 15 mm Hg and a 30° angled scope is used. The short gastric vessels of the greater curvature and retrogastric attachments are divided with the Harmonic Scalpel (Ethicon Endosurgery, Cincinnati, OH) or a sealer/divider instrument (LigaSure, Valleylab, Boulder, CO). The dissection extends proximally to the esophagogastric junction and distally toward the pylorus.

The antrum is preserved and the greater curvature of the stomach divided 8–10 cm from the pylorus. This procedure is performed using two firings of 60-mm green cartridge (4.8-mm staple height) endoscopic linear stapler (Tyco Healthcare, Norwalk, CN). A 40F Maloney bougie is then inserted transorally and aligned along the lesser curvature (a 40F bougie is used for sleeve alone, and a 50–60 one is used if a complete DS is performed).

A vertical subtotal, sleeve gastrectomy is then fashioned along the lesser curvature 1 cm away from the bougie toward the esophagogastric junction. This procedure is performed with multiple firings of a 60-mm blue cartridge (3–5-mm staple height) endoscopic linear stapler. To decrease blood loss from the transected gastric plane, a reinforcement absorbable polymer membrane (Bioabsorbable Seamguard, Gore, Flagstaff, AZ) is used with the stapler.[6] Some authors have used a continuous running suture along the stapler line for this purpose and to prevent leakage.

The authors have discontinued the use of bovine pericardial strips due to an intraluminal migration seen in a patient (Peri-strips, Synovis Life Technologies, St. Paul, MN).[7] The resected stomach is retrieved by way of the right paramedian trocar site with a large plastic impermeable bag (Tyco Healthcare, Norwalk, CN). The bougie is removed and replaced with an orogastric tube for a methylene blue study. The proximal duodenum is compressed with atraumatic instruments to allow stomach distension with dye, which suggests the pouch size to be in the range of 100–150 mL. Fascia closure of all port sites 10 mm or larger is accomplished with a fascia closure device (Karl Storz, Tutlingen, Germany).

RESULTS

In the authors' initial series, from September 2000 to September 2001, 33 patients underwent an LSG as a first-stage procedure. These patients had a good postoperative course with no major morbidity or mortality. The median operative time for LSG in patients with BMI greater than 60 was 97 ± 28 minutes (66 ± 175), with minimal blood loss and no conversions to open surgery. Hospital stay averaged 3 days (range 2–5 days). Of these patients, 23 completed the second stage: laparoscopic duodenoileostomy/ileo-ileostomy (LDI-II). After 6 months of follow-up, the mean BMI dropped from 66 ± 5 to 53. At the time of the second stage, the mean BMI was 51 ± 6 kg/m^2 (excess weight loss was $32\% \pm 10\%$).

These encouraging results have been reproduced by other authors in superobese patients. Almogy and coworkers reported a series of 21 patients who underwent longitudinal gastrectomy for treatment of morbid obesity.[8] The preoperative mean BMI was 56 kg/m^2. Of these 21 patients, 9 were offered the procedure preoperatively due to known high perioperative risks. In 12 of these patients, a laparoscopic BPD/DS was planned, but because of intraoperative findings, or hemodynamic instability, they received a sleeve gastrectomy. Five patients developed complications, but no deaths were reported. With a median follow-up of 18 months, the median weight loss at 12 months was 45%. After a year, 40% of the patients had achieved more than 50% excess weight loss. Baltasar and colleagues reported different indications in 31 patients who underwent LSG: 7 procedures were done as a first stage of the DS, 7 as the only alternative in very high-risk patients, 16 in patients with a BMI from 35 to 43, and 1 sleeve gastrectomy as revisional surgery for gastric banding.[9] One (3%) patient died due to intra-abdominal bleeding. The excess body weight loss (EWL) was 56% (4–27 months after LSG) in the superobese group. However, patients with lower BMI had an EWL of 62%.

Mognol and coworkers performed LSG in 10 patients with a BMI of more than 60 kg/m^2 (Ref. 2). They reported no conversions, no morbidities, and no mortalities. EWL, after 1 year, was 51%. They concluded that LSG was an appropriate first-step procedure and an acceptable one-stage restrictive procedure if long-term results were good.

Indications for LSG have gone further based on the favorable results in superobese patients. Some groups have offered the procedure as a sole restrictive bariatric procedure. In 2002, Moon Han and colleagues, in Korea, reported a series of 130 patients (mean BMI of 37 kg/m^2; range 30–56 kg/m^2) who underwent LSG.[10] They offered this procedure as a first step in all patients with the intention to continue to a second stage dependent on weight regained after 1 year. Their inclusion criteria were a BMI of more than 35, or a BMI of more than 30, with associated comorbid conditions. They performed the LSG using four 12-mm trocars with laparoscopic staplers, resecting the greater curvature and fundus over a 48F bougie. The average operative time was 70 minutes (45–100) with 1 patient who required conversion to open surgery due to a short gastric vessel bleeding. In this series, they reported 5 (4%) postoperative complications, 2 of them, major: 1 leakage and 1 delayed bleeding that required reexploration for drainage and irrigation. Another patient experienced nausea and vomiting for 21 days after surgery. The patient required total parenteral nutrition during this period. One (1%) patient died 21 days after surgery. An autopsy showed peritonitis with no evident leakage. EWL was 55% at 3 months, 72% at 6 months, and 83% at 12 months. In 60 patients with a follow-up of at least 1 year, the appetite continued to be 54% of the preoperative score and the food intake was 41% of the preoperative food intake. At the 1-year follow up, 1 patient failed to achieve satisfactory weight loss (EWL: 21%; BMI: 56–51). This patient underwent a Roux-en-Y gastric bypass as a second stage. After a year, another 4 patients began to regain weight and will likely need a second-stage DS. Most of these patients had an initial BMI of more than 50.

Another interesting experience was published recently by Langer and coworkers.[11] They studied the LSG as a sole bariatric procedure and the rate of success and gastric dilatation in 23 patients. They performed an LSG over a 48F bougie, starting the sleeve opposite to the Vagus nerve branches, resecting the greater curvature and fundus. The staple-line was oversewn using a running suture to prevent bleeding and leakage. A water-soluble contrast swallow was performed routinely on the first day and a liquid diet was then started for the next 4 weeks. BMI at the time of surgery was 49 ± 7 kg/m^2 (range 40–73 kg/m^2). No morbidities and mortalities were reported. EWL after 6 and 12 months was 46% and 56%, respectively. Two patients underwent conversion to gastric bypass: One due to severe gastroesophageal reflux 15 months after surgery (EWL: 98%) and one for poor weight loss at 2 years. After a year of follow-up, 14 patients underwent an upper gastrointestinal series to rule out gastric dilatation. Only 1 patient had radiologic signs of dilatation; however, the patient had achieved an EWL of 59% at the annual follow-up obtained 30 months after the procedure. They concluded that the LSG could be a reasonable approach in patients with a BMI of less than 50 and that gastric dilatation may not be a limiting factor as a single bariatric procedure. However, they provided the patient with explicit information regarding the possible dilatation of the sleeve and need of a second-stage procedure.

DISCUSSION

Why is the LSG successful? The smaller longitudinal gastric pouch restricts food intake mechanically, which prevents overeating in the first 6–12 months postoperatively. The role of the gastric pouch in weight control is complex and involves satiety-regulating mechanisms. The hypothesis that explains the role of the gastric pouch in satiety emphasizes the importance of stretching walls with eating or drinking. The signals from wall receptors in the stomach are relayed by neural pathways to the appetite centers in the brain.[12] Successful maintenance of satiety may depend on the neurohormonal gut-brain axis.

Ghrelin,[13] a recently discovered orexigenic hormone secreted primarily by the fundus of the stomach, has been implicated in both mealtime hunger and in long-term regulation of body weight.[13–16] Sleeve gastrectomy may contribute to weight loss by decreasing ghrelin secretion that increases satiety, as well as by regulating gastric emptying. Langer and colleagues observed a significant decrease of plasma ghrelin at 1 and 6 months after LSG. Ghrelin remained unchanged in the banding patients.[17] LSG patients achieved a 61% EWL compared to 28% in the banding group at 6 months ($p < 0.001$).

Can the LSG be used as a sole bariatric procedure? Recent data has shown good results in patients with BMI less than 50 (Table 19–1). However, all the published studies have a short-term (1 year) follow-up period. It has been evident that a subgroup of patients do regain weight after the year, and the authors speculate that this proportion will rise with a longer follow-up. Dilatation may be the first cause of failure.[18] It may be a result of an excessively large pouch being created at the initial operation because of missed posterior gastric folds.[19] Excessive pressure against the pouch walls by large meals, repeated vomiting, or distal obstruction leads to its dilatation. Increasing proximal pouch diameter may also be a result of hiatal hernia, missed preoperatively or intraoperatively.[20]

An adequate patient selection and appropriate surgical technique may not prevent pouch dilatation. The pouch expansion may be controlled by external wrapping or with an external silastic ring support, as proposed by Fobi and coworkers, in gastric bypass.[21,22] It is unlikely that a laparoscopic adjustable gastric banding will be useful to prevent gastric dilatation, because it is a known frequent complication of this method,[23] and when used in superobese patients, a lesser percent of EWL is achieved at 1 year.[24] The subgroup of patients with a BMI more than 50 kg/m^2 have had less EWL than those with a lower BMI. Most of these patients require a second-stage procedure to assure weight control.

Table 19–1.

Results of Laparoscopic Sleeve Gastrectomy

Studies	n	Preop BMI	Complication (%)	Mortality (%)	EWL (6 months) (%)	EWL (12 months) (%)
Almogy[8] (2004)	21	>50	23	0	42	44
Mognol[2] (2005)	10	64 (61–80)	0	0	41	51
Baltasar[9] (2005)	31	35–74	ND	3	ND	46
Gagner[18] (2002)	33	66	3	0	30	32
Moon Han[10] (2005)	130	37	1	0	72	83
Langer[11] (2006)	23	49 (40–73)	0	0	46	56

BMI, body mass index; EWL, excess body weight loss; ND, none determined.

In comparison, LSG has an advantage over other restrictive procedures. Lower ghrelin plasma levels can enhance weight control. However, the absence of a foreign body avoids distortion of gastric anatomy in case of revisional surgery.

Dapri and coworkers reported a prospective randomized trial in 80 patients which compared laparoscopic adjustable banding and LSG.[25] After 1 year, the mean excess weight loss was 36% for the banding group and 56% for the LSG ($p < 0.002$). They reported a loss of feeling of hunger in 75% of the LSG patients compared to 43% in the banding group ($p < 0.007$). However, they reported gastroesophageal reflux in 22% of the LSG compared to 9% in the banding group. They also observed a higher reoperation rate in the banding patients for complications of the system.

The intragastric balloon was described by Nieben and Harboe to produce food intake restriction in obese patients.[26] With time, new, smooth, spherical saline-filled balloons became available (e.g., Bioenterics intragastric balloon, BIB) and were accepted in some countries as an option for first-stage treatment for weight loss. The BIB seems an appropriate alternative, especially in high-risk patients, because of its simplicity.[27]

The senior author compared a series of LSG with 2 series of BIB retrospectively.[28] The mean BMI was 69 for the LSG series, 60 for the Weiner and colleagues series,[29] and 58 for the Busetto and coworkers' series.[30] No procedure-related complications were reported except for 1 trocar-infection in the LSG. However, 4 (7%) patients had the BIB removed: one for balloon dysfunction, one for abdominal pain, and 2 for noncompliance. One patient had spontaneous elimination of the balloon in the stools. The EWL at 6 months for the LSG was 35% compared to 26% and 21% for the two BIB series. They concluded that LSG allowed a rapid and greater weight loss compared to the BIB, and although it is a procedure that requires a 2–3-day hospital stay, it can be performed safely with only minor complications. However, although the BIB is an ambulatory procedure, it carries a risk of intolerance and bad quality of life.

CONCLUSION

In conclusion, LSG has become an appropriate restrictive procedure with good short-term results and low morbidity rates. It has been adopted increasingly with 2 main indications: as a first-stage procedure in high-risk patients with high BMI and as a restrictive operation in patients with lower BMI. Longer follow-up is required for LSG to prove its efficacy as a sole operation. The possibility to offer a second-stage procedure in case of weight regain with low morbidity and no anatomical distortion precludes an increasing adoption in the bariatric arsenal.

References

1. Regan JP, Inabnet WB, Gagner M, Pomp A: Early experience with two-stage laparoscopic Roux-en-Y gastric bypass as an alternative in the super-super obese patient. *Obes Surg* 13(6):861–864, 2003.
2. Mognol P, Chosidow D, Marmuse JP: Laparoscopic sleeve gastrectomy as an initial bariatric operation for high-risk patients: Initial results in 10 patients. *Obes Surg* 15(7):1030–1033, 2005.
3. Marceau P, Hould FS, Simard S, et al.: Biliopancreatic diversion with duodenal switch. *World J Surg* 22(9):947–954, 1998.
4. Marceau P: Contribution of bariatric surgery to the comprehension of morbid obesity. *Obes Surg* 15(1):3–10, 2005.
5. Carmichael AR, Sue-Ling HM, Johnston D: Quality of life after the Magenstrasse and Mill procedure for morbid obesity. *Obes Surg* 11(6):708–715, 2001.
6. Consten EC, Gagner M, Pomp A, Inabnet WB: Decreased bleeding after laparoscopic sleeve gastrectomy with or without duodenal switch for morbid obesity using a stapled buttressed absorbable polymer membrane. *Obes Surg* 14(10):1360–1366, 2004.
7. Consten EC, Dakin GF, Gagner M: Intraluminal migration of bovine pericardial strips used to reinforce the gastric staple-line in laparoscopic bariatric surgery. *Obes Surg* 14(4):549–554, 2004.
8. Almogy G, Crookes PF, Anthone GJ: Longitudinal gastrectomy as a treatment for the high-risk super-obese patient. *Obes Surg* 14(4):492–497, 2004.
9. Baltasar A, Serra C, Perez N, et al.: Laparoscopic sleeve gastrectomy: A multi-purpose bariatric operation. *Obes Surg* 15(8):1124–1128, 2005.
10. Moon Han S, Kim WW, Oh JH: Results of laparoscopic sleeve gastrectomy (LSG) at 1 year in morbidly obese Korean patients. *Obes Surg* 15(10):1469–1475, 2005.
11. Langer FB, Bohdjalian A, Felberbauer FX, et al.: Does gastric dilatation limit the success of sleeve gastrectomy as a sole operation for morbid obesity? *Obes Surg* 16(2):166–171, 2006.
12. Flanagan L: Understanding the function of the small gastric pouch. In: Deitel M, et al. (eds.): *Update: Surgery for the Morbidly Obese Patients.* FD-Communications, 2000; p. 147–160, Chapter 18.
13. Kojima M, Hosoda H, Date Y, et al.: Ghrelin is a growth-hormone-releasing acylated peptide from stomach. *Nature* 402(6762):656–660, 1999.
14. Cummings DE, Weigle DS, Frayo RS, et al.: Plasma ghrelin levels after diet-induced weight loss or gastric bypass surgery. *N Engl J Med* 346(21):1623–1630, 2002.
15. Date Y, Kojima M, Hosoda H, et al.: Ghrelin, a novel growth hormone-releasing acylated peptide, is synthesized in a distinct endocrine cell type in the gastrointestinal tracts of rats and humans. *Endocrinology* 141(11):4255–4261, 2000.
16. Nakazato M, Murakami N, Date Y, et al.: A role for ghrelin in the central regulation of feeding. *Nature* 409(6817):194–198, 2001.
17. Langer FB, Reza Hoda MA, Bohdjalian A, et al.: Sleeve gastrectomy and gastric banding: effects on plasma ghrelin levels. *Obes Surg* 15(7):1024–1029, 2005.
18. Gagner M, Rogula T: Laparoscopic reoperative sleeve gastrectomy for poor weight loss after biliopancreatic diversion with duodenal switch. *Obes Surg* 13(4):649–654, 2003.
19. Deitel GC (ed.): *Update: Surgery for the Morbidly Obese Patients.* FD-Communications, 2000; Chapter 16, p. 135 and Chapter 20, p. 171.
20. Wilson LJ, Ma W, Hirschowitz BI: Association of obesity with hiatal hernia and esophagitis. *Am J Gastroenterol* 94(10):2840–2844, 1999.
21. Fobi MA, Lee H, Felahy B, et al.: Choosing an operation for weight control, and the transected banded gastric bypass. *Obes Surg* 15(1):114–121, 2005.
22. Fobi MA: Placement of the GaBP ring system in the banded gastric bypass operation. *Obes Surg* 15(8):1196–1201, 2005.
23. de Csepel J, Quinn T, Pomp A, Gagner M: Conversion to a laparoscopic biliopancreatic diversion with a duodenal switch for failed laparoscopic adjustable silicone gastric banding. *J Laparoendosc Adv Surg Tech A* 12(4):237–240, 2002.
24. Dolan K, Hatzifotis M, Newbury L, Fielding G: A comparison of laparoscopic adjustable gastric banding and biliopancreatic diversion in superobesity. *Obes Surg* 14(2):165–169, 2004.

25. Dapri JH, de Bilde D, Leman G, Cadiere GB: A prospective randomized trial between the band gastroplasty and the sleeve gastrectomy: Results after 1 year [abstract]. In: *13 International Congress of the European Association for Endoscopic Surgery.* 2005; p. 112. Oral presentation 0172.

26. Nieben OG, Harboe H: Intragastric balloon as an artificial bezoar for treatment of obesity. *Lancet* 1(8265):198–199, 1982.

27. Genco A, Bruni T, Doldi SB, et al.: BioEnterics intragastric balloon: The Italian experience with 2,515 patients. *Obes Surg* 15(8):1161–1164, 2005.

28. Milone L, Strong V, Gagner M: Laparoscopic sleeve gastrectomy is superior to endoscopic intragastric balloon as a first stage procedure for super-obese patients (BMI > or = 50). *Obes Surg* 15(5):612–617, 2005.

29. Weiner R, Gutberlet H, Bockhorn H: Preparation of extremely obese patients for laparoscopic gastric banding by gastric-balloon therapy. *Obes Surg* 9(3):261–264, 1999.

30. Busetto L, Segato G, De Luca M, et al.: Preoperative weight loss by intragastric balloon in super-obese patients treated with laparoscopic gastric banding: A case-control study. *Obes Surg* 14(5):671–676, 2004.

Laparoscopic Gastric Bypass: Trans-Oral Circular Stapling

Renam Catharina Tinoco, MD, FACS, TCBC • Augusto Claudio Tinoco, MD, TCBC

I. INTRODUCTION

II. ANESTHESIA AND SPECIAL CARE

III. TECHNIQUE

IV. COMMENTS

INTRODUCTION

The Roux-en-Y gastric bypass (RYGP) is considered to be gold standard in the United States for the surgical treatment of morbid obesity. The anastomosis of the gastric pouch to the jejunum can be done manually,[1] with a linear stapler,[2] with a circular stapler with the collocation of an anvil, transgastric, or with the circular stapler passing the anvil through the mouth.[3,4] The latter method of anastomosis has been our preference.

The laparoscopic RYGP was first performed by Wittgrove and Clark, 1994. The gastric-jejunal anastomosis was first performed via retrocolic passage, but nowadays almost all of the surgeons perform this via ante-colic passage. The proximal gastric pouch is narrowed by a silicone ring as suggested by Fobi and Capella.[5,6] However, most surgeons today make a calibrated anastomosis, about 1.2 cm, thereby avoiding the use of foreign material.

To make the jejunal stretch to the gastric pouch, surgeons section the greater omentum, gaining extra centimeters.[7] We use a 10–12-cm devascularization of the jejunum, which is taken to the gastrojejunal anastomosis. The anastomosis with the gastric pouch being completed, the segment of the devascularized jejunum is resected.

ANESTHESIA AND SPECIAL CARE

It is necessary to use an adequate anesthetic considering relaxation and depth, intubations with the patient awake, and the induction of a general anesthesia. The patient walks to the operating room, and at the end of the intervention the patient is already awake and returns to the room on his or her own. After staying in the postanesthetic recovery room for 2 hours, the patient walks to his or her room, without the need to visit intensive care unit (ICU).

Pneumatic calf sequential compression is used for the prevention of thromboembolism. With the patient in supine position, without bending the inferior members, a reduced surgical time (60–90 minutes), the use of pneumatic leggings, being able to walk the same day of surgery, and the application of intense physical therapy, we feel justified in the selective use of prophylactic anticoagulants.

The patient is placed adequately on the surgical table appropriate for the obese patient, which permits reverse and lateral movement without there being dislocation during the surgical procedure. No gastric tube is left in place and the bladder catheter is removed within 24 hours. A balanced diet is begun on the first postoperative day.

TECHNIQUE

The surgeon and the camera are positioned on the right and the assistants on the left of the patient for better use of the circular stapler. Seven trocars, longer ones preferred, are used: One 10/11 mm for optics, three 12 mm for work, and three 5 mm to retract the liver, the stomach and for aspiration (Figure 20–1).

Before starting the surgery, the anvil of the stapler (CEA 25) is removed from the body of the instrument and is connected to the nasogastric tube 22, removing the small spring that is on the anvil so that it will be loose and can be fixed with a wire in the vertical position (Figure 20–2). This way it can be easily passed through the esophagus with the aid of traction.

The access is obtained on the superior margin of the umbilicus with a long Veress needle, creating a pneumoperitoneum of 15 mm Hg. Seven trocars are placed, using #2, #3, and #7 for work. The surgery is begun with downward traction of the stomach with a Babcock grasper and retraction of the liver by a grasper attached to the diaphragm to the

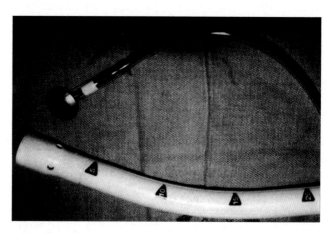

Figure 20–2. Circular stapler and anvil attached to nasogastric tube.

right of the esophageal hiatus, avoiding the use of the liver retractor.

Approximately 3 cm from the esophageal–gastric junction, two veins are located, which are grasped and sectioned with harmonic shears to have access to the posterior wall of the stomach. With blunt dissection on the gastric wall, we reach the greater curvature. Through trocar #3 an endoGIA 45 blue load stapler is introduced and fired (Figure 20–2). In sequence, through trocar #2 this stapler is used once or twice more, completing the section (Figure 20–3).

The anesthetist passed a #22 gastric catheter with an anvil from the CEEA 25 stapler through the mouth. After making a small opening of the gastric pouch with a cautery, the catheter is passed into the abdomen (Figure 20–4). The catheter is removed through the assistant trocar and sectioned with harmonic shears. A suture is placed using a poliglycolic 3.0 suture attaching the anvil of the stapler to the gastric pouch.

The table is in normal position, and the ligament of Treitz is identified after the elevation of the mesocolon. After opening the mesentery with the use of harmonic shears, the jejunum is transected 50 cm from the ligament of Treitz and fixed using endoGIA 45 white load. The distal portion of the jejunum is devascularized for about 10–12 cm. When using the antecolic approach, this stretching of the mesentery decreases tension at the gastrojejunostomy (Figure 20–5).

In the morbid obese, we use a 150-cm Roux limb and 200 cm in the super obese. A jejunojejunal anastomosis is done using endoGIA 45 white load via a small opening with a cautery in each limb. The anastomosis is completed with a manual continuous suture, using 3.0 Vycril.

The table is in right lateral position and trocar #4 is dilated for the introduction of the circular stapler, and at this moment glucagon 1 mg is injected intravenously to relax the jejunum and to make the introduction of the stapler easier. The jejunum is opened with a monopolar hook and the

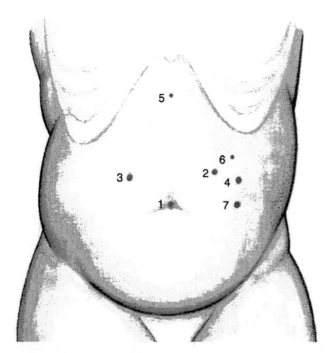

Figure 20–1. Positioning of the trocars. Seven trocars are used, longer ones preferred. One 10-mm long for optic (naval), three 12-mm long for the use of the staplers, harmonic shears, and three 5-mm long to retract the liver and the aspirator.

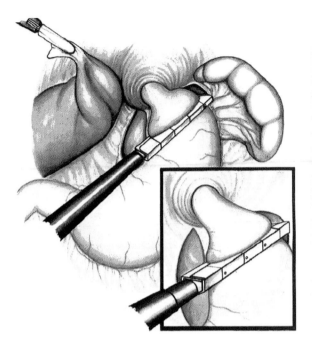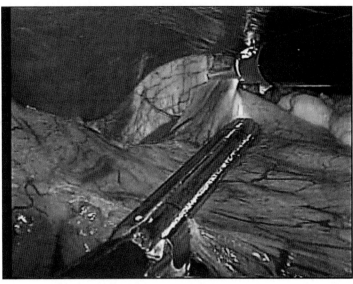

Figure 20–3. High section of the stomach with a linear stapler 45 blue load. Most of the time, three loads of this stapler are used.

stapler penetrates 7–10 cm, perforating it on its antimesenteric side. The perforating plastic portion of the stapler is removed, which is connected to the anvil situated in the gastric pouch (Figure 20–6). The stapler is closed and fired. It is important to observe the position of the anvil, which should mold to the rest of the stapler; the assistant surgeon adequately positions the proximal gastric pouch.

The excess of the jejunum is resected using endoGIA 45 white load (Figure 20–7). Both mesenteric orifices are closed using silk 3-0 suture. An orogastric catheter is passed and 100 mL of methylene blue is injected to test the anastomosis. If

there are no leaks, the catheter is removed. A needle biopsy of the liver is performed and the vacuum drain is placed.

COMMENTS

Nowadays most surgeons are changing from open surgery to laparoscopic bariatric surgery. The learning curve is a really long one, demanding strict training. From 2000 to 2004 we have operated on 942 patients, and the gastrojejunostomy has always been performed with antecolic approach. In the

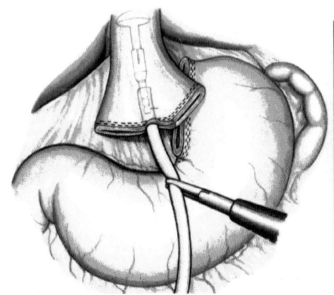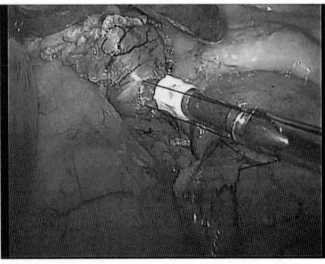

Figure 20–4. An opening is made in the gastric pouch with a cautery and the tube is pulled down through by one of the trocars and sectioned with harmonic shears.

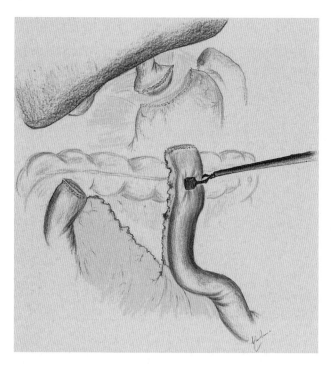

Figure 20–5. A 10–12-cm segment of the jejunum is devascularized with harmonic shears. This facilitates the elevation of the jejunal handle to the gastric pouch for an anastomosis without tension.

first 400 cases, we did not close the mesenteric defects, and similar to what most surgeons find, we have had a high rate of intestinal obstruction. However, we currently close two of the orifices and have not seen this type of complication. The anastomoses made using the stapler are not reinforced with the use of manual sutures.

We have observed fistulas at the gastrojejunostomy, and we believe that these occur due to the injection of the blue dye. Currently 100 mL of methylene blue dye is injected. If leaking occurs, we reinforce the sutures. We also have had some cases of jejunojejunostomy obstructions due to bezoar, including one case of perforation.

We do not routinely use thromboembolism prophylaxis with anticoagulants. The use of supine position, pneumatic calf compression, and early deambulation should suffice in our opinion.

Gastrojejunostomy stenosis, which in the beginning reached 20%, today is only 5%. This has happened because as soon as the patient presented with dysphagia they are submitted to early endoscopic dilation. Nowadays we recommend that the patient with premature dysphagia be maintained on a liquid diet, and generally this symptom disappears within 30 days. Unfortunately, in the cases where we performed premature dilation many of the patients presented a wider anastomosis and consequently began gaining weight. The mean operating time varies between 50 and 90 minutes.

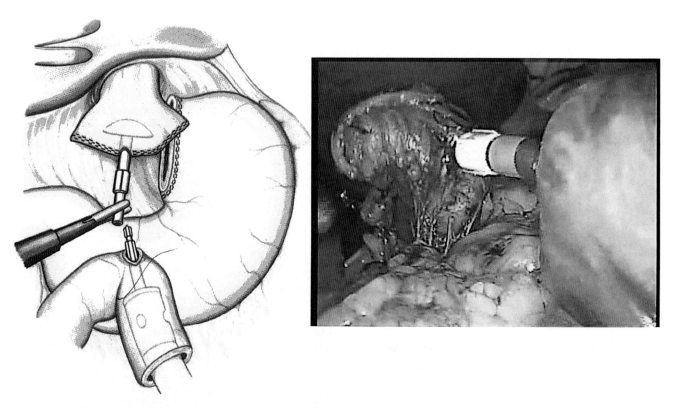

Figure 20–6. After finishing the intestinal portion in which the sectioning of the jejunum is performed at 50 cm from the Treitz angle and the jejunojejunal anastomosis is done, the stapler is introduced through the abdominal wall through one of the orifices made for the trocars in the left flank, then in the jejunal handle. Then the connection of the stapler with the tip of the anvil is done and only after the approximation of the gastric pouch to the jejunum, the stapler is triggered completing the anastomosis.

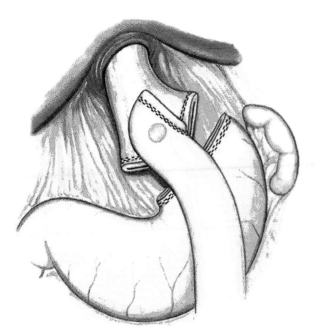

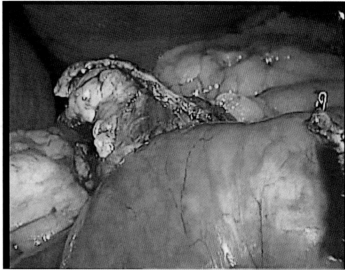

Figure 20–7. A completed gastrojejunal anastomosis and the portion of the devascularized jejunal handle is resected with the application of the linear stapler 45 white load.

References

1. Higa KD, Bone KB, Ho T: Complications of the laparoscopic Roux-en-Y gastric bypass: 1,040 patients—What have we learned? *Obes Surg* 10:509, 2000.

2. Schauer PR, Sayeed I: Laparoscopic surgery for morbid obesity. *Surg Clin North Am* 81:1143, 2001.

3. Wittgrove AC, Clark WO, Tremblay LJ: Laparoscopic gastric bypass Roux-en-Y. *Obes Surg* 4:353, 1994.

4. Tinoco RC, Tinoco ACA: Cirurgia Laparoscópica da Obesidade Mórbida. In: Madureira F (ed.): *Técnicas avançadas de cirurgia laparoscópica.* São Paulo, Editora Atheneu, 2001; p. 197.

5. Fobi MA: Vertical banded gastroplasty VS. Gastric bypass: Ten years follow-up. *Obes Surg* 3:369, 1993.

6. Capella JF, Capella RF: The weight reduction operation of choice: Vertical banded gastroplasty or gastric bypass. *Am J Surg* 171:74, 1996.

7. Gagner M:Roux-en-Y gastric bypass after previous unsuccessful gastric restritive surgery. *J Gastrointest Surg* 7:429, 2003.

Laparoscopic Gastric Bypass: Circular Stapler Technique

Alan Wittgrove, MD, FACS

I. EVOLUTION OF LAPAROSCOPIC GASTRIC BYPASS TECHNIQUE

II. TECHNIQUE FOR CIRCULAR GASTROENTEROANASTOMOSIS

III. MODIFICATIONS OF THE STAPLING TECHNIQUE

IV. RESULTS

V. ALTERNATIVE SURGICAL TECHNIQUES

The gastric bypass operation was described by Mason in 1969[1] and has evolved, with many variations, since the original loop technique. Many investigators, including Dr. Henry Buchwald, abandoned the loop technique because of many complications, such as alkaline gastritis and esophagitis, and the Roux-en-Y technique was brought forward and refined. The Roux en-Y has been the standard for the "hybrid" of bariatric operations for over three decades understanding that the Roux limb needed to be at least 60 cm to eliminate the reflux but many aspects of the operation remained unproven. It has been felt that the size of the gastric pouch, the restriction at the level of the gastroenterostomy, and the maintenance of an adequate length of common channel (to maintain absorption) are important in this operation.

As the laparoscopic era developed in bariatric surgery, three different ways to perform the gastroenterostomy emerged. The circular stapler was first used by me, as the primary author of this chapter, and Dr Champion[2] and Dr Higa[3] spearheaded the linear stapling and hand-sewn techniques, respectively, which will be discussed in other chapters.

In 1993, we developed the laparoscopic gastric bypass, and in 1994 the technique was first reported with results.[4] In this operation, the gastroenterostomy was created with a 21-mm circular stapling device. The first technique of circular stapler anvil placement involved pulling the anvil down from the mouth to the stomach pouch with a wire being placed percutaneously into the peritoneal cavity. This technique was derived from the method used in the percutaneous endoscopic gastrostomy tube placement. The key step was the development of the Endopath Stealth endoscopic/conventional circular stapler, 21 mm, by Ethicon Endo-Surgery.[5] Historically, our group had used a hand-sewn gastroenterostomy of 12 mm since the early 1980s and we were comfortable with the results of that operation. As I was in Belgium, studying techniques for the performance of the Nissen Fundoplication, I was reviewing a study on our postoperative gastric bypass patients. It turned out that our highest complication was incisional hernia, at a rate of about 15%. We discussed various ways to try to decrease this hernia rate and decided to try the operation laparoscopically to decrease our number one complication. We had worked in the laboratory for months trying different techniques and then the 21-mm circular stapler was being readied for release and that seemed to fit nicely with the planned procedure. The 21-mm stapler creates a uniform and reproducible 12-mm anastomosis and that was the size of the gastroenterostomy we were used to creating. This technique also allowed us to preserve the small gastric pouch, which is felt to be essential to long-term weight control.[6] In the animal model, we had tried several methods of anvil placement as we were developing the concept of the laparoscopic gastric bypass but settled on the transoral placement because we had extensive experience in placing Percutaneous Endoscopic Gastrostomy (PEG) catheters and it was a relatively easy adaptation.

Over time, several different surgical groups began to use this technique but changed the type and size of the anvil. As this occurred, some concerns were raised pertaining to possible esophageal injuries and the size of an anvil. In order to avoid complications, surgeons should adhere to basic guidelines and use the device they are familiar with, as circular staplers are not generically equivalent. To avoid injury, any forced maneuvers and pushing the anvil from above are to be avoided as those techniques may lead to esophageal trauma. In addition, elevation of the angle of the jaw, forward, during traction of the pull wire from below, while deflating the endotracheal tube, are important technical details which may avoid injury and facilitate passage of the anvil. A stuck anvil is very rare and can be retrieved using endoscopic techniques.[6] No esophageal injuries were noted in the first 1,400 patients on whom this technique was done, as confirmed by endoscopy in every case.[4]

EVOLUTION OF LAPAROSCOPIC GASTRIC BYPASS TECHNIQUE

Laparoscopic Roux-en-Y gastric bypass was first described in 1993 by Wittgrove et al.[7] The technique involves creation of a 15–30 mL isolated gastric pouch, a 21-mm stapled circular anastomosis, a 75-cm retrocolic, retrogastric Roux limb, and stapled side-to-side jejunojejunostomy. They employed a transoral pull-wire technique to advance the anvil, as will be discussed below. Many surgeons currently follow this technique; however, some prefer to extend the Roux-limb length to 150 or 250 cm for superobese patients. Gagner and colleagues used an antecolic, antegastric Roux limb and a 25-mm circular stapler. This avoids the creation of retrocolic tunnel, though there are suggestions that this may create tension and increase risk of stricture at the gastroenterostomy. Most surgeons agree that mesenteric defect and Petersen's defect should be routinely closed, in some fashion. Internal hernias and bowel obstructions have been reported, which have prompted surgeons to begin closing all mesenteric defects.

There is a debate concerning the formation of the gastrojejunostomy in RYGBP. Before lapaparoscopic era, the gastric anastomosis was commonly performed in hand-sewn fashion. In general, three schools dominated the laparoscopic technique. One, described by my group, uses a circular stapler to perform gastrojejunostomy. On the other hand, Champion reported good results with a linear stapler. The third, some feel more difficult technique, is the hand-sewn anastomosis, as described by Higa. Despite the controversies, most agree that the selection of a particular technique mainly depends on the individual surgeon's preferences, familiarity with the technique, and the expertise. None of these approaches are considered as a *standard* in laparoscopic bariatric surgery but it is recommended that any individual surgeon perform one technique, mainly. This allows for a further development of comfort and expertise and the ability to follow the patients as a series. Whichever technique is chosen, it is not completely free of possible complications. Among other problems, gastrointestinal anastomosis leak remains one of the most important. It is considered prudent (but not standard of care) to check the gastrojejunostomy for leaks, before closing the procedure. Many surgeons instill methylene blue solution in the gastric pouch and observe for any coloring around the anastomosis. Our technique has always been to use the endoscope to insufflate air into the gastric pouch, with the small bowel cross clamped several centimeters distal to the anastomosis. The anastomosis is then visualized while it is under irrigation fluid to see if air bubbles escape, much like doing a patch test on a tire inner tube. This technique allows immediate evaluation of the anastomosis and if problems are noted they can be sutured directly, prior to closing.

TECHNIQUE FOR CIRCULAR GASTROENTEROANASTOMOSIS

The patient is placed in standard supine position on the operating table. Pneumoperitoneum is induced by inserting a Verese needle in the left upper abdominal quadrant, just below the rib margin. (This step is often avoided by surgeons who enter the abdomen with a technique that allows visualization, through the trocar, with the laparoscopy, directly.) The initial operating port is inserted at the umbilicus with the assistance of the laparoscope and subsequent cannulas are introduced under direct, laparoscopic, vision. The trocars at the umbilicus, right upper quadrants, and left upper quadrants are 10/12 mm. We use smooth cannulas but there are ridged cannulas available if the ports come out with repeated instrument movement. A 5-mm port is placed at the subxyphoid area for the liver retractor.

A 5-mm toothed grasper is placed through the subxyphoid port and attached to the diaphragm near the esophagus, to retract the liver. The esophagus is identified and the cardioesophageal junction (angle of His) is brought into view so the adhesions can be taken down under direct vision. A balloon catheter, such as a Baker jejunostomy tube, is inflated in the body of the stomach and snugged into the esophagogastric junction for sizing purposes. The dissection is begun along the lower edge of the balloon, along the lesser curvature, directly on the gastric wall. The anterior wall of the stomach is elevated and a tunnel is created adjacent to the gastric wall around the lesser curvature and extending along the posterior gastric wall. An initial application of the linear (45 mm) stapling device is then made in a horizontal direction. The dissection is then continued, and the direction of the transection line is turned more vertically, aiming for the angle of His. Care should be taken to remove the balloon catheter before the stapling device is fired so as to limit the risk of transfixing these catheters in the staple-line.

The pouch should be vertically oriented and of sufficient size to admit the anvil of the Stealth 21-mm circular stapler (about 15 cc). Two to four applications of the 45-mm linear stapler are generally sufficient to create the proper sized gastric pouch.

The endoscopist then performs flexible endoscopy of the gastric pouch, and a percutaneous venous cannula is used to introduce a loop suture into the lumen of the stomach, where it is grasped by the endoscopic snare and retrieved through the mouth. The loop is easily passed through the stem of the Stealth anvil, and is then used to draw the anvil, stem first, through the oropharynx and esophagus into the stomach pouch. The narrowest area of the anvil's transit is at the level of the balloon on the endotracheal tube and that is why we described the jaw manipulation and endotracheal tube balloon deflation above. The anesthesiologist should maintain control of the endotrachial tube during that maneuver. The anvil is placed under tension and gentle manipulation is applied to create an opening just large enough to bring the stem through the wall of the stomach pouch. Cautery may be used if the loop is wire; however, we currently use a loop *suture* and cautery should be avoided. The anvil is generally placed on the gastric wall, posterior to the staple-line with this technique; however, it may be more advantageous to place the anvil through the linear staple-line to avoid areas of ischemia. Placing the anvil through the posterior wall allows the suture on the anvil to elevate the gastric pouch and retract it anteriorly, which tends to facilitate the completion of the gastroenterostomy.

The hepatogastric omentum is opened into the lesser sac and a Penrose drain is placed behind the stomach. This will be used to bring the small bowel into the upper abdomen after the enteroenterostomy is completed.

The omentum is retracted into the upper abdomen. The colon is retracted anteriorly and cephalad, and a peritoneal incision is made anterior and to the left of the ligament of Treitz. Dissection at this location will lead to penetration of the mesocolon, into the lesser peritoneal sac, through an area which is generally avascular. A pair of blunt grasping forceps, or reticulating forceps, are then passed behind the colon and stomach into the lesser sac, and the Penrose drain is grasped and drawn back into the lower abdominal field.

The small bowel is examined and the proximal jejunum is identified at the ligament of Treitz. The peritoneal reflection must be clearly demonstrated, to avoid misidentification. The small bowel is followed distally for approximately 10–12 cm, to reach a comfortable length of small bowel and mesentery. The small bowel is then transected with the linear 45-mm stapling device with minimal transaction of the

small bowel mesentery and the proximal end is immediately grasped by the assistant surgeon for identification. The distal end of the transected small bowel is then used to construct the 75-cm Roux limb. A side-to-side enteroenterostomy is then constructed. This is accomplished with two applications of the linear 35-mm stapler, and the opening for the introduction of the 35-mm stapler is closed with the linear 45-mm stapler.

The Penrose drain is then sutured to the distal portion of the previously transected small bowel, and a sufficient length of small bowel, approximately 10 cm, is drawn into the upper abdomen. A longitudinal incision is made on the antimesenteric aspect, 5–6 cm from the stapled end. The Stealth is then inserted directly through the skin at the lower port site on the left. The stapler is introduced into the lumen of the small bowel through the enterotomy and advanced to the stapled end. The stem of the anvil is grasped, using the anvil grasping forceps, through the upper right lateral port. The penetrator of the Stealth is then extended and united with the anvil stem. The orientation of the bowel is observed and maintained as the Stealth is closed and discharged to avoid rotation of the small bowel. The Stealth is withdrawn and the enterotomy is closed with an application of the linear 45-mm stapling device. Three sutures are placed from the small bowel to the pouch to involute the gastroenterostomy, anteriorly. This closes any potential crossed staple-lines and buttresses any potential ischemic gastric tissue between the two staple-lines. The small bowel is then cross-clamped and it is at this point that we perform our final endoscopy with air insufflation to check the integrity of the gastroenterostomy.

The small bowel is then returned below the mesocolon, without excess tension, so that the staple-line rests at the transverse colon mesentery. This helps to fixate the small bowel and eliminate the potential space for an internal hernia. We additionally place a suture from the small bowel to the colon mesentery, on the patient's left side, to further fix the Roux limb and avoid potential internal hernias. The small bowel mesentery, at the enteroenterostomy, is then closed to minimize internal hernias at that site as well.

A drain is placed in the sulcus of the liver and diaphragm, cephalad to the gastroenterostomy and into the subdiaphragmatic space on the left.

MODIFICATIONS OF THE STAPLING TECHNIQUE

Since the initial laparoscopic gastric bypass we did in 1993 several modifications have been made by our surgical team. The size of the gastric pouch continues to be 15 cc, sized each time with a sizing balloon and that has been constant for both our laparotomy as well as the laparoscopic operations.

The endoscopy, for the introduction of the 21-mm circular stapler anvil, can be performed immediately after the gastric division, or just prior to performing the gastroenterostomy. The pull wire is grasped by the endoscopic snare either intragastric or by allowing the snare to penetrate the gastric wall and grasp the loop as the snare is in the inraperitoneal space.

As noted above, we currently place more sutures in the mesentery to close the defects rather than the technique we used for the first 1,000 cases or so. Prior to *closing* the defects our internal hernia rate was about 5%. Over the past 2 years we have seen only a rare internal hernia.

The proximal Roux limb is passed retrocolic and retrogastric, at the base of the transverse mesocolon. This approach shortens the path of the Roux limb to the proximal gastric pouch and reduces bowel tension. This pull-through technique is facilitated by using a length of Penrose drain. The Penrose drain is retrieved through the clear area of the lesser omentum, near the caudate lobe of the liver, and the small bowel limb is drawn into the upper abdominal space in relation to the proximal gastric pouch. We have used several different techniques for this maneuver but we find this easy and efficient.

Intraoperative endoscopy, upon completion of the gastroenterostomy, with the proximal small bowel cross-clamped, helps with the early detection of air leakage while the bowel wall is distended with air from the endoscope.[7] Several different techniques had been tried, including instillation of methylene blue, but we find this quite effective and we believe there is benefit in performing an endoscopic evaluation intraoperatively.

The most significant change in technique was placing the circular stapler directly through the skin incision rather than placing it through a 33-mm trocar. Initially, the circular stapler was introduced via a 33-mm port. Several surgeons began using other techniques for the placement of this stapler and we adopted the technique after discussion with Dr. Baltasar. As we first discarded the port, we found our wound infection rate went up since the potentially contaminated stapler was brought directly through the subcutaneous tissue. We tried several methods of protecting the wound from the contaminated anvil of this instrument but the one that worked best for us was simply using the plastic sheath already as a part of the instrument. We loosen the plastic as we are ready to remove the instrument and slide the plastic down over the end of the stapler, into the subcutaneous tissue. With this maneuver our wound infection rate dropped to less than 1%.

RESULTS

Weight loss exceeds 50% of excess body weight (EBW) within 6 months of surgery, and rises steadily to an average EBW loss of 75% at 18 months. Graded, significant comorbidities were reduced or completely resolved in over 91% of the situations. Gastroesophageal reflux disease was completely resolved in 100% of patients. Diabetes mellitus resolved in 92% and was reduced in the remaining patients. Sleep apnea was eliminated in all afflicted patients. Of 18 hypertensive patients, 94% experienced clinical remission, while one remained mildly hypertensive, on medications.[7]

In the first 1,000 cases of the primary author, the complications are as listed below. Leak that required reoperation was 0.8%. Hemorrhage requiring transfusion was 1.2%. Wound infection was 6% and prompted us to change the way we sheathed the circular stapler as noted above. Stricture requiring dilation was 3.8%.

Various techniques of the construction of the gastrojejunostomy were described by many authors with the intention to decrease complications. Among possible early and late complications, anastomotic leaks remain the most considerable, as the outcome may be fatal. Current literature on gastric bypass reports a 2%–5% incidence of leaks. Carrasquilla et al. report very low incidence of leaks: 0.1% (1 in 1,000 cases). This technique involves an antecolic and antegastric approach and the use of a circular stapler for the gastroenterostomy.[8]

Stenosis of the gastroenterostomy after laparoscopic Roux-en-Y gastric bypass is another situation that occurs after either stapled or hand-sewn anastomoses. Prospective analysis of 1,000 patients who underwent LRYGBP with the gastroenteroanastomosis constructed with a linear stapler revealed 3.2% patients with stenosis at the gastroenterostomy. The majority of strictures occur within the first four to six weeks after surgery. Some strictures occur later and are generally related to smoking or medication usage. In our series, endoscopic dilation was quite effective in treating the strictures at the gastrooenterostomy. An experienced endoscopist is needed to dilate the stricture formation as there is the potential for perforation. In my personal series, all early strictures responded to dilation and there were no reoperations. Some series show dilation less effective and emphasize the need for surgical revision.[9] Over dilation may lead to less weight loss secondary to loss of restriction.

Nguyen et al. analyzed the frequency of anastomotic stricture following laparoscopic GBP using a 21-mm versus a 25-mm circular stapler for construction of the gastrojejunostomy and the safety and efficacy of endoscopic balloon dilation in the management of anastomotic stricture. Anastomotic stricture occurred more frequently with the use of the 21-mm compared to the 25-mm circular stapler. Symptoms of stricture are usually presented within 6 weeks after the primary operation Recurrent stricture develops in 17% of patients. The excess body weight loss at 1 year for patients in whom the 21-mm circular stapler was used for creation of the gastrojejunostomy was similar to that for patients in whom the 25-mm circular stapler was used.[10] Longer study is needed to determine if long-term weight loss is similar to using either the 21-mm or the 25-mm circular stapler.

Early gastrointestinal hemorrhage after gastric bypass is an infrequent complication. Nguyen et al. reported that 3.2% of patients who underwent an LRYGBP with creation of the gastrojejunostomy anastomosis with a circular stapler developed postoperative hemorrhage in 24 hours after surgery. Clinical presentations may include hematemesis, bright red blood per rectum, melena, and hypotension. Nuclear scintigraphy is rarely required for identification of hemorrhage site. Conservative management is usually sufficient; however, patients with hemodynamic instability and patients with early onset of hemorrhage may require operative intervention for control of hemorrhage. The sites of hemorrhage include not only the gastrojejunostomy but also the gastric remnant staple-lines.[11]

ALTERNATIVE SURGICAL TECHNIQUES

Majority of technical modifications of circular stapler technique for the creation of the gastroenterostomy involve the anvil placement. Although there are very few reports describing pharyngeal or esophageal injuries, the risk of such injuries and difficulties in maneuvering the anvil from the pharynx to the proximal part of the stomach is still a potential concern. A case of hypopharyngeal perforation after an attempted transoral insertion of an anvil was reported by Nguyen et al.[12] In an effort to overcome this potential risk and to obviate the need for intraoperative endoscopy, alternative techniques of guiding the anvil into its position through a distal gastrotomy have been described. Dr Scott and Dr de la Torre reported placement of the anvil by attaching a suture and directing it toward a chosen site, in the soon to be gastric pouch.[13] Murr et al. described a technique for introducing the anvil of the circular stapler using a totally transabdominal approach.[14] Some optional techniques avoid upper endoscopy for the transoral introduction of the 21-mm circular stapler anvil down to the gastric pouch.[15] Dr Marema and Dr Gagner have popularized an approach whereby they use a nasogastric tube connected to the anvil and introduce the anvil transorally. No endoscopy is used. The integrity of the gastroenterostomy is verified with the injection of methylene blue into the gastric pouch. Modification described by Gould et al. involves the creation of a gastrostomy for transgastric placement of the anvil.[16]

References

1. Mason EE, Ito C: Gastric bypass. *Ann Surg* 170(3):329–339, 1969.
2. Champion JK, Williams MD: Prospective randomized comparison of linear staplers during laparoscopic Roux-en-Y gastric bypass. *Obes Surg* 13(6):855–859, 2003; discussion: 860.
3. Higa KD, et al.: Laparoscopic Roux-en-Y gastric bypass for morbid obesity: Technique and preliminary results of our first 400 patients. *Arch Surg* 135(9):1029–1033, 2000; discussion: 1033–1034.
4. Wittgrove AC, Clark GW: Combined laparoscopic/endoscopic anvil placement for the performance of the gastroenterostomy. *Obes Surg* 11(5):565–569, 2001.
5. Wittgrove AC, Clark GW, Tremblay LJ: Laparoscopic gastric bypass, Roux-en-Y: Preliminary Report of Five Cases. *Obes Surg* 4(4):353–357, 1994.
6. Wittgrove AC, Clark GW: Laparoscopic gastric bypass: Endostapler transoral or transabdominal anvil placement. *Obes Surg* 10(4):376–377, 2000.
7. Wittgrove AC, Clark GW, Schubert KR: Laparoscopic gastric bypass, Roux-en-Y: Technique and results in 75 patients with 3–30 months follow-up. *Obes Surg* 6(6):500–504, 1996.
8. Carrasquilla C, English WJ, Esposito P, et al.: Total stapled, total intra-abdominal (TSTI) laparoscopic Roux-en-Y gastric bypass: One leak in 1000 cases. *Obes Surg* 14(5):613–617, 2004.
9. Schwartz ML, et al.: Stenosis of the gastroenterostomy after laparoscopic gastric bypass. *Obes Surg* 14(4):484–491, 2004.
10. Nguyen NT, Stevens CM, Wolfe BM: Incidence and outcome of anastomotic stricture after laparoscopic gastric bypass. *J Gastrointest Surg* 7(8):997–1003, 2003; discussion: 1003.
11. Nguyen NT, Rivers R, Wolfe BM: Early gastrointestinal hemorrhage after laparoscopic gastric bypass. *Obes Surg* 13(1):62–65, 2003.
12. Nguyen NT and Wolfe BM: Hypopharyngeal perforation during laparoscopic Roux-en-Y gastric bypass. *Obes Surg* 10(1):64–67, 2000.
13. de la Torre RA, Scott JS: Laparoscopic Roux-en-Y gastric bypass: A totally intra-abdominal approach—technique and preliminary report. *Obes Surg* 9(5):492–498, 1999.
14. Murr MM, Gallagher SF: Technical considerations for transabdominal loading of the circular stapler in laparoscopic Roux-en-Y gastric bypass. *Am J Surg* 185(6):585–588, 2003.
15. Borao FJ, Thomas TA, Steichen FM: Alternative operative techniques in laparoscopic Roux-en-Y gastric bypass for morbid obesity. *JSLS* 5(2):123–129, 2001.
16. Gould JC, Garren MJ, Starling JR: Lessons learned from the first 100 cases in a new minimally invasive bariatric surgery program. *Obes Surg* 14(5) 618–625, 2004.

Laparoscopic Gastric Bypass: Transgastric Circular Stapler

Roger de la Torre, MD • J. Stephen Scott, MD • Matthew Fitzer, MD

INTRODUCTION

Numerous techniques have been published for performing laparoscopic Roux-en-Y gastric bypass. Some of the most widely adopted of these techniques are described in other chapters of this book, and each of these techniques has been shown to produce successful outcomes when performed by experienced surgeons.

This chapter describes the authors' preferred technique: antecolic, antegastric, circular-stapled gastrojejunostomy with transgastric anvil placement. We favor a circular-stapled anastomosis because of its efficiency and reproducibility. Transgastric delivery of the anvil has several advan-

tages: It allows precise anvil placement by the operating surgeon, requires no special equipment, and can be performed without the assistance of the anesthesiologist. Furthermore, it eliminates the risk of hypopharyngeal and esophageal trauma, which has been described when the transoral route is used for anvil placement.[1,2]

The choice of the antecolic route for the roux limb is based on the consideration of internal hernias. Two reviews of internal hernias after laparoscopic gastric bypass found that the retrocolic window was the most common site of symptomatic herniation.[3,4] Antecolic placement of the Roux limb avoids creation of a retrocolic defect. Only on rare occasion, such as when a Roux limb has poor mobility and would create anastomotic tension at the gastrojejunostomy, do we prefer the retrocolic route for the Roux limb to reach the gastric pouch.

PROCEDURE

Perioperative Preparation

Preoperatively, the patient is given 5,000 U of heparin subcutaneously, sequential compression devices are placed on the patient's legs, and prophylactic antibiotics are administered. Following induction, a Foley catheter is introduced. A soft, 16 F balloon tipped orogastric tube is placed by the anesthesiologist. The patient lies supine with the arms abducted and secured on arm boards. Because steep reverse Trendelenburg positioning will be required, the patient is secured to the operating room table with a hip belt and footplate.

Trocar Placement

When the draping is complete, the surgeon and camera operator take position on the patient's right side, while the assistant and scrub tech are on the opposite side. To initiate the operation, the xiphoid is identified by palpation, and 15 cm caudad to this and 3 cm to the left of the midline a 1-cm transverse skin incision is made. An optical, bladeless 10-mm trocar (trocar #1) is advanced under vision with a zero degree laparoscope into the abdomen. After insufflation, a 10-mm 45° scope is used, instead of the straight laparoscope, for the operation. Working ports are introduced, as shown in Figures 22–1 and 22–2. A 12-mm trocar (trocar #2) is placed in the

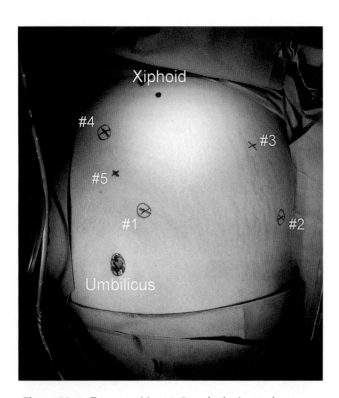

Figure 22–1. Trocar positions 1–5 marked prior to placement.

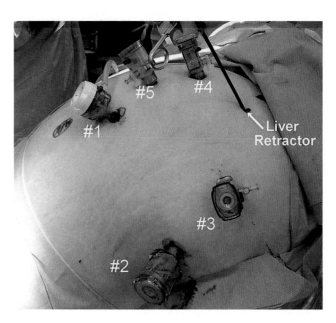

Figure 22–2. Trocars after placement. Note that the liver retractor does not require a trocar.

left anterior axillary line at the same level as the camera port. A 5-mm port (trocar #3) is then placed at the midpoint of the line between the xiphoid and trocar #2. The surgeon then places the right-sided working ports. The first is a 12-mm port, which is positioned 7 cm caudal and 4 cm to the right of the xiphoid (trocar #4). A 5-mm port (trocar #5) is placed 5 cm inferior to trocar #4, just to the right of the midline. Occasionally, liver enlargement requires that some or all of the working ports be shifted caudally.

Dividing the Omentum

Atraumatic graspers are used to elevate the gastrocolic omentum, and it is divided with the ultrasonic shears on high power through trocar #3. The goal is to create a slit in the draping portion of the omentum just to the left of midline, as this is where the Roux limb will lie with least tension. The division begins at the free edge and proceeds toward the transverse colon (Figure 22–3). In patients with prior pelvic surgery, adhesions often fix the omentum in the pelvis. This may prevent the assistant from beginning the omental split on the draping edge. Instead, it should be started laterally and arc toward the midline, ending as usual just left of midline at the transverse colon.

The Jejuno-jejunostomy

The transverse colon is gently swept cephalad by two atraumatic graspers to help expose the ligament of Treitz (Figure 22–4). The surgeon then measures 50 cm from the ligament of Treitz, directing the jejunum in a clockwise fashion as atraumatic graspers are used to run this part of the small bowel distally. A linear cutter stapler with a 2.5 mm leg length cartridge is used to divide the small bowel at the 50-cm mark through trocar #4 (Figure 22–5). The small-bowel mesentery is further divided with the ultrasonic shears for 3–4 cm to achieve more

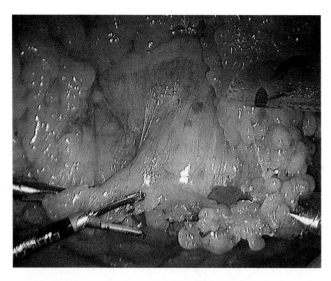

Figure 22–3. Care must be taken to avoid injury to the transverse colon while creating the omental split.

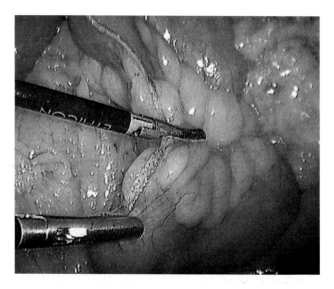

Figure 22–6. The mobility of the Roux limb depends on an adequate mesenteric division.

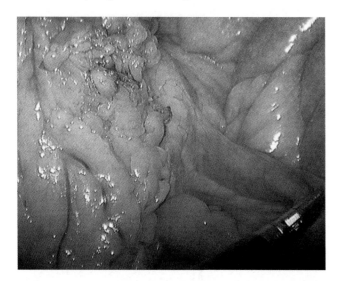

Figure 22–4. The ligament of Treitz is positively identified before measuring out the biliopancreatic limb.

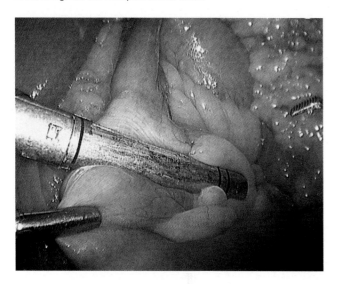

Figure 22–5. Division of the jejunum.

mobility of the Roux limb (Figure 22–6). Although a longer mesenteric split produces better mobility, problematic bleeding may be encountered if the split approaches too close to the base of the mesentery. Also, when dividing the mesentery, care must be taken not to devascularize the biliopancreatic limb. The blood supply to the distal-most Roux limb is less important because several centimeters will be sacrificed at the end of the operation.

With the biliopancreatic limb now created, the Roux limb is measured by the surgeon. While the assistant holds the biliopancreatic limb superiorly, the surgeon measures 100 cm from the distal segment of divided jejunum, guiding the bowel in a counterclockwise direction this time. This distance can be increased to 150 cm if the patient is a diabetic or has a BMI above 50.

The surgeon brings a 76-cm silk 2-0 suture on a taper needle into the abdomen through trocar #4 and uses it to approximate the antimesenteric edges of the Roux and biliopancreatic limbs (see Figure 22–7). Note that the back end of the suture is left dangling out of trocar #4 (Figure 22–8). This traction suture facilitates the subsequent construction of the jejunal anastomosis by bringing the long axis of both bowel limbs parallel with the long axis of the linear stapler. The ultrasonic shears create a 1-cm enterotomy on the antimesenteric aspect of both limbs of the small bowel while in-line countertraction is maintained on the traction suture (Figure 22–9). The assistant also helps to steady the bowel, using atraumatic graspers. The linear stapler is readied with 2.5-mm cartridge and brought into the abdomen through trocar #4. It is opened, and its two arms are guided into the enterotomies. Before the stapler is deployed, it is positioned away from the bowel mesentery to ensure that the anastomosis is made on the antimesenteric aspect of the bowel (Figure 22–10). The stapler is fired and removed. This now leaves a single enterotomy, which the surgeon will close with a 15-cm silk suture 2-0 and the assistant follows (Figure 22–11).

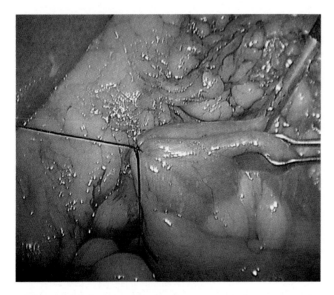

Figure 22–7. The jejunal traction suture greatly facilitates the creation of the small bowel anastomosis.

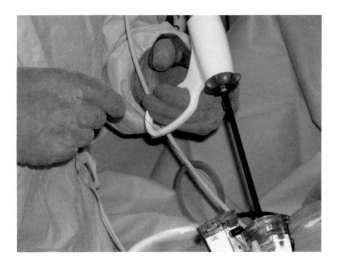

Figure 22–8. The end of the long traction suture hangs out of trocar #4.

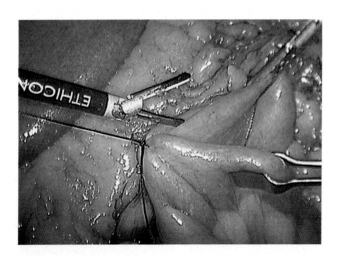

Figure 22–9. The ultrasonic shears create small bowel enterotomies.

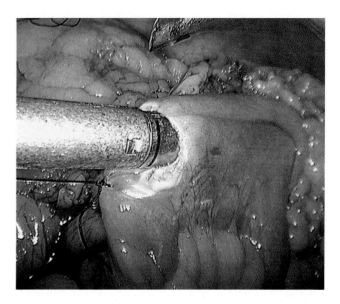

Figure 22–10. Upward traction on the shaft of the linear stapler ensures that the anastomosis is created of the bowel's antimesenteric aspect.

Note that the surgeon sews toward the traction suture and ties to it when the closure is complete. Both sutures are then cut.

Closing the Intermesenteric Space

The intermesenteric space must next be closed to reduce the risk of a subsequent internal hernia. In one of the largest published reviews of internal hernias, the frequency of herniation at this space was second only to that of the retrocolic window.[3] The defect is closed with a 20-cm silk 2-0 suture in a running fashion. The assistant grasps the cut tail of the traction suture and uses it to expose the defect for the surgeon. Closure begins at the bowel with a seromuscular bite of both the Roux limb and the biliopancreatic limb. From there, it is advanced toward the mesenteric end of the defect (Figure 22–12). Bites should be shallow and incorporate serosa and the fibrofatty

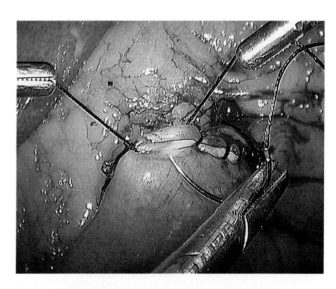

Figure 22–11. Closure of the enterotomy.

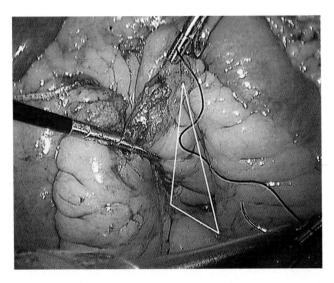

Figure 22–12. Good retraction by the assistant is required to properly close the intermesenteric defect. The triangle denotes the intermesenteric defect.

connective tissue of the mesentery of both limbs. Care must be taken to spare the blood vessels, as injury to these can result in troublesome bleeding or bowel devascularization. As the closure approaches the base of the mesentery, the endpoint of the defect must be identified (Figure 22–13). This is best achieved by swinging the Roux limb clockwise around the defect toward the upper abdomen just prior to completing the closure.

Placing the Liver Retractor

The focus now shifts to the upper abdomen. The patient is in steep reverse-Trendelenburg position. Placement of the liver retractor at this point facilitates exposure of the esophagogastric junction. The site chosen for the retractor is usually just inferior and 1–2 cm to the left of the xiphoid. If the liver is

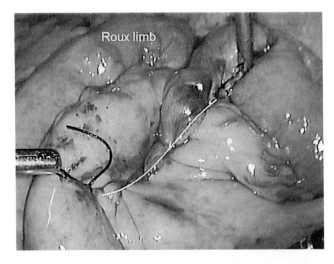

Figure 22–13. Properly positioning the Roux limb reveals the endpoint of the mesenteric closure. The line denotes the now closed intermesenteric defect.

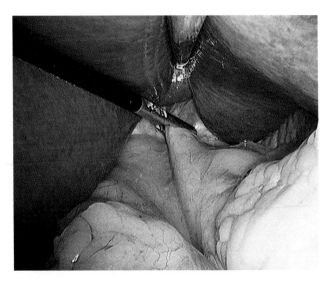

Figure 22–14. Correct positioning of the liver retractor facilitates the gastric dissection.

large, it may need to be lower. A 5-mm stab wound is made at the chosen location. A pointed surgical clamp is pushed through the fascia into the peritoneal cavity thereby creating a passage for the locking atraumatic grasper that will serve as the retractor. When the passage is made, the grasper is placed into the abdomen through the stab incision; no trocar is needed. The grasper is guided under the left lobe of the liver to the esophageal hiatus; here it grasps the right crural muscle and is locked into position (Figure 22–14). The purpose of the grasper thus placed is twofold: It facilitates visualization of the upper stomach, and it serves as a reminder of the location of the esophagus during the division of the stomach.

Dissecting the Angle of His

During the dissection of the angle of His, the gastric fundus is separated from the left crus of the diaphragm. The purpose of this dissection is to help clarify the endpoint of the retrogastric dissection that will be performed when creating the pouch. The angle of His is addressed now because exposure to this area will become more difficult to handle after the anvil to the circular stapler is positioned. The assistant exposes the angle of His for dissection by grasping the fundus high and laterally, and retracting it inferolaterally. The surgeon dissects bluntly with a 10-mm Babcock clamp, beginning in the tissue just superior to the cardia of the stomach. The dissection proceeds posteriorly, gently separating the fundus from the left crus until the retrofundic fat pad is identified (Figure 22–15). This landmark is the endpoint of the dissection.

Sizing the Pouch

The 16 F balloon tipped orogastric tube, which was advanced into the stomach by the anesthesiologist prior to initiation of the case, is now identified within the stomach. The anesthesiologist inflates the balloon with 15 cc of air. To assure that there is no redundant tubing in the stomach, the

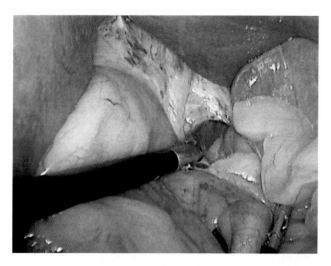

Figure 22–15. The retrofundic fat pad: Endpoint of the angle of His dissection.

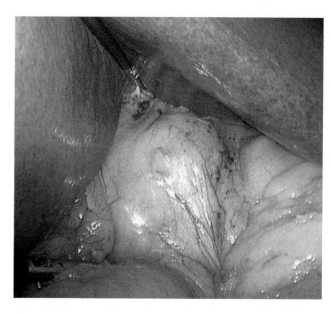

Figure 22–17. The balloon is retracted to the esophageal hiatus.

anesthesiologist is asked to slowly retract the tube while the surgeon grasps it from outside the stomach, adjacent to the balloon using a Babcock clamp through trocar #4 (Figure 22–16). When the anesthesiologist feels resistance, the surgeon releases the tube allowing further retraction of the tube and balloon. The anesthesiologist is asked to stop when there is a second point of resistance, which signals that the balloon is held up at the gastroesophageal junction (Figure 22–17). Visual inspection confirms the position of the balloon, and a site is chosen on the balloon's equator for the placement of the anvil. The anesthesiologist is now asked to mark the tube at the patient's teeth, to deflate the balloon, and then to withdraw it 10 cm back into the esophagus.

Placing the Anvil of the Circular Stapler

The 21-mm anvil is prepared with a traction suture prior to beginning the case. The pointed, plastic anvil dilator is attached to the anvil shaft and a silk 2-0 ligature is threaded

through the eyelet of the dilator. The ligature is tied into two loops: the one most proximal to the eyelet of the anvil dilator is 2 cm and the second loop is 4 cm in length. These loops aid in subsequent intraabdominal manipulations of the anvil. Next, the anvil is placed into the abdomen by the assistant. To achieve this, trocar #2 is removed and the shaft of the anvil to the circular stapler is placed within it (Figure 22–18). Note that the assistant must often dilate the fascia of this trocar site to facilitate insertion of the anvil. The trocar is then replaced into the abdominal incision, pushing the anvil through the abdominal wall as it advances (Figure 22–19). Once inside the abdominal cavity, the surgeon removes the anvil from the trocar and places it to the side.

Attention now turns to the stomach. The greater curvature is positioned by the surgeon so that a small, full-thickness gastrotomy can be made by the assistant with the ultrasonic

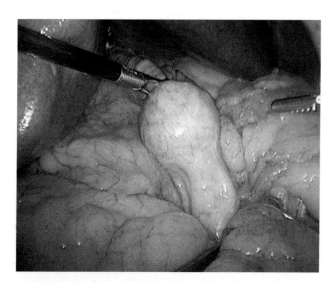

Figure 22–16. Preparing to position the inflated balloon.

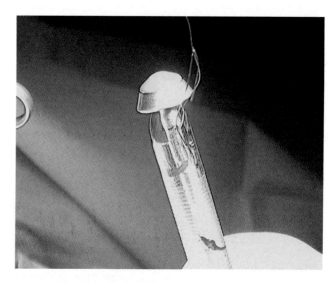

Figure 22–18. Preparing to place the anvil into the abdomen.

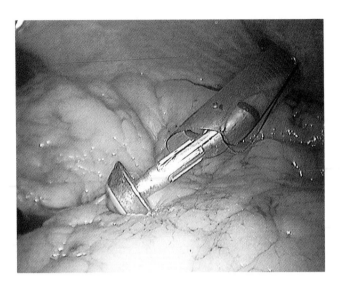

Figure 22–19. The anvil is delivered into the abdomen.

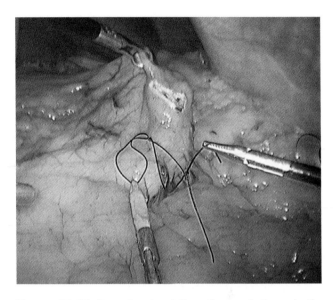

Figure 22–21. Preparing to deliver the anvil through the stomach wall.

shears through trocar #3 (Figure 22–20). The surgeon confirms that it is full thickness by placing a blunt grasper through it and into the stomach. The gastrotomy is dilated slightly with this grasper to permit subsequent passage of the anvil. The assistant places a "dolphin-nose" or other sharply pointed grasper through trocar #2. After grasping the free end of the silk ligature that had been looped through the anvil dilator, the pointed grasper is guided into the gastrotomy (Figure 22–21), from where it is carefully advanced to the location selected earlier on the proximal, anterior stomach. The tip of the pointed grasper is then advanced through the anterior wall of the stomach while the remaining three graspers hold counter tension as shown in Figure 22–22. The surgeon using the grasper in the right hand holds the stomach near the gastrotomy, pulling inferolaterally. With a closed 10-mm

Babcock clamp through trocar #4, posterior traction is maintained on the upper stomach beneath the advancing pointed grasper. The the assistant holds with the right hand an atraumatic grasper, which provides posterolateral traction as the pointed grasper is advanced through the gastric wall. Once through, the surgeon takes the silk ligature from the assistant and the pointed grasper is withdrawn. Cephalad traction on the silk draws the shaft of the anvil into the stomach, through the stomach wall, and places the anvil in the desired position (Figure 22–23).

With the anvil placed, the distal of the two silk loops is cut to shorten the suture. The assistant uses the remaining loop to help position the anvil for the surgeon, who secures it with a purse string of 3-0 vicryl (Figure 22–24). Following

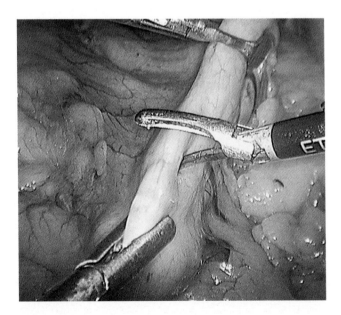

Figure 22–20. The gastrotomy is made on the distal greater curvature, distant from the proposed site of the anvil.

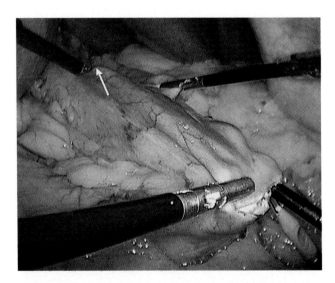

Figure 22–22. Appropriate retraction is essential for delivering the anvil. The arrow denotes the advancing tip of the pointed grasper.

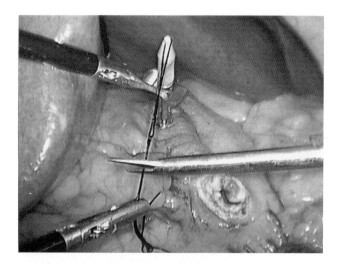

Figure 22–23. The anvil in position after traversing the stomach. The distal silk loop is cut free by the assistant.

this, a running silk 2-0 suture is used to close the gastrotomy (Figure 22–25).

Dividing the Stomach

Dissection of the hepatogastric ligament is now performed in order to create a retrogastric tunnel for subsequent division of the stomach. The dissection is started on the hepatogastric ligament 1-cm distal to the level of the anvil, where the ultrasonic shears are used to open the serosa longitudinally for a distance of 1.5–2 cm (Figure 22–26). The surgeon then carefully negotiates a blunt grasper through the fatty tissue of the ligament toward the lesser sac, taking care not to injure surrounding blood vessels. This process is aided by retraction from the assistant, who should elevate the anvil through trocar #3 while helping to expose the dissection plane in the ligament through trocar #2 with a 10-mm Babcock (Figure 22–27). Once the lesser sac has been entered, the linear stapler is introduced into the abdomen to begin dividing the stomach. Triple-row 3.5-mm stapler cartridges are used for this purpose. Before firing the stapler, it is important to confirm

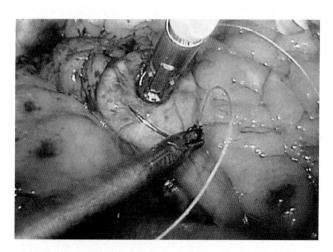

Figure 22–24. The purse string secures the anvil in place.

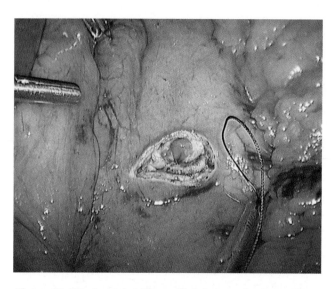

Figure 22–25. A running 20-cm silk 2-0 closes the gastrotomy.

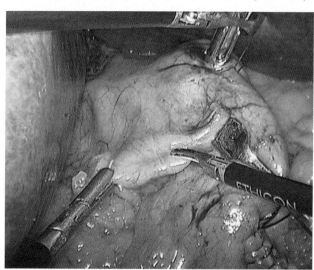

Figure 22–26. Scoring the serosa minimizes bleeding and allows the hepatogastric ligament dissection to proceed with optimal visualization.

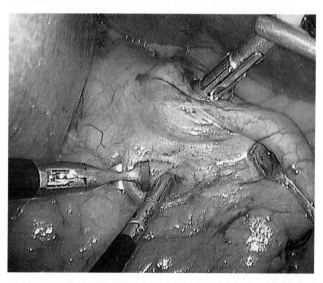

Figure 22–27. Retraction for the hepatogastric dissection.

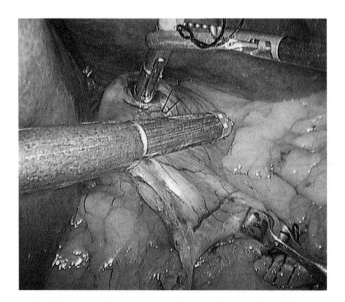

Figure 22–28. The first bite of stomach is divided with the linear stapler.

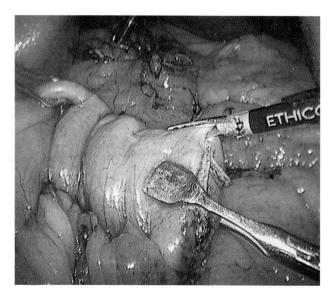

Figure 22–30. An enterotomy is created in the Roux limb to admit the circular stapler.

with the anesthesiologist that the 16 F balloon tipped tube used earlier has been properly withdrawn into the esophagus. The stapler is positioned near the anvil of the circular stapler such that the anvil acts as a template for creating the pouch (Figure 22–28).

After firing the linear stapler, the staple lines should be inspected. Additional blunt dissection is sometimes necessary posterior to the stomach to facilitate stapler positioning for progressive firings. Additional linear stapler firings are performed around the edge of the circular stapler's anvil. Typically, the first two firings are performed through trocar #4, and the assistant finishes the division working toward the dissected angle of His with another 2–3 firings through trocar #2 (Figure 22–29). Care should be taken to completely exclude the fundic tissue from the pouch and to perform complete division of the stomach.

Creating the Gastrojejunostomy

After the pouch is completed, the assistant removes the anvil dilator from the anvil in preparation for stapling the anastomosis. The Roux limb is retrieved from the lower abdomen by the surgeon, who positions it for the assistant so that he can make an enterotomy near the divided edge of the Roux limb with the ultrasonic shears through trocar #3 (Figure 22–30).

The 21-mm circular stapler is now brought into the abdomen (Figure 22–31). To achieve this, the skin incision for trocar #2 must be lengthened slightly. The stapler is then pushed through the abdominal wall and guided into the Roux limb through the enterotomy. It is then advanced for a distance of 10–15 cm. The surgeon then holds traction on the Roux limb so that the trocar of the circular stapler can be extended through the bowel wall on the antimesenteric side (Figure 22–32). The now extended trocar is guided into

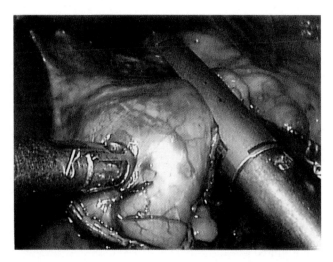

Figure 22–29. The stomach is completely divided to finish the pouch.

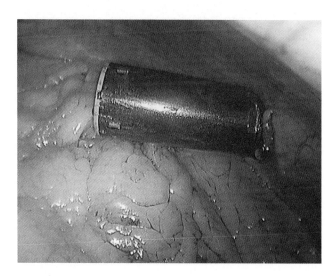

Figure 22–31. The circular stapler is placed within the abdomen.

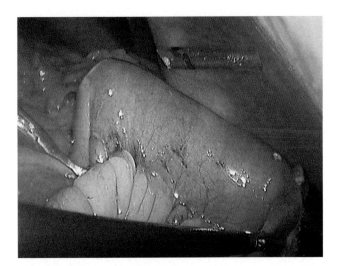

Figure 22–32. The surgeon holds two-handed traction while the circular stapler's trocar is extended by the assistant.

the shaft of the anvil and locked into place (Figure 22–33). The stapler is closed and fired according to the manufacturer's instructions, after which it is very carefully withdrawn from the Roux limb and removed from the abdomen. The tissue rings are then extracted from it and inspected for completeness.

Trocar #2 is now replaced into the abdomen. A towel clamp at the skin is often necessary to keep the pneumoperitoneum from escaping through this somewhat dilated site. Next the blind, distal segment of the Roux limb that contains the enterotomy must be excised. First, the mesentery to that portion of bowel is divided with the ultrasonic shears through trocar #2. This process is facilitated by appropriate exposure from the surgeon (Figure 22–34). When the mesentery is adequately divided, the intestine is resected using the linear cutter with 2.5 mm stapler loads (Figure 22–35). When resecting the extra bowel, a margin of at least 1 cm of intestine should be

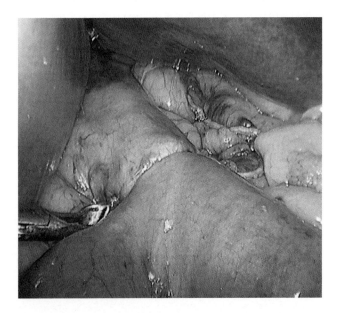

Figure 22–33. The circular stapler is prepared to fire.

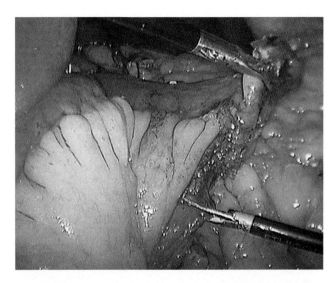

Figure 22–34. Transecting the mesentery of the redundant segment of Roux limb.

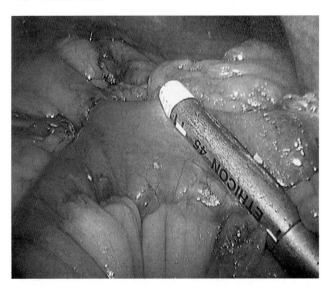

Figure 22–35. The redundant, blind end of the Roux limb is removed.

left between the end of the Roux limb and the circular anastomosis. If the Roux limb is cut closer, an ischemic bridge of tissue may result. The resected Roux segment is removed through the enlarged opening at the site of trocar #2.

Oversewing the Gastrojejunostomy

At this point the surgeon may choose to oversew the gastrojejunostomy to assure adequate hemostasis. This may be done with either continuous or interrupted sutures (Figure 22–36).

Air Insufflation Leak Check

With the anastomosis complete, the operating table is then returned to the flat position. The surgeon gently occludes the Roux limb 6–8 cm distal to the gastrojejunostomy with a Babcock and infuses saline with a suction/irrigation device until the pouch and anastomosis are submerged (Figure 22–37).

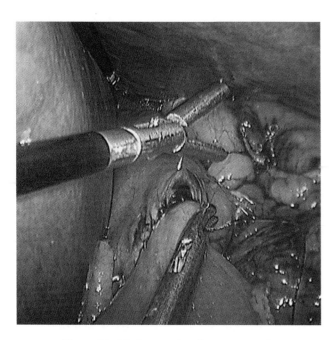

Figure 22–36. Oversewing the anastomosis.

The anesthesiologist advances the 16 F balloon tipped tube, which had been retracted into the esophagus, back to the mark made previously. The balloon is not inflated. Oxygen is then applied through the distal port of the tube at a flow rate of 1 L/min. The surgeons observe the gastric pouch and Roux limb for appropriate distention and to note if any bubbles are visible (Figure 22–38). If the leak check is negative, the catheter is put to suction briefly and then removed. Decisions regarding the appropriate action for a positive leak test must be made on a case-by-case basis. The problem must be identified and appropriate corrective action taken.

With the leak check complete, the irrigation fluid is evacuated. A 1.6 cm wide Penrose drain is placed so that it lies along the lateral staple line of the gastric pouch and the

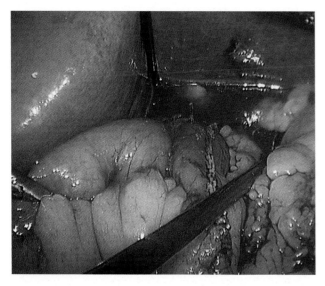

Figure 22–37. The bowel is occluded distal to the anastomosis with a Babcock in preparation for the air insufflation leak lest.

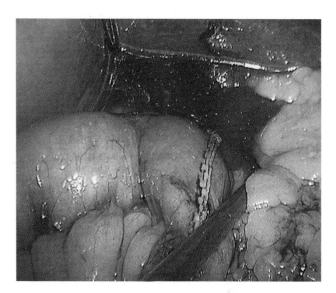

Figure 22–38. A negative leak test is confirmed when the Roux limb distends without the appearance of bubbles.

gastrojejunostomy. The drain is brought out through trocar #2 and secured to the skin with a suture. The liver retractor is carefully removed, and then the working ports are serially pulled out while the camera surveys their sites to confirm the absence of bleeding. The camera is then withdrawn and trocar #1 is removed. The skin edges at all trocar sites are reapproximated and sterile dressings are applied. A gauze dressing is placed over the Penrose site.

POSTOPERATIVE CARE

Patients ambulate with assistance on the day of surgery. With each nursing assessment, they are encouraged to perform calf flexion/extension exercises and incentive spirometry. Pain is controlled with the use of IV narcotics.

On the first postoperative day, patients undergo a water-soluble contrast study of their pouch in radiology. If this exam is negative for leakage or obstruction, the patients undergo a methylene blue dye test: 5 cc of methylene blue dye is mixed with 25 cc of ice water, which the patient is instructed to ingest. An hour after the patient drinks the blue mixture, the dressing over the Penrose drain is inspected. The finding of blue dye indicates the presence of a leak. If the dye test is negative, the patient is allowed sugar-restricted liquids. Appropriate home medications are resumed.

Patients are discharged home on the second postoperative day if they tolerate the liquid diet and no problems are identified. The first follow-up visit is at 7–10 days. At this appointment, patients are queried regarding the output of the Penrose drain. Usually, after 1 week, the output consists of scanty serosanguinous fluid that requires only one or two gauze dressing changes per day. The presence of more copious drainage, output resembling ingested liquids, bile, or saliva, or the presence of concerning symptoms will prompt a contrast study to search for a leak. If there are no such concerns, the drain is removed. The patient is seen again at 1 month. The focus of that and future visits shifts to matters of nutrition, exercise, and maximizing weight loss and well-being.

CONCLUSIONS

There are several effective techniques for performing laparoscopic Roux-en-Y gastric bypass. The transgastric, circular-stapled approach described above is offered as an efficient and reproducible method for performing this operation.

References

1. Nguyen NT, Wolfe BM: Hypopharyngeal perforation during laparoscopic Roux-en-Y gastric bypass. *Obes Surg* 10:64–67, 2000.
2. Scott DJ, Provost DA, Jones DB: Laparoscopic Roux-en-Y gastric bypass: Transoral or transgastric anvil placement? *Obes Surg* 10:361–365, 2000.
3. Higa KD, Ho T, Boone KB: Internal hernias after laparoscopic Roux-en-Y gastric bypass: Incidence, treatment and prevention. *Obes Surg* 13:350–354, 2003.
4. Champion JK, Williams M: Small bowel obstruction and internal hernias after laparoscopic Roux-en-Y gastric bypass. *Obes Surg* 13:596–600, 2003.

23

Laparoscopic Gastric Bypass: Linear Technique

Michael D. Williams, MD, FACS • J.K. Champion, MD, FACS

INTRODUCTION

The laparoscopic Roux-en-Y gastric bypass (LRYGBP) remains the procedure of choice for the treatment of morbid obesity by the majority of bariatric surgeons in the United States. The laparoscopic approach, first described by Wittgrove and Clark,[1] is one of the most significant advances in the surgical treatment of morbid obesity. Variations in construction of the gastrojejunostomy (GJ) include the hand-sewn technique[2] described by Higa as well as the circular stapler technique.[1] We prefer the linear stapler technique[3] to construct our GJ because it is less technically demanding and time saving when compared to the circular or hand-sewn techniques. The skills and technology employed have enabled us to successfully perform over 2,300 hundred cases to date. This chapter describes our linear technique of the GJ during the LRYGBP.

PREPARATION AND SETUP

Case preparation and setup is paramount to performing the procedure in a safe, consistent, and expeditious manner. Patients receive a preoperative dose of low molecular weight heparin, sequential compression device, and antibiotic prophylaxis. A footboard is attached to the operating table in anticipation of steep reverse Trendelenburg position. A supply cart with any potential extra supplies is maintained within the operating room. We use four reusable 5-mm trocars and two disposable 12-mm trocars to perform the procedure. The reusable trocars limit the overall expense of the procedure when compared to disposable trocars. The abdomen is entered using a direct entry approach with a 12-mm direct-view trocar and a zero degree 10-mm laparoscope. The remaining 5-mm trocars and 12-mm trocar are inserted under direct visualization (Figure 23–1). An Allis clamp is placed into the

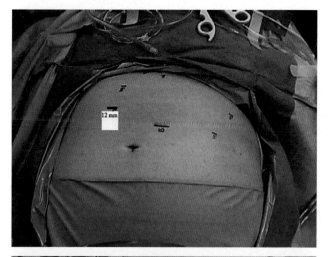

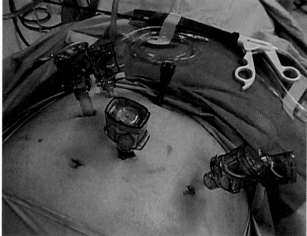

Figure 23–1. Location of trocar sites.

epigastric liver and positioned under the left lobe of the liver and attached to the diaphragm to maintain exposure of the upper stomach. The procedure is divided into three steps: pouch construction, enteroenterostomy, and the gastroenterostomy formation.

Pouch Construction

The construction of the gastric pouch is initiated by dividing the peritoneal attachments along the left crus to expose the angle of His. The angle of His serves as a target point when forming the vertical staple-line during pouch formation. An endoscopic ruler is used to measure 5 cm from the angle of His along the lesser curvature of the stomach. Blunt dissection is used to create a window into the lesser sac, 5 cm from the angle of His, adjacent to the lesser curvature to avoid injury to the vagal nerve branch. A 45-mm linear surgical stapler with a 3.5-mm staple is then positioned and fired horizontally. The lesser sac window allows for precise placement of the stapler jaws onto the stomach. A 50F blunt tip bougie is passed transorally into the upper stomach along the lesser curvature and placed against the horizontal staple-line. The stapler is

nestle repositioned in a vertical position along the bougie and fired to create a vertically oriented pouch. Several firings of the 45-mm linear cartridges may be required to create a totally isolated pouch.

A consistent pouch size is maintained by the use of the 50F bougie and an endoscopic ruler to measure a 5-cm pouch length. The vertical orientation of the gastric pouch minimizes the incorporation of parietal cells and allows creation of an anastomosis on an area of the stomach that is less distensible than the greater curvature. The staple-line is inspected for bleeding and uniform staple formation. Homoclips are placed at any bleeding areas or vulnerable sites such as staple-line crossings. The operating table is then repositioned to a horizontal position and formation of the enteroenterostomy is initiated.

Forming the Enteroenterostomy

The enteroenterotomy is considered the second step in our technique. The omentum and transverse colon is lifted in a cranial position and placed under the left lobe of the liver to maintain exposure of the ligament of Treitz. The small bowel is measured using an endoscopic ruler 40 cm distal to the ligament of Treitz and transected at this location using a linear stapler with a 60-mm cartridge with 2.5-mm staples (Endo GIA II Universal, US Surgical, Norwalk, CN). The small bowel mesentery of the divided bowel is lengthened using the LigasSure (Valleylab, Boulder, CO) device to allow the distal small bowel to reach the gastric pouch without tension. The distal small bowel is then measured, as a general guide, 60 cm if the body mass index (BMI) is 40–47 kg/m^2, 80 cm if the BMI is 48–49 kg/m^2, and 100 cm if the BMI is $\geq$50 kg/m^2. The distal small bowel is then anchored to the proximal small bowel at the measured location using two nonabsorbable anchoring sutures via an extracorporeal technique. The purpose of the anchoring sutures is twofold, it maintains bowel alignment during the stapled anastomosis and prevents kinking of the anastomosis as in the Brolin's antiobstruction stitch.[4]

The enteroenterotomy construction requires a combination of intracorporeal suturing and use of the linear stapler technique. An enterotomy is made on the proximal and distal small bowel between the two anchoring sutures. A linear 45-cm stapler with 2.5-mm staples is inserted into the enterotomies and fired to create a side-to-side anastomosis. The enterotomy is subsequently closed with a 2–0 nonabsorbable continuous suture. The mesenteric defect is then approximated with a nonabsorbable continuous suture to decrease the incidence of internal hernia at this location (Figure 23–2). The end of the Roux limb is then passed antecolic and antegastric and anchored to the end of the gastric pouch using two nonabsorbable sutures. The omentum is divided in the midline with the 10-mm LigaSure device to decrease the tension on the Roux limb due to excess weight and bulk. Occasionally, the omentum may be especially thin and splitting of the omentum may not be necessary.

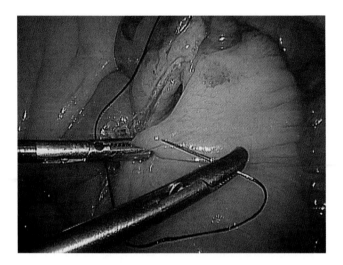

Figure 23–2. Closure of the mesenteric defect.

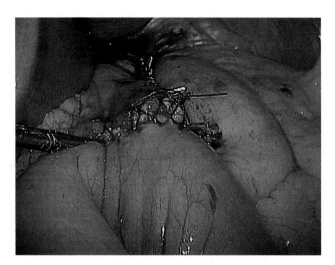

Figure 23–3. The completed gastrojejunostomy.

Patients with an extremely short mesentery will sporadically be encountered. In such cases, the antecolic passage may not be possible due to excessive tension on the GJ anastomosis. This situation requires a retrocolic passage of the Roux limb. In performing a retrocolic passage, a defect in the gastrocolic ligament wide enough to accommodate the small bowel is created. A 4-inch Penrose drain is placed in the lesser sac and directed in a caudal position. The omentum and transverse colon is then lifted cranially to expose the transverse mesocolon and the ligament of Treitz. A defect in the mesocolon is created superior and lateral to the ligament of Treitz. This maneuver allows visualization of the Penrose drain, which is anchored to the end of the Roux limb. The Roux limb is advanced into the lesser sac and subsequently retrieved via the gastrocolic defect. The suture attached to the Penrose drain is transected and the Penrose drain removed from the abdominal cavity. This retrocolic passage creates two additional defects (Peterson's defect and transverse mesocolon defect), which should be closed with a continuous nonabsorbable suture. We have demonstrated a 4.5% incidence of small bowel obstruction in our retrocolic group compared to 0.43% in our antecolic group; therefore, we prefer the antecolic approach when possible.[5]

Forming the Gastrojejunostomy

The third step of our technique is construction of the GJ. The operating table is repositioned to reverse Trendelenburg position and the antimesenteric end of the Roux limb is anchored to the end of the anterior edge of the gastric pouch with two nonabsorbable sutures. A gastrotomy is made between the anchoring sutures, as well as an enterotomy on the adjacent Roux limb. A linear 30-mm stapler with 3.5-mm staples is inserted halfway into the gastrotomy and enterotomy then fired to create an anastomosis between the gastric pouch and Roux limb. A 30F, blunt-tip bougie is passed transorally into the gastric pouch and advanced into the Roux limb. Closure of the GJ is completed by a continuous 2.0 nonabsorbable suture.

Placement of the bougie allows for precise calibration of the GJ and prevents inadvertent incorporation of the "back-wall" of mucosa during the hand sew of the anterior anastomosis. The completed anastomosis is demonstrated (Figure 23–3).

Intraoperative Leak Test

Several techniques may be used to check for a gastrointestinal leak at the GJ. A Glassman clamp is used to occlude the lumen of the alimentary limb distal to the GJ. This allows for distension of the GJ with air or fluid based on the method chosen by the operating surgeon. A nasogastric tube is then advanced to a position just proximal to the GJ and dilute methylene blue is instilled into the nasogastric tube as the anastomosis is inspected for leakage of dye. Some surgeons prefer to insert air into the nasogastric tube as the GJ is submerged with irrigation fluid. A positive leak is manifested as air bubbles at the anastomotic site. We prefer to use intraoperative endoscopy to identify any correctable technical errors at the GJ.[6] An endoscope allows intraluminal visualization of anastomosis and identifies mucosal hemorrhage. Air is instilled via the gastroscope and leak sites are identified as bubbles are produced in the irrigation fluid surrounding the anastomosis. The endoscope is advanced into the alimentary limb to ensure patency of the anastomosis. Any identified leak should be repaired prior to completion of the procedure.

Drain

We use certain criteria to place closed-suction drains adjacent to the GJ. Patients with comorbidities that affect healing such as insulin-dependent diabetes, collagen vascular disease, or steroid dependent patients receive a drain. Drains are also placed after repair of a gastrointestinal leak or in patients who require continuous positive airway pressure for sleep apnea. Some patients who receive a drain and experience a postoperative gastrointestinal leak may be treated conservatively. Conservative management however should be abandoned if the patient develops signs of sepsis or a collection is inadequately drained.

CONCLUSION

The LRYGBP is a reliable method used to treat morbid obesity. Proper surgeon training should include mastering intracorporeal and extracorporeal laparoscopic suturing and two-handed choreography. The linear technique utilizes the laparoscopic linear stapler to construct the gastric pouch and perform the anastomosis of the alimentary limb to the gastric pouch. This technique is relatively easy to reproduce by dividing the procedure into the three steps we described. The laparoscopic linear stapler obviates the concern of port site contamination during retrieval of the circular stapler from the abdominal cavity as well as saves the time required to sew the posterior wall of the GJ during the hand-sewn technique.

Bariatric surgeons, however, generally choose the technique of GJ based on their training and comfort level with the various methods.

References

1. Wittgrove AC, Clark GW, Tremblay LJ: Laparoscopic gastric bypass, Roux-enY: Preliminary report of five cases. *Obes Surg* 4:353–357, 1994.
2. Higa KD, Boone KB, Ho T, et al.: Laparoscopic Roux-en-Y gastric bypass for morbid obesity: Technique and preliminary results of our first 400 patients. *Arch Surg* 135(9):1029–1033, 2000.
3. Champion JK: Laparoscopic Roux-en-Y gastric bypass with a linear endostapler technique. *Obes Surg* 10:13, 2000.
4. Brolin RE: The antiobstruction stitch in staple Roux-en-Y enteroenterstomy. *Am J Surg* 169(3):355–357, 1995.
5. Champion JK, Williams MD: Small bowel obstruction and internal hernias after laparoscopic Roux-en-Y gastric bypass. *Obes Surg* 13(4):596–600, 2003.
6. Champion JK: Role of routine intraoperative endoscopy in laparoscopic bariatric surgery. *Surg Endosc* 16(12):1663–1665, 2002.

24

Laparoscopic Roux-en-Y Banded Gastric Bypass

Thomas Szegö, MD, PhD • Carlos José–Lazzarini Mendes, MD

INTRODUCTION

The advent of videolaparoscopy at the end of the 1980s revolutionized digestive tract surgery. Skepticism of the surgical community was overcome by proof of the real advantages provided by this new abdominal access. Less surgical trauma, shorter length of stay, shorter sick leave from work, less pain, and better esthetic result convinced surgeons they had to learn about and train in the new technique.

Bariatric surgery was not different, particularly gastric bypass, in which surgeons have improved to better master gastric videolaparoscopy, since Wittgrove et al.[1] (see Chapter 14) described the applicability of laparoscopy to perform this complex procedure. However, laparoscopic approach should not substantially change the principles that guide the technique to be employed. The technique already proven by laparotomy must be reproduced through a minimally invasive procedure.

On the basis of these assumptions, we initiated our experience with bariatric surgery reproducing the technique extensively used by the San Diego Group, coordinated by Dr. Allan Wittgrove and Wesley Clark.[1] It consists of no banding,

performing gastrojejunal anastomosis with a no. 21 circular stapler; the anvil is introduced through the mouth and the stapler through the abdomen, not closing the defects (mesentery, mesocolon, and "Petersen") created by the surgery. Since it is difficult to introduce the anvil through the mouth and there is an additional cost of the stapler, we decided to perform a totally manual two-layer gastrojejunal anastomosis. Because of the high incidence of bowel loop sliding to the supramesocolic area, we carefully close the intracavitary spaces to avoid formation of internal hernias.[2] The manual anastomosis is a cheaper procedure; however, it takes longer and is not completely reproducible.

On the basis of the experience of Ken Champion (Atlanta, GA), we started performing gastrojejunal anastomosis with a linear stapler[3,4] and transposing the jejunum by an antecolic and antegastric approach. The purpose was to reduce the incidence of internal hernias, which are more frequent in laparoscopic surgeries than in laparotomies.[2,3,5]

After the initial experience with this technique, we observed that patients submitted to laparoscopy with no banding, as compared with the historic group with banding, had a smaller and inconsistent weight loss.[6] On the basis of this finding we decided to perform the following routine: Laparoscopic Roux-en-Y banded gastric bypass.[7–10]

TECHNIQUE DESCRIPTION

The surgery is performed with the patient in supine position, under general anesthesia, and the surgical team is displaced as follows: The surgeon and the camera are on the right and the assistant surgeon and the scrubbing nurse are on the left.

One 10-mm portal is used for the camera and one 12-mm portal is used for the staplers. Four 5-mm portals are used for the other forceps. A 15-mm Hg pneumoperitoneum is used to initiate the operation.

The first step consists of releasing the angle of His and sectioning the gastrophrenic ligament. This maneuver makes gastric section easier. Then, the smaller gastric curvature is dissected at approximately 2-cm cranially to the incisura angularis. The dissection is performed close to the gastric wall, between the vascular and nervous bundle of the smaller omentum and the gastric wall.

The vertical section is done under the guide of a 12-mm diameter probe introduced by the anesthesiologist. Close to the probe, the stomach is sectioned with a linear stapler with six staple lines, checking if the stomach has been completely divided and determining an excluded gastric chamber and another small chamber continuing with the esophagus, with no communication between them.

A 3-0 PDS continuous seromuscular suture is made invaginating the staple-line of the excluded stomach. This suture is intended to increase safety of the procedure, thus reducing the risk of leakage and postoperative adherences. A 6.5-cm long silicon band with a 2-0 Ethibond suture inside is used. The band is passed with a Mixter forceps. This maneuver requires special care since there is a risk of perforating the stomach when passing the forceps behind it. The band wire is tied up and we make a reinforcement suture in the gastric pouch, starting from the angle of His and trying to invaginate the corner of the mechanical suture, up to roughly 2 cm above the band. The needle remains in the cavity and will be used to fix the jejunum to the gastric stump.

Now we move to inframesocolic phase. The first jejunal loop is identified (angle of Treitz) and we measure 100 cm of jejunum. By antecolic and antegastric approach, we transpose the loop close to the gastric pouch. In about 10% of patients it is necessary to extensively open the greater omentum to enable approximating the loop with no tension.

The needle previously left to fix the loop is used and a continuous seromuscular suture is made between the jejunum and gastric stump. The aim of this suture is to cover the staple-line with jejunum and to efficiently fix the band to the left with the pouch; on the right, the fixation is made with the gastrohepatic ligament. The jejunal loop is cut very close to the stomach and approximately 1 cm of the mesentery is released. Then, 100-cm of jejunum is measured in order to make the alimentary loop.

The jejunojejunal anastomosis is made with a 45-mm linear stapler in anisoperistaltic position. The jejunal orifice is closed with a 3-0 PDS continuous two-layer suture. The laterolateral gastrojejunal anastomosis is performed with a 45-mm linear stapler and the orifice is closed with a PDS continuous two-layer suture, similar to the jejunojejunal anastomosis.

In order to test the anastomosis, the anesthesiologist introduces the probe through it and infuses a methylene blue solution in the loop clamped with a forceps. If the anastomosis is patent and there is no leakage, the mesenteric defect is closed with an Ethibond continuous suture.

The first 700 patients of our series used laminar or tubulolaminar drains. Assessing the efficacy of this procedure, we concluded that routine drainage is not necessary and should be reserved for specific indications. In the next 400, we used selective drainage (less then 1%) and we had no complications due to the drain or the lack of it. The cutaneous incisions are intradermally closed with a fast absorption suture (4-0 rapid Vycril). Patients are re-fed the next day and discharged from hospital on the second postoperative day.

COMMENTS

The advances in operative technique have allowed tactic changes, thus improving short- and long-term results. As of 1998, after operating over 1,100 patients by laparoscopic Roux-en-Y banded gastric bypass, we could reduce the operative time from an average of 6 hours (first experiences) to 70 minutes. Silicon banding showed better results in weight loss and lower incidence of short-term failure in up to 18 months of follow-up. The evaluation of patients followed up for over 5 years is ongoing; hence, there are no conclusive results.

The transposition of the antecolic, antegastric jejunal loop has so far eliminated internal hernias. However, it has not avoided intestinal obstruction due to adherences or kinking of the jejunojejunal anastomosis. We observed three cases of intestinal obstruction, in which 2 (0.6%) were due to kinking and 1 (0.4%) was due to adherence in the last 300 patients submitted to the antecolic technique. We found four fistulas in the free peritoneum in the first 200 patients (2%) but the next 900 patients had no fistula; in the whole series, the incidence of fistulas was 0.4%. Only one of these patients died (0.1%).

Pulmonary embolism prophylaxis was made with anticoagulant agents, pneumatic compression stockings, and early ambulation. There were 2 (0.2%) nonfatal cases of pulmonary embolism. We did not close the fascia in the orifices. Five (0.5%) patients had hernia in some incision and one of them presented hernia in two incisions. The total was 6 hernias in 5 patients.

The surgical treatment of morbid obesity has been under reevaluation of managements and techniques. The best, or perfect, technique has not been developed yet. Any new alteration should be carefully studied, analyzed, and tested according to the most strict clinical research standards. Each group should use the technique(s) that better fits their needs and possibilities, provided they perform a usual and already proven technique. The careful selection of patients, techniques, and management will lead to better results.

References

1. Wittgrove AC, Clark W, Tremblay LJ: Laparoscopic gastric bypass, Roux-en-Y: Preliminary report of five cases. *Obes Surg* 4:353–357, 1994.

2. Higa KO, Ho T, Boone KB: Internal hernias after laparoscopic Roux-en-Y gastric bypass: Incidence, treatment and prevention. *Obes Surg* 13:350–354, 2003.

3. Champion JK, Williams M: Small bowel obstruction and internal hernias after laparoscopic Roux-en-Y gastric bypasss. *Obes Surg* 13:596–600, 2003.

4. Shope TR, Cooney RN, McLeod J, Miller CA, Haluck RS: Early results after laparoscopic gastric bypass: EEA *vs.* GIA stapled gastrojejunal anastomosis. *Obes Surg* 13:355–359, 2003.

5. Szego T, Mendes CJL, Bitran A: Derivação gastrojejunal por laparoscopia com e sem anel.– In: Garrido. AB Jr (ed.): *Cirurgia da Obesidade.* St. Paulo, Editora Atheneu, 2002.

6. Schauer P: Gastric bypass for severe obesity: Approaches and outcomes. *Surg Obes Relat Dis* 1:297–300, 2005.

7. Capella JF, Capella RF: The weight reduction operation of choice: Vertical banded gastroplasty or gastric bypass. *Am J Surg* 171:74–79, 1996.

8. Capella RF, Capella JF: Open transected banded gastric bypass with jejunal interposition without gastrostomy Capella Pouch Operation. In: Szego T (ed.): *Video Atlas of Obesity Surgery.* St. Paulo, Editora Atheneu, 2002.

9. Fobi MAL, Lee H, Holness R, Cabinda D: Gastric bypasss operation for obesity. *World J Surg* 22:925–935, 1998.

10. Fobi MAL, Lee H, Igwe D, Felahy B, Stanczyk M, Fobi N: Open transected banded gastric bypass with jejunal interposition and gastrostomy Fobi Pouch Operation (FPO). In: Szego T (ed.): *Video Atlas of Obesity Surgery.* St. Paulo, Editora Atheneu, 2002.

25

Laparoscopic Gastric Bypass: Hand Sewn

Kelvin D. Higa, MD, FACS • Jennifer Elizabeth Higa

INTRODUCTION

Wittgrove, Clark, and Tremblay performed the first laparoscopic gastric bypass in 1993.[1] Since then, there has been a dramatic increase in the number of bariatric procedures worldwide.[2] Although improved outcomes and the dissemination of knowledge through the Internet have increased the awareness of the public of the benefits of bariatric surgery, the minimally invasive approach is primarily responsible for the increased demand.[3] The laparoscopic/endoscopic anvil placement for creation of a circular-stapled gastrojejunal anastomosis remains one of the most ingenious applications of available technology to date. However, with initial anastomotic leakage rates of up to 5%,[4] similar to leakage rates reported by colorectal surgeons[5] using the circular stapler, we concluded that failure was probably related more to the limitations of the endomechanical device rather than surgical technique.

We had no anastomotic leaks in our open gastric bypass experience (<500 patients), similar to others using manual suturing techniques.[6] Therefore, it seemed logical to use manual suturing for the gastrojejunal anastomosis in our laparoscopic operation.[7] Michele Gagner was the first to describe the hand-sewn gastrojejunal anastomosis, but abandoned it for the transoral circular stapler technique.

Novice surgeons often evaluate new procedures based on the speed at which they can learn and master the technique as well as the total operative time. Safety and long-term outcomes are often secondary to the objective of completing the task at hand. Seasoned bariatric surgeons understand the importance of consistent anatomic construct for weight optimization, weight maintenance, and avoidance of secondary complications.[8,9] Early laparoscopic solutions for the gastric bypass adopted methods of gastric pouch formation based more on a horizontal orientation[4,10,11] rather than a true lesser curve based pouch, vertical in orientation that we advocate.[9] Fortunately, it now appears that weight loss, weight maintenance, and complications are similar among the various pouch configurations and are probably related more to overall volume rather than orientation.

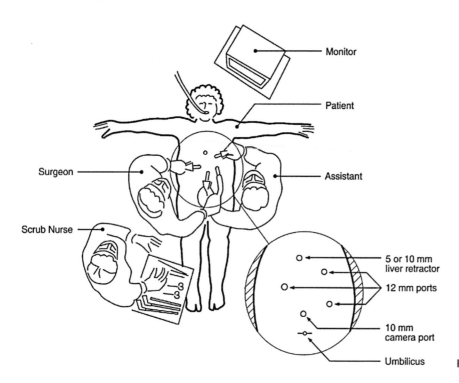

Monitor

Patient

Surgeon

Assistant

Scrub Nurse

5 or 10 mm liver retractor

12 mm ports

10 mm camera port

Umbilicus

Figure 25–1. Position and port placement.

We performed our first laparoscopic gastric bypass in 1998, and our team has performed over 5000 procedures as of 2006. The basic orientation and approach has remained the same with few modifications based on experience and outcomes. For example, we now use continuous nonabsorbable sutures to close all mesenteric defects to decrease the incidence of postoperative internal hernias.[12] Our laparoscopic approach to the gastric bypass is very familiar to that of the veterans of bariatric surgery. We have tried to incorporate the principles learned over decades of research and anecdotal experience and have tried not to violate those principles just to perform it laparoscopically. Our approach is serviceable, reproducible, and revisable, although perhaps the most technically demanding of procedures. However, it is useful as a platform for more advanced bariatric procedures, including revision operations.

PREPARATION FOR SURGERY AND POSITIONING

A multidisciplinary team consisting of a surgeon, psychologist, nutritionist, anesthesiologist, and medical bariatrician evaluates each patient. In addition, a cardiac evaluation and directed weight management is advised on an individual basis. Weight loss prior to surgery has not only been shown to decrease the size of the liver and volume of intra-abdominal fat,[13] but patient education may also improve overall performance.[14]

Bowel preparation is unnecessary. A liquid diet 24 hours prior to surgery will prevent the possibility of retained food in the stomach from obstructing the jejunojejunal anastomosis immediately after surgery—a potential cause of acute gastric distension.[15]

Bariatric patients are a moderate risk for perioperative venous thromboembolism.[16] Prophylaxis in the form of mechanical (sequential compression boots and early ambulation) and pharmacological (subcutaneous fractionated or unfractionated heparin) is advised. Traditional parenteral antibiotic prophylaxis is standard. Catheterization of the bladder allows the anesthesiologist to be liberal with intraoperative fluids—an important consideration in postoperative nausea management.[17]

Positioning of the patient in the operating room must include attention to the prevention of pressure sores and neuropathy (Figure 25–1). Dedicated operative tables must be weight rated appropriately with lateral extensions to accommodate the larger patients. Protocols for patient transfer and other safety issues should be included as part of a hospitalwide awareness program. The patient is supine and maintained in a gentle reverse Trendelenburg position that helps with mechanical ventilation and allows for a more natural angle of attack of the laparoscopic instruments. Dramatic changes in orientation or the split leg scenario are unnecessary and time consuming to set up.

SURGICAL PROCEDURE

The original model for this operation was the laparoscopic Nissen fundoplication. This port arrangement allows for excellent exposure of the proximal stomach and surprisingly good exposure of the ligament of Treitz. Extremes of size can be challenging: adequate space to allow the formation of the Roux limb in smaller patients can be as problematic as the inadequate length of instrumentation and difficulties associated with visualization of the proximal stomach in the larger patients (Figure 25–2). However, this five-port arrangement

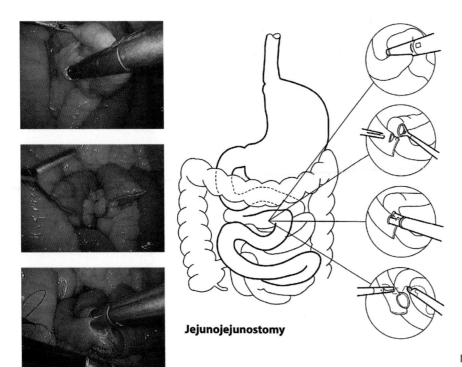

Jejunojejunostomy

Figure 25–2. Formation of the Roux limb and jejunojejunostomy.

is applicable to almost every patient and body type. This arrangement also allows for concomitant cholecystectomy if indicated.

The epigastric port is used for liver retraction. This is unnecessary in some patients, but most will require either lifting the liver anteriorly or displacing it to the patient's right in larger individuals. The left upper quadrant port is used for retraction and vertical pouch stapling, while the right upper quadrant port and left lower port are used for suturing both the jejunojejunostomy as well as the gastrojejunostomy. The left lower port is also the site of introduction of the linear stapler for the formation of the Roux limb.

Initial entry is performed without insufflation utilizing a nonbladed optical trocar system. The camera is placed midline, 8–12 cm from the xyphoid, while other ports are placed to allow creation of the Roux limb, formation of the gastric pouch, and performance of the gastrojejunal anastomosis (Figure 25–3). Attention to the angle of entry of the port can reduce the resistance of the abdominal wall to the instrumentation allowing for a more precise and less fatiguing operation. The ports can be "redirected" by creation of a new fascial pathway preserving the original skin entry site. These specific ports do require fascial closure, which greatly improves operative efficiency and also reduces a potential source of postoperative pain.

The omentum is displaced cephalad to expose the ligament of Treitz. In patients whose omentum is adherent to pelvic structures or involved in an incarcerated ventral hernia, we prefer to incise the gastrocolic omentum and open the transverse mesocolon from above, thus exposing the ligament of Treitz directly. Ventral hernias are repaired at a later date when optimal weight loss and nutrition insure a greater degree of primary success and the use of prosthetic mesh is not

compromised by contamination of enteric contents. However, if a hernia is reduced, then it must be repaired at this time.[18]

The proximal jejunum is transected with a 2.5-mm linear stapler, and the mesentery is divided with another firing of the instrument or with the harmonic scalpel. The Roux limb is measured and a side-to-side linear anastomosis is performed. Typically, the length of the Roux limb can be up to 150 cm without an associated increased incidence of malabsorptive complications.[19] However, there is no convincing evidence that extending Roux limb lengths in this range is of any benefit, especially in patients with BMI < 50 kg/m^2.[20] The enterotomy is closed with a single layer of absorbable suture. The mesenteric defect must be closed with a continuous, nonabsorbable suture to limit the possibility of internal herniation. This modification has effectively reduced our internal hernia rate from 4–5% to less than 0.5%.

The Roux limb is passed through a retrocolic tunnel and fixed to the transverse mesocolon with nonabsorbable sutures, which also includes closing the Petersen's space. Alternatively, some surgeons prefer an antecolic route for the Roux limb claiming a lower incidence of postoperative bowel obstructions.[21]

There are times when the mesocolon is uncomfortably short and will not allow for the safe passage of a retrocolic Roux limb. In these rare instances, the decision to route the Roux limb antecolic should be made prior to the transection of the jejunum. This site must be more distal from the ligament of Treitz, typically 50–100 cm, to limit the tension on the gastrojejunal anastomosis. By lengthening the biliopancreatic limb, iron and calcium absorption may be less efficient and the incidence of these deficiencies may be theoretically

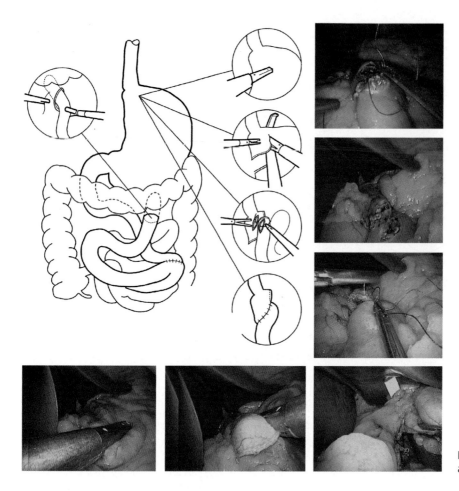

Figure 25–3. Formation of gastric pouch and gastrojejunostomy.

increased or more difficult to manage with oral supplementation alone. Also, it is more difficult for the endoscopist to access the common bile duct or the gastric remnant.

Controversy exists as to whether the large resultant Petersen's space associated with an antecolic Roux limb requires closure. Clearly, these patients are still at risk for intestinal volvulous.[22,23] Therefore, our philosophy as well as others[24] is to eliminate the risk of postoperative bowel obstruction rather than simply settling for a reduction in the incidence. Therefore, we strongly advocate closing all mesenteric defects. However, the long-term stability of suture closure of these defects is as yet to be determined.

The liver retractor is now placed to allow dissection of the proximal stomach. Occasionally, a very large liver will not allow for sufficient visualization—an indication for open conversion. However, displacement of the liver to the right, rather than anterior, will allow sufficient exposure in the largest of patients. Alternatively, the surgeon may decide to abort the procedure, evaluate the cause of hepatic enlargement (usually steatosis), and institute therapy (medical weight reduction) in anticipation of performing the procedure at a later time under more ideal circumstances. Alternatively, a sleeve gastrectomy may be an option if the patient has been properly counseled and consented.[25] In this way, surgical restraint and proper judgment may reduce the morbidity associated with these operations.

Perigastric dissection along the lesser curve of the stomach is performed 3–5 cm distal to the gastroesophageal junction and continues until the retrogastric space is reached. At times, dense adhesions to the pancreas are encountered. Visualization is enhanced by opening a gastrocolic window and approaching this area from behind the stomach. Care is taken to avoid thermal injury to the adjacent viscera and vagus nerves.

A six row—3.5 mm—linear cutter stapler is used to form the lesser curve based, proximal gastric pouch. Four row staplers have been unreliable, in our experience. It is essential to exclude the distensible gastric fundus in order to obtain optimal long-term weight management. This requires meticulous dissection behind the stomach at the level of the angle of His and also helps to prevent injury to the esophagus or spleen. The gastric pouch is estimated to be 10–15 mL in volume.

The inferior aspect of the pouch is determined with the first horizontal stapler brought in via the right upper quadrant port. All subsequent firings are vertically oriented through the left upper quadrant port. High, subcostal placement of this port will allow the standard length stapling instrument to reach the angle of His in every instance. It is preferable to divide the fat pad at the hiatus to better visualize the gastroesophageal junction prior to stapling. Occasionally, a 4.5-mm stapler is required for exceptionally thick tissue. Care must be taken in order to avoid stapling across the inferior aspect of the esophagus in an attempt to eliminate all of the distensible gastric fundus. This is an area of potential leak as the esophagus does not hold staples well and is a particularly difficult area to repair or manage nonoperatively.

The 34F orogastric tube is advanced into the stomach after the first horizontal stapling, and it assists in the estimation of pouch size. It is imperative to completely separate the gastric pouch from the gastric remnant. An esophageal retractor or "gold-finger" type instrument can greatly assist in this maneuver.

The retrocolic Roux limb is brought anterior to the gastric remnant to lie in close approximation to the newly formed gastric pouch. Although some surgeons prefer a retrogastric route, subsequent access and visualization of the anastomosis is more difficult if revision surgery is necessary. A two-layer, hand-sewn anastomosis completes intestinal continuity.

The formation of the gastrojejunostomy begins with a running posterior, exterior layer of 3-0 polyglactin (Vicryl) sutures. Beginning distally and sewing proximally, the antimesenteric side of the Roux limb is approximated to the inferior staple line of the gastric pouch—incorporating the staples in the suture line. Enterotomies are performed on the gastric pouch and Roux limb adjacent to the suture line. A second posterior, full thickness, running suture line is performed and continued anterior beyond the termination of the first posterior suture.

Two anterior suture lines are run from the distal anterior aspect of the enterotomy, the first being full thickness and the second seromuscular. Prior to completion of the anastomosis, the 34F tube is carefully inserted across the anastomosis to help calibrate the opening as well as providing assurance of a patent anastomosis. The anterior sutures are tied with their respective posterior counterparts.

The anastomosis and proximal staple lines can be tested with blue dye, air insufflation via the orogastric tube, or with operative endoscopy. However, we do not employ routine testing or drainage of the anastomosis unless dictated by clinical suspicion.

The port sites are inspected for bleeding upon withdrawal of the trocars, and the skin is closed with simple absorbable monofilament sutures.

POSTOPERATIVE MANAGEMENT

Perioperative antibiotic is continued for 24 hours, while thromboembolism prophylaxis continues until the patient is discharged. Analgesia is in the form of patient-controlled narcotic delivery systems and intravenous ketoralac. Oral narcotics are offered when clear liquids are tolerated. Metoclopramide is administered routinely, and a variety of antiemetic pharmacological agents are available for the nurses to use at their discretion.

Routine postoperative contrast studies add little to the management of these patients and serve only to delay

discharge secondary to nausea.[26] A normal postoperative upper gastrointestinal study should not preclude the surgeon from intervening based on clinical suspicion of a leak.[27]

The patients are started on clear liquids the day of surgery and are required to ambulate with assistance. Preoperative oral medications can be resumed as soon as the patient can tolerate clear liquids. Most patients are discharged by the second postoperative day.

Patients are continued on a clear liquid diet for 1 week and slowly advanced to solids over a 3–4-week period. Patients are instructed to take either an H2 blocker or proton pump inhibitor for 30 days. Routine follow-up visits are at 1 week, 3 weeks, and quarterly for the first year, then on a yearly basis. Ongoing nutritional, emotional, and exercise counseling as well as support groups are provided. Complete nutritional assessment occurs on a yearly basis or when symptoms or clinical suspicion dictates.

RESULTS

Wittgrove's 8-year data[28] suggests long-term weight loss equivalent to or better than 5-year data for open gastric bypass reported by MacLean et al.[29] and 14-year data reported by Pories.[30] Our data suggests the same. More importantly, reduction in medical morbidities is quite remarkable, underscoring the impact and importance of surgical weight reduction in health care maintenance.

Early complication rates and operative times suffer from a very steep learning curve. This is not only dependent on the initial experience of the surgeon but also on his or her ability to organize a systematic method of approaching this complex operation. Efficiency as a result of preparedness of the operative team is critical. Our data suggests that more than 100 procedures, as primary surgeon, may be necessary for this process and correlates with the experience of others.[31]

Short-term percent excessive weight loss, reduction in medical comorbidities, and improvement in quality of life have been well documented for the open as well as the laparoscopic gastric bypass. However, and just as importantly, definitive 5–10-year data is lacking for but a few selective series. Interestingly, short-term data appears to be superior to "open" standard gastric bypass series suggesting a subtle difference in the anatomical construct of the laparoscopic procedures.

COMMENTS

The laparoscopic gastric bypass is one of the most challenging surgical procedures performed today. The distortion and obscuration of anatomy by intra-abdominal fat in combination with limitations of instrumentation has led to many ingenious solutions in an attempt to emulate proven, standard techniques. Although current endomechanical staplers have proven to be reliable, initial designs were less forgiving in this application. Despite reliable anastomotic stapling techniques, experts agree that advanced laparoscopic suturing skills are still required in order to perform this operation safely.

Current procedural refinements have allowed for operative efficiencies surpassing the open gastric bypass. The patient benefits of minimally invasive surgery in terms of wound morbidity, cardiovascular compromise, and immune function have been demonstrated.[32–35] However, the learning curve is a long and tedious endeavor. In addition, the bariatric patient presents more than just a technical challenge. Ultimately, the treatment of obesity requires a multidisciplinary team dedicated to life-long management of this serious disease process. Morbid obesity, unlike its associated comorbidities, cannot be cured—only controlled. Surgeons unable to appreciate the management of obesity beyond just the surgical procedure should not venture into this specialty. However, there is no more powerful therapy for the treatment and prevention of disease than weight reduction. There is no more effective a method of initial weight reduction and long-term weight control than bariatric surgery. The laparoscopic Roux-en-Y gastric bypass with hand-sewn gastrojejunostomy has proven itself in this regard.

References

1. Wittgrove AC, Clark GW, Tremblay LJ: Laparoscopic gastric bypass, Roux-en-Y: preliminary report of five cases. *Obes Surg* 4:353–357, 1994.
2. Buchwald H, Williams S: Bariatric Surgery Worldwide 2003. *Obes Surg* 14:1157–1164, 2004.
3. Nguyen NT, Root J, Zainabadi K, et al.: Accelerated growth of bariatric surgery with the introduction of minimally invasive surgery. *Arch Surg* 140(12):1198–202, 2005.
4. Wittgrove AC, Clark GW, Schubert KR: Laparoscopic gastric bypass, Roux-en-Y: technique and results in 75 patients with 3–30 month follow-up. *Obes Surg* 6:500–504, 1996.
5. Vignali A, Fazio VW, Lavery IC, et al.: Factors associated with the occurrence of leaks in stapled rectal anastomoses: a review of 1,014 patients. *J Am Coll Surg* 185(2):185–186, 1997 Aug.
6. Jones KB Jr, Afram JD, Benotti PN, et al.: Open versus Laparoscopic Roux-en-Y Gastric Bypass: A Comparative Study of Over 25,000 Open Cases and the Major Laparoscopic Bariatric Reported Series. *Obes Surg* 16: 721–727, 2006.
7. Higa KD, Boone KB, Ho T, Davies OG: Laparoscopic Roux-en-Y gastric bypass for morbid obesity: technique and preliminary results of our first 400 patients. *Arch Surg* 135(9):1029–1033, 2000.
8. Mason EE, Maher JW, Scott DH, et al.: Ten years of vertical banded gastroplasty for severe obesity. Problems in general surgery series. In: Mason EE, Nyhus LM (eds): *Surgical Treatment of Morbid Obesity*. Vol. 9. Philadelphia, PA, JB Lippincott, 1992; p. 280–289.
9. MacLean LD, Rhode BM, Forse RA: Surgery for obesity: an update of a randomized trial. *Obes Surg.* 5:145–150, 1995.
10. Wittgrove AC, Clark GW, Schubert KR: Laparoscopic gastric bypass, Roux-en-Y: technique and results in 75 patients with 3–30 month follow-up. *Obes Surg.* 6:500–504, 1996.
11. de la Torre RA, Scott JS: Laparoscopic Roux-en-Y gastric bypass: a totally intra-abdominal approach: technique and preliminary report. *Obes Surg.* 9:492–498, 1999.
12. Schauer PR, Ikramuddin S, Hamad G, et al.: Laparoscopic gastric bypass surgery: current technique. *J Laparoendosc Adv Surg Tech A.* 13(4):229–239, 2003.
13. MacLean LD, Rhode BM, Forse RA: Surgery for obesity: an update of a randomized trial. *Obes Surg.* 5:145–150, 1995.
14. Higa KD, Ho T, Boone KB: Internal hernias after laparoscopic Roux-en-Y gastric bypass: incidence, treatment and prevention. *Obes Surg* 13(3):350–354, 2003.
15. Lewis MC, Phillips ML, Slavotinek JP, Kow L, Thompson CH, Toouli J: Change in liver size and fat content after treatment with optifast? very low calorie diet. *Obes Surg.* 16(6):697–701, 2006.
16. Giusti V, De Lucia A, Di Vetta V, et al.: Impact of preoperative teaching on surgical option of patients qualifying for bariatric surgery. *Obes Surg.* 14(9):1241–1246, 2004
17. Higa KD, Boone KB, Ho T: Complications of the laparoscopic Roux-en-Y gastric bypass: 1040 patients – what have we learned? *Obes Surg* 10: 509–513, 2000.
18. Westling, A, Bergvist D, Bostrom A, et al.: Incidence of deep venous thrombosis in patients undergoing obesity surgery. *World J Surg.* 26:470–473, 2000.
19. Ali SZ, Taguchi A, Holtmann B, Kurz A: Effect of supplemental preoperative fluid on postoperative nausea and vomiting. *Anaesthesia* 58(8):780–784, 2003.
20. Eid GM, Mattar SG, Hamad G et al.: Repair of ventral hernias in morbidly obese patients undergoing laparoscopic gastric bypass should not be deferred. *Surg Endosc.* 18(2):207–210, 2004.
21. Brolin RE, Kenler HA, Gorman JH, Cody RP: Long-limb gastric bypass in the super obese: a prospective randomized trial. *Ann Surg.* 215:387–395, 1991.
22. Inabnet WB, Quinn T, Gagner M, Urban M, Pomp A: Laparoscopic Roux-en-Y gastric bypass in patients with BMI <50: a prospective randomized trial comparing short and long limb lengths. *Obes Surg.* 15(1):51–7, 2005.
23. Champion JK: Small bowel obstruction after laparoscopic Roux-en-Y gastric bypass. *Obes Surg.* 12:197–198, 2002 (Abstract 17).
24. Khanna A, Newman B, Reyes J, Fung JJ, Todo S, Starzl TL: Internal hernia and volvulus of the small bowel following liver transplantation. *Transpl Int* 10(2): 133–136, 1997.
25. MacLean LD, Rhode BM, Nohr CW: Late outcome of isolated gastric bypass. *Ann Surg.* 231:524–528, 2000.
26. Coleman MH, Awad ZT, Pomp A, Gagner M: Laparoscopic closure of the petersen mesenteric defect. *Obes Surg* 16(6):770–772, 2006.
27. Cottam D, Qureshi FG, Mattar SG, et al.: Laparoscopic sleeve gastrectomy as an initial weight-loss procedure for high-risk patients with morbid obesity. *Surg Endosc.* 20(6):859–863, 2006.
28. Singh R, Fisher B: Sensitivity and specificity of postoperative upper gi series following gastric bypass. *Obes Surg.* 13:73–75, 2003.
29. Sims TL, Mullican MA, Hamilton EC, et al.: Routine upper gastrointestinal gastrografin swallow after laparoscopic Roux-en-Y gastric bypass. *Obes Surg.* 13:66–72, 2003.
30. Wittgrove AC, Endres JE, Davis M et al.: Perioperative complications in a single surgeon's experience with 1000 consecutive laparoscopic Roux-en-Y gastric bypass operations for morbid obesity. *Obes Surg* 12:457–458, 2002 (Abstract L4).
31. MacLean LD, Rhode BM, Forse RA: Results of the surgical treatment of obesity. *Am J Surg* 165: 155–162, 1993.
32. Poires WJ, Swanson MS, MacDonald KG: Who would have thought it? An operation proves to be the most effective therapy for adult-onset diabetes mellitus. *Ann Surg* 222: 339–352, 1995.
33. Schauer PR, Ikramuddin S, Hammad G, et al.: The learning curve for laparoscopic Roux-en-Y gastric bypass in 100 cases. *Surg Endosc.* 17:212–215, 2003.
34. Schauer PR: Physiologic consequences of laparoscopic surgery. In: Eubanks WS, Soper NJ, Swanstrom LL (eds.) *Mastery of Endoscopic Surgery and Laparoscopic Surgery*. Philadelphia, PA, Lippincott Williams and Wilkins, 2000; p. 22–38.
35. Nguyen NT, Lee SL, Goldman C, et al.: Comparison of pulmonary function and postoperative pain after laparoscopic vs open gastric bypass: a randomized trial. *J Am Coll Surg.* 192:469–476, 2001.

26

Laparoscopic Gastric Bypass: Evolution, Safety, and Efficacy of the Banded Gastric Bypass

Robert T. Marema, MD, FACS • RoseMarie Toussaint, MD, FACS •
Michael Perez, MD, FACS • Cynthia K. Buffington, PhD

INTRODUCTION

The banded gastric bypass (BGBP), also known as a *silastic ringed gastric bypass*, is a combination of a Roux-en-Y GBP and a vertical banded or ringed gastroplasty. The procedure involves inclusion of a ring or band proximal to the gastro-jejunostomy to simulate the pylorus and assist in restriction of stoma enlargement. The long-term weight loss success of patients who have had the banded or silastic ringed GBP suggests that the procedure may be more effective in weight-loss maintenance than the GBP alone. However, there are currently no long-term, randomized comparative studies of the benefits or complications of the banded versus nonbanded GBP procedures.

This chapter discusses (1) the evolution of the BGBP to its more common form, the laparoscopic banded or ringed transected GBP, (2) our technique and that of others in inclusion of the restrictive band or ring to the GBP, (3) complications associated with BGBP and the treatment or prevention, thereof, and (4) data available pertaining to the procedure's effectiveness in the short- and long-term maintenance of weight loss.

EVOLUTION OF THE BANDED GASTRIC BYPASS

Prosthetic devices have been used in bariatric operations to control the outlet of the gastric pouch for maintenance of weight loss for more than a quarter of a century. Mason,[1] for instance, improved the efficacy of gastroplasty through the use of a band that restricted the outflow of food from the pouch and increased feelings of satiety. The procedure was known as the vertical banded gastroplasty (VBG) and was found in a short-term study[1] (1 year) to be as effective in inducing weight loss as the GBP. Based upon these early observations, a number of surgeons abandoned the GBP for the less invasive VBG procedure. Longer-term comparative studies[2-4] (2 and 3 years postoperatively) of the two procedures showed that the VBG, over time, produced significantly less weight loss than did the GBP and the rate of recidivism of the VBG was considerably higher. Many bariatric practices, thereafter, abandoned the VBG and converted any failed VBG surgeries to GBP.

The BGBP evolved out of such conversions. In the process of converting the VBG to a GBP, the removal of the mesh band proved technically difficult. In most instances, the original band had to be left intact, requiring that the gastroenterostomy anastomosis be constructed distal to the band. The initial BGBP was, therefore, a VBG containing a malabsorptive component.[5]

Fobi was among the first to recognize that BGBP produces superior weight loss to that of the nonbanded GBP procedure.[5,6] At the 1988 meetings of the American Society for Bariatric Surgery, Fobi presented data showing that VBG–GBP conversion patients not only have superior weight loss to primary nonbanded GBP patients but also demonstrate significantly greater long-term (5 years or more) weight-loss maintenance. Other investigators[7] confirmed these findings and found that excess weight loss with the VBG–GBP is comparable to that of more malabsorptive procedures, such as the biliopancreatic diversion.[8] These observations gave birth to the BGBP as a primary procedure.[5,9-11]

The initial BGBP described by Fobi and associates[5] consisted of a silastic ring placed no more than 2 cm proximal to the gastrojejunostomy of a stapled GBP procedure. The ring circumference of the procedure was 5.0 cm but was later enlarged for improved food tolerance. In a series of revisions designed to reduce the incidence of staple-line dehiscence and fistula formation, Fobi et al.[12-15] converted their BGBP procedure from a silastic ring stapled GBP to a silastic ring transected GBP and finally to a transected bypass with the efferent limb of jejunum interposed between the bypassed stomach and pouch, a procedure presently known as the "Fobi Pouch."

In ongoing studies, Fobi et al.[10,12-19] demonstrated the safety and long-term effectiveness of the silastic ring BGBP. The data show that the procedure is safe and highly effective in inducing weight loss, not only for the routine morbidly obese population but also for patients with super morbid obesity, older surgical candidates, and individuals with moderate obesity. The data further show that the band is particularly effective in long-term weight-loss maintenance. The investigators found that 90% of BGBP patients 10 years postsurgery maintain 50% or more of their excess weight loss.[18-19]

Capella and Capella[11,20] also found that BGBP is highly effective in inducing exceptional weight loss and long-term maintenance. Similar to Fobi, the surgery evolved from the investigators' observations of improved weight loss with VBG–GBP conversion. The primary BGBP of Capella and Capella, similar to that of Fobi, went through a series of modifications to eventually involve a banded transected pouch with interposition of the jejunum between the pouch and bypassed stomach for reduced risk of fistula formation. The band used by Capella and Capella is a 7.5×1.3 cm polypropylene band placed around the distal pouch approximately 1.5 cm proximal to the gastrojejunostomy. The final circumference of the band is 5.5 cm.

In a population of 652 patients having had the BGBP operation of Capella and Capella, exceptionally low incidence rates for either early or late complications were observed.[20] Weight loss success with BGBP 5 years postsurgery was more than 90%. Based upon these observations, Capella and Capella[20] concluded that BGBP is safe and efficacious and produces weight loss superior to that reported for nonbanded GBP[21] and comparable to the weight loss that occurs with more malabsorptive procedures.[22]

Our own studies[23-24] have, likewise, found highly successful weight loss with the laparoscopic BGBP procedure, i.e., 82% 2–3 years postsurgery. The BGBP of our procedure is similar to that described by Fobi[12-14] but with a rectangular pouch (see next section). To our knowledge, our center was the first to routinely perform the BGBP laparoscopic, with development of technique that allows for ring placement in two additional minutes of operative time.

A report[25] published nearly a decade ago estimated that approximately 25% of American bariatric surgeons select the BGBP as their primary procedure. Today, the number of surgeons performing the BGBP is believed to be considerably higher. Surgeons who choose the procedure are convinced that maximal weight loss and long-term weight loss success are much improved. However, there are currently no published data of the results of long-term randomized, comparative trials pertaining to the weight loss or the complications of banded versus nonbanded GBP procedures. Such trials are currently in progress.

BANDED GASTRIC BYPASS TECHNIQUES FOR POUCH FORMATION AND RING PLACEMENT

Most surgeons performing the BGBP use a variation of either the Fobi or Capella procedures for pouch formation and ring materials or placement. In the Fobi procedure, the pouch (<25 mL) is transected from the bypassed stomach and the proximal section of the Roux limb is interposed between the pouch and bypass stomach. The stoma is supported by a silastic ring fashioned by the surgeon. According to the investigators' technique, the stomach is transected obliquely to the left of the gastroesophageal junction (GEJ) down and across to a point 6–7 cm from the GEJ on the lesser curvature to a point approximately 1 cm to the left of the GEJ using a linear cutter (Endo-Surgical). An 8F silastic tube is placed around the pouch, approximately 2 cm from the inferior tip of the pouch. The ends of the tubing, overlapped by 1 cm, are tied with a 2-0 Prolene suture, creating a ring circumference of 6–6.5 cm around the pouch.

Recently, Fobi[26] reported on the safety and efficacy of a premanufactured lock-in-place ring. This report denotes that the GaBP Ring System is a set containing a prosthetic autolocking band and a radiopaque gastrostomy marker. The band is placed around the transected vertical gastric pouch, approximately 2 cm proximal to the tip of the pouch. Less than 5 minutes is required to place and secure the premanufactured band.

The operation of Capella and Capella[11,20] also involves creation of a transected vertical pouch with interposition of the jejunum between the pouch and bypassed gastric segment. The pouch of the Capella procedure, however, is trapezoidal and the distal width approximates that of the jejunum. According to their technique, a 7.5 cm × 1.3 cm polypropylene band is placed around the distal portion of the pouch approximately 1.5 cm from its distal margin. The band is marked with 1-cm stitches for a final circumference of 5.5 cm when closed. The mesh is then closed around the pouch with metal clips and the excess band is excised. In the Capella operation, the flared distal portion of the pouch and an intact gastrohepatic ligament through which the ring transverses keep the ring from descending toward the anastomosis, reducing the risk for ring migration and associated leaks or ulceration.

The Marema BGBP Surgery (Our Procedure)

The laparoscopic technique for a ringed GBP was first attempted by Marema.[23] To create the pouch, mobilization of tissues begins at the GEJ and along the lesser curvature using the harmonic scapel. The stomach is transversely divided with the endoscopic linear cutter for a length of 4 cm at a point 5 cm distal to the GEJ. Subsequently, vertical transections from the first transverse division are performed with sequential firing of the linear cutter toward the angle of His. The size of the pouch created is 15–20 mL with a 32F Hurst bougie. The transoral placement of the anvil of a 21-mm circular stapler (EES) into the distal gastric pouch is performed.

A silastic tubing 3 mm in diameter (Heyer-Schulte Silicone Elastomer) is used. This comes in a presterilized package 20 cm in length. The tubing is cut to a length of 7 cm and is introduced through the middle port of the patient's left side. A tunnel is created behind the gastric pouch, through the gastrohepatic mesentery, 1 cm above the proposed gastrojejunostomy. The tunneling is done by blunt dissection in order to limit the trauma and keep the gastrohepatic ligament virtually intact. This avoids interference with the blood supply to the gastric pouch and assists in preventing migration of the ring. A curved grasper is passed through the tunnel and is attached to the silastic ring, which is then advanced through the tunnel.

A preformed loop of silk is prepared with a slipknot, and a grasper is passed from the patients' left, through the loop, to receive the end of the silastic ring (Figure 26–1). This

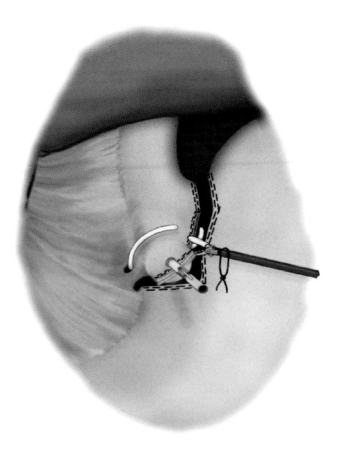

Figure 26–1. Introduction of preformed loop of silk.

end is pulled through the loop to the patient's left. A second grasper is then advanced from the patient's right side, through the loop, to secure the end of the silastic ring. It is pulled back through the loop, advancing to the right (Figure 26–2).

The ends of the silastic tubing are overlapped by 1 cm to give a 6-cm circumference to the ring (Figure 26–3). The knot of the silk is then set around both ends of the ring and stabilized with an additional knot (Figure 26–4). The ring usually leads to a soft tissue reaction or scar tissue that isolates the band. The silastic ring is held in this site by the soft tissue tunnel; it is seen to lie with no compression on the stomach wall. The usual time required for this additional procedure is 2 minutes.

SAFETY OF THE BANDED GASTRIC BYPASS PROCEDURE

Presently, there are no available data from randomized, comparative studies of the incidence rates of short- or long-term complications with the banded versus nonbanded GBP procedures. However, several studies[13,14,19,20,24,27,28] report that the incidence rates for complications with open or laparoscopic BGBP are similar to those of other GBP procedures. Incidence rates for perioperative complications, i.e., atelectasis, DVT, PE, outlet stenosis, leaks, wound infection, pulmonary problems, or early mortality, do not exceed those reported either for GBP procedures or the incidence rates for

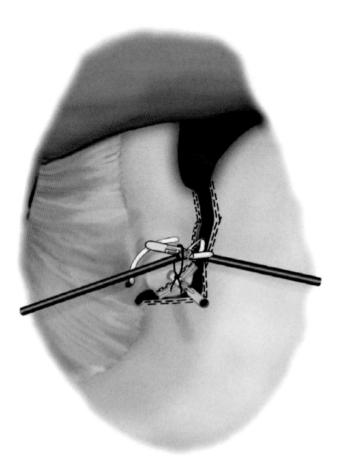

Figure 26–2. Second grasper through the preformed silk loop.

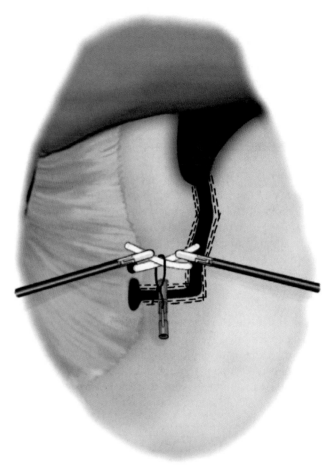

Figure 26–3. Overlapped ends of the Silastic tubing.

late complications, such as incisional hernias, small-bowel obstruction, anemia and vitamin deficiencies, protein malnutrition, anorexia, transient hair loss, hypoglycemia, gastrogastric fistulas, and strictures. Ring erosion[16,27] is an additional complication of the BGBP procedure, as is the increased risk for food intolerance.[16,27–29]

Ring Migration and Erosion

Ring erosion with BGBP, according to Fobi et al.,[16] is more likely to occur in revision and conversion operations than for primary procedures. In a series of nearly 3000 BGBP patients, the investigators found that the incidence of ring erosion was 1.6% for all patients, 0.9% for primary patients, 5.5% in secondary operations, and 28.6% for patients who had band replacement after erosion. The incidence of ring erosion for our own series of 3544 primary BGBP patients was 1.07%. In a more recent series[18] Fobi and associates reported a ring erosion incidence only 0.48% and, in their trials of the premanufactured autolock band system, the investigators[26] found no band erosions over a period of up to 27 postoperative months. White and associates[28] also found an exceptionally low incidence of ring erosion over a postoperative period of up to 14 years. Out of their series of 342 BGBP patients, only 2 cases of ring erosion occurred, both in the context of staple-line disruption and ulceration.

The design of the pouch with the Capella BGBP procedure[11,20] may reduce the risk for band migration. In the Capella procedure, the distal portion of the pouch is trapezoidal. This flared portion of the ring, coupled with an intact gastrohepatic ligament through which the ring traverses, prevents the ring from descending toward the anastomosis. In their series of more than 650 patients followed for greater than 5 years postoperatively, not a single episode of ring migration occurred and band erosion was rare.

As discussed by Fobi,[13,16,19] ring erosion can present as an intraluminal erosion and as a gastric bezoar. Erosion can also present as a migrating ring with or without an associated bezoar formation obstructing the gastrojejunal outlet or obstructing distally in the GI tract. Possible causes for band erosion, as discussed by Fobi,[16] are (1) a band that is too constrictive, (2) suturing of the band to the stomach, (3) imbricating the band with stomach, or (4) infection. Symptoms of band erosion may include those similar to outlet stenosis or obstruction, dysphagia, weight regain, epigastric pain, dyspepsia, anemia, hematemesis, or melena. Endoscopic evaluation is the most effective tool for diagnosis and treatment of band erosion, although spontaneous extrusion of the band may occur in some instances. Surgical removal of the band may be required in certain cases but only as a last resort.

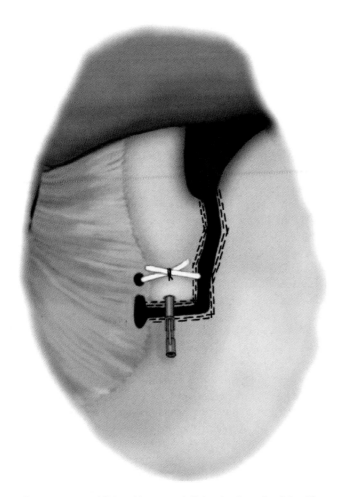

Figure 26–4. Additional knots stabilizing both ends of the Silastic tubing into the SR.

Food Intolerance and Chronic Regurgitation

The occurrence of vomiting and food intolerance is often higher for the banded, as compared to nonbanded, GBP procedure because of the reduced size of the exit point of the pouch. The condition, in fact, may be so severe as to warrant ring removal or ring circumference enlargement. Ideally, the band or ring should reduce the gastric lumen to a size that allows a variety of foods to be eaten while, at the same time, provides for successful weight loss.

The ring circumference of the early primary BGBP procedures averaged 5–5.5 cm.[5,9,11] In a comparative study of ring size circumference, Crampton and associates[30,31] found that a 6-cm ring caused a significantly lower incidence of food intolerance than did a ring circumference of 5.5 cm while providing equivalent weight loss. The investigators found, over a period of up to 24 months after surgery, that 28% of patients with a ring size of 5.5 cm had food intolerance and 14% of patients had to have their rings removed to improve their quality of eating. In comparison, only 12.5% of patients having a 6-cm ring experienced food intolerance and only 1 individual required ring removal. Based on these findings, the investigators recommended a ring size of 6 cm and a larger ring for patients experiencing

difficulty postsurgery or for those at high risk for food intolerance preoperatively.

The initial BGBP procedure of Fobi et al.[5,9] was performed with a 5-cm silastic ring. Fobi, however, found that this ring circumference was associated with a high incidence of food intolerance that could be largely resolved by increasing the ring circumference. Presently, these investigators use a 6-cm ring for women and a 6.5-cm ring for males. According to Fobi, the 6 and 6.5 cm rings lower the risk for food intolerance to rates similar to other short-limb GBP procedures.[19] Our own series show a relatively low incidence of food intolerance in association with a standard ring size of 6.0 cm in circumference.

White and associates[28] in a series of more than 350 BGBP patients studied the association between ring size and the need for ring removal to improve eating. The data show an inverse relationship between ring size and the percentage of patients requiring ring removal. According to the study results, 15% of patients with a ring size of 5.5 cm required ring removal to allow for appropriate eating, as did 6% of patients with a ring of 6.0 cm. However, only 2% of individuals whose ring size was 6.5 cm needed to have their rings removed. Based on these findings, the investigators suggested that a ring size of 6.5 cm may be most appropriate for lowering the risk of food intolerance while maintaining optimal weight-loss success.

Arasaki et al.[29] found that the occurrence of lower esophageal sphincter (LES) hyptonia, in addition to ring size, is an important prognostic factor for chronic regurgitation with BGBP. In their studies, all preoperative patients had an esophageal manometry examination with diagnosis of hypotonia of the LES for 31% of the study population. All study patients were divided into two groups according to ring length, 6.2 or 7.2 cm. Over the course of six postoperative months, those patients who experienced chronic regurgitation were identified. According to the findings, patients who had the smaller, 6.2 cm rings were 4.5 times more likely to suffer from chronic regurgitation than those with the larger ring. The incidence of chronic regurgitation among patients with LES hypotonia was seven times greater than for those with normal LES pressure. The investigators concluded that both ring size and LES hypotonia are prognostic factors for chronic regurgitation, and that preoperative manometry may be helpful in predicting patients requiring a larger ring size.

Future prospective studies of other prognostic indicators of food intolerance may prove extremely valuable in helping surgeons more appropriately adapt ring size to the patient. Other prognostic indicators of food intolerance may include specific psychological and behavioral issues, metabolic aberrations, dentition, ethnicity, or even aging. White and associates,[28] in their series of BGBP patients, used age as a predictor of ring size. They believed that the motility of the esophagus and gastric pouch above the ring are likely to be reduced in older individuals, necessitating a larger ring size. Although the investigators did not directly study the association between esophageal motility and ring size, they did find a significant reduction in the number of patients requiring ring removals after putting their "aging policy" into practice. Knowledge of the effects of age, along with the other possible prognostic factors, on food tolerance with BGBP may prove extremely valuable in helping surgeons to select the most appropriate ring size for maximal weight loss without the additional risk of food intolerance.

EFFICACY OF BGBP

Although there are presently no comparative, randomized trials pertaining to the effectiveness of BGBP, it is generally recognized that the procedure produces greater weight loss than either the short- or long-limb nonbanded GBP procedures.[32] Our own data show an average EWL of 82% with BGBP.[23,24] Others have, likewise, reported EWL with BGBP that exceeds or approaches 80%.[18–20,28,33,34] Such weight loss is equivalent to that of more malabsorptive bariatric surgical procedures.[8,22] Unlike the malabsorptive surgeries, however, the procedure has a far lesser incidence of diarrhea, gas bloating syndrome, pungent body odor, protein malnutrition, and vitamin and mineral deficiencies.

Not only does BGBP seem to produce superior weight loss compared to nonbanded procedures but, more importantly, superior weight loss maintenance, as well. With other GBP procedures, some weight regain occurs around the time that the dumping syndrome diminishes at 2–3 years postsurgery. The pouch dilates and there is less restriction at the anastomosis, reducing feelings of satiety and allowing for greater intake of food.[35,36] The restrictive nature of the BGBP surgery is maintained, decreasing stoma enlargement and associated weight regain.

Fobi and associates[18,19] found that their BGBP patients maintain maximal EWL achieved at weight loss nadir (average = 77%) for as long as 5 years postsurgery. Over 7–10 years postsurgery, more than 90% of patients maintain an EWL of at least 50% or higher, with an EWL of nearly 70% after 10 postoperative years. Other investigators have also demonstrated the long-term effectiveness of the BGBP procedure. Howard et al.[34] found 5 years postsurgery an average EWL of 77% and a success rate (>50% EWL) of 90% among their BGBP patients. Capella and Capella[20] also found after five postoperative years an average EWL of 77% and a success rate of 93%.

White and associates[28] studied the weight loss effectiveness of the BGBP for a postoperative period of up to 14 years. The investigators found that their BGBP patients achieved maximal EWL (87%) at 18 months postsurgery with exceptional weight loss maintenance long term. After 10 and 14 postoperative years, EWL averaged 75% and 59%, respectively. In these same studies, White et al.[28] found that patients whose rings had to be removed lost far less weight long-term. Fobi and associates,[16] likewise, found significantly more weight regain over time for patients whose restrictive rings had to be removed, i.e., average regain of weight approximately 14% EWL. These findings provide further evidence

of the role of the restrictive band in long-term weight-loss maintenance.

BGBP may also help to improve the weight-loss outcomes of subgroups of patients who generally fail to lose as much weight with surgery as do the general bariatric population, such as the elderly or super morbidly obese. The weight-loss failure rate (<50% EWL) of morbidly obese patients having had a nonbanded GBP procedure has been reported to be as high as 43%.[21] The failure rate for the super morbidly obese patients (average BMI = 60) of the Capella BGBP series,[20] however, was only 3% after 5 years postsurgery and their average EWL was 74%. Fobi et al.[18,19] also found highly significant and long-term weight-loss success (~65% EWL at five postoperative years) among patients with super super morbid obesity (>500 pounds), and our own studies[37] found that our super morbidly obese BGBP patients lose even more total body weight than their less-obese cohort over a study period of three postoperative years.

Advanced age is another predictor of reduced weight-loss success with bariatric procedures. Our studies,[38] as well as those of Fobi and associates,[18,19,39] show that BGBP is highly effective in inducing weight loss among older bariatric patients (age ≥ 60 years). Excess weight loss of our older BGBP patients 2–3 years postsurgery averages to 74%. These findings are nearly identical to those of Fobi and associates[18,19,39] who found an average EWL of 72–73% among their older bariatric patients 2–3 years postsurgery. The studies of Fobi et al.[18,19,39] further show that the older BGBP patients have excellent weight-loss outcomes long term, i.e., average EWL = 66% and 62% after 5 and 9 years postoperatively. BGBP is, therefore, highly effective in inducing and sustaining weight loss of older bariatric patients.

SUMMARY

The BGBP, as a primary procedure, evolved out of the findings that VBG patients, whose band was left intact during conversion to a GBP, had greater sustained weight loss than those who had a nonbanded GBP. Over time, surgeons have found that the BGBP produces weight loss that is comparable to that of more malabsorptive procedures and is highly effective in sustaining weight loss long term (10–14 years). The BGBP is performed both laparoscopic and open, and placement of the ring with either access approach generally requires only about 2 minutes. Incidence rates for complications (short- and long-term) with BGBP are similar to those reported for nonbanded GBP surgeries. Band erosion is a complication inherent to the BGBP, although the incidence of band erosion for primary procedures is generally less than 1%. Today, it is believed that greater than 25% of bariatric surgeons use the BGBP as their primary bariatric procedure.

References

1. Mason EE: Vertical banded gastroplasty for obesity. *Arch Surg* 193:334–337, 1982.

2. Sugerman HJ, Starkey JV, Birkenhauer R: A randomized prospective trial of gastric bypass versus vertical banded gastroplasty for morbid obesity and their effects on sweets versus non-sweets eaters. *Ann Surg* 205:613–624, 1987.

3. Sugarman HJ, Wolper JL: Failed gastroplasty for morbid obesity: revised gastroplasty versus Roux-en-Y gastric bypass. *Am J Surg* 148:331–336, 1987.

4. Deitel M, Jones B, Petrov I, et al.: vertical banded gastroplasty: Results in 233 patients. *Can J Surg* 29:322–324, 1986.

5. Fobi MA, Lee H, Fleming AW: surgical techniques of the banded R-Y gastric bypass. *J Obesity Weight Reg* 8:99–103, 1989.

6. Fobi MAL: Paper presented at the American Society of Bariatric Surgery, 1988.

7. Salmon PA: Gastroplasty with distal gastric bypass: A new and more successful weight loss operation for morbidly obese. *Can J Surg* 31:111–114, 1988.

8. Scopinaro N, Adami GF, Marinari GM et al.: Biliopancreatic diversion. *World J Surg* 22:936–946, 1998.

9. Fobi MAL: Why the operation I prefer is silastic ring vertical banded gastric bypass. *Obes Surg* 1:423–426, 1991.

10. Fobi MAL, Lee H: Silastic ring vertical banded gastric bypass for treatment of obesity, two years follow up in 84 patients. *J Natl Med Assoc* 86:125–128, 1994.

11. Capella RF, Capella JF, Mandac H, et al.: Vertical banded gastroplasty–gastric bypass: Preliminary report. *Obes Surg* 1:389–395, 1991.

12. Fobi MAL, Lee H: The surgical technique of the Fobi-pouch operation for obesity (the transected silastic vertical gastric bypass). *Obes Surg* 8:283–288, 1998.

13. Fobi MAL, Lee H, Holness R, Cabinda D: Gastric bypass operation for obesity. *World J Surg* 22:925–935, 1998.

14. Fobi MAL, Lee H, Igwe D, Stanczyk M, Tambi JN: Transected silastic ring vertical gastric bypass with jejunal interposition, a gastrostomy and a gastrostomy site marker (Fobi Pouch operation for obesity). In: Deitel M, Cowan GSM, Jr, (eds): *Update: Surgery for the Morbidly Obese Patient*. Toronto, FD-Communications, 2000, p. 203–226.

15. Fobi MA, Lee H, Igwe D Jr, Stanczyk M, Tambi JN: Prospective comparative evaluation of stapled versus transected silastic ring gastric bypass: 6-year follow-up. *Obes Surg* 11:18–24, 2001.

16. Fobi M, Lee H, Igwe D, et al.: Band erosion: incidence, etiology, management and outcome after banded vertical gastric bypass. *Obes Surg* 11:699–707, 2001.

17. Fobi MAL, Lee H, Igwe D, et al.: Gastric bypass in patients with BMI <40 but >32 without life-threatening co-morbidities: Preliminary report. *Obes Surg* 12:52–56, 2002.

18. Fobi MA, Lee H, Felahy B, et al.: Choosing an operation for weight control and the transected banded gastric bypass. *Obes Surg* 15:114–121, 2005.

19. Fobi MA: The banded gastric bypass. BariMD ask the experts. January, 1996. Available at //www.barimd.com.

20. Capella JF, Capella RF: An assessment of vertical banded gastroplasty-Roux-en-Y gastric bypass for the treatment of morbid obesity. *Am J Surg* 183:117–123, 2002.

21. McLean LD, Rhode BM, Norh CW: Late outcome of isolated gastric bypass. *Ann Surg* 23:524–528, 1999.

22. Marceau P, Hould FS, Simard S, et al.: Biliopancreatic diversion with duodenal switch. *World J Surg* 22:947–954, 1998.

23. Marema RT: Laparoscopic Roux-en-Y gastric bypass: a step-by-step approach. *J Am Coll Surg* 200:979–982, 2005.

24. Marema RT, Perez M, Buffington CK: Comparison of the benefits and complications between laparoscopic and open Roux-en-Y gastric bypass surgeries. *Surg Endosc* 19:525–530, 2005.

25. Talich J, Kirgan D, Fisher BL: Gastric bypass for morbid obesity: A standard surgical technique by consensus. *Obes Surg* 7:198–202, 1997.

26. Fobi MAL: Placement of the GaBP ring system in the banded gastric bypass operation. *Obes Surg* 15:1196–1201, 2005.

27. Salinas A, Santiago E, Yeguez J, Antor M, Salinas H: Silastic ring vertical gastric bypass: Evolution of an open surgical technique, and review of 1588 cases. *Obes Surg* 15:1403–1407, 2005.

28. White S, Brooks E, Jurikova L, Stubbs RS: Long-term outcomes after gastric bypass. *Obes Surg* 15:155–163, 2005.

29. Arasaki CH, Del Grande JC, Yanagita ET, Alves AKS, Riccioppo D, Oliveira CF: Incidence of regurgitation after the banded gastric bypass. *Obes Surg* 15:1408–1417, 2005.

30. Crampton NA, Isvornikov V, Stubbs RS: Silastic ring gastric bypass: Results in 64 patients. *Obes Surg* 17:74–79, 1997.

31. Crampton NA, Izvornikov V, Stubbs RS: Silastic ring gastric bypass: A comparison of two ring sizes: A Preliminary Report. *Obes Surg* 7:495–499, 1997.

32. Fisher BC, Barber AE: Gastric bypass procedures. *Eur J Gastroenterol Hepatol* 11:93–97, 1999.

33. Zorrilla PG, Salinas RJ, Salinas-Martinez AM: Vertical banded gastroplasty-gastric bypass in Mexican patients with severe obesity: 1 year experience. *Obes Surg* 7:322–325, 1997.

34. Howard L, Malone M, Michael A, et al.: Gastric bypass and vertical banded gastroplasty—a prospective randomized comparison and 5 year follow-up. *Obes Surg* 5:55–60, 1995.

35. Halverson JD, Koehler RE: Assessment of patients with failed gastric operation for morbid obesity. *Am J Surg* 145:357–363.

36. Halverson JD, Koehler RD: Gastric bypass: analysis of weight loss and factors determining success. *Surgery* 90:446–455, 1981.

37. Marema RT, Buffington CK: Are the surgical risks of laparoscopic or open gastric bypass greater for patients with super-obesity? *Obes Surg* 15:950 (Abstract). Paper presented at the 2005 IFSO meetings in Maastrich, Netherlands.

38. Toussaint R-M, Marema RT, Buffington CK: Safety and efficacy of gastric bypass for patients 62 years and older. Paper presented at the 2006 meetings of the ASBS in San Francisco, CA.

39. Fobi MAL: Paper presented at the 2003 IFSO Meetings in Salamanca, Spain.

27

Laparoscopic Gastric Bypass: Silastic Ring

Daoud Nasser, MD • Adriana Sales Finizola, MD

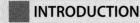 INTRODUCTION

The *Roux-en-Y Gastric Bypass* with ring had already been popularized by Capella and Fobi[1,2] through the open technique for the treatment of morbid obesity.[3] It started being performed by laparoscopy in 1994 by Wittgrove and Clark.[4]

The videolaparoscopic benefits have been shown by many authors,[5–9] including less postoperative pain, less incisional hernias and adhesions incidence, less cardiopulmonary repercussion, lower trauma stimuli, and shorter hospital stay.

These data show a description of the videolaparoscopic gastric bypass with ring and Roux-en-Y diversion, with hand-sewn gastrojejunal anastomosis.

OPERATIVE TECHNIQUE

Patient Care

Patients go to the hospital the night before surgery. Two hours before the procedure, they receive instructions from the surgical team, prophylactic low-weight heparin, and sedation. During surgery, the patients are submitted to leg sequential compression devices, antibiotic prophylaxis, and total venous anesthesia.

Trocars and Team Position

The trocar sites are very important to carrying out the procedure in an ergonomic and comfortable position.)[10] The surgeon stays on the right side of the patient. Five trocars are used (Figure 27–1). The *Verres* needle is inserted on the left hypochondrium to start the pneumoperitoneum.

Trocar A—The first 10-mm trocar punction is made in the umbilicus on the female and brevilineal patients. In other patients, this trocar is inserted at 15 cm from the Xifoid appendix, on the midline. A 30°–40° laparoscope is inserted through this trocar.

Trocar B—The second port is 5 cm to the left and parallel to trocar A in the hemiclavicular line, with a 12-mm trocar.

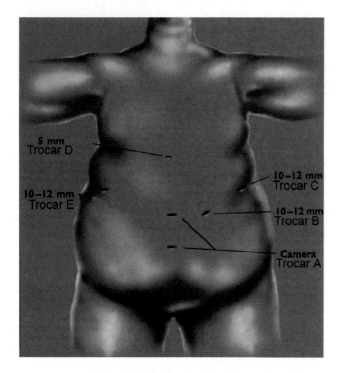

Figure 27–1. Trocar placement.

Trocar C—The third puncture is done at the left anterior axillary line, under the costal margin, with a 12-mm trocar.

Trocar D—The fourth port is positioned under the Xifoid appendix, where a 5- or 10-mm trocar is inserted for liver retraction.

Trocar E—The fifth puncture is done at the right hemiclavicular line, under the costal margin.

We use Trocar B and E as working ports; eventually, trocar C can be used for that purpose. The operating table is turned right to improve ergonomics. The five ports were enough for the great majority of patients, but in superobese, longilineal patients, or with severe steatotic liver, other punctures may be necessary for a safe surgery.

Gastric Pouch and Enteroenteric Anastomoses

The first step is the dissection of the His angle and the perigastric (cardia) fat tissue removal, which improves the pouch final stapling.

The lesser curvature of the stomach is opened 8–10 cm far from the esophagogastric junction to reach the retrogastric space, and that is where gastric transection starts with an endoscopic linear stapler, through trocar E, in an oblique and ascending way. During this step, it is important to cut the retrogastric adhesions and pull the posterior gastric wall laterally to the left side of the patient using trocar B, in order to perfectly adjust the pouch size. The second staple cartridge is passed through trocar C, headed cranially (longitudinally) parallel to the lesser curvature and immediately

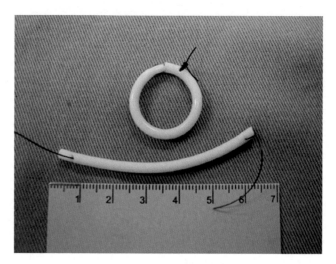

Figure 27–2. Silastic ring.

lateral to a 30F *Fouchet* catheter passed through the mouth into the upper stomach along the lesser curvature. The third staple load for gastric transection is through trocar C, at the cranial way, parallel to the orogastric catheter and following the way of the last fire to the His angle. The next step is to dissect the retrogastric part of the angle of His and to position the "Gold Finger" instrument, which will retract caudally and laterally the stomach, using trocar B. The fourth staple unit through trocar C heads toward the *His* angle and completes the gastric transection. Care should be taken not to staple the esophagus. We use blue loads (3.5-mm length staples) in these steps.[10]

The gastric pouch becomes thin and tubular. We prepare a silastic ring catheterr with a diameter of 3.2 mm and length of 6–6.2 cm using a mononylon inside it (Figure 27–2), which is tied around the gastric pouch, 3 or 4 cm from the esophagogastric junction (Figure 27–3). We reinforce all the staple lines with a Prolene 3-0 stich, and a soft fixation of the ring at the anterior-lateral pouch wall is done. The omentum is transected with the ultrasonic scalpel. We then measure 50 cm of the small intestine from the Treitz ligament; the bowel is pulled up in an antecolic and antegastric fashion,

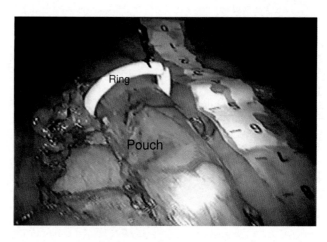

Figure 27–3. Gastric pouch.

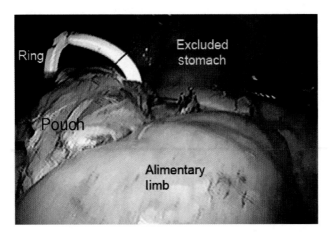

Figure 27–4. Gastric bypass with ring.

and the gastrojejunal anastomoses is performed, hand sewn in two layers with PDS 3-0 before the transection of the small intestine (Figure 27–4). This transection is done near the gastrojejunal anastomoses with stapler. We measure 100–120 cm the alimentary limb, where the jejunojejunostomy is to be made with the transected bowel with stapler through trocar E in a side-to-side fashion; the intestinal orifice is closed with a one layer PDS 3-0, hand sewn. We use white stapling loads (2.5-mm length staples) this time. The mesenteric defect is closed with a Prolene 3-0 continuous suture. The Metilen Blue test is done in all patients routinely. The *Petersen* space is closed afterwards. The proximal alimentary limb is fixed to the excluded stomach. All patients received abdominal drainage (Figure 27–5).

COMMENTS

The first gastric bypass with a *Roux-en-Y* surgery was performed in January 2000, and until March 2006, 512 procedures were done. We had one patient (0.19%) with pulmonary embolism, one pneumonia, one esophageal lesion, one intestinal perforation who had a lethal evolution, and three patients (0.58%) with gastric fistula who had good clinical resolution. Complications related to the ring were as follows: three patients (0.58%) had slippage with stenosis (Figure 27–6); two of those patients had the ring removed by laparoscopy, and both are keeping stable weight; the third patient was submitted to a degastrectomy with gastric bypass without ring. Two patients (0.38%) had ring erosion (Figure 27–7), and the rings were removed by endoscopic procedure. Both patients keep stabilized in weight, because the gastrojejunal anastomosis was good enough. Our statistics confirm the literature data.[5,11–14]

Based on our results, we routinely use some steps to improve the technique:

- Long and slim (8–10 cm) gastric pouch
- Staple line invagination of both pouch and excluded stomach
- Fixation of the alimentary limb at the excluded stomach

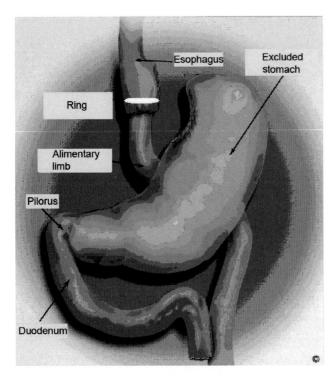

Figure 27–5. Gastric bypass with ring and Roux-en-Y diversion.

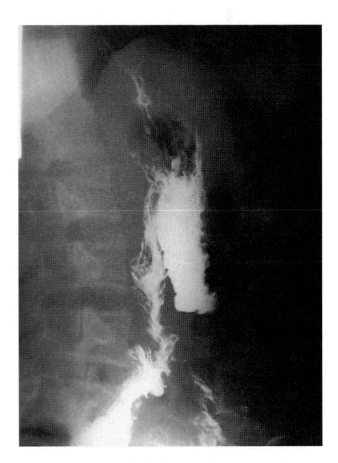

Figure 27–6. Blind loop slippage.

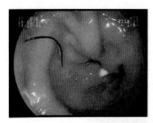
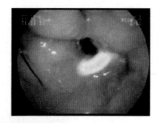
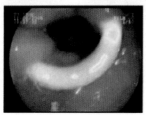

Figure 27–7. Ring erosion.

About the ring

- Positioned 3–4 cm from the esophagogastric junction
- Good flexibility
- Located 3–4 cm from the gastrojejunal anastomoses
- Soft fixation on the anterior gastric wall
- Protect the inside ring stitch knot

Five years after, the excess weight loss is 73%. After a technical improvement in 2005, we hope for better result as in the next follow-up analyses of that technique, which has already proven to be effective in the treatment of the morbid obese patients.[3,9,15]

References

1. Capella RF, Capella JF, Mandac H: Vertical banded gastroplasty-Gastric bypass: preliminary reprt. *Obes Surg* 1:389, 1991.
2. Fobi MAL, Lee H, Holness R, Cabinda D: Gastric bypass operation for obesity. *World J Surg* 22:925–935, 1998.
3. Nasser D, Elias AA: Indication of surgical treatment in severe obesity. *Cirurgia da Obesidade. Atheneu* 10(1):45–46, 2003.
4. Wittgrove AC, Clark GW, Tremblay LJ: Laparoscopic gastric Bypass, Roux-en-Y: Preliminary report of Five cases. *Obes Surg.* 4(4):353–357, 1994.
5. Marema RT, Perez M, Buffington CK: Comparison of benefits and complications between laparoscopic and open Roux-en-Y gastric bypass series. *Surg End* 3, 2005.
6. Nguyen NT, Ho HS, Palmer LS, Wolfe BM: A comparison study of laparoscopic versus open gastric bypass for morbid obesity. *J Am Coll Surg* 191(2):149–157, 2000.
7. Nguyen NT, Lee SL, Goldman C, et al.: Comparison of pulmonary function and pos operative pain after laparoscopic versus open gastric bypass: a randomized trial. *J Am Coll Surg* 192(4):469–477, 2001.
8. Podnos YD, Jimenez JC, Wilson SE, Stevens CM, Nguyen NT: Complications after laparoscopic gastric bypass: a review of 3464 cases. *Arch Surg* 138(9):957–961, 2003.
9. Rosenthal R, Simpfendeorfer CH, Szomstein S: Laparoscopic gastric bypass for refractory morbid obesity. *Surg Clin N Am* 85:119–127, 2005.
10. Nasser D: Pre and pos operative care in Obesity Surgery. *AGE editora* 195–201, 2005.
11. Higa KD, Boone HB, Ho T: Comparison of the laparoscopic Roux-en-Y gastric bypass: 1.040 patients what have learned? *Obes Surg* 10(6):509–513, 2000.
12. Nguyen NT, Huerta S, Gelfand D, Stevens CM, Jim J: Bowel obstruction after laparoscopic Roux-en-Y gastric bypass. *Obes Surg* 14(2):190–196, 2004.
13. Schauer PR, Ikramuddin S, Gourash W, Ramanatha R, Luketich J: Outcomes after laparoscopic Roux-en-Y gastric bypass for morbid obesity. *Ann Surg.* 232(4):515–529, 2000.
14. Higa KD, Ho T, Boone KB: Internal Hernias after laparoscopic Roux-en-Y gastric bypass: incidence, treatment and prevention. *Obes Surg.* 13(3):350–354, 2003.
15. Wittgrove AC, Clark GW: Laparoscopic gastric bypass, Roux-em-Y-500 patients: technique and results, with 3–60 month follow-up. *Obes Surg* 10(3): 233–239, 2000.

Laparoscopic Biliopancreatic Diversion: Approach

Dyker Santos Paiva, MD • Lucinéia Bernardes Lima, MD

INTRODUCTION

Nicola Scopinaro introduced the biliopancreatic diversion in 1976, when he started studies in dogs, aiming at reducing or preventing serious complications from the jejunoileal bypass, such as unstable diarrhea, electrolyte disturbance, hypovitaminosis, protein malnutrition, hepatic insufficiency, nephrolithiasis, nausea, vomiting, and polyarthritis.[1] (Please see Chapter 13.)

Due to the lack of blind-loop syndrome and malabsorption being selective as to starch and fat, the biliopancreatic diversion is free of those complications pertaining to the jejunoileal bypass.[1,2]

From the surgical model proposed at first by Scopinaro, several modifications were made in the length, at times of the alimentary limb, now in the biliopancreatic limb or the common channel, and also in the size of the remaining stomach, always in an attempt to achieve the best weight-loss results with minimal nutritional complications.[3] After 1984

a standard was set consisting of a gastrectomy with the remaining stomach with a volume from 200 to 500 mL, a 2.5-m alimentary limb, and a 50-cm common channel. It is crucial for the measurement of the intestinal loops to be taken always on the antimesenteric side with maximum traction (please see Chapter 10) (Figure 28–1).[4]

Cholecystectomy was added to the procedure due to the high rate of biliary stones, probably due to a failure of the enterohormonal stimulus, with dismotility of the gallbladder associated with an increase in cholesterol biliary excretion.[3]

Laparoscopic surgery for the treatment of morbid obesity began in the 1990s with the implantation of lap bands, both adjustable or not, by Catona, Belachew, Forsell, and Cadiére,[5–7] and by Clark and Wittgrove, who introduced the first laparoscopic gastric bypass.[8] (Please see Chapters 14 and 16.)

In 1999, Gagner did the first biliopancreatic diversion with duodenal switch laparoscopically.[9] In 2000, Paiva did the

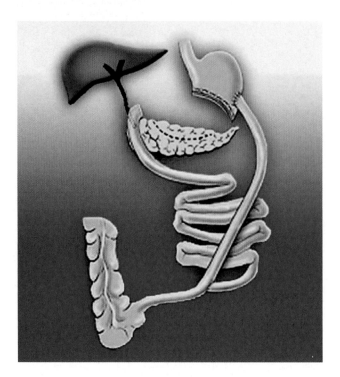

Figure 28–1. BPD standard.

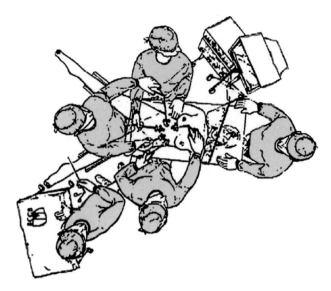

Figure 28–2. Positioning of the team during the first and third stages of the surgery.

first biliopancreatic diversion—as described by Scopinaro—through laparoscopy.[10]

It is apparent that laparoscopic surgery has many advantages compared to conventional surgery. These include reduced postoperative recovery time and return to normal activities, decrease in the rate of cardiopulmonary complications, lower hypermetabolic response, and a decrease in complications related to the abdominal wall, including infections, herniae, and postoperative dehiscence. It also has the advantage of reducing adhesions and decreasing postoperative ileus.[9,11–16]

Indications for laparoscopic surgery are the same as those for open surgery, and these benefits certainly are extensive in the obese population. Every bariatric surgical can conceivably be done by laparoscopic surgery.[17]

The presence of previous procedures is not a contraindication to laparoscopic surgery; actually, the mobilization of adhesions with delicate dissection and minimum mobilization of structures represents advantages in relation to conventional surgery—it may provide good exposure alternatives without compromising visualization.[17]

The proper positioning of the trocars and the ability of using several suture techniques are important things to take into account. This is especially true for patients who had previous surgery with intra-abdominal adhesions, thus presenting a further challenge to the surgeon.[17]

TECHNICAL ASPECTS

Patient Position

The positioning of the patient requires an adequate surgical table capable of safely bearing the weight and must also be

capable of changing position during the procedure. We must pay especially close attention to the pressure areas, since due to the patient's weight, there is a greater risk of ischemic, vein, and nervous injuries.

The patient is placed supine with abducted legs; right upper member abducted and left upper arm along side the body. The anesthesiologist is at the patient's head.

The laparoscopy monitor should be placed to the right of the patient, next to the head of the table.

The surgery is divided into three distinctive stages. In the first stage, the surgical table is placed in a moderate reverse *Trendelenburg.* During this stage, the surgeon stands between the legs of the patient. The first assistant, who also operates the camera, is placed to the left of the surgeon, the second assistant on the right, and the scrub nurse holder next to the second assistant (Figure 28–2).

During the second stage of the surgery, the table is placed in moderate *Trendelenburg.* The laparoscopy monitor is moved toward the trunk of the patient; the surgeon is at the left of the patient, close to the patient's shoulder, having the first assistant to his left. The second assistant should be placed to the right of the patient (Figure 28–3).

During the third and last stage of the surgery, the whole team should return to the start position.

Positioning of the Trocars

The pneumoperitoneum is done using the *Veress* needle into the left upper quadrant, close to the costal margin, at the level of the mid-clavicular line. CO_2 pressure should be maintained at 15 mm/Hg during the procedure.

A total of six[6] trocars are used (Figure 28–4):

Trocar 1 (10 mm) is introduced in the midline, supraumbilically and about 20 cm below the xiphoid process. In morbidly obese patients, the umbilical scar should never be used as an anatomic point of reference for the introduction of the trocars.

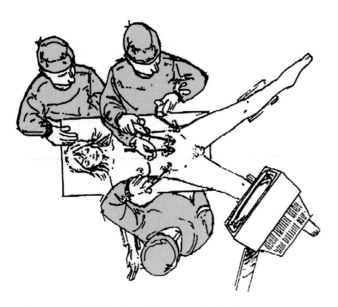

Figure 28–3. Positioning of the team during the second stage.

Trocar 2 (12 mm) is positioned on the outer border of the left abdominal rectus close to the costal margin, at the level of the mid-clavicular line.

Trocar 3 (10 mm) is introduced close to the xiphoid process.

Trocar 4 (5 mm) is introduced in the right upper quadrant, close to the costal margin, at the level of the right axillary line.

Trocar 5 (12 mm) is introduced halfway up an imaginary line traced between trocars 1 and 4.

Trocar 6 (10 mm) is introduced about 10 cm below trocar 2, at the same level of that one.

The procedure is entirely done with a 10-mm and 30° optical system.

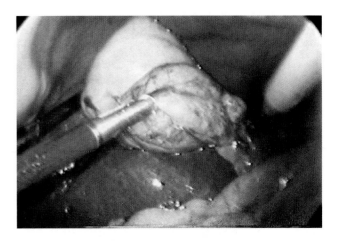

Figure 28–5. Cholecystectomy.

First Stage of the Surgery

Cholecystectomy

The first stage of the surgery is the cholecystectomy and the gastrectomy.

During the cholecystectomy, optical system is placed at portal 1, and the grasping forceps at portal 4 so that the assistant can lift the falciform ligament, thus exposing the gallbladder. The surgeon then works with a grasping forceps at portal 5 and a dissection forceps at portal 2. The exposure of the liver is made by means of portal 3 by using the liver retractor. The cholecystectomy is made by sectioning the cystic artery and ducts with a metallic clip and later dissection with a harmonic scalpel. The gallbladder is left in the right hypochondrium over the liver to be removed from the abdominal cavity at the end of the surgery (Figure 28–5).

Gastrectomy and Duodenal Section

During the gastrectomy, the optical system stays in portal 1; the first assistant uses the grasping forceps in portal 4 to expose the stomach. The surgeon uses portal 2 for the harmonic

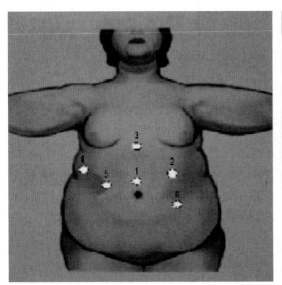

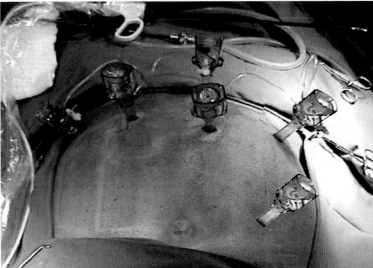

Figure 28–4. Positioning of the trocars.

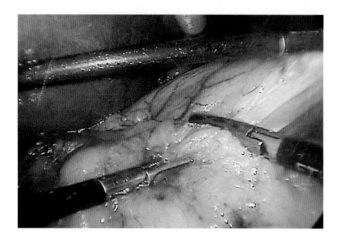

Figure 28–6. Dissection of the great curvature.

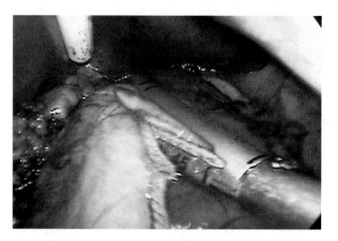

Figure 28–8. Gastrectomy.

scalpel and portal 5 for the grasping forceps, thus exposing and dissecting the stomach. The second assistant pushes the liver away by means of portal 3.

The gastrectomy is made in the cranium-caudal direction following the great curvature and starting about 15 cm below the angle of His. This dissection is always made with the harmonic scalpel, and close to the gastric wall, aiming at reducing bleeding, and it extends down to 2 cm distal from the pylorus (Figure 28–6).

After the greater curve is freed by means of a small hole in the lesser gastric curvature, about 3 cm above the pylorus, from this point on the lesser curvature is dissected in the caudal direction, down to 2 cm distal to the pylorus in order to fully free the proximal duodenum. After this stage, the duodenal transaction is done with a linear endostapler (Figure 28–7).

After the duodenal transection, the stomach is cranially pulled in order to facilitate the dissection of the lesser gastric curvature, which is made up to the level of the left gastric artery, always close to the gastric wall, so as to prevent bleeding.

Once the level of the left gastric artery is reached, the full gastric transaction from the greater curve is done with the linear endostapler (Figure 28–8).

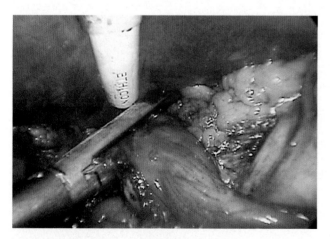

Figure 28–7. Section of the duodenum.

At this point the orogastric catheter is removed. The remaining stomach is left with a volume of approximately 400 mL.

The divided stomach is left in the patient's left hypochondrium to be removed at the end of surgery together with the gallbladder.

Second Stage of the Surgery

During this stage, the surgeon positions himself at the level of the patient's left shoulder, having the first assistant on his left and the second assistant on the right of the patient.

The surgical table is placed in a moderate *Trendelenburg* position. The optical system is placed in portal 2 by the first assistant.

The surgeon uses portals 5 and 6 by grasping forceps for measuring the intestinal loops, and one of them has a mark cut 10 cm from the distal extremity. Via portal 3, the introduction of the needle holder for stitches is done when necessary. The second assistant uses portal 4 for exposing the loops and helping with the stitches.

Measurement of the Loop and Enteroanastomosis

In the second part of the operation, the ileocecal junction is identified, and the ileal loop is measured from this point. The measurement is made with two forceps, measuring at 10 cm increments on the antimesenteric margin, completely stretched in order to obtain a correct measurement. When the 50 cm measurement is completed, a stitch is applied, and the enteroanastomosis will be performed at this point (Figure 28–9).

The measurement of the loop continues up to 250 cm from the ileocecal valve, at which level it is divided using the linear endostapler, which is introduced into the cavity through portal 5 (Figure 28–10).

Thus, we have already defined the alimentary limb, which will later be anastomosed to the stomach.

At this point of the surgery, a Penrose drain is stitched to the margin of the alimentary limb to help in passing it through the orifice made on the mesocolon (Figure 28–11).

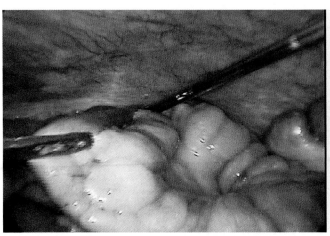
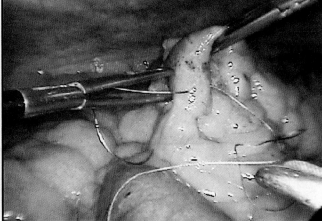

Figure 28–9. Measurement of the intestinal loop.

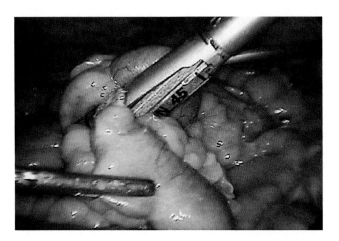

Figure 28–10. Section of the ileum.

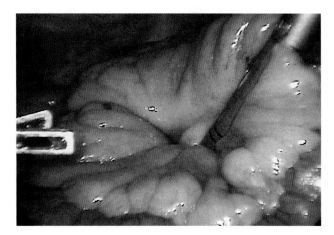

Figure 28–12. Opening of the mesentery.

We proceed now to the opening of the mesentery down to its root, which can be done with the linear endostapler or by using the harmonic scalpel. At this point, one can sporadically use metallic clips to improve hemostasis (Figure 28–12).

Care is taken to run grasping forceps along the entire alimentary limb and to arrange it on the right side of the ab-

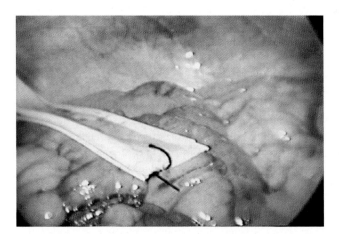

Figure 28–11. Alimentary limb.

dominal cavity, thus identifying the stitch left 50 cm from the ileocecal valve. We have already identified the alimentary limb and the biliopancreatic limb; at this time, therefore, the enteroanastomosis in isoperistatic position is done. This is done first by opening a small orifice into both loops with the harmonic scalpel and passing a linear endostapler through this orifice. The orifice of the endostapler is closed in a running seromuscular suture (Figure 28–13).

Once the anastomosis is concluded, the mesenteric opening should always be closed with running suture (Figure 28–14).

Third Stage of the Surgery

At this point, the entire surgical team returns to the position of the first stage of the surgery, as well as the laparoscopy set.

The first assistant is responsible for the optical system, which is introduced into portal 1 and, by means of a grasping forceps, into portal 4. The surgeon uses portals 2, 5, and 6 for exposure, mesocolon opening, and gastroenteroanastomosis. And the second assistant uses portal 3 to expose the liver.

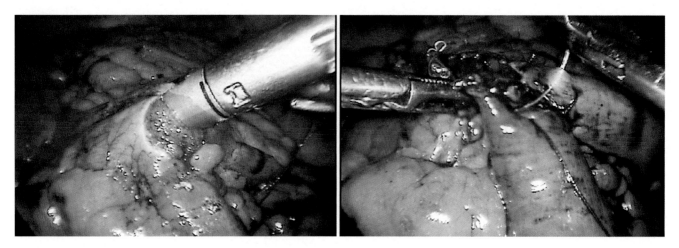

Figure 28–13. Enteroanastomosis.

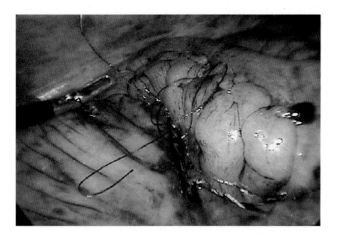

Figure 28–14. Mesenteric suture.

Opening of the Mesocolon

The transverse colon is pulled cephalic in order to identify the ligament of Treitz, and about 2 cm above it the mesocolon is opened about 3 cm in order to pass the alimentary limb (Figure 28–15).

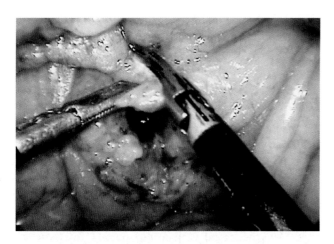

Figure 28–15. Opening of the mesocolon.

Gastroenteroanastomosis

After the proper positioning of the alimentary limb through the transverse mesocolon, the continuous seromuscular suture between the posterior wall of the stomach and the alimentary limb is made. This suture is made so as to facilitate the simultaneous introduction of the linear endostapler into the stomach and the loop in order to perform the gastroenteroanastomosis. The orifice of the endostapler is closed by means of a running seromuscular suture (Figure 28–16).

After the gastroenteroanastomosis is finished, the mesocolon opening is closed. The gastroenteroanastomosis can also be done in the same way described above, but with the alimentary limb in a precolic position, at the surgeon's option.

After the surgical procedure is finished, portal 2 is widened to 2 cm, and through it gallbladder and the stomach are removed. In this place, the aponeurosis is closed with separate stitches.

POSTOPERATIVE CONTROL

After discharge from the hospital, the patients are instructed by a weekly control during the first month. During this period, diet is at first restricted to liquids, and then gradually evolving to viscous liquids, and at the end of the first month a solid diet, always respecting the maximum volume of 200 mL per meal. The need for the ingestion of protein and calcium is emphasized, and all kinds of fat should be avoided.

Hematological tests are run every 3 months during the first year, then every 6 months during the second and third years. These tests aim at an advanced diagnosis for anemia, protein deficiency, calcium disturbances, and any tendencies toward hypovitaminosis.

All patients are recommended to daily ingest polyvitamins, omeprazole, and iron during the first postoperative year; the use of this medication should be revised after this time, depending on the patient's evolution.

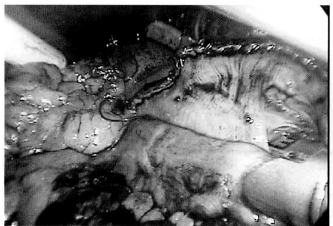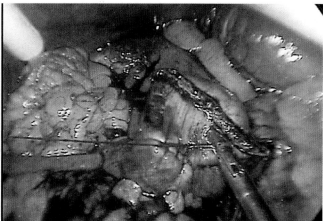

Figure 28–16. Gastroenteroanastomosis.

CONCLUSIONS

Biliopancreatic diversion is an excellent procedure because it offers the patients advantages in relation to restrictive procedures, since they can continue to eat normally,[18] besides being a more effective surgery with better maintenance of long-term weight loss,[18] and with a very large satisfaction rate of the patient as to the procedure.[19]

As to the issue of postoperative control and supplementing of iron, calcium, or vitamins for a long term, it is no different from other procedures.

The greater risk of malabasortive procedures is protein malnutrition, which Scopinaro reports being of 2.7%, with 1.0% of recurrence in a minimum segment of 2 years (see Chapter 10). This rate can differ for different kinds of populations. This represents an acceptable level for a serious complication, but can be solved by the elongation of the common channel, thus providing the patient with a larger absorption area and a definitive solution for the problem.

The objective of the biliopancreatic diversion is not only the loss of excess weight or the healing of comorbidities, but especially the maintenance of long-term weight loss, which this malabsortive surgery has already proven capable of providing. As shown by Scopinaro, the surgery maintains more than 70% of the excess weight loss during a follow-up of 20 years.

Laparoscopic surgery is an important technological advancement that allows complex and much less invasive procedures to be done with significant reduction of trauma to the abdominal wall.

The current stage of the laparoscopic surgery allows for increasingly complex techniques to be done this way with increasingly auspicious results. The biliopancreatic diversion can be done by laparoscopy with no need for modifications of the technical principles proposed by Scopinaro.

The technique presents a high level of complexity and can be safely done as long as the surgeon is experienced in advanced laparoscopic surgery, has a well-trained team, and has the adequate material.

The harmonic scalpel is indispensable for the safe undertaking of the surgery. The measurement of the intestinal loop, an important factor for the good result of the surgery, can be done by precision by laparoscopy. This measurement is done between two forceps, being thus equivalent to manual traction. By following the standardization presented, our results reproduce the ones described in the literature.

All advantages of the laparoscopic surgery are confirmed when applied to the morbid obese patient. Besides being an achievement, the accomplishment of a technique for the treatment of morbid obesity by laparoscopy is the certainty of the decrease of risks and complications in this group of patients.

We can conclude that the biliopancreatic diversion is feasible by laparoscopy, without changes in the original technique: it does not increase either risks or complications, and especially, it does not compromise the results.

References

1. Scopinaro N, Gianetta, Civalleri D, et al.: Biliopancreatic by-pass for obesity: I. An experimental study in dogs. *Br J Surg* 66:613, 1979.
2. Scopinaro N, Gianetta, Civalleri D: Biliopancreatic bypass for obesity: II. Initial experience in man. *Br J Surg* 66:619, 1979.
3. Scopinaro N, Gianetta, Civalleri D, et al.: Two years of clinical experience with biliopancreatic bypass for obesity. *Am J Clin Nutr* 33:506, 1980.
4. Scopinaro N, Gianetta, Friedman D, et al.: Evolution of biliopancreatic bypass. *Clin Nutr* 5:137, 1986.
5. Cadiere GB, Bruyns J, Himpens J, et al.: Laparoscopic gastroplasty. *Br J Surg.* 81:1524, 1994.
6. Catona A, Gossemberg M, La Manna A, et al.: Laparoscopic gastric banding: preliminary series. *Obes Surg* 3:207, 1993.
7. Buchwald H, Buchwald JN: Evolution of operative procedures for the management of morbid obesity 1950–2000. *Obs Surg* 12:705, 2002.
8. Wittgrove AC, Clark GW, Tremblay LJ: Laparoscopic gastric bypass, Roux-en-Y: Preliminary report of five cases. *Obes Surg* 4: 353, 1994.
9. Ren CJ, Patterson, Gagner M: Early results of laparoscopic biliopancreatic diversion with duodenal switch: A case series of 40 consecutive patients. *Obes Surg* 10: 514, 2000.
10. Paiva D, Bernardes L, Suretti L: Laparoscopic biliopancreatic diversion for the treatment of morbid obesity: Initial experience. *Obes Surg* 11:619, 2001.

11. Westling A, Gustavsson S: Laparoscopic vs. open Roux-en-Y gastric bypass: A prospective, randomized trial. *Obes Surg* 11:284, 2001.

12. Fried M, Krska Z, Danzig V: Does the laparoscopic approach significantly affect cardiac functions in laparoscopic surgery? *Pilot study in non-obese and morbidly obese patients. Obes Surg* 11(3):293–296, 2001.

13. Schauer PR, Sirineke KR: The laparoscopic approach reduces the endocrine response to elective cholecystectomy. *Am Surg* 61:106, 1995.

14. Wittgrove AC, Clark GW, Schulort KR: Laparoscopic gastric bypass: 5 years prospective study of 500 patients followed from 3–60 moths. *Obes Surg* 10:233, 2000.

15. Schauer PR, Sayeed I: Laparoscopic surgery for morbid obesity. *Surg Clin North Am* 81:1145, 2001.

16. Nguyen NT, Lee SL, Anderson JT, Palmer LS, Canet F, Wolf BM: Evolution of intra-abdominal pressure after laparoscopic and open gastric bypass. *Obes Surg* 11:40, 2001.

17. Higa KD, Boone KB: Tienchin Ho: Complications of the laparoscopic Roux-en-Y gastric bypass: 1040 patients—what have we learned? *Obes Surg* 10:509, 2000.

18. Scopinaro N, Adami GF, Marinari GM et al.: Biliopancreatic diversion. *World J Surg* 22:936, 1998.

19. Marceau P, Hould FS, Simard S, et al.: Biliopancreatic diversion with duodenal switch. *World J Surg* 22:947, 1998.

29

Laparoscopic Biliopancreatic Diversion: Duodenal Switch

Aniceto Baltasar, MD

SUMMARY

- The biliopancreatic diversion (BPD) with duodenal switch (DS) is a mixed, hybrid surgery to treat morbid obesity.
- The vertical sleeve gastrectomy with a >50 cc pouch is the restrictive part.
- The biliopancreatic diversion of the DS is the malabsorptive part.
- Technically difficult but with excellent weight loss and quality of life.

INTRODUCTION

The duodenal switch (DS) is one alternative to the Scopinaro biliopancreatic diversion (BPD). Hess[1] did the first case in March 1988 (in a woman with BMI = 60 and she has BMI = 29 17 years later), and Marceau[2] made the first publication. Baltasar[3,4] showed more cases. Gagner[5] performed the first LDS in July 1999, and Baltasar[6,7] published the second world experience.

LDS is (1) *vertical sleeve gastrectomy* (VSG) with pyloric preservation of less than 60 cc and (2) BPD of *common channel* (CC) of 65 cm, a *alimentary loop* (AL) of 235 cm, and the remaining *biliopancreatic loop* (BPL) as the proximal small bowel.

SURGICAL TECHNIQUE

General endothracheal anesthesia is given. The patient is supine with the separated legs. Three surgeons perform the operation, one in between the legs and the other two on the sides. Direct vision approach is always used for the first trocar with an Ethicon Endopath#12 on the lateral border of the right rectus muscle, 3–4 fingerbreadths below the right costal margin. This is the only large trocar, the working trocar (WT). Trocars are positioned. The camera is 30° and placed in the midline, and the other four trocars are 5 mm. A silk suture passed from the right costal margin around the round ligament brings the liver and round ligament to the right and leaves the antro and duodenum well exposed. Cholecystectomy is done at this time.

The *harmonic ultrasound* (HUS) is used to cut the vessels at the greater curvature of the stomach, starting opposed from the *incisure angularis,* and progressing to the top and freeing the stomach from the left *crura.* Sometimes adhesions from the posterior stomach wall and pancreas have to be separated.

The left-side-placed surgeon cuts the vessels the distal stomach down and passes the pylorus, for at least 3 cm, and he creates a tunnel posterior to the pylorus and in between duodenum and the pyloric artery.

The right-side-placed surgeon passes the stapler by the WT, divides the duodenum with a linear white stapler with a single 6-cm cartridge firing.

The surgeon in between the legs places a seroserosa continuous running suture of 3-0 PDS to prevent duodenal leaks.

The anesthetist inserts a #12-mm nasogastric tube (RUSCH) in the antrum with a guide wire inserted within and to the tip. The right-placed surgeon divides the antrum by the WT, starting 1 cm proximal to the pylorus and firing a blue 4.5 cm cartridge twice very close to the gastric stent. Starting at the *incisure angularis,* he uses a 6-cm-long blue cartridge to divide sequentially and very close to the stent up to and lateral to the His angle fat pad.

The anesthetist removes the stent, leaves the guide wire inside, and then passes a small 7-mm regular nasogastric (NG) tube, under guidance, to the antrum. This maneuver saves time since sometimes without a guide it is very cumbersome to try to pass a NG tube. The surgeon who is between the legs places a continuous running seroserosa suture of 3-0 PDS from the esophageal gastric junction (EGJ) to the middle of the suture line and then a second one to the distal. This suture effectively controls bleeding at the pouch suture line and prevents leakages. The remaining lesser-curvature-based pouch is tested for leaks with less than 50 cc of diluted Methylene blue.

The surgical team changes position to the head of the patient. The patient is placed in a *Trendelenburg.* The greater omentum is split in the middle up to the transverse colon with the HUS.

Measurements of the first 65 cm of the CC are done by using marked, curved, smooth clamps in 5 cm steps. One clip is placed to mark the place for the CC–BPL anastomosis and two proximal. The rest of the bowel is measured up to 300 cm from the ileocecal valve. The mesentery of the small bowel is divided with a bloodless field by the HUS. The bowel is divided transversally with a linear white 45 mm cartridge passed through the only WT. The distal AL is held by a clamp from the xiphoid and kept identified and superior to the transverse colon.

The BPL is divided transversally with the HUS, the distal bowel identified again, and the union on the BPL–CC divided longitudinally. The BPL–CC anastomosis is a single layer, end-to-side, hand sewn with two PDS threads united in the middle with knots. One is used for a continuous running suture of the posterior wall and the other for the extramucous anterior wall. The mesenteric defect is closed by a running 3-0 suture.

The patient and surgical team change position to reverse *Trendelenburg* situation as in the beginning. The duodenoileal anastomosis (DIA) is always done end-to-end in two layers. The first layer brings together the posterior wall of the duodenum to the posterior one of the ileum by interrupted stitches of silk to release tension at the suture line. The sutures can include the end of both bowel staples to increase holding strength. Both anterior loops, ileum and duodenum, are divided transversally with the HUS. A double PDS 3-0 suture is used for a whole-wall, watertight, continuous suture of the posterior first and then the anterior wall. A second anterior suture line of interrupted silk or continuous PDS adds the final second layer to the DIA.

The pouch is tested for leaks with the nasogastric tube placed in the antrum using Methylene blue or air. Revision of the cavity and aspiration is done. The stomach is removed by enlarging the #12 WT, directly and without any bag. Two drains are placed under vision posterior and anterior to the stomach and the DIA. The WT opening is closed with Maxon by one suture and the skin with silk.

Operating times range from 2.15 to 4 hours but with a mean of 2.45 hours.

Patients are extubated in the recovery room and usually transferred to a regular ward, where they sit 2 hours after surgery and incentive spirometry and active leg exercises are encouraged.

They have a control GI series with Gastrografin next day and are discharged with drains.

Patients drink a diluted Methylene blue everyday to rule out leaks, and the drains are removed on the 7th POD (postoperative day). They are allowed to drink liquids starting next day for 2 weeks, mashed food for another week, and then a free diet. Supplementation with calcium, iron, and fat-soluble vitamins (A, D, E and K) are recommended for life.

Patients

Two hundred and ninety-nine MO patients have been treated with the Laproscopic Duodenal Switch (LDS) hand-sewn technique starting May 10, 2000. Mean BMI is 50.6 (38–71). Conversion was required in 12 out of the first 60 patients. No conversions have been done in the last 100 cases.

Two patients died within 30 days due to a duodenal stump leak (without seroserosa reinforcement) and a pulmonary emboli (0.66% mortality). Another patient (BMI 69) died at home 34 days after surgery due to pulmonary emboli also.

There were 21 leaks (6%), 10 of them at the GEJ, 9 at the DIA, and 1 duodenal stump leak in a patient who died.

The GEJ leaks required: four of them several surgeries and two of them a total gastrectomy. Two of them had a patch of ascended BPL and both healed. The DIA leaks were four asymptomatic, three well drained and cured conservatively, and two required resection and new DIA.

One patient had Roux-O and required reoperation. One patient had gastroparesis and did not respond to any therapy and finally had a total gastrectomy. Two patients had functional stenosis at the jejunojejunostomy and were treated by interventional radiology by decompression of the whole AL with a long tube.

There were three patients with intestinal obstructions who required laparotomy and two of them bowel resection. None of them had internal hernias.

Three patients developed protein-caloric malnutrition and one had a lengthening procedure by laparoscopy.

One patient died of undiagnosed acute appendicitis in a different community.

This is a short-term follow-up, and percentages of EWL and EBMIL[8] are expected to be similar than in the open surgery. Our long-term OPEN DS patients have an EWL percentage of 69 and EBMIL percentage of 73 at 5 years.

CONCLUSION

The hand-sewn LDS is a very complex procedure with a very difficult learning curve (more than with the LRNYGBP). Early complications are expected at the beginning of the experience, but it can be an excellent procedure with quality of life and weight loss.

References

1. Hess DS, Hess DW: Biliopancreatic diversion with a duodenal switch. *Obes Surg* 8:267–282, 1998.
2. Marceau P, Biron S, Bourque RA, Potvin M, Hould FS, Simard S: Biliopancreatic Diversion with a New Type of Gastrectomy. *Obes Surg* 3(1):29–35, 1993 Feb.
3. Baltasar A, del Río J, Bengochea M, et al.: Cirugía híbrida bariátrica: Cruce duodenal en la derivación bilio-pancreática. *Cir Esp* 59:483–486, 1996.
4. Baltasar M, Bou R, Bengochea M, Serra C, Pérez N: Mil operaciones bariátricas. *Cir Esp Mayo* 79(6):349–355, 2006.
5. Ren CJ, Patterson E, Gagner M: Early results of laparoscopic biliopancreatic diversion with duodenal switch: a case series of 40 consecutive patients. *Obes Surg* 10(6):514–523, 2000 Dec.
6. Baltasar A, Bou R, Miró J, Pérez N: Cruce duodenal por laparoscopia en el tratamiento de la obesidad mórbida: técnica y estudio preliminar. *Cir Esp* 70(2):102–104, 2001.
7. Baltasar A, Bou R, Miro J, Bengochea M, Serra C, Perez N: Laparoscopic biliopancreatic diversion with duodenal switch: Technique and initial experience. *Obes Surg* 12(2):245–248, 2002.
8. Deitel M, Greenstein RJ: Editorial recommendations for reporting weight loss. *Obes Surg Apr* 13:159–160, 2003.

30

Two-Stage Approach for High-Risk Patients

Camilo Boza, MD • Michel Gagner, MD, FRCSC, FACS

BACKGROUND

During the past decade, bariatric surgery has evolved into multiple forms characterized by restriction, limited absorption, or both. Roux-en-Y gastric bypass has become the "gold standard" for obesity surgery.[1] MacLean, Sugerman, and their colleagues, however, have reported that construction of a small gastric pouch with proximal small-bowel bypass has not yielded comparable weight-loss results in patients in the higher end of the spectrum of obesity.[2,3] These super-obese (body mass index, BMI > 50) and super-superobese (BMI > 60) patients lose more weight, but stabilize at a BMI considered to be obese or even morbidly obese. Therefore, these proximal-bypass procedures may decrease the actuarial mortality risk in superobese patients.

Biliopancreatic diversion with duodenal switch (BPD/DS) is often regarded as the most extreme obesity surgery practiced currently. A vertical, subtotal, laparoscopic sleeve gastrectomy (LSG) is fashioned along the lesser curvature, and with the pylorus preserved, the duodenum is transected to form the biliopancreatic limb. The distal ileum is transected 250 cm from the ileocecal valve and distal end is brought up to create a duodenoileostomy. This alimentary limb then joins the biliopancreatic limb in the distal ileum with a 100-cm common channel.[4–6]

In one study, review of the historical cohort of open BPD–DS in the super super obese patients ($N = 28$) showed a 17.0% morbidity and 3.5% mortality rate.[7] A minimally invasive approach could potentially offer better postoperative pulmonary function, earlier return of physical activity, better wound healing, and in turn, reduced morbidity and mortality, because this population of patients often has underlying cardiovascular, pulmonary, and metabolic diseases that put them at adversely increased surgical risks.[8,9]

The authors began performing laparoscopic BPD–DS (LBPD–DS) in 1999.[10,11] The following year, the technical approach was reported and results of the early series of 25 and 40 patients with a mean BMI of 60 kg/m^2 were noted. An overall 15.0% major morbidity and 2.5% mortality rates were achieved. When the data were stratified to patients with BMI greater than 65 kg/m^2, a 38.0% versus 8.3% complication rate was noted in patients with BMI less than 65 kg/m^2. More recent review of the unpublished 138 LBPD–DS experience (mean BMI: 54 kg/m^2) showed excellent excess body weight loss (EBWL) of 68.0% at 6 months. Overall 13.0% major morbidity and 1.4% mortality rates were noted. In the super super morbidly obese patients with BMI > 60 kg/m^2 ($N = 31$), the morbidity (23.0%) and mortality (6.5%) rates of LBPD–DS were significantly higher.

For the surgeons, LBPD–DS is technically difficult, physically demanding, and requires advanced laparoscopic skills. For the super-superobese patients who carry much of their weight in the neck, torso, and abdomen, the various positions of the operative table to facilitate exposure may compromise their ventilation and preclude them from extended anesthesia. At times, increased pneumoperitoneum to 20 mm Hg may be necessary to counter the excessive weight of the abdominal wall. A large, fatty liver—as well as heavily laden omentum and mesentery—also could jeopardize the anastomosis. Tremendous and sustainable weight loss is desirable, but should not compromise patient safety. Given the preliminary results, it became apparent that an alternative approach to LBPD–DS was necessary in the super-superobese patients. From the authors' experience of more than 100 LBPD–DS procedures, a two-stage procedure was offered to the super-superobese patient—stage one: LSG and stage two: laparoscopic duodenoileostomy/ileoileostomy (LDI–II). Early weight loss in any bariatric procedure is suspected to be a result of decreased caloric intake because of a smaller gastric capacity. By separating the restrictive and malabsorptive procedures, these patients were postulated to lose approximately 100 lbs in 6–9 months. However, the concern was that patients might begin regaining weight as the stomach adapts and expands after this period of time. The authors' algorithm was to bring patients back into this window of opportunity for the second-stage malabsorptive surgery to create limited absorption of food by way of a shortened common channel and alimentary limb.

The authors hypothesized that, with a relatively lower BMI and an improved pulmonary and cardiovascular status, as well as other medical comorbidities,[12] the patients would have a reduced morbidity and mortality rate. Findings of the first series of super-superobese patients who completed this novel concept of a two-stage LBPD–DS are reported herein.

OPERATIVE TECHNIQUE

First Stage: Laparoscopic Sleeve Gastrectomy

The surgical technique of a complete LBPD–DS has been described previously.[13,14] Patients are positioned with the legs split in reverse, the Trendelenburg position, with assurance of proper support to the extremities. The surgeon stands between the legs, with the assistants on both sides. Seven ports are inserted routinely. Pneumoperitoneum is established to 15 mm Hg and a 30° angled scope is used. The short gastric vessels of the greater curvature and ret-

rogastric attachments are divided with a sealer/divider instrument (LigaSure, Valleylab, Boulder, CO). The dissection extends proximally to the esophagogastric junction and distally toward the pylorus. The antrum is preserved and greater curvature of the stomach is divided 8–10 cm from the pylorus. This procedure is performed using two firings of 60 mm, green cartridge (4.8-mm staple height) endoscopic linear stapler (Tyco Healthcare, Norwalk, CO). A 60F Maloney bougie is then inserted transorally and aligned along the lesser curvature. A vertical subtotal, sleeve gastrectomy is then fashioned along the lesser curvature 1 cm away from the bougie toward the esophagogastric junction. This procedure is performed with multiple firings of a 60-mm blue cartridge (3–5-mm staple height) endoscopic linear stapler. To decrease blood loss from the transected gastric plane, a reinforcement absorbable polymer membrane (Seamguard, Gore, Flagstaff, AZ) is used with the stapler.[15] Use of bovine pericardial strips is then discontinued because of an intraluminal migration seen in the patient (Peristrips, Synovis Life Technologies, St. Paul, MN).[16] The resected stomach is retrieved by way of the right paramedian trocar site with a large plastic impermeable bag (Tyco Healthcare, Norwalk, CO). The bougie is removed and replaced with an orogastric tube for a methylene blue study. The proximal duodenum is compressed with atraumatic instruments to allow stomach distension with dye, which suggests the pouch size to be in the range of 100–150 mi. Fascia closure of all port sites 10 mm or larger is accomplished with a fascia closure device (Karl Storz, Tutlingen, Germany).

Second Stage: Laparoscopic Duodenoileostomy/Ileoileostomy

Patients return for the second-stage procedure after significant weight loss with a minimal interval time of 6 months. Operative setting, trocar placement, and surgical instruments are similar to that of the first stage; however, some incisions have to be created lower because of the rapid loss of abdominal fat following the first procedure. The gastrocolic ligament from the distal antrum to the proximal duodenum is divided using ultrasonic dissector (LCS, Ethicon-endosurgery, Cincinnati, OH). The operative plane is immediately adjacent to the stomach to avoid injury to the duodenal vessels. A small window is opened in the inferior border of the proximal duodenum and a retroduodenal plane developed. This step is critical and the most distal dissection of the duodenum is stopped when the anterior pancreatic tissue joins the duodenal wall. Superiorly, this dissection is performed between the common bile duct, laterally, and hepatic artery, medially. The superior arterial arcade is preserved to prevent a severe ischemia of the duodenopyloric area. A 45-mm white cartridge (2.5-mm staple height) linear stapler is used to transect the duodenum. Surgical clips for hemostasis are avoided at the proximal stump to prevent interference with the circular stapler, often used to fashion the duodenoileostomy. Using a transoral technique, the anvil of a 25-mm circular end-to-end anastomosis (CEEA) (Tyco Healthcare, Norwalk, CO) device is placed in a flip-top position, anchored to a transected 18F nasogastric tube and advanced using techniques described previously. The anvil is brought out through a small enterotomy made in the midduodenal stump and advanced gently beyond the pylorus. Using a 50-cm umbilical tape measured previously, the ileum is measured 100 cm proximally and marked with a suture on the antimesenteric border. An additional 150 cm is measured and the bowel divided with a 60-mm white cartridge linear stapler. Using an ultrasonic dissector (LCS), the mesenteric fat of the transected ileum is partially divided between vessels and the distal stump opened. The skin and fascia of the right paramedian port is enlarged to accommodate insertion of a 25-mm CEEA device stapler. A sterile camera bag is placed routinely around this device to protect the wound from the contaminated stapler upon removal. The circular stapler is advanced into the lumen at a minimum of 10 cm, and the unit is brought antecolic in a clockwise manner toward the anvil. The spike is advanced under mild tension on the antimesenteric side and removed. The stapler is then coupled with the spike of the anvil and fired. The sterile camera bag is advanced over the entire stapler, then removed. The opened distal stump is closed with several firings of the 45-mm white cartridge (2.5-mm staple height) linear stapler. Alternatively, a linear stapler with primary closure of the enterotomy can be used to fashion the proximal anastomosis. A methylene blue test is then performed with occlusion of bowel distal to the anastomosis. The alimentary limb is followed to the marking suture or clip placed previously. The transected proximal ileum can be located easily by following the mesentery. A side-to-side ileoileostomy is then performed with a 60-mm white cartridge linear stapler (USSC, Norfolk, CO). The enterotomy is then closed with running #2-0 silk sutures. Both mesenteric defects (ileoileostomy and Petersen's space) are closed with a running #2-0 silk suture.

RESULTS

Patients

From September 2000 to September 2001, 33 patients underwent first-stage LBPD–DS with LSG. Of these patients, 23 completed the second stage: LDI–II. Data from 18 patients with BMI greater than, or equal to, 60 kg/m^2 completing the two-stage LBPD–DS were collected prospectively and reviewed retrospectively.

Eighteen patients completed the two-stage LBPD–DS. The patients were 13 women and 5 men, with a mean age of 41 years (range 25–56 years). Preoperative BMI was 65.8 $\pm$ 4.7 kg/m^2 (range 60.2–75.7 kg/m^2), weight was 187 $\pm$ 26 kg (range 154–227 kg), and percentage above ideal body weight was 305% $\pm$ 24.0% (range 281%–365%). Cardiopulmonary or metabolic comorbidities existed in 12 patients (66.7%). Three patients had a previous cholecystectomy—two with a laparoscopic and one with an open approach. In addition to a large right subcostal incision, the latter patient also had a midline ventral hernia repair, which necessitated extensive laparoscopic lysis of adhesions at surgery. Two additional patients had secondary procedures performed at the time of LSG—one cholecystectomy with intraoperative cholangiogram and one hysterectomy for chronic anemia due to menorrhagia. The median operative time for LSG, excluding the three patients with secondary procedures, was 97 $\pm$ 28 minutes (range 66–175 minutes). Blood loss was minimal. No conversions to laparotomy were noted. Hospital stay averaged 3 days (range: 2–5 days). A 20.0% decrease in BMI and 30.5% EBWL was noted during 6 months. No deaths and no major complications followed LSG. One patient developed a superficial wound infection at a port site and was treated with a course of oral antibiotics.

The second-stage procedure was performed between 71 and 321 (median 196) days after the first. The data at the time of the second stage was BMI 50.7 $\pm$ 5.9 kg/m^2, weight 144 $\pm$ 21 kg, EBWL 31.5% $\pm$ 9.7%, and the percentage above was 239.0% $\pm$ 31.0%. Minimal adhesions to the stapled stomach were noted after the first-stage procedure. The median operative time was 141 $\pm$ 37.7 minutes. No conversions to laparotomy were noted. The mean hospital stay was 3 days (range 2–9 days). Analysis of the data disclosed that 56.0% ($N = 10$) of patients had a 3-month follow-up and 22.0% ($N = 4$) had a 6-month follow-up. Again, no morbidity or mortality was noted. One late major complication was that one patient developed deep vein thrombosis (DVT) of the

Table 30–1.

Laparoscopic Sleeve Gastrectomy Versus Intragastric Ballon

Author		N	Preop BMI (kg/m^2)	Follow-up (months)	Mean Weight (kg)	% EWL	BMI Loss (kg/m^2)	Final BMI (kg/m^2)
Busetto[10]	BIB	43	58.4	5.4	171	26.1	9.4	49
Weiner[8]	BIB	17	60.2	4	195	21	6.4	53.8
Gagner	LSG	20	68.9	6	200	34.9	15.9	53.0

BMI, body mass index; BIB, bioenterics intragastric balloon; LSG, laparoscopic sleeve gastrectomy.

posterior tibial vein 3 months after the second-stage procedure and was hospitalized for systemic heparinization and empiric caval filter placement. He became rapidly deconditioned, hypoproteinemic, and required parenteral nutrition. Otherwise, this series showed no wound infection, anastomotic leakage, or incision hernia.

Comorbidities were improved overall. All four patients who required diabetes management before were off hypoglycemic medications, insulin, or both. One patient had intermittent biliary colic without evidence of cholelithiasis. She was placed on ursodiol (Actigall, Ciba-Geigy, Summit, NJ) for gallstone prophylaxis, and her symptoms disappeared. An overall 46.8% decrease in BMI and 68.5% change of EBWL were noted from the first stage to 6 months after the second stage. When data were combined from a total of 36 procedures in 18 patients, no mortality, one minor complication of wound infection (2.8%), and a major late complication of deep vein thrombosis with subsequent transient hypoproteinemia were noted in the same patient.

DISCUSSION

Although impressive EBWL is seen, BPD patients have significant nutritional and metabolic complications that warrant modifications of the original Scopinaro procedure.[17,18] BPD–DS is a hybrid bariatric procedure of restriction and malabsorption. In the 1990s, Hess, Marceau, and colleagues published their experiences with BPD–DS with modifications, which included a vertical subtotal gastrectomy, pylorus-preserving DS, and elongation of the common channel length.[4–6] Again, excellent and sustainable weight loss was achieved and, in properly selected patients, the morbidity and mortality rates were acceptable and compatible to that of the more commonly performed Roux-en-Y gastric bypass.

Super-superobese patients (BMI > 60 kg/m^2) are on the extreme end of the spectrum of morbid obesity with all its ramifications. Although BPD–DS could achieve excellent weight loss with acceptable risks in obese patients, review of the authors' open BPD–DS patients with BMI greater than 60 kg/m^2 ($N = 28$) showed 17.0% morbidity and 3.5% mortality rates.[7] A laparoscopic approach in this population is potentially beneficial from the cardiovascular, pulmonary, infectious, and wound-healing point of view.[8,9] However, the authors' review of more than 30 super-superobese patients who underwent LBPD–DS showed 7 (23.0%) morbidities and 2 (6.5%) deaths among these patients.[7] Neither open nor laparoscopic one-stage approaches have been satisfactory in this group of patients.

Gratifying to see is that these dreadful statistics drastically reduced to zero mortality and 5.6% total morbidity rates by separating the operative procedures based on its two distinctive components—restriction and malabsorption. Patients did not encounter any increased anesthesia risks by having the procedure staged into two operations. In fact, many of these patients returned with improved or cured comorbidities and significant EBWL. Patients were able to better tolerate pneumoperitoneum and operative-table positioning adjustments without hemodynamic compromise. Operative exposure was greatly improved because of the significant weight loss in the anterior abdominal wall, which facilitated pneumoperitoneum. Each procedure seems to pose a smaller risk for the patient. An early convalescence without complications allowed the patients to be motivated in their dietary change and attitude toward weight loss. When they returned for the second stage, patients often reported improved comorbidities that would otherwise have added extra risk to their surgery. These patients have almost no reserve for any type of physiologic challenge and a minor problem could rapidly develop into major morbidity and mortality. Could these improved results be an effect of the learning curve? Possibly, the learning curve is a complex phenomenon that includes not only technical improvement but also better judgment in selecting appropriate patients. Perhaps the two-stage operation in itself is the result of this maturation process.

Recently, Almogy et al. reported a series of 21 patients who underwent longitudinal gastrectomy for treatment of morbid obesity.[19] Preoperative mean BMI was 56 kg/m^2. Of these patients, 9 were offered the procedure preoperatively because of known high perioperative risks, and in 12 an LBPD–DS was planned but because of intraoperative findings or hemodynamic instability they received an LSG. Five patients developed complications, but no deaths occurred. With a median follow-up of 17.5 months, the median weight loss at 12 months was 45.1%. After a year, 40.0% of the patients had achieved more than 50.0% excess weight loss. Baltasar reported different indications in 31 patients who underwent LSG: 7 procedures were done as a first stage of the DS, 7 cases as the only alternative in very high risk patients, 16 cases of patients with a BMI from 35 to 43, and 1 LSG as revisional surgery for gastric banding.[20] One patient died due to intra-abdominal bleeding (3.2%). The EBWL was 56.0% (4–27 months after the LSG) in the superobese group. However, patients with lower BMI had an EWL of 62.0%. Mognol et al. performed LSG in 10 patients with a BMI more than 60 kg/m^2.[21] They reported no conversions, no morbidity, or no mortality. EWL after 1 year was 51.0%. They concluded that LSG was an attractive first-step procedure and an acceptable one-stage restrictive procedure if long-term results are good.

Why is the LSG so successful? The smaller longitudinal gastric pouch restricts food intake mechanically, which prevents overeating in the first 6–12 months postoperatively. In fact, the role of the gastric pouch in weight control is complex and involves satiety-regulating mechanisms. The hypothesis that explains the role of the gastric pouch in satiety emphasizes the importance of stretching walls with eating or drinking. The signals from wall receptors in the stomach are relayed by neural pathways to the appetite centers in the brain.[22] Successful maintenance of satiety may depend on the neurohormonal gut–brain axis. Ghrelin, a recently discovered orexigenic hormone secreted primarily by the fundus of the stomach, has been implicated in both mealtime hunger and long-term regulation of body weight.[23–26] LSG may contribute to weight loss by decreasing ghrelin secretion, increasing satiety, and regulating gastric emptying.[27] Increased weight lost with the LSG with DS suggests that gastrectomy contributes to weight loss itself.[28] The role of longitudinal gastrectomy in weight control has also been confirmed in an animal model.[29]

Other authors have used different methods to achieve initial weight loss in high-risk patients. The intragastric balloon was described by Nieben and Harboe to produce food intake restriction in obese patients.[30] With time, new, smooth, spherical saline-filled balloons became available (Bioenterics Intragastric Balloon, BIB) and accepted in some countries as an option for first-stage treatment for weight loss. The BIB seems to be an attractive alternative, especially in high-risk patients, because of its simplicity.[31] Milone et al. compared a series of LSG retrospectively with two series of BIB.[32] The mean BMI was 68.8 kg/m^2 for the LSG series, 60.2 kg/m^2 for the Weiner et al.[33] series, and 58.4 kg/m^2 for Busetto et al.[34] series. No procedure-related complications were reported except for 1 trocar infection in the LSG. However, four (7.0%) patients had the BIB removed: one for balloon dysfunction, one for abdominal pain, and two for noncompliance. One patient had spontaneous elimination of the balloon in the stools. The EWL at 6 months for the LSG was 34.9% compared to 26.0% and 21.0% for the two BIB series. They concluded that LSG allowed a more rapid and greater weight loss compared to the BIB, and although it is a procedure that requires a 2–3-day hospital stay it can be performed safely with one minor complication. However, although the BIB is an ambulatory procedure, it carried a risk of intolerance and bad quality of life. However, they concluded that both procedures were effective as a first stage for patients.

Dapri et al. presented a prospective randomized trial in 80 patients that compared laparoscopic adjustable banding and LSG.[35] After 1 year, the mean excess weight loss was 36.0% for the banding group and 56.0% for the LSG group ($p < 0.002$). They reported a loss of feeling of hunger in 75.0% of the LSG patients compared to 42.5% in the banding group ($p < 0.007$). However, they reported gastroesophageal reflux in 22.0% of the LSG compared to 9.0% in the banding group. They also observed a higher reoperation rate in the banding patients for complications of the system. Langer et al. observed a significant decrease of plasma ghrelin at 1 and 6 months after LSG.[27] Ghrelin remained unchanged in the banding patients. LSG patients achieved a 61.0% EWL compared to 28.0% in the banding group ($p < 0.001$) at 6 months.

Why not just stop there after a successful LSG and cancel the second stage, the LDI–II? Similar to vertical-banded gastroplasty, gastric pouch dilatation is anticipated. Dilatation may be a result of an excessively large pouch created at the initial operation because of missed posterior gastric folds.[36] Excessive pressure against the pouch walls by large meals, repeated vomiting, or distal obstruction leads to its dilatation. Increasing proximal-pouch diameter may also be a result of hiatal hernia, missed preoperatively or intraoperatively.[37] An adequate patient selection and appropriate surgical technique may not prevent pouch dilatation. The pouch expansion may be controlled by external wrapping, or with an external silastic ring support as proposed by Fobi in gastric bypass.[38,39] It is unlikely that a laparoscopic adjustable gastric banding will be useful to prevent gastric dilatation, because it is known as a frequent complication of this method,[40] and when used in superobese patients, a lesser percent of EWL is achieved at 1 year.[41]

Despite the impressive weight-loss data with BPD–DS for the super morbidly obese patients, many surgeons and patients are cognizant of the potentially life-threatening hypoproteinemia and metabolic derangement like hypocalcemia. This risk is decreased in BPD–DS compared to BPD. Protein malnutrition is the main early problem with BPD, and gastric volume greatly influences the incidence of hypoproteinemia: the smaller the stomach, the greater the risk.[18] Malnutrition states have been measured and identified in the "very little stomach" biliopancreatic bypass, and persist even 1 year after surgery.[18]

A recent report by Marceau and colleagues has confirmed that bone demineralization is not encountered 10 years later when patients are supplemented with regular oral calcium and when parathyroid hormone levels are maintained below 100.[42] Nonetheless, for the severely morbidly obese patients, a less-extreme measure of weight loss has been explored. Brolin et al. showed that the long limb Roux-en-Y gastric bypass results in better weight loss than the standard Roux-en-Y bypass without an increased morbidity and mortality in the superobese.[43] Recently, Sugerman and colleagues published their experience with malabsorptive distal gastric bypass (DGB) for failed standard gastric bypass, in 27 superobese patients.[44] Five had a common channel of 50 cm, and 22 had a common channel of 150 cm, with an alimentary limb of 250 cm. All of the former 5 patients had to be reversed due to severe malnutrition, of whom 2 died of hepatic failure. In addition, 3 of the 22 patients who had the longer common channel had to be reversed and needed nutritional support for protein malnutrition. These results show that DGB has a worse protein deficiency rate (14.0%) than BPD–DS (1.0–2.0%), with a higher long-term complication rate. In 3 adolescents who underwent a DGB, 1 had to be reversed to a standard gastric bypass due to severe malnutrition. Even Sugerman and colleagues, long-time proponents of gastric bypass, stated recently in the same paper that late weight regain after gastric bypass is a concern in this study and perhaps the DS procedure may provide longer-lasting benefit.[45]

CONCLUSION

In conclusion, the staged procedures of LSG and LDI–II is our preferred surgical option in the super-superobese patients, because this alternative is both safe and effective. It has resulted in a drastic reduction of morbidity and mortality compared to the traditional one-stage approach for super-superobese patients.

References

1. Gentileschi P, Kini S, Catarci M, Gagner M: Evidence-based medicine: Open and laparoscopic bariatric surgery. *Surg Endosc* 16(5):736–744, 2002.

2. MacLean LD, Rhode BM, Nohr CW: Late outcome of isolated gastric bypass. *Ann Surg* 231(4):524–528, 2000.

3. Sugerman HJ, Londrey GL, Kellum JM, et al.: Weight loss with vertical banded gastroplasty and Roux-en-Y gastric bypass for morbid obesity with selective versus random assignment. *Am J Surg* 157(1):93–102, 1989.

4. Hess DS, Hess DW: Biliopancreatic diversion with a duodenal switch. *Obes Surg* 8(3):267–282, 1998.

5. Marceau S, Biron S, Lagace M, et al.: Biliopancreatic diversion, with distal gastrectomy, 250 cm and 50 cm limbs: long-term results. *Obes Surg* 5(3):302–307, 1995.

6. Marceau P, Hould FS, Simard S, et al.: Biliopancreatic diversion with duodenal switch. *World J Surg* 22(9):947–954, 1998.

7. Kim WW, Gagner M, Kini S, et al.: Laparoscopic vs. open biliopancreatic diversion with duodenal switch: A comparative study. *J Gastrointest Surg* 7(4):552–557, 2003.

8. Nguyen NT, Ho HS, Palmer LS, Wolfe BM: A comparison study of laparoscopic versus open gastric bypass for morbid obesity. *J Am Coll Surg* 191(2):149–155, 2000; discussion: 155–157.

9. Nguyen NT, Goldman C, Rosenquist CJ, et al.: Laparoscopic versus open gastric bypass: A randomized study of outcomes, quality of life, and costs. *Ann Surg* 234(3):279–289, 2001; discussion: 289–291.

10. Ren CJ, Patterson E, Gagner M: Early results of laparoscopic biliopancreatic diversion with duodenal switch: A case series of 40 consecutive patients. *Obes Surg* 10(6):514–523, 2000; discussion: 524.

11. de Csepel J, Burpee S, Jossart G, et al.: Laparoscopic biliopancreatic diversion with a duodenal switch for morbid obesity: A feasibility study in pigs. *J Laparoendosc Adv Surg Tech A* 11(2):79–83, 2001.

12. Rubino F, Gagner M: Potential of surgery for curing type 2 diabetes mellitus. *Ann Surg* 236(5):554–559, 2002.

13. Ren CJ, Cabrera I, Rajaram K, Fielding GA: Factors influencing patient choice for bariatric operation. *Obes Surg* 15(2):202–206, 2005.

14. Feng JJ, Gagner M: Laparoscopic biliopancreatic diversion with duodenal switch. *Semin Laparosc Surg* 9(2):125–129, 2002.

15. Consten EC, Gagner M, Pomp A, Inabnet WB: Decreased bleeding after laparoscopic sleeve gastrectomy with or without duodenal switch for morbid obesity using a stapled buttressed absorbable polymer membrane. *Obes Surg* 14(10):1360–1366, 2004.

16. Consten EC, Dakin GF, Gagner M: Intraluminal migration of bovine pericardial strips used to reinforce the gastric staple-line in laparoscopic bariatric surgery. *Obes Surg* 14(4):549–554, 2004.

17. Scopinaro N, Adami GF, Marinari GM, et al.: Biliopancreatic diversion. *World J Surg* 22(9):936–946, 1998.

18. Gianetta E, Friedman D, Adami GF, et al.: Etiological factors of protein malnutrition after biliopancreatic diversion. *Gastroenterol Clin North Am* 16(3):503–504, 1987.

19. Almogy G, Crookes PF, Anthone GJ: Longitudinal gastrectomy as a treatment for the high-risk super-obese patient. *Obes Surg* 14(4):492–497, 2004.

20. Baltasar A, Serra C, Perez N, et al.: Laparoscopic sleeve gastrectomy: A multipurpose bariatric operation. *Obes Surg* 15(8):1124–1128, 2005.

21. Mognol P, Chosidow D, Marmuse JP: Laparoscopic sleeve gastrectomy as an initial bariatric operation for high-risk patients: Initial results in 10 patients. *Obes Surg* 15(7):1030–1033, 2005.

22. Flanagan L: Understanding the function of the small gastric pouch. In: Deitel M, et al. (ed.): *Update: Surgery for the Morbidly Obese Patients*. Toronto, ON, FD-Communications, 2000;pp. 147–160, Chapter 18.

23. Cummings DE, Weigle DS, Frayo RS, et al.: Plasma ghrelin levels after diet-induced weight loss or gastric bypass surgery. *N Engl J Med* 346(21):1623–1630, 2002.

24. Date Y, Kojima M, Hosoda H, et al.: Ghrelin, a novel growth hormone-releasing acylated peptide, is synthesized in a distinct endocrine cell type in the gastrointestinal tracts of rats and humans. *Endocrinology* 141(11):4255–4261, 2000.

25. Kojima M, Hosoda H, Date Y, et al.: Ghrelin is a growth-hormone-releasing acylated peptide from stomach. *Nature* 402(6762):656–660, 1999.

26. Nakazato M, Murakami N, Date Y, et al.: A role for ghrelin in the central regulation of feeding. *Nature* 409(6817):194–198, 2001.

27. Langer FB, Reza Hoda MA, Bohdjalian A, et al.: Sleeve gastrectomy and gastric banding: Effects on plasma ghrelin levels. *Obes Surg* 15(7):1024–1029, 2005.

28. Lagace M, Marceau P, Marceau S, et al.: Biliopancreatic diversion with a new type of gastrectomy: Some previous conclusions revisited. *Obes Surg* 5(4):411–418, 1995.

29. Papachristou D, Fotiadis C, Baramily B, et al.: Prevention of obesity in swine by longitudinal gastrectomy. *Ann Chir* 42(5):357–359, 1988.

30. Nieben OG, Harboe H: Intragastric balloon as an artificial bezoar for treatment of obesity. *Lancet* 1(8265):198–199, 1982.

31. Genco A, Bruni T, Doldi SB, et al.: BioEnterics intragastric balloon: The Italian experience with 2515 patients. *Obes Surg* 15(8):1161–1164, 2005.

32. Milone L, Strong V, Gagner M: Laparoscopic sleeve gastrectomy is superior to endoscopic intragastric balloon as a first stage procedure for super-obese patients (BMI) > or = 50). *Obes Surg* 15(5):612–617, 2005.

33. Weiner R, Gutberlet H, Bockhorn H: Preparation of extremely obese patients for laparoscopic gastric banding by gastric-balloon therapy. *Obes Surg* 9(3):261–264, 1999.

34. Busetto L, Segato G, De Luca M, et al.: Preoperative weight loss by intragastric balloon in super-obese patients treated with laparoscopic gastric banding: A case-control study. *Obes Surg* 14(5):671–676, 2004.

35. Dapri JH, de Bilde D, Leman G, Cadiere GB: A prospective randomized trial between the band gastroplasty and the sleeve gastrectomy: Results after 1 Year. In: *13 International Congress of the European Association for Endoscopic Surgery*. 2005; p. 112. Oral presentation 0172.

36. Deitel GC (ed.): *Update: Surgery for the Morbidly Obese Patients*. FD-Communications, 2000; Chapter 16, p. 135 and Chapter 20, p. 171.

37. Wilson LJ, Ma W, Hirschowitz BI: Association of obesity with hiatal hernia and esophagitis. *Am J Gastroenterol* 94(10):2840–2844, 1999.

38. Fobi MA, Lee H, Felahy B, et al.: Choosing an operation for weight control, and the transected banded gastric bypass. *Obes Surg* 15(1):114–121, 2005.

39. Fobi MA: Placement of the GaBP ring system in the banded gastric bypass operation. *Obes Surg* 15(8):1196–1201, 2005.

40. de Csepel J, Quinn T, Pomp A, Gagner M: Conversion to a laparoscopic biliopancreatic diversion with a duodenal switch for failed laparoscopic adjustable silicone gastric banding. *J Laparoendosc Adv Surg Tech A* 12(4):237–240, 2002.

41. Dolan K, Hatzifotis M, Newbury L, Fielding G: A comparison of laparoscopic adjustable gastric banding and biliopancreatic diversion in superobesity. *Obes Surg* 14(2):165–169, 2004.

42. Marceau P, Biron S, Lebel S, et al.: Does bone change after biliopancreatic diversion? *J Gastrointest Surg* 6(5):690–698, 2002.

43. Brolin RE, Kenler HA, Gorman JH, Cody RP: Long-limb gastric bypass in the superobese. A prospective randomized study. *Ann Surg* 215(4):387–395, 1992.

44. Sugerman HJ, Kellum JM, DeMaria EJ: Conversion of proximal to distal gastric bypass for failed gastric bypass for superobesity. *J Gastrointest Surg* 1(6):517–525, 1997.

45. Sugerman HJ, Sugerman EL, DeMaria EJ, et al.: Bariatric surgery for severely obese adolescents. *J Gastrointest Surg* 7(1):102–107, 2003; discussion: 107–108.

Laparoscopic Reoperative Surgery

31

Restrictive Procedures: Adjustable Gastric Band

Mitiku Belachew, MD

BACKGROUND

In its early days, bariatric surgery proved it could generate effective weight loss.[1,2] Conventional laparotomic surgery, however, presented a greater risk of morbidity and mortality in severely obese patients.[1,3] Then, with the laparoscopic explosion, came the challenge: Laparoscopy created the hope of a minimally invasive solution to these at-risk patients but laparoscopic surgery was still considered a contraindication for this group of patients due to a deep operative field, massive visceral fat, hypertrophic and steatotic liver, and inadequate instrumentation. So, the challenge—and the opportunity— became overcoming the technical difficulties to create a surgical treatment that would be both effective and safe.

Thus, laparoscopic banding for the treatment of morbid obesity was born in 1991. Along with the manufacturer, Inamed Health, we worked through the first phase, the Animal Model phase, where we gradually refined the operative technique to the point of standardization and succeeded in creating the laparoscopic adjustable gastric band. Satisfied that the first phase was complete, we presented a video of laparoscopic banding in pigs at the June 1993 meeting of the American Society for Bariatric Surgery. The concept was received with great enthusiasm and we moved on to the second phase.[4]

We submitted a protocol for the device's application in human models to the Ethics Committee of the Centre Hospitalier Hutois in Huy, Belgium, where the project was approved unanimously. We then performed the first human laparoscopic adjustable gastric banding (LAGB) on September 1, 1993, in a procedure that lasted 3 hours, with no intra- or postoperative complications.[5] The patient has had good long-term weight loss and is still followed regularly.

From 1993 to 1994, 25 patients underwent this new procedure in the clinical trial program and in March 1994 we conducted the First International Workshop in Belgium with 30 surgeons in attendance. We developed the workshop in conjunction with the manufacturer to include live operations with complete interaction and training in the animal lab to give the participants the opportunity to learn the technique. At this time we also formulated our Ten Commandments (Table 31–1).[6] Since that first training, hundreds of workshops have been held internationally and in the United States. The LAP-BAND was approved in the United States by the Food and Drug Administration in June 2001 and over 200,000 LAP-BANDs have been sold worldwide to date.

The design of the band has changed very little since 1993. Modifications to the access port and evolutionary and technical changes to the surgical procedure have been made, which have significantly reduced the complication rate.

OTHER ADJUSTABLE GASTRIC BANDS

The author's practical experience with LAGB involved the development and implementation of a single device—the LAP-BAND System.[7] Therefore, the main focus of the chapter is on this particular system, although the management of complications after laparoscopic banding is the same for all of the banding systems. Hence, the chapter also applies to the following laparoscopic adjustable gastric bands:

- LAP-BAND, Inamed Health, USA (formerly BioEnterics Corporation).
- Swedish Adjustable Gastric Band, Obtech Medical AG, Switzerland (acquired by Ethicon Endo-Surgery, Inc.—Johnson & Johnson).
- MIDBAND, Médical Innovation Développment, France.
- Heliogast Adjustable Gastric Ring, Hélioscopie, France.
- Others.

INTRODUCTION

Reported complications specific to the adjustable gastric band are early or late.

Early complications

- Gastrointestinal perforation;
- bleeding (hepatic or spleen injury or gastric vessels).

These complications have become very rare.

Late complications

- Pouch dilatation due to over-inflation of band and/or excessive food intake;
- band slippage (gastric prolapse, herniation);
- a combination of pouch dilatation and band slippage;
- band erosion;
- port leakage or migration.

As with any surgical procedure, the incidence of complications decreases with individual surgeon experience (the "learning curve").[8] Additionally, complication rates have generally decreased over the years with improvements in surgical technique.[9,10] Thus, initial rates of band slippage (gastric prolapse) have decreased from the early reported rates of around 22% to less than 5%.[8,11–13] For example, Dargent reported that changing from a perigastric to the pars flaccida procedure produced a decrease in band slippage from 5.2% to 0.6%.[14] This surgeon stated that he had benefited from previous surgeons' experience and was able to achieve low rates of band slippage by placing the band higher from the beginning of his series. Similarly, by changing to the pars flaccida technique, another bariatric surgery group reduced the incidence of gastric prolapse from 15% to 1.8%.[13]

Improper placement of the access port can lead to rotation of up to 180° or to fracture at the tube junction. Satisfactory placement, with suturing to the fascia, ensures access for adjustments, patient comfort and convenience, and stabilization.[10,15] Complications with the access port affect the integrity of the LAP-BAND system and mitigate effective weight loss. However, many problems are preventable.[16]

LAP-BAND erosion is rare and may occur months after placement. One possible cause is minute injury to the gastric wall during the initial procedure.[17] Mortality following LAP-BAND placement is virtually nonexistent and is zero in many series, both large and small.[11,18–28]

It is also noteworthy that reoperation in laparoscopic banding does not have the same significance as in other bariatric surgery procedures. Actually, in more than 80% of the patients the complications can be corrected by minimally invasive (laparoscopic) surgery.[29] Operations such as band removal, band repositioning, and conversion to Roux-en-Y gastric bypass (RYGBP) may be performed laparoscopically after LAP-BAND complications.

ADVANTAGES AND DISADVANTAGES OF THE LAPAROSCOPIC BANDING SYSTEMS

Advantages

The advantages of LAP-BAND are many: It is the safest bariatric surgery in the world today.[30] Its most important effect may be its satiety mechanism that causes patients to feel full after a small meal without becoming hungry between meals, easily facilitating compliance with new dietary rules.

Table 31–1.

Ten Commandments

The recommendations which concerned at least the first 10 procedures the surgeons undertook after their participation at the LAGB workshop were termed the *Ten Commandments*:

1. Make a good patient selection. Avoid dealing with superobese patients. The ideal patient during the learning curve is a female with BMI 40–45 kg/m^2 with gynoid-type obesity.

2. Know all the details of the operation. Study again and again the real-time video of the procedure. Follow the protocol strictly, including patient positioning, surgical technique, and instrumentation.

3. Go back to the animal lab if necessary to improve your laparoscopic skill.

4. Train your surgical colleagues, residents, anesthesiologists, and nurses who are working with you in the operating room. They also should know all the details of the procedure before it starts.

5. Be sure to have adequate instrumentation—a good liver retractor, good cautery hook, a good suction-irrigation.

6. Make sure that a Company's advisor is present. They know the technical details of the operation and can be of help.

7. Do not take any unreasonable risk by persisting in the laparoscopic approach when there is danger. In any of the following conditions, convert to laparotomy:

   Inadequate laparoscopic image where anatomic landmarks of the stomach cannot be well defined; huge fatty liver covering the whole upper abdomen (invisible stomach);

   important and/or uncontrollable bleeding;

   danger of stomach perforation (risky posterior dissection);

   if 2 hours after placement of trocars, establishment of retraction, and position of instruments no progress can be seen in the dissection of the retrogastric space. Have pity on the patient, anesthesiologist, and nursing staff. Avoid marathon operations.

8. If the dissection of the retrogastric space has been difficult and if you have any doubt concerning gastric integrity, ask the anesthesiologist to inject methylene blue through the nasogastric tube. A gastric perforation looked for, discovered, and well managed during the operation may avoid insurmountable problems postoperatively.

9. In the early postoperative days, if a patient complains of abnormal abdominal pain or respiratory problems or if the chart shows moderate fever and/or tachycardia, suspect gastric perforation. We have learned from our conventional bariatric surgery that obese patients do not behave in the same way as nonobese patients in the presence of intra-abdominal sepsis. They often do not complain of pain or show high fever. Abdominal palpation does not show the usual signs of peritonitis. Indirect and nonspecific signs such as respiratory distress and/or tachycardia should be considered seriously as they may mean perforation evolving toward peritonitis. Peritonitis in an obese patient, not managed in time and properly, can result in death. Hence, never hesitate to request a Gastrografin study whenever there is a doubt and ask the radiologist to look for a leak.

10. Do not leave the balloon of the silicone band over-inflated at the operation because this may result in early food intolerance due to postoperative edema. It may also result in pouch dilatation and/or stomach slippage in the postoperative weeks because of high pressure inside the pouch and repeated vomiting. Reduce by half the volume of saline needed to achieve the fourth light on the sensor if used, or leave the balloon empty after calibration. Because of the postoperative edema induced by the use of the cautery hook, the stomach wall may be thicker and the stoma diameter too narrow in the postoperative period. Wait for a capsule to develop around the band before inflation (about 2 months) to obtain an optimal size stoma.

The LAP-BAND is adjustable to the patient's needs and the procedure is completely reversible. Eighty percent of the complications can be managed laparoscopically and, in case of failure, the band can be removed with no adverse sequelae. Mortality is approximately 0.05%.[30]

Intra- and Perioperative Advantages

The procedure is minimally invasive and standardized. Surgeons are trained and fully proctored in the procedure so learning curve issues are minimized and operative complications are infrequent. Pain is minimal, with early ambulation and fast recovery. Hospital stay is short and may be performed as day surgery.

Additionally, gastric banding is purely restrictive so there are none of the nutritional issues that accompany malabsorptive procedures.

Disadvantages

Because adjustable gastric banding is purely restrictive, weight loss may take place more slowly than with procedures that contain a malabsorptive element (RYGBP and biliopancreatic diversion, BPD).[22] This slower weight loss, however, is often mischaracterized as "less weight loss," though in the longer term ($\geq$3 years) LAP-BAND weight loss has been shown to rival the weight loss yielded by RYGBP.[22,30] In fact, there is some evidence to indicate that as time goes on gastric bypass (and vertical banded gastroplasty, VBG) patients begin to regain weight,[31–33] whereas LAP-BAND patients tend to maintain their weight loss or continue to lose.

In addition to the risks inherent in all surgical procedures, there are complications specific to the LAP-BAND procedure. Some can be serious, requiring reoperation and removal of the band or the access port. The most common of these are stomach slippage with dilatation of the pouch, band erosion into the lumen of the stomach, and access port complications. In this chapter we will discuss the causes of these problems and address their remedies.

▮ COMPLICATIONS OF LAP-BAND

How to Avoid Complications

Before talking about the management of complications after Lap-Banding I would like to highly emphasize the importance of taking all available precautions to avoid complications. "Prevention is better than cure."

Good patient and surgeon selection, as well as good surgical technique and follow-up procedures, can go a long way to prevent and minimize complications and to recognize problems before they become serious.

Good Patient Selection

Choosing appropriate candidates for the procedure is crucial to achieving optimal results and avoiding unsatisfactory outcomes.[34]

The first duty of a surgeon is to not harm the patient. We must identify issues early and choose not to operate if there is a significant chance we can do more harm than good or when undesirable outcomes are likely. At the same time, we must be reluctant to exclude anyone from reaping the benefits of this surgery in terms of weight loss, health, and quality of life. A sound and practical balance must be achieved.

The guidelines for bariatric surgery established by the National Institutes of Health[35] and the inclusion criteria set forth by the LAP-BAND's manufacturer and the FDA serve as the basis for patient selection. Essentially, the inclusion

criteria stipulate BMI $\geq$ 40 or 35 kg/m^2 with comorbidities related to the obesity and a documented history of morbid obesity with a number of failed weight loss attempts.

Above all, patients must understand that successful outcomes with LAP-BAND surgery require the partnership of patient, surgeon, and multidisciplinary team. Patients must understand the procedure, have realistic expectations and full comprehension of their role in effecting outcomes—good or bad. Complete information must be disseminated and full discussion must take place to allow the surgeon and the multidisciplinary team to properly assess the patient's understanding of the process and his or her commitment to it. Patients who do not or cannot understand this, or those who see the operation as a "magic bullet" without appreciating the responsibilities involved, over the short term and the long term, are not candidates for this surgery.[34]

Multidisciplinary Approach

Preoperative

The multidisciplinary team is, minimally, made up of primary care physician, surgeon, dietician, and psychologist/psychiatrist. All team members possess expertise not only in their particular fields, but also in the management of obesity. Additional requirements for team members include sensitivity to the special needs of morbidly obese individuals and commitment to the multidisciplinary approach.[36]

Patients meet with each team member individually for evaluation and counseling prior to surgery. A thorough physical examination that includes medical evaluation and diagnostic workup is performed, weight history is taken, and food preferences are recorded. Because life-long changes will be required, the dietician and psychologist begin the diet and behavior modification process prior to surgery. Team conferencing following individual evaluations serves to determine the patient's appropriateness for the surgery and identify individual needs to be considered.

Postoperative

Patients are discharged from the hospital with complete dietary, activity, and medication instructions that are important both in the immediate postoperative period and over the long term. Firm dietary guidelines are crucial in the immediate postoperative period. During the first 2–4 weeks following surgery, the patient is instructed to take only liquids as undue fullness or vomiting while the band is settling into position and the membrane is forming around it could cause a strain on the proximal pouch and contribute to slippage.[37]

Because the capacity for food is substantially reduced, the dietician aids the patient in formulating a diet plan to include all essential nutrients and counsels the patient regarding how to eat to avoid obstruction and other problems. And, as weight loss increases the patient's mobility, enhancing the ability and desire to be more physically active, an exercise therapist may be called upon to assist with an exercise regimen. With such physical and lifestyle changes taking place, patients are encouraged to participate in individual and/or group psychological counseling and in support groups.

The primary physician continues to oversee the patient's physical condition and medication, monitoring co-morbidities and heeding signs of potential complications. The initial surgeon follow-up visit normally takes place 5–8 weeks after surgery, and the first adjustment (addition of saline to the band) may take place at that time. However, if weight loss up to that point has been good and the patient is still experiencing satiety, this first adjustment may be postponed until necessary.[37]

Life-Long Follow-Up

As we have previously noted, successful outcomes from LAP-BAND surgery require the long-term commitment of patient, surgeon, and multidisciplinary team. All parties must remain resolute that the evaluation and care that began preoperatively be continued after surgery and extended indefinitely.

Follow-up requires continuing supervision of weight loss and the appropriate administration of band adjustments. Special circumstances, such as pregnancy and illness, must be accommodated and the band emptied if necessary. Comorbidities and metabolic and nutritional status must be monitored. Food choices, exercise, and behavioral modification must be overseen and modified when necessary. It is the ongoing collaboration with all multidisciplinary team members that provides the comprehensive care necessary for optimal patient outcomes.

Good Technique

Good technique must begin with good surgeon selection and training. This surgery requires both mastery of laparoscopic surgical technique and the ability to manage obese patients for a long term.[38]

Since we began the surgeon training workshops in 1993, it has been the policy of the LAP-BAND's manufacturer (Inamed Health, Santa Barbara, CA) to make the product available only to surgeons who have participated in an approved workshop. And only surgeons with advanced laparoscopic skills and experience (such as Nissen Fundoplication or RYGBP) are invited to attend. Additionally, surgeons must have extensive experience dealing with morbidly obese patients. As a further safeguard, all newly trained surgeons are proctored by an expert LAP-BAND surgeon in their first procedures. The manufacturer takes seriously the imperative to properly prepare surgeons for performing this surgery on such high-risk patients. Advanced workshops are held several times a year for surgeons to improve their skills and to address issues that may arise. The technique taught in the LAP-BAND surgeon training workshops has been modified over the years to render the procedure simple, safe, reproducible, and easily teachable.[13]

Early on, we used the perigastric technique and placed the band somewhat low on the stomach. We subsequently found the dissection rather difficult and plagued by a too-high slippage rate. The now-standardized pars flaccida dissection we teach involves minimal dissection and placement of the band out of the lesser sac, leading to a higher position of the band away from the body of the stomach. The technique is straightforward and has proved to be one of the most important factors in significantly reducing the slippage rate. Other factors we teach to help prevent complications are strict attention to gastric-to-gastric suturing and leaving the band empty for at least 6 weeks after surgery.

Guidelines for Stoma Adjustment

Unlike other bariatric procedures in which the amount of restriction achieved at operation is fixed, the key benefit of the LAP-BAND is its adjustability. Optimal use of this adjustability feature is fundamental to weight loss success. The principle is simple—a properly placed and adjusted band produces prolonged satiety after a small meal, facilitating a major reduction in food intake leading to weight loss. If the band is not properly adjusted, weight loss outcomes will suffer. Therefore, we place a heavy emphasis on proper follow-up and adjustment in our LAP-BAND surgeon workshops.

The simplest and least expensive adjustment is the "in-office," where the surgeon makes adjustment decisions based on weight loss and symptoms. This procedure can be performed by simple palpation and passing a noncoring needle into the port.[37] Radiographic adjustment is less cost effective but permits viewing of the status of esophagus, pouch, outlet, and the entire system. This way, the presence of a complication is immediately apparent and the surgeon is ready to take corrective steps.[37] Determinants of the need for adjustment are the rate of weight loss, the degree to which satiety has been induced, and the presence of symptoms that may suggest obstruction.

Overfilling of the device can lead to complications and underfilling thwarts weight loss. The importance of proper stoma adjustment is taught and emphasized in the surgeon training workshops and recommended adjustment schedules have been published by several expert LAP-BAND surgeons.[37,39,40]

Early Complications

Bleeding and Other Reasons to Discontinue Laparoscopy

The intraoperative section of the instruction I provided in my Ten Commandments for surgeons (the seventh commandment) in their first 10 procedures continues to apply for all procedures and merits (restating here):

Do not take any unreasonable risk by persisting in the laparoscopic approach when there is danger. In any of the following conditions, convert to laparotomy:

- *Inadequate laparoscopic image where anatomic landmarks of the stomach cannot be well defined;*
- *huge fatty liver covering the whole upper abdomen (invisible stomach);*
- *important and/or uncontrollable bleeding;*

- *danger of stomach perforation (risky posterior dissection);*
- *if 2 hours after placement of trocars, establishment of retraction, and position of instruments no progress can be seen in the dissection of the retrogastric space. Have pity on the patient, anesthesiologist, and nursing staff. Avoid marathon operations.*

Perforation and Sepsis

Both gastric and esophageal perforations are possible during gastric banding surgery. The gastric perforation/injury rate for LAP-BAND surgery is approximately 0.8%.[30] Intraoperative perforation, especially on the posterior wall, is an extremely serious complication that, if overlooked, causes leakage, sepsis, and eventual death.[7] Therefore, if the dissection has been difficult and if there is any doubt concerning gastric integrity, methylene blue should be injected through the nasogastric tube. A gastric perforation looked for, discovered, and well managed during the operation may avoid insurmountable problems postoperatively.

Fortunately, the pars flaccida dissection is some distance away from the stomach wall, thus reducing the risk of intraoperative damage to the posterior wall. A Gastrografin swallow performed prior to food or water intake can rule out gastric or esophageal injury.[7] If perforation of the posterior wall is found with the contrast medium, reoperation must be undertaken immediately to suture the perforation and remove the band. It is not advisable to put the band after suturing the perforation as this will enhance septic complications and later be responsible for erosion.

Esophageal perforation can be caused by passage of the orogastric calibration tube during laparoscopic placement of the band. Diagnosed immediately, however, it may be successfully treated laparoscopically with band removal, drainage, and parenteral nutrition.[41]

Acute Obstruction

The major perioperative complication associated with the LAP-BAND placement is acute obstruction immediately after surgery, usually caused by a band that is too tight.[42] In the "old days" of banding we used the Gastrostenometer for perioperative calibration to avoid the outcome of a too-tight stoma. This device, however, is no longer available. The use of the pars flaccida technique may actually have increased the incidence of this complication due to the incorporation of perigastric fat, particularly in patients with greater visceral obesity.[43] Esophagograms performed the day after surgery to document band position and pouch size will also detect the presence of both perforation and obstruction.

Acute esophageal or stoma obstruction can appear with or without gastric slippage. If there is no slippage, the obstruction can usually be managed conservatively. If slippage has occurred, laparoscopic reintervention will be required to remove and replace the band.

Preventing these types of obstructions, however, is highly preferable and can be accomplished during the surgical procedure. The team of Shen and Ren[43] has modified the surgical technique to incorporate the routine removal of the perigastric fat pad during LAP-BAND placement. They have since seen a drastic reduction in their obstruction rate. And Bernante et al.[42] now use the newer, larger 11-cm LAP-BAND for their higher BMI patients and have seen no obstructions since adoption of this practice.

Late Complications

Slippage and Dilatation

Gastric slippage has historically been the most frequently occurring complication associated with LAP-BAND placement.

Two different types of slippage can be identified: anterior and posterior. Anterior slippage occurs when higher pressure in the upper pouch pushes the band downward over the anterior aspect of the stomach. Posterior slippage is the upward herniation of the posterior stomach wall through the band.

Modification of the surgical technique from the perigastric dissection to the pars flaccida has significantly reduced the rate of posterior slippage because the technique of creating the retrogastric tunnel no longer involves the excessive dissection posterior to the stomach.[13,44–49] Dissection is through the pars flaccida, away from the stomach. This allows the band to fit snugly to the posterior aspect of the stomach, without much room for slippage. Chevallier et al.[50] in a study of 1,000 patients saw their slippage rate drop from 24% with the perigastric approach to 2% after adopting the pars flaccida dissection. Dolan and Fielding[51] report a band removal rate of 5.9%. Since the change to pars flaccida from perigastric dissection, the slippage rate has dropped from 14.2% to 1.3%. Still, the complication is not likely to disappear completely.

Slippage should be suspected when a patient who has had a normal postoperative course begins to experience symptoms such as food intolerance, dysphagia, reflux, vomiting, and upper abdominal or back pain.[52,53]

Slippage is accompanied by pouch dilatation. Dilatation, however, may be present without slippage and can be managed conservatively by deflation of the band and dietary instructions. If there is no significant improvement or if symptoms resume after deflation, an esophagogram will confirm or rule out slippage. A true slip is not amenable to conservative treatment and requires surgical intervention, most often laparoscopically, where the band can be removed and replaced. Some surgeons have managed to laparoscopically salvage the LAP-BAND and reposition it, although this tactic is not recommended by the manufacturer. Another alternative is conversion to RYGBP.

Erosion

Erosion is defined as the partial or complete movement of the band into the gastric lumen of the stomach. It is a well-known yet uncommon complication of adjustable gastric banding, with a rate of occurrence that has remained at approximately 1%–2%[54] since development of the band over 12 years ago.

Band erosion is a serious complication, however, as it always requires reoperation and removal of the band.

Symptoms are almost always benign, nonurgent, and non-life-threatening and the erosion may only be found by gastroscopy.[55] A problem may first present as lack of satiety and cessation of weight loss, even after induction of additional saline into the band. At times, the condition may manifest as back or shoulder pain, with or without fever. The first indication may be an infected port site, especially if it is protracted and unresponsive to drainage or antibiotics.

One of the causes of gastric erosion may be undetected intraoperative microperforation or other surgical damage to the gastric wall. A port site infection traveling up the tube to contaminate the band may also cause erosion. And anything that places excessive stress on the upper pouch—overeating, vomiting, or overfilling of the band—may be a causative or contributory factor.

Again, the key to managing erosion is prevention. Surgeons must have the necessary laparoscopic skill and experience; strict attention to the technical details of the surgical procedure is critical in order to prevent intraoperative injury or detect and repair it immediately, should it occur; correct band placement is essential—it must be left empty, not be too tight, and there must be no suturing to stomach. Of course, regular and long-term follow-up will prevent and diagnose problems early.

Erosion always requires revisional surgery, although rarely on an urgent basis. In the past, management involved band removal and suturing of the stomach wall, followed by several months' healing time and delayed replacement at a third operation.[56] More recently, surgeons have found that the erosion can be treated safely with simultaneous laparoscopic band removal, gastric wall suturing, and immediate replacement of the band, thereby averting weight gain, the reappearance of comorbidities, and the need for additional surgery.[55] And, because the LAP-BAND procedure has not altered the anatomy and there has been no cutting or stapling, even an immediate conversion to another procedure such as RYGBP can be accomplished with low morbidity rates.[57]

Port-Related Complications

Correct placement of the port and its secure fixation are important aspects of the surgical procedure.[58] After band placement is completed, the reservoir is fixed to the anterior abdominal wall in the subcutaneous space and is connected by a radiopaque tube to an inflatable band that is placed around the proximal part of the stomach. Its purpose is to be punctured percutaneously postsurgery at fixed intervals to inject or withdraw normal saline in order to adjust the diameter of the band, thus the degree of gastric restriction.[59] The access port is an essential part of the LAP-BAND system as it enables one of its major benefits—adjustability.

Access port complications are usually minor but can be serious enough to negate the procedure's purpose, which is, of course, weight loss. The inability to adjust the band may result in failure of the operation.[60] Most port complications are considered minor because they are rarely life threatening and usually do not require an abdominal reoperation. Sometimes, however, they do necessitate a reoperation at the port site, and occasionally at the level of the band, which may require removal. Reoperation at the port site creates new risks of port site infection, and port repair/replacement may require general anesthesia, which exposes the patient to new risks.[61]

Prevention of access port complications must include strict attention to correct placement and anchoring of the port as well as the meticulous maintenance of sterility during surgery and adjustments. The most frequently reported complications related to the port site are port site infection, tubing disconnection with port dislodgement, and tubing leaks.

Port Site Infection

Infection of the injection port must be diagnosed promptly in order to prevent the infection from diffusing to the rest of the device, which may lead to the removal of the entire band. Again, sterility cannot be overemphasized. Additionally, port site infection may be an early sign of band erosion.[61]

Tubing Disconnection and Port Dislodgement

Incorrect placement of the port could be the cause of port disconnection from the band and connecting tube.[62] According to Spivak,[58] tunneling the access port along the left subcostal area is an important technique to protect the port system from breaking. And, by changing the access port tube position from vertical to horizontal in relation to the abdominal wall movement protects from "wear and tear" forces. Plus, the addition of fixation at the subxiphoidal location helps maintain a straight orientation of the access port for easier adjustments.

Tubing Leaks

Puncture of the tube can lead to a leak at the level of the connections. A leaking tube may be suspected with cessation of weight loss in a patient who had previously been losing weight. Change of the port may be required but can usually be accomplished under local anesthesia.

REOPERATIONS

Expertise in performing reoperations for complications or insufficient weight loss is an essential part of any bariatric surgery practice. Even as all appropriate steps are taken preoperatively, intraoperatively, and postoperatively, procedures will sometimes fail and surgeons must become skilled at both repairing complications and in converting to other procedures when the need arises.

The rate of revisional surgery following LAP-BAND is similar to that of other forms of bariatric surgery.[51] LAP-BAND failure can be defined as band removal due to lack of weight loss or a complication. The LAP-BAND failure rate is approximately 5%, similar to other forms of bariatric surgery.[51] The most common reasons for reoperation are intraoperative injury/perforation, slippage/dilatation, insufficient weight loss, persistent dysphagia, persistent port infection, and patient request.

Because the LAP-BAND as a primary bariatric operation is minimally invasive and leaves the anatomy intact, most reoperations can be accomplished laparoscopically with low increased risk to the patient. Should the primary LAP-BAND procedure fail, the available remedies are: band removal, band repositioning (when appropriate), band removal with replacement, and band removal with conversion to another procedure. Most times the removal and the replacement can take place within the same laparoscopic procedure. Patients who have undergone successful revision after complications from LAP-BAND have scored highly in the Moorehead-Ardelt part of the BAROS quality-of-life test.

Techniques of Laparoscopic Reoperations After Lap-Band

The basic techniques of laparoscopic reoperations after laparoscopic banding may be summarized as follows.

1. *Laparoscopic access to the operation site*: The importance of adhesion is variable from one patient to the other. The adhesion could be very loose and easy to remove in some cases and tough and organic in others, especially if there has been sepsis (erosion). It is essential to proceed methodically and have good exposure at all times. Cautery hook and scissors may suffice in most cases but the use of ultrasonic dissector may be useful. Adhesiolysis with the liver, the omentum, the stomach, and the diaphragm should be undertaken carefully until the band is visualized.
2. *Removal of the band*: Once the adhesion has been freed up to the buckle of the band, removal of the band and the tubing is relatively easy. The band is cut anywhere on its body and pooled out of the capsula. Some surgeons have managed to open the LAP-BAND laparoscopically and reposition it, although this tactic is not recommended by the manufacturer. The reason for reusing the band is based on the fact that in many places the patient must pay for the new band, a sometimes unbearable burden.
3. *Perform a new bariatric procedure*: Once the LAP-BAND is safely and successfully removed, another bariatric procedure may be considered. Whatever the procedure, the new site on the stomach (band placement or stomach transaction) should be outside the initial band site. It is essential to make sure that the integrity of the organs (the stomach) has been respected after the extensive dissection prior to the new procedure. Again I would like to reiterate the Ten Commandments (number 8): *If the surgeon has any doubt concerning gastric integrity, he/she should ask the anesthesiologist to inject methylene blue through the*

nasogastric tube. A gastric perforation looked for, discovered, and well managed during the operation may avoid insurmountable problems postoperatively. If there has been perforation and/or the procedure is nonfeasible with safety, conversion to laparotomy or a two-step operation may be envisaged. The type of bariatric procedure will depend on the surgeon's/patient's preference and the character of the complication as well as the local perioperative anatomy.

Band Removal

A procedure to remove the band due to a complication or patient request can almost always be accomplished laparoscopically and the anatomy will return to its original form. Patients must be advised, however, that without rebanding or conversion to another procedure, the lack of restriction will likely result in the regain of all lost weight.

Band Replacement

The first line of treatment for many complications is removal and replacement of the band. In the past, the usual practice consisted of a procedure to remove the band and repair the stomach wall (perforation), then, after some months of healing, initiating another procedure to place another band. In recent times, however, the more common process involves just one revisional procedure to perform both band removal and replacement. This one-step revision/replacement serves to avoid the weight gain that occurs between procedures and to prevent the risk associated with an additional surgery.[14,55,56]

Conversions to Other Procedures

LAP-BAND failures due to insufficient weight loss, persistent dysphagia, reflux, esophageal dilatation/motility disorders, or persistent food intolerance may dictate the decision to convert to a bariatric procedure with malabsorption such as RYGBP or BPD.

Patient compliance with the necessary changes in eating behavior is an important aspect of gastric restrictive procedures, including the LAP-BAND, and these types of failures highlight the imperative of intense preoperative counseling and communication so patients understand the role they are to play. Patients who overeat, sabotage the band with high calorie liquids, or otherwise violate the *eating rules* on a consistent basis will be at high risk for failure. These noncompliant individuals may do well when converted to a procedure in which their active participation is not necessary. Malabsorptive procedures such as RYGBP use a kind of aversion therapy, called *dumping syndrome*, to compel compliance.

Conversion to Vertical Banded Gastroplasty

Conversion from LAP-BAND to VBG is highly unusual today. Both are gastric restrictive procedures, although VBG has a history of higher complication rate. In addition, VBG involves cutting and stapling of the stomach and has a much higher mortality rate than gastric banding. In truth, VBG has become all but obsolete, having been essentially replaced in the bariatric world by LAP-BAND. Conversion to a procedure other than VBG seems much more likely.

Conversion to GBP

Because of the malabsorptive element, conversion to RYGBP is most commonly performed when LAP-BAND failure has been the result of insufficient weight loss. However, it is also performed after the occurrence of other complications such as pouch dilatation/slippage, esophageal motility issues, and band erosion.

The conversion can be accomplished as a one-step (band removal plus conversion in the same operation) or two-step (conversion to gastric bypass delayed for healing time after band removal) process. In the case of banding failure due to proximal pouch dilatation, the two-step operation may be chosen to avoid gastric pouch staple-line insufficiency on a thin, dilated stomach.[63]

Laparoscopic Roux-en-Y gastric bypass (LRYGBP) is a complex procedure even when performed as a primary operation. Performed as revisional surgery, it is especially challenging[63] and early morbidity may be fairly high.[57] For the most part, however, results have been good and it has been deemed safe and effective in most patients. Before attempting to perform LRYGBP as a revisional procedure, however, surgeons must be well past the learning curve for laparoscopic Roux-en-Y.

Conversion to BPD

Because BPD is a mostly malabsorptive procedure, some surgeons prefer its use for revision of failed restrictive operations—especially when that failure has been due to insufficient weight loss. Like revisional RYGBP, it can be performed simultaneous with band removal and can be performed laparoscopically or laparotomically. Weight loss is reportedly good after revisional BPD, with or without duodenal switch, but is less than that after primary BPD.[51] For surgeons with the proper skills and experience, this revisional procedure can be performed laparoscopically and safely.

Laparoscopic Versus Open Reoperations

The advantages of laparoscopy compared with open surgery are well known. This applies also to reoperations. The possibility of performing reoperations by laparoscopy would make the procedure minimally invasive. The big challenge is overcoming the technical difficulties as they relate to adhesions and anatomical modifications. This is advanced laparoscopy and should be reserved only for surgeons with high expertise and long experience in advanced laparoscopic surgery. Even then, there could be situations where this will not be possible, especially if the new procedure is complex per se. Then conversion to laparotomy may be envisaged without shame. Again the Ten Commandments (number 7): *Do not*

take any unreasonable risk by persisting in the laparoscopic approach when there is danger. Under insurmountable conditions, convert to laparotomy.

DISCUSSION AND CONCLUSION

The introduction of LAGB into bariatric surgery on September 1, 1993, was a considerable breakthrough. Besides the innovations of total reversibility and adjustability, it introduced the notion of minimal invasiveness. It is not by mere chance that the laparoscopic band gave a new boon to bariatric surgery in general and to laparoscopic surgery in particular for the treatment of morbid obesity. The overall complication rate is lower with LAGB than VBG and much lower than gastric bypass or other highly invasive bariatric procedures. In addition, the types of complications associated with gastric banding are, on the whole, less severe than those following gastric bypass and are rarely life threatening.

Actually, in more than 80% of the patients the complications can be corrected by minimally invasive (laparoscopic) surgery.[29] Reoperations such as band removal, band repositioning, and conversion to RYGBP may be performed laparoscopically after LAP-BAND complications. Conversion to BPD is much more challenging and perhaps its relevance is a matter of discussion.

References

1. Buchwald H, Buchwald J: Evolution of operative procedures for the management of morbid obesity 1950–2000. *Obes Surg* 12:705–717, 2002.
2. Mason EE: Vertical banded gastroplasty for obesity. *Arch Surg* 117:701–706, 1982.
3. Kral JG: Surgical treatment of obesity. *Med Clin North Am* 73(1):251–264, 1989.
4. Belachew M, Legrand M, Jacquet N: Laparoscopic placement of adjustable silicone gastric banding in the treatment of morbid obesity: An animal model experimental study. A video film. A preliminary report. *Obes Surg* 3:140, 1993.
5. Belachew M, Legrand M, Defechereux TH, Burtheret MP, Jacquet N: Laparoscopic adjustable silicone gastric banding in the treatment of morbid obesity. A preliminary report. *Surg Endosc* 8:1354–1356, 1994.
6. Belachew M: Les Dix Commandements pour Eviter les Complications de la Chirurgie Bariatrique sous Laparoscopie. *Le journal de coelio-chirurgie* 29:58–60, 1999.
7. Belachew M, Legrand M, Vincent V: History of LAP-BAND: From dream to reality. *Obes Surg* 11:297–302, 2001.
8. O'Brien PE, Brown WA, Smith A, McMurrick PJ, Stephens M: Prospective study of a laparoscopically placed, adjustable gastric band in the treatment of morbid obesity. *Br J Surg* 86(1):113–118, 1999.
9. Fielding GA, Rhodes M, Nathanson LK: Laparoscopic gastric banding for morbid obesity. Surgical outcome in 335 cases. *Surg Endosc* 13(6):550–554, 1999.
10. Spivak H, Favretti F: Avoiding postoperative complications with the LAP-BAND system. *Am J Surg* 184(6B):31S–37S, 2002.
11. Favretti F, Cadiere GB, Segato G, et al.: Laparoscopic adjustable silicone gastric banding (Lap-Band): How to avoid complications. *Obes Surg* 7(4):352–358, 1997.

12. Belachew M, Legrand M, Vincent V, Lismonde M, Le Docte N, Deschamps V: Laparoscopic adjustable gastric banding. *World J Surg* 22(9):955–963, 1998.

13. Fielding GA, Allen JW: A step-by-step guide to placement of the LAP-BAND adjustable gastric banding system. *Am J Surg* 184(6B):26S–30S, 2002.

14. Dargent J: Surgical treatment of morbid obesity by adjustable gastric band: The case for a conservative strategy in the case of failure—a 9-year series. *Obes Surg* 14:986–990, 2004.

15. Gambinotti G, Robortella ME, Furbetta F: Personal experience with laparoscopic adjustable silicone gastric banding in the treatment of morbid obesity. *Eat Weight Disord* 3(1):43–45, 1998.

16. Susmallian S, Ezri T, Elis M, Charuzi I: Access-port complications after laparoscopic gastric banding. *Obes Surg* 13:128–131, 2003.

17. Abu-Abeid S, Szold A: Laparoscopic management of Lap-Band erosion. *Obes Surg* 11:87–89, 2001.

18. Rosenthal RJ, Szomstein S, Kennedy CI, Soto FC, Zundel N. Laparoscopic surgery for morbid obesity: 1001 consecutive bariatric operations performed at the bariatric institute, cleveland clinic Florida. *Obes Surg* 16:119–124, 2006.

19. Burhop JW, Chiang MC, Engstrand DJ, O'Driscoll M: Laparoscopic bariatric surgery can be performed safely in the community hospital setting. *WMJ* 104(5):48–53, 2005.

20. Parikh MS, Shen R, Weiner M, Siegel N, Ren CJ: Laparoscopic bariatric surgery in super-obese patients (BMI>50) is safe and effective: A review of 332 patients. *Obes Surg* 15:858–863, 2005.

21. Spivak H, Hewitt MF, Onn A, Half EE: Weight loss and improvement of obesity-related illness in 500 U.S. patients following laparoscopic adjustable gastric banding procedure. *Am J Surg* 189(1):27–32, 2005.

22. Jan JC, Hong D, Pereira N, Patterson EJ. Laparoscopic adjustable gastric banding versus laparoscopic gastric bypass for morbid obesity: A single-institution comparison study of early results. *J Gastrointest Surg* 9(1):30–39, 2005; discussion: 40–41.

23. Fielding GA: Laparoscopic adjustable gastric banding for massive superobesity (>60 body mass index kg/m2). *Surg Endosc* 17(10):1541–1545, 2003.

24. Weiner R, Blanco-Engert R, Weiner S, Matkowitz R, Schaefer L, Pomhoff I. Outcome after laparoscopic adjustable gastric banding—8 years experience. *Obes Surg* 13:427–434, 2003.

25. Zinzindohoue F, Chevallier JM, Douard R, et al.: Laparoscopic gastric banding: A minimally invasive surgical treatment for morbid obesity. Prospective study of 500 consecutive patients. *Ann Surg* 237(1):1–9, 2003.

26. Favretti F, Cadiere GB, Segato G, et al.: Laparoscopic banding: Selection and technique in 830 patients. *Obes Surg* 12:385–390, 2002.

27. Doldi SB, Micheletto G, Lattuada E, Zappa MA, Bona D, Sonvico U. Adjustable gastric banding: 5-year experience. *Obes Surg* 10:171–173, 2000.

28. Lucchese M, Alessio F, Valeri A, Cantelli G, Venneri F, Borrelli D. Adjustable silicone gastric banding: Complications in a personal series. *Obes Surg* 8:207–209, 1998.

29. Belachew M, Belva PH, Desaive C. Long-term results of laparoscopic adjustable gastric banding for the treatment of morbid obesity. *Obes Surg* 12:564–568, 2002.

30. Chapman A, Kiroff G, Game P, et al.: Laparoscopic adjustable gastric banding in the treatment of obesity: A systematic literature review. *Surgery*, 135(3):326–351, 2004.

31. Kalarchian MA, Marcus MD, Wilson GT, Labouvie EW, Brolin RE, LaMarca LB: Binge eating among gastric bypass patients at long-term follow-up. *Obes Surg* 12:270–275, 2002.

32. Hsu LK, Benotti PN, Dwyer J, et al.: Nonsurgical factors that influence the outcome of bariatric surgery: A review. *Psychosom Med* 60(3):338–346, 1998.

33. Kolanowski J: Surgical treatment for morbid obesity. *Br Med Bull* 53(2):433–444, 1997.

34. Dixon JB, O'Brien PE: Selecting the optimal patient for LAP-BAND placement. *Am J Surg* 184(6B):17S–20S, 2002.

35. NIH conference. Gastrointestinal surgery for severe obesity. Consensus Development Conference Panel. *Ann Intern Med* 115:956–961, 1991.

36. Ferraro D: Preparing patients for bariatric surgery. *Patient, Clinician Rev* 14(1):57–64, 2004.

37. Favretti F, O'Brien PE, Dixon JB: Patient management after LAP-BAND placement. *Am J Surg* 184(6B):38S–41S, 2002.

38. Belachew M, Zimmermann JM: Evolution of a paradigm for laparoscopic adjustable gastric banding. *Am J Surg* 184(6B):21S–25S, 2002.

39. Shen R, Dugay G, Rajaram K, Cabrera I, Siegel N, Ren CJ: Impact of patient follow-up on weight loss after bariatric surgery. *Obes Surg* 14:514–519, 2004.

40. Belachew M, Ernnould D: Directives pour l'ajustement de l'anneau modulable laparoscopique. *Le journal de coelio-chirurgie* 42:5–11, 2002.

41. Soto FC, Szomstein S, Higa-Sansone G, et al.: Esophageal perforation during laparoscopic gastric band placement. *Obes Surg* 14:422–425, 2004.

42. Bernante P, Francini Pesenti F, Toniato A, Zangrandi F, Pomerri F, Pelizzo MR: Obstructive symptoms associated with the 9.75-cm Lap-Band in the first 24 hours using the pars flaccida approach. *Obes Surg* 15:357–360, 2005.

43. Shen R, Ren CJ: Removal of peri-gastric fat prevents acute obstruction after Lap-Band surgery. *Obes Surg* 14:224–229, 2004.

44. Zimmermann JM: LAP-BAND: Changes in surgical technique: Outcome of 1410 surgeries performed from July 1995 through April 2001. Presented at the 6th *World Congress of the International Federation for the Surgery of Obesity*, Crete, Greece, September 5–8, 2001.

45. Rubin M, Benchetrit S, Lustigman H, Lelcuk S, Spivak H. Laparoscopic gastric banding with Lap-Band for morbid obesity: Two-step technique may improve outcome. *Obes Surg* 11:315–317, 2001.

46. Weiner R, Bockhorn H, Rosenthal R, Wagner D: A prospective randomized trial of different laparoscopic gastric banding techniques for morbid obesity. *Surg Endosc* 15(1):63–68, 2001.

47. Fielding GA: LAP-BAND persisting good result with slipped band by modified technique. Presented at the 6th *World Congress of the International Federation for the Surgery of Obesity*, Crete, Greece, September 5–8, 2001.

48. Fielding GA, Rhodes M, Nathanson LK: Laparoscopic gastric banding for morbid obesity. Surgical outcome in 335 cases. *Surg Endosc* 13(6):550–554, 1999.

49. Dargent J: Pouch dilatation and slippage after adjustable gastric banding: Is it still an issue? *Obes Surg* 13:111–115, 2003.

50. Chevallier JM, Zinzindohoue F, Douard R, et al.: Complications after laparoscopic adjustable gastric banding for morbid obesity: Experience with 1000 patients over 7 years. *Obes Surg* 14:407–414, 2004.

51. Dolan K, Fielding G: Bilio pancreatic diversion following failure of laparoscopic adjustable gastric banding. *Surg Endosc* 18(1):60–63, 2004.

52. Tran D, Rhoden DH, Cacchione RN, Baldwin L, Allen JW: Techniques for repair of gastric prolapse after laparoscopic gastric banding. *J Laparoendosc Adv Surg Tech A* 14(2):117–120, 2004.

53. Keidar A, Szold A, Carmon E, Blanc A, Abu-Abeid S: Band slippage after laparoscopic adjustable gastric banding: Etiology and treatment. *Surg Endosc* 19(2):262–267, 2005.

54. Msika S: Surgery for morbid obesity: 2. Complications. Results of a technologic evaluation by the ANAES, *J Chir (Paris)* 140(1):4–21, 2003.

55. Abu-Abeid S, Bar Zohar D, Sagie B, Klausner J: Treatment of intragastric band migration following laparoscopic banding: Safety and feasibility of simultaneous laparoscopic band removal and replacement. *Obes Surg* 15(6):849–852, 2005.

56. Niville E, Dams A, Van Der Speeten K, Verhelst H: Results of lap rebanding procedures after Lap-Band removal for band erosion—a mid-term evaluation. *Obes Surg* 15:630–633, 2005.

57. Suter M, Giusti V, Heraief E, Calmes JM: Band erosion after laparoscopic gastric banding: Occurrence and results after conversion to Roux-en-Y gastric bypass. *Obes Surg* 14:381–386, 2004.

58. Spivak H, Gold D, Guerrero C: Optimization of access-port placement for the lap-band system. *Obes Surg* 13:909–912, 2003.

59. Ammori BJ: A simple technique to fix the reservoir in laparoscopic gastric banding. *J Laparoendosc Adv Surg Tech A* 14(4):250–252, 2004.

60. Susmallian S, Ezri T, Elis M, Charuzi I: Access-port complications after laparoscopic gastric banding. *Obes Surg* 13:128–131, 2003.

61. Fabry H, Van Hee R, Hendrickx L, Totte E: A technique for prevention of port complications after laparoscopic adjustable silicone gastric banding. *Obes Surg* 12:285–288, 2002.

62. Zieren J, Menenakos C, Paul M, Muller JM: Prevention of catheter disconnection after laparoscopic adjustable gastric banding. *J Laparoendosc Adv Surg Tech A* 14(2):77–79, 2004.

63. Mognol P, Chosidow D, Marmuse JP: Laparoscopic conversion of laparoscopic gastric banding to Roux-en-Y gastric bypass: A review of 70 patients. *Obes Surg* 14:1349–1353, 2004.

32

Restrictive Procedures: Utilization of Adjustable Gastric Banding for Failed Stapled Operations

Paul E. O'Brien MD, FRACS

INTRODUCTION

Bariatric surgical procedures are now well established as effective in achieving major weight loss in the severely obese. In particular, gastric stapling procedures have been in common usage now for over 35 years and considerable data on their benefits and their hazards are now available. They are highly effective in achieving strong weight loss in the first 2 years after operation and several systematic reviews have documented this impressive effect.[1]

However, there are failures. There are patients who fail to lose sufficient weight to solve the problems caused by their obesity. There are patients who have an initial successful outcome only to find there is a progressive regain of weight after 2 or 3 years. And there are patients who suffer side effects and complications of the gastric stapling procedure that leads to the need for its reversal or revision.

In this chapter we look at the prevalence of failed gastric stapling, including gastric bypass and gastroplasty and the option of conversion to laparoscopic adjustable gastric banding (LAGB). We will review the appropriate selection of patients and their preoperative assessment, review the surgical options for these patients, and seek to determine what is a realistic expectation of outcomes.

EXPERIENCE OF REVISION OF STAPLING TO STAPLING

Gastric bypass is commonly regarded as the most effective form of gastric stapling and yet nearly 50% of the RYGBP patients will have lost less than 50% of the excess weight at 5 years after surgery. In a systematic review which looked at the medium-term (3–10 years) outcomes after all current bariatric procedures, the published reports of RYGBP patients showed mean excess weight loss of 58%, 45%, 55%, and 53% at 5, 6, 7, and 10 years after surgery. The patient doing poorly is most likely to cease attending follow-up clinics and generally by 5 years less than 50% of patients are still attending follow-up. Rarely do published reports gave figures for loss to

Table 32–1.

Indication for Revision in 310 Patients in a Randomized Controlled Trial of Three Forms of Gastric Stapling[4]

Indications	Gastroplasty	Gastrogastrostomy	Gastric Bypass	Total
Stomal dilatation	8	22	5	35 (11%)
Stomal stenosis	12	5	2	19 (6%)
Staple-line dehiscence	3	6	3	12 (12%)

follow-up. The true %EWL for all patients is therefore almost certainly below the published figures.

Multiple randomized controlled trials have shown that gastroplasty patients do less well than do RYGBP patients[2,3] and this group of operations is now becoming of historic interest only. Nevertheless, there are many tens of thousands of patients who were treated by gastroplasty in the 1980s and 1990s and who are now seeking relief of their symptoms of maladaptive eating or better weight loss or both. It could therefore be estimated that, on the basis of 30,000 bariatric procedures in the United States alone per year during the last two decades of the twentieth century and an expectation of less than 50% of them have achieved loss of half of their excess weight, there are likely to be 300,000 patients from that era in that country alone who would benefit by better weight loss.

However, the principal reason for revisional surgery is not failure of weight loss but the presence of complications. In the Adelaide obesity trial, a randomized controlled trial testing three different forms of gastric stapling, Roux-en-Y gastric bypass, gastroplasty, and gastrogastrostomy,[4] we reported on a total of 63 revisional procedures that were performed on the 310 patients of the trial (20%) at a median of 32 months after the original surgery, all for complications of the procedures. Table 32–1 lists the reasons for revisional surgery. Revision rates were highest for gastrogastrostomy at 30%, mostly for stomal dilatation, 22% for gastroplasty, usually for stomal stenosis, and 10% for gastric bypass. Overall, the outcome of the revisional surgery, always to the same or another form of stapling, was disappointing with only 23% of patients finally judged to have had a worthwhile outcome. This was achieved at significant cost, including one potentially life-threatening complication due to an anastomotic leak, 3 reversals, 10 further revisions, and 44 endoscopic dilatations. Not surprisingly, the enthusiasm for revision to stapling has not thrived.

Others have reported similar outcomes. Benotti and Forse[5] reported a complication rate of 16% and a modest but statistically significant weight reduction from a BMI of 39 to 34 kg/m^2 in 63 patients who had had a range of previous bariatric procedures. Behrns et al.[6] performed revisional procedures on 61 patients, with one death, serious morbidity in 11%, and a mean weight loss of 16 kg. Conversion to

Roux-en-Y gastric bypass leads to better outcomes than conversion to gastroplasty.

EXPERIENCE OF REVISION OF STAPLING TO LAGB

The LAGB procedure became available in 1993 and extensive subsequent study has shown it to be safe and effective in achieving weight loss, improved heath, and improved quality of life.[7,8] Inevitably, soon after its introductions, patients who had had a poor result from stapling procedures asked if a better outcome for them could be achieved with the LAGB. We commenced treating such patients after July 1994 and to date have performed LAGB placement as a revisional procedure from other bariatric procedures in 135 patients. We formally reviewed and reported our experience in the late 1990s[9] at which time 50 patients had been treated. The initial procedure for these patients was gastroplasty in 35, gastric bypass in 2, fixed gastric banding in 11, and jejunoileal bypass in 2. The predominance of gastroplasty reflects the activity of the surgical community in the state of Victoria in the 1980s when very few gastric bypass procedures were being performed.

The reasons for seeking revision are listed in Table 32–2. Most patients had failure to lose weight even when stomal stenosis was present. The maladaptive eating caused by the stomal stenosis induced an eating pattern that led to weight

Table 32–2.

Reasons for Conversion From Gastric Stapling to LAGB in 50 Patients[9]

Indication	Total
Failure of weight loss or weight regain alone	32 (64%)
Maladaptive eating and weight regain	14 (28%)
Maladaptive eating with adequate weight loss	3 (6%)

gain in the presence of severe difficulties with normal food. They therefore suffered the worst of both outcomes—an intolerable restriction on eating and yet weight gain and severe obesity.

There were three particular outcomes from that study that deserve emphasis. First, there were more complications in the perioperative period than occurred with the primary LAGB patients. LAGB is one of the safest procedures in surgery, especially given the high-risk status of the patients. In over 3,000 patients treated by our group, there has not been a death and the complications are almost always minor and present in less than 2% of patients. The revisional LAGB patients however had a complication rate of 17%. Partly this reflected the use of open surgery, which was standard for revisional procedures at that time. However clearly the risk of the procedure is higher and therefore the gains need to be scrutinized to ensure that the risk was worthwhile.

The second feature of this group of patients was their total lack of late problems. The principal problem with LAGB as a primary operation for obesity had been the need to do additional surgery late after primary placement for prolapse of stomach through the band or erosion of the band into the gastric lumen. Neither problem occurred in the 50 patients we had followed for up to 6 years. What was lost in the perioperative period with a higher incidence of perioperative complications was regained in the follow-up period with the total absence of late complications.

The third particular feature of this group of revisional patients was that their outcomes in terms of weight loss, resolution of comorbidities, and improvement in quality of life was very good. The weight loss of 46% ± 18% EWL was not different to that achieved in our primary LAGB group at that time (53% ± 19% EWL). There was documented improvement in hypertension, diabetes, dyslipidemia, gastroesophageal reflux, and sleep apnea. Quality of life was measured using the SF-36 and showed highly statistically significant improvement in seven of the eight scaled scores.[9] We therefore concluded that, contrary to our experience with revision to further gastric stapling, revision to LAGB achieved worthwhile outcomes while retaining the safety of LAGB as a primary operation.

SELECTION AND ASSESSMENT OF PATIENTS

Not all patients who are failing a bariatric procedure should be considered for revisional surgery. There are always reasons for failure—patient factors, doctor factors, and operation factors. If, after careful analysis, you feel that patient factors are a significant contributor, careful consideration should be given before proceeding with revision. However, it is important to recognize the maladaptive eating pattern of the gastric stapling patient, i.e., the tendency to eat sweet foods such as ice cream and chocolate, as a feature of the stenosis of the gastroplasty or gastric bypass and not a weakness of the patient.

Assessment of the Patient

All patients should undergo a full clinical assessment as would occur for any bariatric patient. In addition, on history, it is important to identify the cause for the failure. Technical errors with the original procedure, failure of staple-lines, or stenosis, or dilatation of the stoma, are all problems that can be addressed by revision. Noncompliance by the patient or a belief by the patient that it is someone else's problem or fault are more difficult to repair. In general, if a good weight loss had occurred initially followed by failure the prognosis of a revision is better than if weight loss never occurred.

All patients should have a barium meal and an upper gastrointestinal endoscopy to delineate the anatomy as completely as possible. The ideal structure for revision to LAGB has a medium sized or large gastric pouch with the stoma at some distance from the esophagogastric junction. This provides room for placement of the band and usually sufficient tissue for anterior fixation. Particular attention needs to be paid to the size of the stoma. Any stenosis will need to be reversed as a part of the revisional procedure. The reason for failure should be evident from these studies.

We would order further specific investigations such as sleep studies, respiratory function tests, etc., on their merit from the clinical assessment.

TECHNIQUES OF REVISION

In our initial experience, we performed all revisional procedures by open surgery. More recently, we have used a laparoscopic approach if there have not been more than two previous bariatric procedures and we do not need to reverse a stenosis by division of a staple-line. All attempted laparoscopic procedures have been successful but you must be prepared to spend time dividing adhesions.

All adhesions should be divided up to the diaphragm, completely mobilizing the lateral segment of the left lobe of liver from the anterior wall of the stomach. In open procedures, we also divide the left triangular ligament sufficient to allow retraction of the liver across to the right. Otherwise good exposure of the distal esophagus is not possible.

Any reversal of the existing procedure is then undertaken. This is almost always for stomal stenosis as gastric pouch enlargement, staple-line dehiscence, or stomal dilatation are an advantage at this stage. To reverse stomal stenosis, we perform a gastrotomy immediately distal to the stoma and use heavy curved Mayo scissors to divide the staple-line sufficient to create a 4-cm diameter pathway. The divided margins of gastric wall are sealed closed with a running suture of 2/0 vicryl. The gastrotomy is then closed also with 2/0 vicryl.

The pathway for placement of the band is then dissected using the standard pars flaccida approach. Be careful to measure the path before determining if a LAP BAND VG or 10-cm band is indicated. If in doubt, use the larger band. Anterior fixation can be more difficult than with primary placement due to the abnormal anatomy present. Achieve fixation as best you can using the tissues adjacent to the band, with the reassurance that prolapse has proved to be very unlikely in this setting.

If laparotomy has been performed and particularly, if a gastrotomy was needed, it is strongly advised to place the access port through a incision separate from the laparotomy as risk of infection of the main wound is real and would be made more likely by the presence of the port. Initial adjustment of the band is performed at 4 weeks after placement and subsequent schedule of adjustments and support is identical to that used for our primary LAGB patients.

CONCLUSIONS

All bariatric procedures are subject to possible failure. If this occurs in gastric stapling patients due to technical problems with the procedure, revision to LAGB has been shown to be feasible, safe, and effective. Most revisions can be done laparoscopically and patients can then be expected to follow a path not different from the primary LAGB patient.

References

1. Buchwald H, Avidor Y, Braunwald E, et al.: Bariatric surgery: A systematic review and meta-analysis. *JAMA* 292(14):1724–1737, 2004.
2. Hall JC, Watts JM, O'Brien PE, et al.: Gastric surgery for morbid obesity. The adelaide study. *Ann Surg* 211(4):419–427, 1990.
3. Sugerman HJ, Starkey JV, Birkenhauer R: A randomized prospective trial of gastric bypass versus vertical banded gastroplasty for morbid obesity and their effects on sweets versus non-sweets eaters. *Ann Surg* 205(6):613–624, 1987.
4. Hunter R, Watts JM, Dunstan R, et al.: Revisional surgery for failed gastric restrictive procedures for morbid obesity. *Obes Surg* 2(3):245–252, 1992.
5. Benotti PN, Forse RA: Safety and long-term efficacy of revisional surgery in severe obesity. *Am J Surg* 172(3):232–235, 1996.
6. Behrns KE, Smith CD, Kelly KA, et al.: Reoperative bariatric surgery. Lessons learned to improve patient selection and results. *Ann Surg* 218(5):646–653, 1993.
7. O'Brien PE, Dixon JB, Brown W, et al.: The laparoscopic adjustable gastric band (Lap-Band): A prospective study of medium-term effects on weight, health and quality of life. *Obes Surg* 12(5):652–660, 2002.
8. Chapman A, Kiroff G, Game P, et al.: Laparoscopic adjustable gastric banding in the treatment of obesity: A systematic review. *Surgery*135:326–351, 2004.
9. O'Brien P, Brown W, Dixon J: Revisional surgery for morbid obesity—conversion to the Lap-Band system. *Obes Surg* 10(6):557–563, 2000.

Restrictive Procedures: Laparoscopic Revision of Vertical Banding to Gastric Bypass

Daniel Gagné, MD, FACS

I. INTRODUCTION AND BACKGROUND

II. INDICATIONS FOR REVISION OF VBG TO RYGBP
Unsatisfactory Weight Loss
Stomal Stenosis/Dysfunction
Reflux Symptoms and Complications
Band Erosion

III. PREOPERATIVE EVALUATION

IV. OPERATIVE TECHNIQUE OF LAPAROSCOPIC
REVISION OF VBG TO RYGBP

V. RESULTS AND OUTCOMES

VI. SUMMARY

INTRODUCTION AND BACKGROUND

The vertical banded gastroplasty (VBG) was first described by Mason in 1982.[1] It is a restrictive procedure that consists of a vertically oriented proximal small pouch (less than 30 mL) that drains through a narrow (10–12 mm) gastric channel. The outlet channel is reinforced with a band of polypropylene (Marlex) mesh, PTFE (Gore-tex), or a silastic ring. The 1991 NIH Consensus Conference for the treatment of morbid obesity endorsed both the Roux-en-Y gastric bypass (RYGBP) and VBG.[2] Although VBG was commonly performed in the 1980s and 1990s for the treatment of morbid obesity,[3] it has largely been abandoned in the United States due to poor long-term results.[4] The VBG was still mentioned as an option in the 2004 ASBS Consensus Conference Statement[5]; however, in February 2006, the US Department of Health and Human Services Centers for Medicare and Medicaid Services announced "that the evidence [for VBG] is not adequate to conclude that it is reasonable and necessary; therefore, it is non-covered for all Medicare beneficiaries"[6]; other private insurers in the United States may follow suit.

Balsinger et al. reported the Mayo clinic 10 year results after VBG and demonstrated a 79% failure rate.[7] Failure after VBG is most commonly due to poor long-term weight loss, which can result from staple-line dehiscence or from maladaptive diet behavior.[7,8] A shortcoming of purely restrictive operations is that bulky solid meals are limited, and patients have a tendency to adopt a high-calorie liquid diet which can pass rapidly through the stoma, leading to regain of weight. Only 26% of the patients in the Mayo study have maintained a weight loss of at least 50% of their excess body weight at 10 years. Other complications that commonly occur after VBG that may require reoperation include stomal obstruction, persistent vomiting, solid food intolerance, pouch dilatation, gastroesophageal reflux disease, aspiration pneumonia, and erosion of the prosthetic band.[9]

Reoperation rates reported in larger VBG series range from 6% to 44%.[4,10–15] Although revision of VBG to VBG has been reported,[9,12] almost all of the bariatric surgical literature supports the conversion to RYGBP as the operation of choice after failed restrictive procedures.[16–19] Multiple studies have demonstrated that RYGBP has a weight loss success rate superior to that seen in VBG.[20–26] VBG is also not as effective as gastric bypass for control of type 2 diabetes mellitus. Several studies have reported conversions of VBG to RYGBP via an open technique, with results of improved weight loss, comorbidities, and correction of complications.[18,27–32] There are several reports of laparoscopic revision of VBG to RYGBP.[15,33–39] Though feasible, revisional bariatric surgery is technically complicated, whether performed open or laparoscopic, and has a higher complication rate than primary bariatric surgery.[40]

INDICATIONS FOR REVISION OF VBG TO RYGBP

Revision of VBG to RYGBP should be considered if a patient has any of the following conditions or complications:

1. Inadequate or unsatisfactory weight loss
   a. with or without staple-line dehiscence
   b. without resolution of obesity-related health problems (BMI ≥ 35 kg/m^2)
   c. weight regain after initial weight loss.
2. Stomal stenosis or stomal symptoms
   a. solid food intolerance
   b. stomal dysfunction
   c. frequent or persistent vomiting
   d. protein malnutrition
3. Gastroesophageal reflux symptoms and complications
   a. Barrett's esophagus
   b. aspiration & aspiration pneumonia
4. Band erosion

Unsatisfactory Weight Loss

Inadequate weight loss or weight regain after VBG may occur with or without staple-line dehiscence. VBG staple-line breakdown has been reported to occur in almost 50% of patients.[22,41,42] Dehiscence of the vertical stapled partition eliminates the restrictive nature of the surgery, leading to ingestion of larger portions and subsequent weight gain.

An anatomically intact VBG may be a more common cause of weight gain in patients. Patients are prone to develop a maladaptive eating behavior due to the restrictive nature of the band. Nutritious foods such as solid protein and vegetables are not tolerated comfortably. Patients substitute with high-calorie soft foods such as ice cream, cookies, sweets, non-diet beverages, or potato chips, which are easily ingested. This maladaptive eating behavior results in persistent weight gain and an "overfed but undernourished" patient.

Stomal Stenosis/Dysfunction

Gastric outlet obstruction of the pouch can result from the band. Mechanical symptomatic stomal stenosis may result from a band that is too tight, an external fibrosing reaction to the band, or chronic ulceration of the stomal channel. Patients usually present with intolerance of solids or persistent vomiting. This occurs in up to 40% of VBG patients. Endoscopy may be required to push a bezoar of food through the channel for temporary relief if there is outlet obstruction. Endoscopic dilatation of the stenotic stoma is usually temporary due to the permanent nature of the band. Physicians and gastroenterologists should refer patients with recurrent problems to a bariatric surgeon to prevent further nutritional complications such as Wernicke's encephalopathy or severe protein calorie malnutrition.

As a pouch enlarges over time due to the fixed band stenosis, a functional stomal stenosis and poor pouch emptying can occur.[9,43] Patients will have symptoms of vomiting, intolerance of solids, and gastroesophageal reflux. In endoscopy, a mechanical narrowing at the level of the band may not be evident, as the endoscope can be maneuvered and can easily traverse the stoma.[43] An upper gastrointestinal (GI) radiological study may demonstrate a dilated, or floppy, pouch and *normal* VBG stoma. A barium meal or gastric emptying study may demonstrate poor pouch emptying or kinking of the outlet. The contribution of pouch volume enlargement to pouch emptying failure, functional obstruction, and reflux symptoms can be explained by the law of LaPlace.[44]

Reflux Symptoms and Complications

Up to 40% of patients will have reflux symptoms that may be persistent. This may be due to mechanical stenosis or functional stenosis, both of which lead to poor pouch emptying. Also, acid-secreting mucosa may be present in large pouches. Barrett's esophagus has been observed in patients with long-standing reflux after VBG.[43] Other complications of severe reflux after VBG that we have observed include distal esophageal stricture as well as recurrent aspiration pneumonia. Revision of VBG to RYGBP improves these symptoms and complications.

Band Erosion

Band erosion into the wall of the stomach may result in stricture, obstruction, ulceration, bleeding, or perforation. The chronic scarring and inflammation associated with erosion of the band usually requires surgical removal, though endoscopic removal has been performed.

PREOPERATIVE EVALUATION

The preoperative office evaluation of patients presenting for revisional bariatric surgery needs to be extremely thorough.

Evaluation of these patients needs to include the comprehensive multidisciplinary evaluation of the routine morbidly obese patient as well as full evaluation of the complications or failure of the VBG. A systematic approach should be undertaken in these potentially difficult and frustrated patients who, for one reason or another, have failed surgical treatment of their morbid obesity.

- *Medical history*: Full evaluation of the obesity-related health problems (type 2 diabetes mellitus, hypertension, sleep apnea, GERD, etc.). Were these present before VBG? Did they resolve after weight loss? Did they recur with weight gain? Did they worsen after VBG? Most of these obesity-related health problems will improve after revision.
- *Operative reports* of the previous surgery should be obtained whenever possible. Operative reports of revisions attempted, hernia repair, and abdominal surgery may also be used as a guide to help determine the GI tract anatomy, laparoscopic access issues, and plan for surgery. The primary bariatric operative note should contain the information about the type of band, dissected tissue planes, use of Seprafilm, gastrostomy tube, as well as any complications or difficulties.
- *Weight history*: A detailed history of the patient's weight gain(s) and loss(es) includes weight-age time-line, highest weight, weight at time of VBG, weight loss results after VBG, and time of weight regain.
- *Dietician consult & history*: All patients should obtain a consultation with a dietician. The patient's diet history should be reviewed and should include dietary compliance since VBG, portion sizes tolerated (Can patients eat a "normal-sized" meal without difficulty?), meal frequency and choices, foods not tolerated, foods that are avoided for fear of vomiting or dysphagia, grazing/foraging habits, frequency of vomiting, hospital visits for endoscopic push-through of obstructed food. Patients with a vertical staple-line dehiscence usually will tolerate a "normal-sized" meal. Dietary counseling, education, and recommendations are instituted along with the patient assignment of a daily food diary that the patient is to bring to each preop visit. Postoperative diet instructions (emphasis on protein, avoidance of dumping syndrome, etc.) are reviewed as well. Serum albumin and vitamin levels should be checked. Patients with stomal obstructive symptoms, as well as the "overfed and undernourished" poor weight loss patients, may be malnourished. These patients are started on multivitamin supplements and liquid protein supplementation prior to surgery to improve their nutritional status. For patients that present with poor weight loss or significant weight regain, an attempt at preoperative weight loss is used as a test of patient compliance.
- *Upper GI x-ray series*: Radiological studies are needed in all patients to evaluate the anatomy and anatomical complications: "normal" VBG anatomy, vertical staple-line dehiscence (Figure 33–1), intact VBG anatomy with stomal stricture (Figure 33–2), pouch size, pouch emptying, and reflux. Staple-line dehiscence with resultant gastrogastric

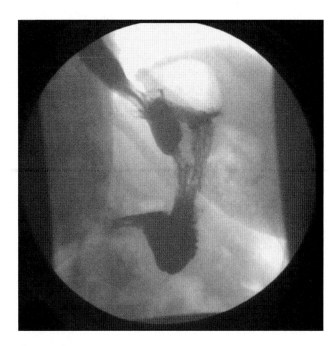

Figure 33–1. Upper GI x-ray demonstrating vertical staple-line dehiscence.

fistula is often small and located proximally near the GE junction. The upper GI series provides a "road map" for planning surgery.

- *Upper endoscopy*: All patients should undergo upper endoscopy to evaluate the VBG anatomy for staple-line dehiscence (gastrogastric fistula) not apparent on upper GI x-ray, size of stoma, stricture, gastroesophageal reflux disease (GERD), esophagitis, stricture from GERD, Barrett's changes, retained food, and band erosion.

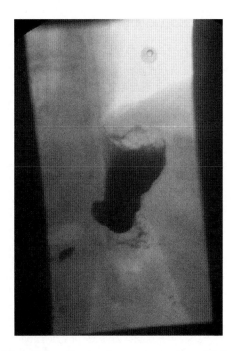

Figure 33–2. Upper GI x-ray demonstrating intact VBG anatomy with stomal stricture.

• *Psychology consult*: Routine psychologist consultation is required in all patients to determine the patient's ability for behavior modification, coping, and support.

• *Informed consent, patient expectations, and compliance* need to be discussed and communicated with the patient and their family. Informed consent needs to be honest and full, including the increased risk of complications compared to primary bariatric surgery, possible prolonged ICU stay, and use of drains and tubes. It is important that the patient demonstrate motivation and compliance with assignments (food diary, preop appointments, no continued weight gain) prior to surgery before being considered candidates for revisional bariatric surgery. Patients noncompliant prior to surgery will most likely be noncompliant afterwards and doomed to fail again. Patient expectations about weight loss, diet, exercise, and follow-up need to be realistic and discussed at length. Patients need to understand their own role in the long-term results of weight loss after surgery.

OPERATIVE TECHNIQUE OF LAPAROSCOPIC REVISION OF VBG TO RYGBP

Several papers and publications have described the approach, necessary steps, and technical "pearls" required in the revision of VBG to RYGBP via an open technique.[27,28,31,33,43] A laparoscopic approach has also been described.[45] Many of the steps and goals of the laparoscopic revisional operation are the same as a primary laparoscopic RYGBP in regards to perioperative care, operating room equipment, patient positioning, trocar placement, creation of a small divided gastric pouch, and Roux limb alignment. The issues more specific to revision of VBG to RYGBP are as follows:

• Careful lysis of adhesions, adequate visualization, identification of tissue planes, hemostasis, and avoiding injury to liver and spleen;

• attention to staple-lines, care when stapling across staple-lines, and avoiding ischemic or devascularized tissue;

• avoid undrained stomach segments in-between staple-lines (gastric sequestration);

• large caliber bougie to help identify proximal stomach and band;

• liberal use of gastrostomy tube placement or gastropexy (for gastric remnant decompression or nutrition);

• liberal use of drains.

The patient is initially placed in the supine position with the arms abducted 60°. The surgeon stands on the patient's right side with assistants on the patient's left. Modified rapid sequence intubation is performed by anesthesia as these patients are at high risk of reflux and aspiration due to their band. Anesthesia then passes an oral-gastric tube to decompress the pouch and stomach, with care not to perforate the pouch.

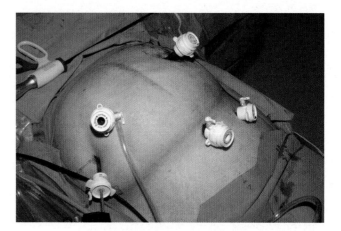

Figure 33–3. Trocar position.

The patient's abdomen is widely prepped and draped. Pneumoperitoneum and access may need to be performed in a few manners, depending on the patient's previous surgeries and incisions. The first choice for Veress needle access, if possible, is in a location similar to a primary LRYGBP—usually in the periumbilical area, measured about 20 cm away from the right costal margin, depending on the size of the patient. Many VBG patients have an upper midline incision with a "free space" caudally. Pneumoperitoneum is achieved at 15 mm Hg pressure; a 12-mm Visiport optical trocar and 0° laparoscope are used to enter the abdominal cavity initially. If the patient's previous midline incision extends to the lower abdomen, then the initial access incision is placed in the right upper quadrant (if there is no previous open cholecystectomy incision) or, alternatively, in the left upper quadrant if there is no evidence of an old gastrostomy tube site.

Once laparoscopic and camera access into the abdominal cavity is gained, an attempt is made to place additional trocars into the same positions as used during a primary LRYGBP (Figure 33–3). Most patients will have adhesions of the omentum, transverse colon, and stomach to the abdominal wall. After initial periumbilical camera port placement, space may be available in the left upper quadrant or right upper quadrant for additional trocars, in positions similar to primary LRYGBP. The camera is also placed into the right and left subcostal 12-mm ports and omental adhesions are taken down using scissors and blunt dissection through the other trocar sites. Working counterclockwise around the abdomen, the adhesions are divided; sometimes a 5 mm right lower quadrant trocar is placed. The omental adhesions are then taken down from the abdominal wall with scissors, blunt dissection, and harmonic scalpel as necessary, from caudal to cephalad. An additional trocar (5 mm) is placed in the left lower quadrant.

The 0° scope is used initially and then changed to the 45° angled scope once the adhesions in the upper abdomen between the stomach and liver are approached. The patient is also placed into a steep reverse Trendelenburg position to help exposure. If the left lobe of the liver is stuck to the diaphragm and abdominal wall, these adhesions are usually not divided. The interface of the undersurface of the liver and anterior wall

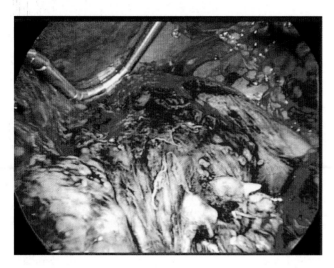

Figure 33–4. Dissected proximal stomach demonstrating pouch, vertical staple-line, and band.

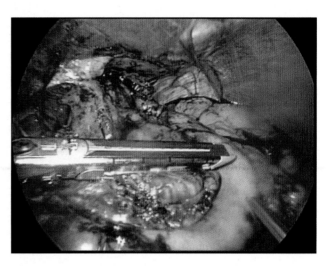

Figure 33–6. Stapler above band during formation of new gastric pouch.

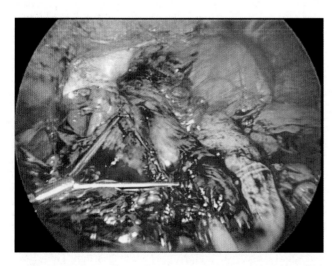

Figure 33–5. Large, blunt-tipped bougie passed into pouch.

of the stomach is identified. Sharp dissection or ultrasonic shears are used initially, and then blunt dissection will usually free most of the stomach away from the liver. The area of the band, band sutures, and staple-lines tend to be densely scarred to the liver. Careful dissection is used at this portion of the procedure, separating the liver away from the lesser curvature of the stomach, hepatogastric ligament, and vessels. The liver "capsule" may tear, causing slight ooze that soon stops. The anatomy of the stomach is often distorted and normal landmarks are obscured. Greater omental adhesions to the anterior stomach, band, and staple-lines need to be divided in the proper plane to better visualize the anatomy of the band and vertical staple-line (Figure 33–4).

Once the stomach is dissected free from adhesions, anesthesia then passes a 32F blunt-tip bougie orally, which is guided into the proximal stomach to delineate the anatomy in the area of the GE junction, the gastric pouch, and the band (Figure 33–5). The angle of His and vertical staple-line are dissected away from the diaphragm with care to avoid splenic in-

jury. Opening the gastrocolic ligament to enter into the lesser sac helps gain access to the posterior stomach, band, vertical staple-line, and pouch to divide adhesions. This will help during the creation and mobilization of the new gastric pouch as well as for Roux limb passage later. A flexible liver retractor can be placed into this space to elevate the stomach anteriorly.

Creation of the new gastric pouch is then performed by using perigastric blunt dissection along the lesser curvature of the stomach, 4 cm distal to the gastroesophageal junction. This is about 1.5–2 cm above the band. The bougie is used as a guide to identify the lesser curvature of the proximal stomach as well the banded area. The perigastric approach is used to help preserve the vasculature and branches of the vagus nerve. Care needs to be taken to avoid an inadvertent gastrostomy. If this occurs, the dissection can resume just cephalad to the gastrostomy site, and the gastrostomy can be resected with staplers. Pouch creation can also be performed by opening the gastrohepatic ligament and stapling with a 2.5-mm height (white load) up to the lesser curvature of the stomach. Once a space is created into the lesser sac, the bougie is pulled back into the esophagus, and an endoscopic-GIA stapler (45-mm length, 3.5-mm staple blue load) is fired transversely across, above the band and up to the vertical staple-line (Figure 33–6). If this portion of the stomach is not soft and pliable, or thicker and scarred, then a green (4.8-mm staple) stapler cartridge is used. The distal portion of the old VBG pouch needs to be below the new staple-line to allow the old retained pouch to drain into the distal stomach through the VBG stoma. If there is a vertical staple-line dehiscence, then the old retained stomach segment of pouch may drain through the dehiscence. When the stoma is stenotic and the VBG staple-line is intact, a gastrogastrostomy between the distal pouch of the VBG and the distal stomach may be needed to help drainage of the distal part of the VBG pouch; this is crucial to prevent any "undrained" area of the stomach to prevent a gastric sequestration. The banded area and the vertical staple-lines may need to be resected.

Blunt dissection is then performed in the lesser sac, medially along the old vertical staple-line up to the angle of His. The proximal stomach is mobilized from the adhesions in the lesser sac and diaphragm, with care taken to avoid injury to the splenic vessels and pancreas. Once the proximal stomach and angle of His are freed and a retrofundic tunnel is created, endoscopic GIA (4.8-mm staple height) staplers are fired to create the pouch, with the bougie as a guide within the pouch and the staplers fired medial to the old vertical staple-line. The left upper quadrant trocar is removed and an endoscopic GIA green load is placed directly through the abdominal wall, coordinating and choreographing the steps needed to (1) remove the trocar, (2) plug the abdominal incisional to avoid escape of pneumoperitoneum, (3) placing and firing the stapler, (4) removing the stapler, and (5) replacing the trocar. This is repeated for each application of the stapler. Usually two to three green staple loads 60 mm in length are needed to create a small (20 mL) divided gastric pouch. The bougie is advanced and withdrawn for each staple fire to help guide with the anatomy. The staple-lines are inspected and reinforced with suture if necessary. In my series of 52 patients, the band was PTFE (Gortex) in 49 patients and polypropylene (Marlex) in 3, so the band was left in place due to the dense inflammatory reaction to the stomach.

The omentum and transverse mesocolon are then elevated cephalad to expose the proximal small bowel. The colon and omentum are retracted by a bowel grasper through the left upper quadrant trocar. The small bowel is then measured from the ligament of Treitz for a length of 45 cm and divided with a 60-mm endoscopic-GIA white (2.5-mm) staple load. The small bowel mesentery is then divided 2–3 cm with the ultrasonic shears. A Penrose drain is sutured to the distal small bowel stump to identify this as the Roux limb. The hepatobiliary limb of bowel is kept to the patient's right side and the Roux limb is measured to the patients left upper quadrant to a length of 90–150 cm. Enterotomies are created with ultrasonic shears to allow passage of the 60-mm endoscopic-GIA white (2.5-mm) staple load, which is fired to create the jejunojejunostomy. The resulting enterotomy defect is then closed with a running 2.0 Vicryl (absorbable) suture. A 2.0 silk suture is used just distal to the anastomosis as an antiobstruction stitch; this same suture is then used in a running fashion to close the mesenteric defect between the two limbs of small bowel.

Ultrasonic shears and blunt dissection are used to create a defect in the transverse mesocolon near the ligament of Treitz to gain access into the lesser sac. The Penrose drain and Roux limb are then passed behind the colon and bypassed portion of stomach. The drain and Roux limb stump are brought anteriorly and aligned with the gastric pouch with stay sutures of 2-0 absorbable suture. The bougie is advanced by anesthesia to help identify the pouch anatomy. Ultrasonic shears are used to create a gastrotomy in the pouch and enterotomy in the Roux limb stump. The mucosa of the revised gastric pouch is often thick and hypertrophied. An endoscopic-GIA stapler (3.5-mm staple) is then passed to a length of 2 cm and fired to create the posterior wall of the gas-

trojejunostomy. Anesthesia then advances the bougie across the anastomosis and the gastrojejunostomy is completed with a running 2-0 absorbable suture over the bougie. This running suture usually incorporates the inferior staple-line of the pouch. A hand-sewn double layer over a bougie, instead of the linear stapled anastomosis, may be required in some patients if there is limited mobility of the gastric pouch. The bougie is removed and an oral-gastric tube is advanced for an air-insufflation test using O_2. Intraoperative endoscopy may be required on occasion to help identify the anatomy and test the anastomosis.

The oral-gastric tube, Penrose drain, and liver retractor are removed. The transverse colon is elevated again to expose the small bowel. A single suture of 2-0 silk is placed just proximal to the jejunojejunostomy staple-line to prevent tension. A running 2-0 silk suture is used to close the space behind the Roux limb mesentery up to the transverse mesocolon. The transverse mesocolon defect around the Roux limb is closed circumferentially with a running, interlocking 2-0 silk suture. The transverse colon and omentum are then placed back to their normal anatomical position.

A gastrostomy is then made in the gastric remnant for suction and decompression. G-tube placement should be considered at this point. Alternatively, a gastropexy can be performed by suturing the bypassed stomach to abdominal wall and marking the site with clips for radiological guidance if a G-tube is needed in the future for drainage or nutrition. Unfortunately, it is not always possible to mobilize the bypassed portion of stomach to reach the abdominal wall due to adhesions, even after releasing the pneumoperitoneum to a pressure of 8–10 mm Hg.

The camera is placed through the left upper quadrant trocar to visualize the umbilical port-site. This is closed with a 0-0 absorbable suture using an Endoclose device. The camera is then placed back into the umbilical trocar. A 10-mm Jackson-Pratt drain is placed into the lesser sac along the gastric remnant staple-line and gastrojejunal (GJ) anastomosis, and brought out through the left upper quadrant trocar site.

The pneumoperitoneum is then released, trocars are removed, and skin incisions are approximated with subcuticular 4-0 absorbable suture. The drain is sutured to the skin with 2-0 Prolene. The operating room table is leveled off. Benzoine, steri-strips, and Band-Aids are applied. The patient is then extubated in the operating room and transported to the recovery room.

Postoperatively, patient management is similar to that of a primary LRYGBP patient. The drain output and character need to be monitored. A water-soluble swallow study should be obtained. Patients are started on clear liquids, multivitamins, and advanced as usual. Leaks after revisional surgery can occur up to 10 days after surgery so the drain is left in at the time of discharge of the patient and removed 10–14 days later. If the patient is "not perfect" clinically, then imaging studies or diagnostic laparoscopy should be considered.

The incidence of ventral incisional hernia from the primary VBG surgery in this group of patients is high. These have been repaired electively after weight loss, though may need to be repaired concurrently. Postoperative care and follow-up are similar to primary LRYGBP. Patients need to be educated about the slightly higher risk of stricture and the need for early and aggressive dilatation.

RESULTS AND OUTCOMES

Several series of open revision of VBG to RYGBP have been reported.[7,18,27–32] The results have uniformly demonstrated improvement in weight loss, comorbidities, and resolution of band-related complications. But there is also a higher rate of complications. Small series and case reports of laparoscopic revision of VBG to RYGBP have yielded similar results.[33–39] The laparoscopic operative times were slightly longer compared to open, and one series had a high rate of conversion to open.[38]

In my recent (unpublished) series of 52 laparoscopic revisions of VBG to RYGBP patients, operative time has averaged about 4 hours, there have been no conversions, no mortalities, and median length of stay was 2 days. Early complications (leaks = 2, abscess = 2, strictures = 3) were more common than in our primary LRYGBP patients. Weight loss has averaged 60% of excess weight at 1 year and 50% at years 2, 3, and 4. Patients with obesity-related health problems had resolution or improvement in most of these conditions. Type 2 diabetes mellitus resolved completely in 7 of 10 patients (70%) and improved in 3 (30%). Hypertension resolved or improved in all; sleep apnea resolved in 3 of 3 (100%). Gastroesophageal reflux resolved or improved in 78%. All patients were able to tolerate solid foods and protein, and had resolution of VBG stomal-related symptoms.

SUMMARY

Long-term results of VBG have been disappointing. Laparoscopic revision of failed open VBG to RYGBP is a challenging but feasible procedure. It provides acceptable weight loss, improvement of obesity-related comorbidities, and improvement in VBG-related complications.

References

1. Mason EE: Vertical banded gastroplasty for obesity. *Arch Surg* 117:701–706, 1982.
2. Consensus Development Conference Panel: Gastrointestinal surgery for severe obesity. *Ann Intern Med* 115:956–961, 1991.
3. Trus TL, Pope GD, Finlayson SR: National trends in utilization and outcomes of bariatric surgery. *Surg Endosc* 19(5):616–620, 2005.
4. Nightengale ML, Sarr MG, Kelly KA: Prospective evaluation of vertical banded gastroplasty as the primary operation for morbid obesity. *Mayo Clin Proc* 66:773–782, 1991.
5. Buchwald H, Consensus Conference Panel: Bariatric surgery for morbid obesity: Health implications for patients, health professionals, and third-party payers. *J Am Coll Surg* 200(4):593–604, 2005.
6. Decision Memo for Bariatric Surgery for the Treatment of Morbid Obesity. Available at: http://www.cms.hhs.gov/mcd/viewdecisionmemo.asp?id=160. Accessed March 1, 2006.
7. Balsinger BM, Poggio JL, Mai J, et al.: Ten and more years after vertical banded gastroplasty as primary operation for morbid obesity. *J Gastrointest Surg* 4:598–605, 2000.
8. Brolin RE, Robertson LB, Kenler HA, et al.: Weight loss and dietary intake after vertical banded gastroplasty and Roux-en-Y gastric bypass. *Ann Surg* 220:782–790, 1994.
9. Mason EE, Cullen JJ: Management of complications in vertical banded gastroplasty. *Curr Surg* 60:33–37, 2003.
10. Ashley S, Bird DL, Sugden G, et al.: Vertical banded gastroplasty for the treatment of morbid obesity. *Br J Surg* 80:1421–1423, 1993.
11. Baltasar A, Bou R, Arlandis F, et al.: Vertical banded gastroplasty at more than 5 years. *Obes Surg* 8:29–34, 1998.
12. Mason EE, Maher JW, Scott DH, et al.: Ten years of vertical banded gastroplasty for severe obesity. *Prob Gen Surg* 9:280–289, 1992.
13. Naslund E, Backman L, Granstrom L, et al.: Seven-year results of vertical banded gastroplasty for morbid obesity. *Eur J Surg* 163:281–286, 1997.
14. Suter M, Jayet C, Jayet A: Vertical banded gastroplasty: Long-term results comparing three different techniques. *Obes Surg* 10:41–46, 2000.
15. Wang W, Yu PJ, Lee YC, et al.: Laparoscopic vertical banded gastroplasty: 5-year results. *Obes Surg* 15:1299–1303, 2005.
16. Yale CE: Conversion surgery for morbid obesity: Complications and long term weight control. *Surgery* 106:474–480, 1989.
17. Linner JH, Drew RL: Reoperative surgery-indications, efficacy, and long-term follow up. *Am J Clin Nutr* 55(Suppl 2):606S–610S, 1992.
18. Behrns KE, Smith CD, Kelly KA, et al.: Reoperative bariatric surgery: Lessons learned to improve patient selection results. *Ann Surg* 218(5):646–652, 1993.
19. Hunter RA, Watts JM, Dunstan RE, et al.: Revisional surgery for failed gastric restrictive procedures for morbid obesity. *Obes Surg* 2:245–252, 1992.
20. Balsiger BM, Murr MM, Poggio JL, et al.: Bariatric surgery. Surgery for weight control in patients with morbid obesity. *Med Clin North Am* 84:477–489, 2000.
21. Kral JG: Surgery for obesity. *Curr Opin Gastroenterol* 17:154–161, 2001.
22. MacLean LD, Rhode BM, Sampalis J, et al.: Results of the surgical treatment of obesity. *Am J Surg* 165:155–162, 1993.
23. Meyer JH: Nutritional outcomes of gastric operations. *Gastroenterol Clin North Am* 23: 227–260, 1994.
24. Sugerman HJ, Starkey JV, Birkenhauer R: A randomized prospective trial of gastric bypass versus vertical banded gastroplasty for morbid obesity and their effects on sweets versus non-sweets eaters. *Ann Surg* 205:613–624, 1987.
25. Capella JF, Capella RF: The weight reduction operation of choice: Vertical banded gastroplasty or gastric bypass? *Am J Surg* 171:74–79, 1996.
26. Sugerman HJ, Londrey GL, Kellum JM, et al.: Weight loss with vertical banded gastroplasty and Roux-Y gastric bypass for morbid obesity with selective versus random assignment. *Am J Surg* 157:93–102, 1989
27. Jones KB: Revisional bariatric surgery—safe and effective. *Obes Surg* 11, 183–189, 2001.
28. Jones KB: Revisional bariatric surgery—potentially safe and effective: *Surg Obes Relat Dis* 1:599–603, 2005.
29. Balsiger BM, Murr MM, Mai J, et al: Gastroesophageal reflux after intact vertical banded gastroplasty: Correction by conversion to Roux-en-Y gastric bypass. *J Gastrointest Surg* 4(3):276–281, 2000.
30. Sugerman HJ, Kellum JM Jr, DeMaria EJ, et al.: Conversion of failed or complicated vertical banded gastroplasty to gastric bypass in morbid obesity. *Am J Surg* 171(2):263–269, 1996.
31. Cordera F, Mai JL, Thompson GB, et al.: Unsatisfactory weight loss after vertical banded gastroplasty: Is conversion to Roux-en-Y gastric bypass successful? *Surgery* 136(4):731–737, 2004.
32. Gonzalez R, Gallagher SF, Haines K, et al.: Operative technique for converting a failed vertical banded gastroplasty to Roux-en-Y gastric bypass. *J Am Coll Surg* 201:366–374, 2005.

33. de Cespel J, Nahouraii R, Gagner M: Laparoscopic gastric bypass as a reoperative bariatric procedure for failed restrictive procedures. *Surg Endosc* 15:393–397, 2001.

34. Gagner M, Gentileschi P, de Csepel J, et al.: Laparoscopic reoperative bariatric surgery: Experience from 27 consecutive patients. *Obes Surg* 12:254–260, 2002.

35. Bloomberg RD, Urbach DR: Laparoscopic Roux-en-Y gastric bypass for severe gastroesophageal reflux after vertical banded gastroplasty. *Obes Surg* 12:408–411, 2002.

36. McCormick JT, Papasavas PK, Caushaj PF, et al.: Laparoscopic revision of failed open bariatric procedures. *Surg Endosc* 17(3):413–5, 2003.

37. Cohen R, Pinhero JS, Correa JL, et al.: Laparoscopic revisional bariatric surgery: Myths and facts. *Surg Endosc* 19:822–825, 2005.

38. Khaitan L, Van Sickle K, Gonzolez R, et al.: Laparoscopic revision of bariatric procedures: Is it feasible? *Am Surg* 71(1):6–10, 2005.

39. Gagné DJ, Goitein D, Papasavas PK, et al.: Laparoscopic revision of vertical banded gastroplasty to Roux-en-Y gastric bypass: An outcomes analysis. *Surg Obes Relat Dis* 1:243, 2005.

40. Cendán JC, Abu-aouf D, Gabrielli A, et al.: Utilization of intensive care resources in bariatric surgery *Obes Surg* 15:1247–1251, 2005.

41. MacLean L, Rhode BM, Forse RA: Late results of vertical banded gastroplasty for morbid and super obesity. *Surgery* 107:20–27, 1990.

42. Svenheden KE, Akesson LA, Holmdahl C: Staple disruption in vertical banded gastroplasty. *Obes Surg* 7:136–138, 1997.

43. Gallagher SF, Sarr MG, Murr MM: Indications for revisional bariatric surgery. In: Inabnet WB, DeMaria EJ, Ikramuddin S (eds.): *Laparoscopic Bariatric Surgery*. Philadelphia, Lippincott Williams & Wilkins, 2005; p. 153–173.

44. Mason EE: Law of LaPlace and obesity surgery. *ISBR Newsletter.* 1998;13:2. Accessed at: http://aboutplastic.surgery.uiowa.edu/ibsr/summer98.htm.

45. Kellogg TA, Ikramuddin S: Laparoscopic conversion of vertical banded gastroplasty to Roux-en-Y gastric bypass, in Inabnet WB, DeMaria EJ, Ikramuddin S (eds.): *Laparoscopic Bariatric Surgery*. Philadelphia, Lippincott Williams & Wilkins, 2005; p. 174–176.

34

Biliopancreatic Diversion: Revisional Surgery

Nicola Scopinaro, MD, FACS

With the exception of eight cases of higher gastrectomy required for GEA stenosis following stomal ulcer, nearly all specific late reoperations after biliopancreatic diversion (BPD) consisted of elongations of the common limb (CL) or restorations of intestinal continuity, protein malnutrition (PM) (with or without additional problems) being the condition to be cured in the vast majority of cases.[1] As both the reoperations are generally implemented to correct an excess of effect of the original operation, and they entail a permanent modification of intestinal absorption, it is critical to ensure that intestinal adaptation mechanisms have been substantially completed, what requires at least 1 year. If the problems persist and reoperation is then indicated, the risk of reoperating prematurely with resultant overcorrection and undue weight regain is minimal.

The elongation of the CL is indicated whenever a recurrent PM occurs in a BPD subject with normal food intake. In this case, PM is due to insufficient protein intestinal absorption, either absolute (insufficient absorption capacity per unit of intestinal length, too rapid intestinal transit due to excessively little stomach) or relative (insufficient protein content of ingested food, excessive loss of endogenous nitrogen). In both cases the aim of the surgical revision is to increase protein absorption, and this, keeping in mind the physiology of the operation, would not be obtained by elongating the CL along the alimentary one. Since, as said above, protein absorption after BPD substantially depends on the total intestinal length from the GEA to the ileocecal valve (ICV), the elongation of the CL for correction of a recurrent PM must be performed at the expense of the biliopancreatic

limb, the length which in our experience has proven effective in all cases being 150 cm, with the result of a total of 400 cm of small bowel in the food stream (Figure 34–1). Similar to what happens with the ad hoc stomach–ad hoc alimentary limb (AHS–AHAL) BPD, this type of revision has a double mechanism of action. In fact, by also increasing fat and starch absorption, it reduces the loss of endogenous nitrogen and the colonic bacteria overgrowth, with the result of a decreased protein requirement and an increased protein absorption in the colon. Incidentally, the fact that mean alimentary protein absorption after elongation is still reduced to ∼80%[2,3] indicates that (1) colonic protein absorption is fully exploited also after elongation; (2) the amount of protein absorbed in the colon after BPD is probably greater than that absorbed in the small bowel; and (3) increasing the length of small bowel between the GEA and the ICV most probably acts by increasing protein absorption more in the colon than in the small bowel.

On the basis of the same rationale, this type of elongation is also indicated in case of excessive weight loss in presence of a normal food intake, as well as to reduce problems of foul-smelling stools and flatulence. Since water absorption capacity is also increased, another indication is the presence of diarrhea due to excessive fluid intake.

Rarely, diarrhea is due to excessive reduction of ileal bile salt absorption. This condition can be easily diagnosed by cholestyramine administration, and it represents the only indication to the elongation of the CL along the alimentary one (two cases in our experience), 100 cm being sufficient in our experience (Figure 34–2).

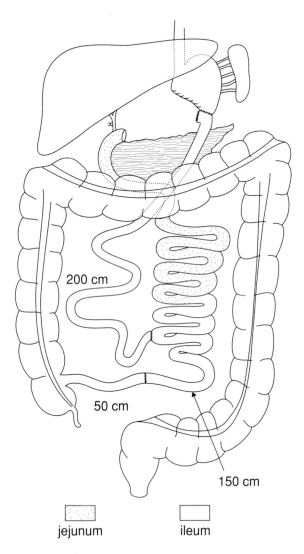

Figure 34–1. Elongation of the common limb along the biliopancreatic limb.

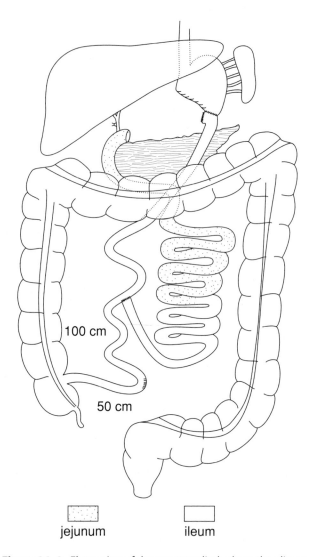

Figure 34–2. Elongation of the common limb along the alimentary limb.

Restoration of the intestinal continuity is specifically indicated in presence of a recurrent PM and/or an excessive weight loss due to permanence of the food limitation effect with or without poor protein intake. The goal in these cases is to restore a normal intestinal absorption capacity in a subject who will maintain his/her weight reduction because of the permanently reduced food intake. This can be obtained with different operations, from a simple high side-to-side enteroenterostomy to the complete reconstruction of the gastrointestinal tract, with a 50-cm ileal loop being interposed between the stomach and the duodenum (Figure 34–3). We prefer to section the alimentary limb (AL) immediately proximal to the enteroenterostomy (EEA) and join the ileal stump to the jejunum, immediately distal to the ligament of Treitz. This type of restoration allows the resumption of a normal protein-energy absorption, still partially preserving both the specific effects of BPD on glucose and cholesterol metabolism (Figure 34–4).

Restoration may be necessary if a disease occurs whose consequences would be worsened by malabsorption, e.g., a

liver cirrhosis, a nephrotic syndrome, a chronic inflammatory bowel disease, a malignancy, or a psychosis. It may also be requested by the BPD subject instead of the elongation after a long period of recurrent PM, or for different reasons, e.g., intolerance of the stool/gas problems, or psychological intolerance of the environmental problems originated by the changed body shape, or what we simply call "intolerance of the operation." These latter subjects do not have one major problem. They seem to magnify a series of minor discomforts just in order to justify their desire of not having the operation anymore, which is often due to fear caused by the negative attitude of the environment.

Only in case of untractable severe bone demineralization (no cases in our experience), or of moderate bone demineralization associated with the condition that indicates the restoration (four cases in our experience), we accept the sacrifice of the effect on glucose metabolism by putting the duodenum in the alimentary continuity, which can be accomplished as shown in Figure 34–3, or, if the effect on cholesterol metabolism is to be preserved, by keeping the

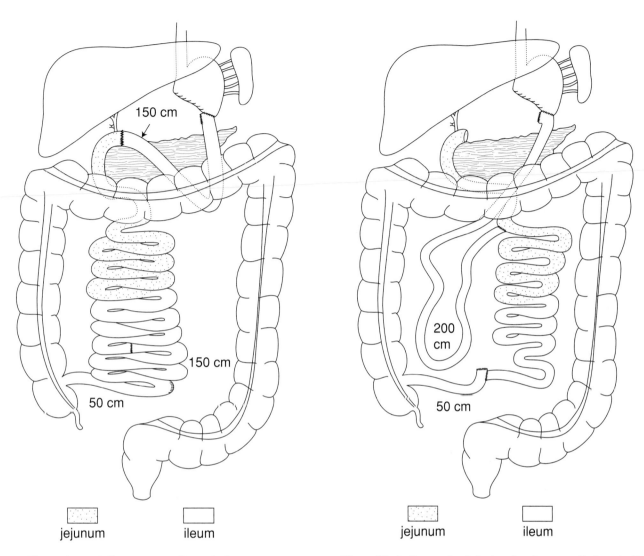

Figure 34–3. Full restoration of intestinal continuity.

Figure 34–4. Restoration bringing the alimentary limb to the ligament of Treitz.

entire AL interposed between the stomach and the duodenum (Figure 34–5).

Exceptionally, a shortening of the intestinal limbs may be considered. The most common cause for weight regain after BPD is excessive intake of simple sugar. Only in case this type of patient's noncompliance can be reasonably excluded, an excess of the adaptive phenomena leading to late energy absorption increase may be suspected. A preliminary measurement of alimentary protein intestinal absorption is, in our opinion, mandatory. A more than 90% absorption on the one hand confirms the excessive adaptation, on the other hand it means that there is a wide margin for shortening without causing excessive protein malabsorption. In two cases, both with 370-cm AL, we resected the proximal part of the AL exceeding the 240 cm which, as a mean of the intestinal measurements taken at late reoperations for any cause, result after adaptation, with redo of GEA. Since these two patients failed to lose weight, we thought it could be due to the highly consuming small bowel removed, which compensated for the decreased absorption. In a third case, with 520-cm AL and 80-cm CL, we sectioned the AL 240 cm distal to the GEA, de-

tached the biliopancreatic limb (BPL) from the distal ileum, and then anastomosed the BPL to the distal stump of the AL section and the proximal stump to the distal ileum, thus creating a CL of 70 cm (mean CL length after adaptation), as shown in Figure 34–6. The patient slowly lost all the excessive weight previously regained. The same operation was subsequently successfully used in another case who had been submitted to BPD elsewhere and had had minimal weight reduction. Both the CL and the AL were excessively long, and this most probably was due to wrong intestinal measurement, even if a rapidly occurring excessive intestinal adaptation could not be ruled out.

The total number of revisions in the 1,639 AHS BPD subjects with a minimum follow-up of 1 year was 112 or 6.8%, 77 (4.7%) being elongation of the CL and 35 (2.1%) restoration of intestinal continuity. If the percentage of reoperations per year in the population at risk is considered (Table 34–1), it is interesting to note that, though almost half of both the reoperations were done in the second and third year, the frequency decreases with time but still exists in the seventeenth

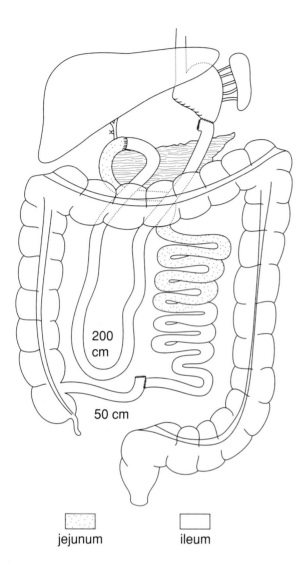

Figure 34–5. Restoration bringing the alimentary limb to the duodenum.

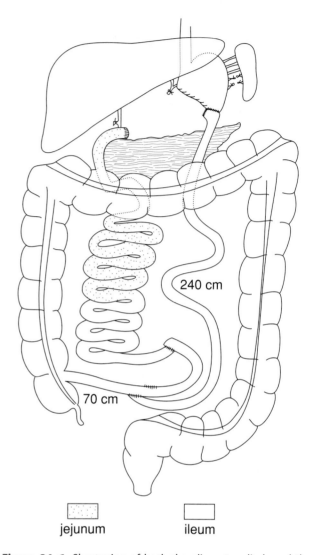

Figure 34–6. Shortening of both the alimentary limb and the common limb.

year after BPD, the no incidence in the last 2 years being evidently due to the paucity of the populations. This is easily explained considering that, since the operation is active indefinitely, the risks associated with it, though progressively reduced, also persist indefinitely. Elongations were still done until the seventeenth year and this is surprising if we consider that the latter operation is requested in 90% of cases to correct a recurrent PM with or without excessive weight loss, both conditions which, being due to insufficient intestinal absorption, are not likely to appear at long term. Actually, on the one hand in some BPD subjects the first episode of PM occurs in the third year or later and the recurrence can also be very delayed, on the other hand BPD subjects are often very reluctant to accept an operation that is expected to cause at least some weight regain. Furthermore, in some cases the recurrent PM does not present with severe episodes but rather with a continuous status of submalnutrition, which is compatible with an acceptable quality of life. Finally, recurrent PM may also be due to insufficient protein content of ingested food, and this, due to changes in eating habits,

may, even if exceptionally, occur in any time of the subject's life.

When the three groups defined in Chapter 8 in the evolution of AHS BPD are considered, the revision rate in the first group of 192 operated subjects was 10.4% (elongations 8.3%, restorations 2.1%). In the second group, the first 430 subjects had a revision rate of 11.2% (elongations 7.9%, restorations 3.3%), and the subsequent 429 had a revision rate of 8.1% (elongations 5.5%, restorations 2.6%), in spite of the reduced incidence of PM. The fact that the frequency of elongation, which is 90% required for recurrent PM, was higher than the incidence of this complication, is explained considering that in that period, thanks to facilities offered by our national health system, we had the possibility of operating on a great number of obese patients of low economical status. In 12 occasions, when the PM episode occurred in the second or third year, after full resumption of eating, and thus it had great probability of recurring, the patients expressed their will of not taking the risk of a second long hospital stay with the consequent loss of income. In those cases, contrarily

Table 34–1.

Revision Rate in a 19-Year Follow-Up in AHS BPD Subjects

Year of Follow-up	Number of Subjects at Risk	Total Revisions	Elongations	Restorations
Second	1639	28 (1.7%)	16 (1.0%)	12 (0.7%)
Third	1555	19 (1.2%)	15 (1.0%)	4 (0.3%)
Fourth	1486	16 (1.1%)	12 (0.8%)	4 (0.3%)
Fifth	1423	12 (0.8%)	9 (0.6%)	3 (0.2%)
Sixth	1372	8 (0.6%)	6 (0.4%)	2 (0.1%)
Seventh	1347	12 (0.9%)	9 (0.7%)	3 (0.2%)
Eighth	1316	2 (0.2%)	1 (0.1%)	1 (0.1%)
Ninth	1280	5 (0.4%)	4 (0.3%)	1 (0.1%)
Tenth	1240	1 (0.1%)	1 (0.1%)	—
Eleventh	1120	2 (0.2%)	—	2 (0.2%)
Twelfth	1031	2 (0.2%)	2 (0.2%)	—
Thirteenth	839	1 (0.1%)	—	1 (0.1%)
Fourteenth	648	1 (0.2%)	1 (0.2%)	—
Fifteenth	417	1 (0.2%)	—	1 (0.2%)
Sixteenth	192	—	—	—
Seventeenth	146	1 (0.7%)	1 (0.7%)	—
Eighteenth	122	—	—	—
Nineteenth	87	—	—	—

to our rule, the elongation was done after a single episode of PM. The same applies for three cases of late sporadic PM. In the third group of 293 BPD subjects with a minimum follow-up of 7 years (and maximum of 13 years), as said above, only three elongations (1.0%) and two restorations (0.7%) were performed, with an overall revision rate of only 1.7%. The revision rate was further reduced (0.8%) in the 392 AHS–AHAL BPD patients operated on from March 1999 to February 2004 (minimum 2-year follow-up).

Out of the total number of 77 elongations, 55 (71%) were required for recurrent PM alone (11 after a single PM episode), 13 (17%) for recurrent PM with excessive weight loss (1 after a single PM episode), 3 for excessive weight loss alone, 3 for diarrhea due to excessive fluid intake, 2 for diarrhea due to excessive bile salt malabsorption (elongation along the AL), and 1 for intolerance of stool/gas problems.

Of the 35 restorations, in 7 cases (19%) the indication was permanence of the food-limitation effect (1 case with recurrent PM, 2 cases with excessive weight loss, and 4 cases

with both conditions). One of these patients, rejecting our advice, had previously asked to be elongated for fear of weight regain. As expected, the elongation was inadequate to cure her recurrent PM and she was eventually restored. Eight subjects with recurrent PM (1 with diarrhea from excessive fluid intake) and normal food intake preferred to be restored instead of elongated. In 6 cases (16%), restoration was required because of liver cirrhosis (1 concomitant with liver transplantation) and in 2 because of psychosis. Five subjects (1 with sporadic PM) requested restoration because of "intolerance of the operation," 2 because of intolerance of stool/gas problems, and 2 because of intolerance of problems due to the changed body shape. Recurrent PM with kidney cancer was the indication in one case and with ovarian cancer in another one. One subject, in total well-being, requested restoration, refusing to explain why.

All problems of recurrent PM, excessive weight loss, diarrhea, stool/gas, and bone demineralization permanently disappeared after revisions. While no recurrences of

Table 34–2.

Weight Changes (%IEW, mean ± SD) Following Surgical Revisions of BPD

Type and Cause of Revision	Elongation for Recurrent PM and/or Excessive WL (71 s.)	Elongation for Other Causes (6 s.)	Restoration for Permanence of Food Limitation Effect (7 s.)	Restoration for Other Causes (28 s.)
Mean % IEW	121 ± 39	90 ± 30	146 ± 47	107 ± 40
At revision	92 ± 12	96 ± 10	77 ± 16	85 ± 16
At 1 year	80 ± 26 (71 s)	74 ± 11 (6 s.)	62 ± 9 (7 s.)	73 ± 14 (28 s.)
At 2 years	71 ± 15 (65 s.)	76 ± 24 (6 s.)	56 ± 14 (7 s.)	65 ± 16 (26 s.)
At 5 years	68 ± 21 (49 s.)	61 ± 22 (6 s.)	60 ± 14 (7 s.)	51 ± 19 (25 s.)
At 10 years	63 ± 21 (41 s.)	48 ± 21 (5 s.)	53 ± 20 (5 s.)	40 ± 20 (20 s.)
Mean GV (mL)	375 ± 95	400 ± 55	335 ± 98	420 ± 80
Mean FI before revision	Slightly increased	Greatly increased	Greatly reduced	Equal
Mean FI after revision	Equal	Moderately increased	Moderately reduced	Equal

GV, gastric volume; FI, self-reported food intake compared with preoperatively.

hypercholesterolemia were ever observed, there were two cases of mild hyperglycemia recurrence in previously diabetic patients after elongation. Mean postrevision changes in body weight, together with mean %IEW at BPD and at revision, are reported in Table 34–2, where mean gastric volumes and pre- and postrevision food intake are also related.

Since protein and starch digestion/absorption occur in the entire small bowel between the GEA and the ICV, and fat absorption in the intestinal segment between the EEA and the ICV, the elongation of the CL along the BPL which is necessary to increase protein absorption also causes an increase of starch and fat absorption. This obviously results in a higher energy absorption threshold, which explains the restabilization at a higher body weight of the subjects undergoing elongation of the CL for recurrent PM and/or excessive weight loss.

The reason why, on the contrary, the subjects elongated for other reasons kept gaining weight until the tenth year is most probably an excessive and uncontrolled intake of simple sugar due to the profound noncompliance of these subjects, proved by the persisting diarrhea from excessive fluid intake and by the fact that mean food intake in these subjects was and remained higher than that of all the other groups. Actually, the two subjects in this group who were elongated along the AL because of diarrhea from excessive bile salt malabsorption had and maintained a food intake equal to the preoperative one, and they did not gain any weight in a 6- and 11-year follow-up, respectively.

Comprehensibly, the subjects restored for permanence of the food limitation effect had a preoperative mean excess weight sharply higher than that of the other groups. Con-

sequently, they had a smaller mean gastric volume and thus an increased risk of the above condition. In fact, their mean self-reported food intake was halved in comparison with the preoperative one, and it remained reduced after revision. The indication to restoration of the intestinal continuity is evidently in keeping with the physiology of BPD. These subjects were actually eating less than the maximum they could absorb, so they were suffering the negative effects of the malabsorption without taking any benefit by it. The restabilization on a higher weight is explained by the fact that on the average they increased their food intake after restoration.

Conversely, and as expected, the subjects with normal food intake who asked for restoration without having the indication to it, as well as those who had to be restored for other diseases, showed postoperatively a progressive weight regain without any change of food intake.

Anyway, the weight changes after BPD revisions indicate that, when the indication was correctly given by us according to the physiology of the operation, the revised subjects had a moderate weight regain with restabilization, the success being maintained, while in the other cases they regained weight progressively toward failure.

Interestingly, in both the second and the fourth group, where the majority of subjects requested a revision which was not indicated by medical problems, the mean pre-BPD excessive body weight was significantly lower than the average initial excess weight (IEW) in our series. This could mean that the subjects who had a smaller weight problem, and thus a smaller benefit by the procedure, are less inclined to accept the side effects of it.

A final consideration regards the mean weight loss at the time of revision, which was in all groups lower than the average in our series. Any degree of weight reduction can be obtained with BPD, but, as we learned at our expenses, the greater the mean weight loss, the greater the number of problems. Unless a surgeon has an experience sufficient to enable him to tailor the operation on each single subject, any mean reduction of the IEW greater than 70% should be considered potentially dangerous. Weight maintenance, not weight loss, is the real magic of BPD.

References

1. Scopinaro N, Gianetta E, Friedman D, et al.: Surgical revision of biliopancreatic bypass. *Gastroenterol Clin North Am* 16:529–531, 1987.
2. Friedman D, Caponnetto A, Gianetta E, et al.: Protein absorption (PA) and protein malnutrition (PM) after biliopancreatic diversion (BPD). *Proceedings of the Third International Symposium on Obesity Surgery*, Genoa, Italy, September, 20–23, 1987, p. 50.
3. Scopinaro N, Marinari GM, Gianetta E, et al.: The respective importance of the alimentary limb (AL) and the common limb (CL) in protein absorption (PA) after BPD. *Obes Surg* 7:108, 1997

35

Biliopancreatic Diversion: Duodenal Switch

João Batista Marchesini, MD, PhD, FACS

I. INSUFFICIENT WEIGHT LOSS AND WEIGHT REGAIN

II. MALNUTRITION

III. INTESTINAL OBSTRUCTION

IV. PERSISTENT SYMPTOMS

V. PERINEAL COMPLICATIONS

VI. DUODENAL *SWITCH* AS AN ALTERNATIVE

Morbid obesity has become a worldwide pandemic and has been treated by different means according to surgeon and/or patient preferences. It encompasses 1.7 billion people and bariatric surgery is the only effective treatment of morbid obesity.[1,2] The formal indications for surgical treatment are still based on body mass index above 40 kg/m^2 or above 35 kg/m^2 associated with comorbidities.[3] The surgical techniques applied for bariatric surgeries are essentially restrictive, malabsorptive, or combined.[4]

Among restrictive procedures, the most commonly described are the vertical banded gastroplasty, the laparoscopic silicone adjustable gastric band, and the sleeve gastric resection.[4,5] Gastric pacemaker that produces early satiety may be considered restrictive as well.[6,7] Intragastric balloon, which is restrictive, is not a formal surgical intervention.[8]

Malabsorptive procedures that have been used for many years, mainly in the United States, have now been abandoned due to their side effects. Jejunoileal bypass and all its variants are still used by some surgeons, but are not recommended because there are better methods available with lower incidence of long-term complications.[3,9]

The combined procedures may be more restrictive or more malabsorptive.[4] Gastric bypass with or without banding is more restrictive.[2,4] The malabsorptive part of these operations is minimal and needs to be better investigated. Among the combined malabsorptive interventions are the biliopancreatic diversion with distal gastrectomy (BPD), biliopancreatic diversion with duodenal switch (BPD–DS), and the distal roux-en-Y gastric bypass (RYGBP). Other techniques are variations of these three.[10–17]

The most popular BPDs are those proposed by Scopinaro,[17,18] including distal gastrectomy with gastroileal anastomosis and its variant, the duodenal switch, which is a vertical gastrectomy with pyloric preservation and duodenoileal anastomosis.[12,13,14,19] The gastric sleeve resection is a restrictive component and the jejunoileal bypass is the malabsorptive one. The method proposed by Hess,[12,13] which has been initially well studied and published by Marceau and coworkers,[14,20] carries the name *duodenal switch* (DS) different from the procedure of duodenal diversion proposed by DeMeester et al.[21] for the surgical treatment of duodenogastric reflux and alkaline gastritis. Variations also occurred with the DS, e.g., Gagner proposed a method wherein a laparoscopic adjustable gastric banding (LAGB) was added to the BPD–DS, avoiding the vertical gastrectomy.[22]

There is no consensus as to what constitutes success or failure after a weight loss procedure, and the long-term results remain a subject of controversies.[20] The ideal weight loss surgery should allow significant durable weight loss, relief of obesity-related associated diseases, and should have low surgical morbidity and mortality rates.[23] It is not possible to separate the amount of weight loss, the presence or absence of comorbidities, and changes in quality of life when evaluating the success of a bariatric treatment. This subject is beyond the scope of this chapter, but deserves special attention.

The main purpose of the present chapter is to study DS from two different viewpoints as far as revision operations are concerned:

1. As a procedure that needs correction or repair due to poor results or side effects.
2. A procedure that is used to correct others that are not reaching their goals.

DS is a very effective weight loss surgical procedure and it is among the most aggressive treatments for morbid obesity as far as weight loss and sustained results are concerned.[3,19] Its effectiveness is, however, defeated by its complications. When it is not possible to control them medically, a revision operation is imposed. We now review these short- and long-term complications and the different choices for their surgical correction.

DS may interfere with the oral intake of foods and supplements, the intestinal pathway integrity and function, the absorption of proteins, vitamins, minerals, and other nutrients, and also the bowel habits. It depends very much on the patient's compliance.[24] The conditions that may require special medical attention and eventual surgical revisions are related to weight regain or insufficient weight loss as well as malnutrition and other complications. These complications may be particular to the DS or common to other bariatric procedures that need also to be mentioned as follows:

1. Insufficient weight loss and weight regain
   a. gastric pouch too big
   b. common channel too long
   c. uncontrolled eating disorders
   d. wrong choice of operation
   e. alcohol addiction or drug side effect
2. Malnutrition
   a. protein malnutrition
   b. vitamin deficiency
   c. mineral deficiency
3. Intestinal obstruction
   a. internal hernias
   b. adhesions

4. Persistent symptoms
   a. diarrhea
   b. vomiting
   c. foul-smelling flatus
5. Anal complications

INSUFFICIENT WEIGHT LOSS AND WEIGHT REGAIN

When the sleeve gastrectomy is performed, the resection may leave a bigger gastric antrum or a fundic pouch too big. The restrictive part of this operation may not be complete and the weight loss may not be sufficient. When this occurs, it becomes necessary to perform a revision operation to trim the stomach and to decrease its volume capacity (Figures 35–1 and 35–2). The same may happen for a longer common channel. It has been established that there are three classical lengths of common channels: 50, 75, and 100 cm. To choose the right length for the right patient may become the problem, leading to insufficient weight loss or weight regain. McConnell has demonstrated, in a comparative study, a relationship between common channel lengths and weight loss.[23]

There is no uniform method for measuring the length of the intestine. When measured if it is loose, the results are

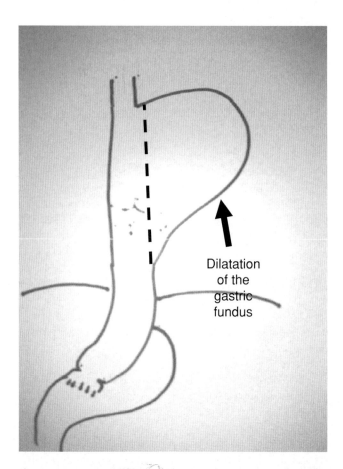

Figure 35–1. Gastric fundus dilatation found in a patient who had regained weight. Nonresponsive to medical treatment, she was submitted to a revision operation.

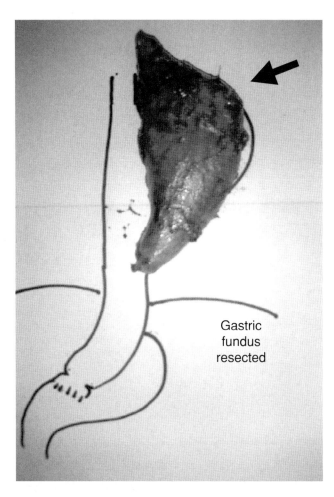

Figure 35–2. The gastric fundus was resected creating a tube-like gastric remnant, which was followed by adequate and sustained weight loss.

microvilli as well as their absorptive surface. It depends also on the blood flow and the functionality of the cells. Measuring of the intestine needs to be reviewed from an anatomical and physiological basis. Hess has proposed to perform common channels and alimentary limbs according to the total length of the small bowel.[25] For common channels, he recommended around 10% of the total length of the small intestine, but this statement needs to be tested by others under more rigid protocols. Scopinaro disagrees with making the intestinal lengths proportional to total bowel length.[17]

Bariatric operations deal with gastrointestinal tract. They do not interfere with the brain's function and little with eating disorders. There are a great number of patients that try to cheat on the weight loss surgery because the eating disorder is not adequately treated.[26] High-risk eating behavior needs to be identified preoperatively in order to prevent postoperative unsuccessful outcome such as insufficient weight loss or weight regain. Grazing[26] and bingeing may be controlled with medication such as the mood modulators, antidepressant agents, medications for anxiety, and others.

Bariatric surgery ameliorates the affective disorders by recovering the self-esteem, but is not the solution for psychiatric or psychological diseases.[27] Sometimes drug treatment for psychiatric conditions is responsible for the weight regain.[28] In certain situations, medical treatment is not effective and complementary revision surgery is necessary.

Interventions such as resizing the stomach and shortening the common channel may be applied, but other choices are also valid. Adding an LAGB to the DS[29,30] or converting DS to GBP may be a choice. Sometimes the wrong choice of an operation is the explanation of unsuccessful weight loss or weight regain. Restrictive procedures, for instance, are a bad operation for sweet eaters. Changing from an LAGB to a DS is the answer for many patients unhappy with their previous operation (Figures 35–3 and 35–4). To change from a GBP to a DS or a BPD may be a good choice for fat eaters. Alcohol abuse goes along with a high caloric intake. Alcohol is one of the main enemies of weight loss surgery. It is very

different from those when measuring it stretched. For sure, the absorptive area will be different with different lengths of intestine. Besides this, absorption depends on the width of the intestine and the mucosal area, and the number of villi and

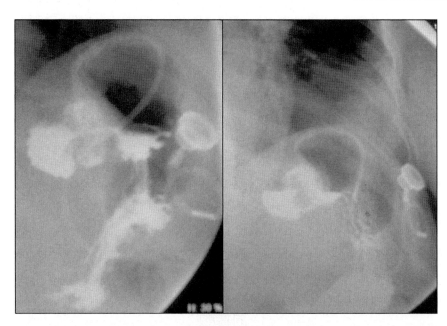

Figure 35–3. Unsuccessful laparoscopic silicone gastric banding placed 7 years before that was deflated due to malfunctioning. Slippage detected through an upper GI series. Patient maintaining morbid obesity.

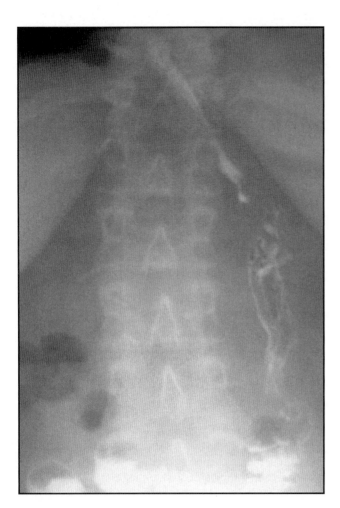

Figure 35–4. Final aspect of the gastric sleeve resection and duodenal switch from the revised LASGB.

important to quit drinking or to have alcohol addiction duly treated.

MALNUTRITION

Malnutrition needs to be treated medically before having surgical revision. Patients submitted to DS may develop protein malnutrition due to poor intake or due to poor absorption. The same may happen with other nutrients, vitamins, minerals, and oligoelements. Compliance is very important.[24] When surgical revision is imposed for DS malnutrition, patients may be treated in two different ways: Increasing the length of the common channel at the expense of the biliopancreatic limb or by enteroenterostomy between the alimentary limb and the jejunum (biliopancreatic limb), close to the Treitz ligament (Figure 35–5). By increasing the absorptive area, protein malnutrition and deficiency of other nutrients are easily corrected.

Scopinaro[17] recommends transferring the alimentary limb from its original position to the biliopancreatic limb higher up, around 200–250 cm from the ileocecal valve (Figures 35–6 and 35–7). One has to pay attention to do it

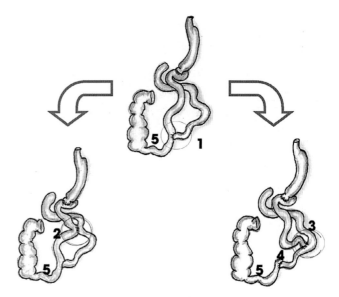

Figure 35–5. Revision operations for postoperative malnutrition after duodenal switch: 1. Roux-en-Y intestinal bypass; 2. Proximal jejunoileostomy; 3. GBP anastomosis transferred proximally; 4. Section of the alimentary limb; and 5. Common channel.

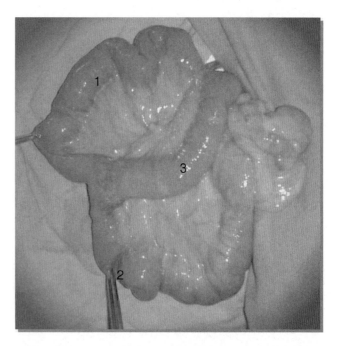

Figure 35–6. Revision operation for malnutrition due to a 50 cm common channel. Anatomic positioning: 1. Alimentary limb; 2. Common channel; and 3. Biliopancreatic limb.

correctly. Transferring the biliopancreatic limb to a higher portion of the alimentary limb in order to increase the length of the common channel is not enough to solve the problem.

Postoperative malnutrition may be related to strictures of the duodenoileal anastomosis or somewhere else in the food pathway. Restriction is imposed by the obstructive pathologic component. This may occur due to suturing reasons such as bad technique, healed leakages, inadequate

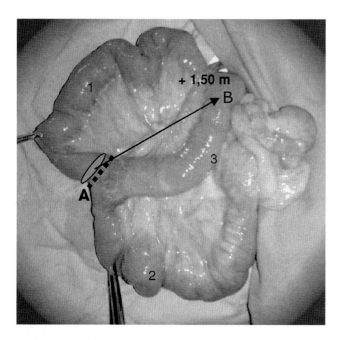

Figure 35–7. Alimentary limb (a) transected at the level of the RNY anastomosis and (b) transferred proximally to 200 cm far from the ileocecal valve.

stapling, etc., or due to secondary diseases such as postoperative peptic ulcers or inflammatory diseases among others.[24,31]

INTESTINAL OBSTRUCTION

This is a complication that is common to all bariatric surgery, and also occurs sometimes in DS patients. Internal hernias and adhesions need emergency surgical intervention, but rarely does the DS anatomy itself need to be modified. Closure of the mesenteric defects to avoid new internal hernias and lysis of adhesions are usually enough to solve these problems. Internal hernias have been described mostly in GBPs.[32]

PERSISTENT SYMPTOMS

Patients submitted to DS as in other malabsorptive procedures may have persistent symptoms of diarrhea and/or foul-smelling flatus due to excessive fatty food intake and excessive anaerobic bacterial growth as well. Besides medical treatment and diet orientation, some patients do not accept these annoying conditions and require surgical correction. Taking down the intestinal biliopancreatic bypass usually solves the problem. The patient ends up solely with a gastric sleeve resection. Weight regain is a risk after such revision surgery. Vomiting may be related to mechanical obstruction of the stomach outlet or proximal partial intestinal occlusion. Stomal ulcers may cause nausea and vomiting. Medical treatment is usually enough. Surgical revisions are seldom required.

PERINEAL COMPLICATIONS

Liquid or acidic stools may cause anal fissure, anal ulcer, and anal bleeding besides triggering a hemorrhoidal crisis of pain and bleeding. Changing bowel habits by changing diet and eventually adding drugs for diarrhea may improve anal conditions. Severe anal fissures may become chronic and difficult to treat. They may require local surgical treatment. When these anal conditions become intractable, DS may need revision and eventually may be modified to GBP, SGR, or simply taken down.

DUODENAL *SWITCH* AS AN ALTERNATIVE

Duodenal *switch* will be now considered as a revisional operation for other bariatric interventions that have not accomplished acceptable weight loss. According to the initial classification of the bariatric procedures, it may be applied to correct previous restrictive, malabsorptive, and combined procedures:
1. vertical banded gastroplasty (VBG)
2. laparoscopic adjustable gastric band (LAGB)
3. sleeve gastric resection (SGR)
4. jejunoileal bypass (JIB)
5. Roux-en-Y gastric bypass (banded and nonbanded) (RYGBP)
1. VBG, as proposed by Mason or MacLean,[3] and its variants as well may be unsuccessful due to poor weight loss or weight regain. The bad result of the VBG may be related to high caloric intake of liquids or semiliquid meals or due to the disruption of the gastrogastric septum and a gastrogastric fistula. The shortcut of the foods through the communication between both gastric chambers may be the explanation for the bad results. Otherwise, stricture at the food pathway may lead to excessive weight loss, repeated vomiting, and nutrient deficiencies.

The high rate of surgical revisions and the inconsistent postoperative weight loss no longer supports the recommendation for VBG as a treatment for morbid obesity.[10] DS is a good alternative for revision operations for unsuccessful VBGs.[33] A conversion from a VBG to a DS starts by cutting the gastric septum through and communicating both gastric chambers. This maneuver is followed by an SGR.

Mucocele of the gastric tube after conversion of a VBG to a DS has been described.[34] It is a consequence of entrapping gastric mucosa between the old and the new stapling lines and should be avoided. This is a very important reason to cut the gastric septum before proceeding with the sleeve gastrectomy.

From this point on, the DS intestinal Roux-en-Y bypass is performed. As this procedure is done with mechanical suturing devices, one has to pay attention to the thickness of the gastric wall in order to apply the proper staples. Duodenal switch without SGR plus restoration of the original gastric capacity has been proposed as a revisional

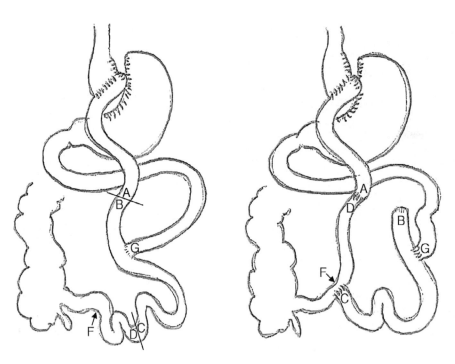

Figure 35–8. Conversion from an RYGBP to a BPD-like procedure.

procedure after failed VBG or LAGB.[35] The advantage of this gastric preserving operation is to avoid gastric resection thereby decreasing surgical morbidity; however, this method needs better evaluation.

2. Laparoscopic silicone adjustable gastric banding is the new version of a VBG. It is a restrictive procedure complying with the principles of Mason's operation. The weight loss is usually insufficient or the weight is regained as time goes by. The weight regain is also secondary to an adaptation for caloric liquid intake. Compliance to restriction is another pitfall. Patients may not tolerate restriction and repeated vomiting. DS is a good alternative for these patients. They will be able to eat better and lose more weight, which will be sustained for a longer period of time.[36]

Conversion from an LAGB to a BPD or BPD–DS may be done successfully by laparoscopic approach.[37] It is a good option to treat unsuccessful gastric banding. It is important to remove the band and dissect free all the adhesions, leaving the gastric anatomy close to the original one in order to perform a correct DS. An incomplete dissection may lead to abnormal rotation of the stomach or excessive gastric fundus may be left in place. This condition is responsible for malfunctioning and poor results for the DS.

3. Only sleeve gastric resection, which is used primarily as the first step for a DS in superobese patients or as a restrictive method for patients with borderline bariatric surgical indications, may need to be completed to a full DS in case of weight regain.[5,22,38]

4. Patients who had a JIB and need conversion due to nutritional or metabolic complications may have the JIB modified to a DS. However, it is necessary to consider that once a patient has not adapted himself or herself to

a malabsorptive procedure it may not be wise to change it to another one.

5. Patients submitted to RYGBP, those regaining or not losing enough weight or those not adapted to dumping syndrome, to excessive vomiting, or other conditions, need to be adequately treated.[39]

Keshishian and coworkers propose DS as the solution for other Weight Loss Surgery (WLS) procedures that have failed.[39] The same proposal is found in Rabkin's publication.[2] This has been our preference too, when possible. In these series, the main reasons for revision to DS are weight regain or inadequate loss, significant dumping syndrome, solid food intolerance, persistent nausea and vomiting, and severe gastroesophageal reflux.

Like other patients undergoing different procedures, these RYGBP patients need to undergo medical treatment. Psychological orientation, diet programming, exercising, and drug treatment consist in the first approach to these patients. Controlling grazing and bingeing is very important. Besides medication for anxiety, depression, panic, or other psychiatric condition, the use of mood modulators may be helpful. When all the attempts fail, a revision operation may be imposed.

To modify an RYGBP to a DS may not be that simple. To anastomose a dilated and/or functioning proximal gastric pouch to the distal stomach that is nonfunctioning, smaller than normal or atrophic, may lead to complications. Malfunction of the new gastric reservoir or leakages may occur. Once this is accomplished, patients will have a better quality of life.

The compromised blood supply of the proximal stomach when dissected free from the short gastric vessels may be a reason for not proceeding with a DS. The left gastric arterial blood supply may be interrupted during the original gastric bypass operation and now, in the absence of the short gastric vessels (interrupted for the DS), this gastric pouch may become dependent only on the esophageal blood vessels.[39] This poor vascular condition may become a contraindication to such technical choice. Transforming a proximal gastric bypass to a distal bypass[40] may be the answer to the problem of uncontrolled body weight.

Another choice for weight regain or insufficient weight loss is to change an RYGBP in a BPD by working only in the intestinal part of the RYGBP as we previously proposed.[40,41] Cutting the intestine just proximal to the gastroenterostomy, below the mesocolon if transmesocolic, anastomosing the ileum to the proximal transected end of the jejunum, and following with a Roux-en-Y ileoileal anastomosis one may reproduce a BPD, which fills the principles of a combined malabsorptive operation (Figure 35–8). The clinical results will be similar to a DS without the technical difficulties imposed by the previous gastric operation. If the previous surgery is a banded RNY, this restriction needs to be removed.[41]

Combining a restrictive procedure with a malabsorptive one has been criticized in the medical literature[42,43]; but as a revisional operation for insufficient weight loss or weight regain it needs to be better studied by different groups. Duodenal switch is an operation to be performed by skillful bariatric surgeons acquainted with all nutritional issues, aware that the postoperative care is for life, well trained in open and laparoscopic approaches, and sustained by a multidisciplinary team. It is one of the most difficult bariatric procedures, and if done, laparoscopically is one of the most difficult operations as well. When DS is used for revision operation, it becomes a defeat for the bariatric surgeon.

Finally, we need to remember that there is always the right patient for the right surgery. It has not been determined so far how to "fit" the patient to the "right size" operation. Compliance, however, is responsible many times for the success or bad results of a bariatric procedure.

The patient who does not understand the importance of, or cannot afford, having correct protein intake is prone to develop severe protein malnutrition. A similar situation is created by inadequate replacements of vitamins, minerals, and other nutrients. If a patient is to benefit from weight loss surgery, he or she has to realize that there will be a cost for it. Tolerance and acceptance for some side effects is very important. The cost and benefit analysis needs to be perfectly understood preoperatively in order to guarantee good or at least acceptable results from a bariatric operation. Compliance is a prime condition for a patient yet to undergo malabsorptive procedure. The socioeconomic status and eating habits of the patient do interfere many times with the end results.

References

1. Buchwald H, Williams SE: Bariatric surgery worldwide 2003. *Obes Surg* 14(9):1157–1164, 2004.
2. Rabkin RA: The duodenal switch as an increasing and highly effective operation for morbid obesity. *Obes Surg* 14:861–865, 2004.
3. DeMaria EJ, Jamal MK: Surgical options for obesity. *Gastroenterol Clin North Am* 34:127–142, 2005.
4. Marchesini JB, Marchesini JCDM: Insucesso terapêutico, complicações tardias e reoperações In: Garrido AB, Ferraz EM, Barroso FL, Marchesini JB, Szego T, Cirurgia da Obesidade. Sociedade Brasileira de Cirurgia Bariátrica, Ed Atheneu, São Paulo, 2002; p. 227–244.
5. Baltasar A, Serra C, Perez N, Bou R, Bergonchea M, Ferri L: Laparoscopic sleeve gastrectomy: A multipurpose bariatric operation *Obes Surg* 15:1124–1128, 2005.
6. Chen J: Mechanisms of action of the implantable gastric stimulator for obesity. *Obes Surg* 14(Suppl):28–32, 2004.
7. Shikora SA: Implantable gastric stimulation—The surgical procedure: Combining safety with simplicity. *Obes Surg* 14(Suppl 1):9–13, 2004.
8. Doldi SB, Micheletto G, Perrini MN, Librenti MC, Rella S. Treatment of morbid obesity with intragastric balloon in association with diet. *Obes Surg* 12:583–587, 2002.
9. Requarth JA, Burchard KW, Colacchio TA, et al.: Long-term morbidity following jejunoileal bypass. The continuing potential need for surgical reversal. *Arch Surg* 130:318–325, 1995.
10. Brolin RL, Robertson LB, Kenler HA, Kody RP: Weight loss and dietary intake after vertical banded gastroplasty and Roux-en-Y gastric bypass. *Ann Surg* 220(6): 782–790, 1994.
11. Gagner M, Matteotti R: Laparoscopic biliopancreatic diversion with duodenal switch. *Surg Clin North Am* 85:141–149, 2005.
12. Hess DS, Hess DW: Biliopancreatic diversion with a duodenal switch. *Obes Surg* 8:267–282, 1998.
13. Hess DS, Hess DW, Oakley RS: The biliopancreatic diversion with the duodenal switch: Results beyond 10 years. *Obes Surg* 15:408–416, 2005.
14. Marceau P, Simard S, Lebel S, Bourque RA, Potvin M, Biron S: Biliopancreatic diversion with duodenal switch. *World J Surg* 22:947–954, 1998.
15. Murr MM, Balsiger BM, Kennedy FP, Mai JL, Sarr MG: Malabsorptive procedures for severe obesity: Comparison of pancreaticobiliary bypass and very very long limb Roux-en-Y gastric bypass. *J Gastrointest Surg* 3:607–612, 1999.
16. Scopinaro N, Gianetta E, Civalleri D, Bonalumi U, Bachi V: Biliopancreatic bypass for obesity: II. Initial experience in man. *Br J Surg* 66:618–620, 1979.
17. Scopinaro N, Adami FG, Marinari GM, Traverso E, Papadia F, Camerini G: Biliopancreatic diversion: Two decades of experience In: Dietel M, Cowan GSM Jr (eds.): *Update: Surgery for the Morbid Obese Patient.* Toronto, Canada, FD Communications; 2000; p. 227–265.
18. Scopinaro N: Limb lengths in BPD-invited commentary. *Obes Surg* 14:333, 2004.
19. Anthone GJ, Lord RV, DeMeester TR, Crookes PF: The duodenal switch operation for the treatment of morbid obesity. *Ann Surg* 238:618–628, 2003.
20. Biron S, Hould FS, Lebel S, et al.: Twenty years of biliopancreatic diversion. What is the goal of the surgery? *Obes Surg* 14:160–164, 2004.
21. DeMeester TR, Fuchs KH, Ball CS, et al.: Experimental and clinical results with proximal end-to-end duodenojejunostomy for pathologic duodenogastric reflux. *Ann Surg* 206:414–426, 1987.
22. Gagner M, Steffen R, Biertho L, Horber F: Laparoscopic adjustable gastric banding with duodenal switch for morbid obesity: Technique and preliminary results. *Obes Surg* 13:444–449, 2003.
23. McConnell DB, O'Rourke RW, Deveney CW: Common channel length predicts outcomes of biliopancreatic diversion alone and with duodenal switch surgery. *Am J Surg* 189:536–540, 2005.
24. Rabkin RA, Rabkin JM, Metcalf B, Lazo M, Rossi M, Lehman-Becker LB: Nutritional markers following duodenal switch for morbid obesity. *Obes Surg* 14:84–90, 2004.
25. Hess DS: Limb measurements in duodenal switch—Correspondence. *Obes Surg* 13:966, 2003.

26. Saunders R: "Grazing": A high-risk factor. *Obes Surg* 14:98–102, 2004.

27. Herpertz S, Kielmann R, Wolf AM, Langkafel M, Senf W, Hebebrand J: Does obesity surgery improve psychosocial functioning? A systematic review. *Int J Obes Relat Metab Disord* 27:1300–1314, 2003.

28. Hamoui N, Kingsbury S, Anthone GJ, Crookes PF: Surgical treatment for morbid obesity in schizophrenic patients. *Obes Surg* 14:349–352, 2004.

29. Slater GH, Fielding GA: Combining laparoscopic adjustable gastric banding and biliopancreatic diversion after failed bariatric surgery. *Obes Surg* 14:677–682, 2004.

30. Sotirios G, Karaindros CA, Papaioannou, et al.: Biliopancreatic diversion with duodenal switch combined with laparoscopic adjustable gastric banding. *Obes Surg* 15(4):517–522, 2005.

31. Petrolesi F: Crohn disease obstruction of the biliopancreatic limb in a patient operated for morbid obesity. *Emerg Radiol* 12:116–118, 2006.

32. Champion JK, Williams M: Small bowel obstruction and internal hernias after laparoscopic Roux-en-Y gastric bypass. *Obes Surg* 13:596–600, 2003.

33. Yashkov YI, Oppel TA, Shishlo LA, Vinnitsky LI: Improvement of weight loss and metabolic effects of vertical banded gastroplasty by an added duodenal switch procedure. *Obes Surg* 11:635–639, 2001.

34. Sanchez-Pernaute A, Perez-Aguirre E, Talavera P, Robin A, et al.: Mucocele of the gastric tube after conversion of vertical banded gastroplasty to duodenal switch: Not just a radiological image. *Obes Surg* 16:524–527, 2006.

35. Di Betta E, Mittempergher F, Di Fabio F, Casella C, Terraroli C, Salerni B: Duodenal switch without gastric resection after failed gastric restrictive surgery for morbid obesity. *Obes Surg* 16:258–261, 2006.

36. De Csepel J, Quinn T, Pomp A, Gagner M: Conversion to a laparoscopic biliopancreatic diversion with a duodenal switch for failed laparoscopic adjustable silicone gastric banding. *J Laparoendosc Adv Surg A* 12(4):237–240, 2002.

37. Dolan K: Biliopancreatic diversion following failure of laparoscopic adjustable gastric banding. *Surg Endosc* 18:60–63, 2004.

38. Gagner M, Rogula T: Laparoscopic reoperative sleeve gastrectomy for poor weight loss after biliopancreatic diversion with duodenal switch. *Obes Surg* 13:649–654, 2003.

39. Keshishian A, Zahriya K, Hartoonian T, Ayagian C: Duodenal switch is a safe operation for patients who have failed other bariatric operation. *Obes Surg* 14:1187–1192, 2004.

40. Pareja JC, Pilla VF, Callejas Neto F, Coelho-Neto JS, Chaim EA, Magro D: Gastroplastia redutora com bypass gastrojejunal em Y-de-Roux: Conversão para bypass gastrointestinal distal por perda insuficiente de peso—experiência em 41 casos. *Arq Gastroenterol* 42:196–200, 2005.

41. Marchesini JB, Marchesini JC, Marchesini SD. "Scopinarização"—uma proposta para correção de operações bariátricas mal sucedidas (resumo). São Paulo, Anais do Congresso Brasileiro de Cirurgia Bariátrica—1991. (Marchesini JB, Marchesini JC, Marchesini SD. "Scopinarização"—a proposal for correction of bariátricas operations badly-succeeded [summary]. Brazilian congressional records of Surgery Bariátrica, São Paulo, 1991)

42. Papadia F: Biliopancreatic diversion and gastric restriction—Correspondence. *Obes Surg* 14:145–146, 2004.

43. Papadia F: Combining gastric banding and biliopancreatic diversion. *Obes Surg* 14:1141–1142, 2004.

44. Cowan GSM Jr, Buffington CK, Hiler ML: Enteric limb lengths in bariatric surgery. In: Dietel M, Cowan GSM Jr (eds.): *Update: Surgery for the Morbid Obese Patient.* Toronto, Canada, FD Communications, 2000; p. 267–276.

45. Cowan GSM Jr, Hiler ML, Buffington CK: Reoperative bariatric surgery. In: Dietel M, Cowan GSM Jr (eds.): *Update: Surgery for the Morbid Obese Patient.* Toronto, Canada, FD Communications, 2000; p. 417–425.

Postoperative Management

36

Infection in Obesity Surgery

Álvaro Antônio Bandeira Ferraz, MD, PhD, TCBC • Edmundo Machado Ferraz, MD, PhD, TCBC

INTRODUCTION

In spite of the worldwide effort to decrease and treat obesity, the increasing prevalence rates have been concerning many countries.[1–6] This preoccupation rises especially when severe obesity is analyzed. In this type of obesity, the only long-term effective treatment is surgery.[7–10]

Despite the low rates of infectious complications, the exponential increase of numbers of bariatric surgery makes us deal more and more with this kind of patient. Postoperative infections continue to represent a great challenge for surgeons and health professionals. The incidence rate of surgical infection varies from surgeon to surgeon, from hospital to hospital, from one kind of surgery to another, and, especially, from patient to patient.[11–13] The aim of this chapter is to discuss some features of essential importance in the physiopathology, prophylaxis, and treatment of postoperative infection in bariatric surgery.

RISK FACTORS

The attempt to prevent the real risk of the patient to develop a postoperative infectious complication has been a reason for a big effort by the scientific community. Patients with a high risk for postoperative infection could be submitted to different types of surgical preparation and management.

In this way, the SENIC Project (Hooton and colleagues[14]) published, in 1981, the result of a multicentric analysis of 58,498 operated patients, identifying risk factors, to develop a valuation index. Evaluating risk factors, the authors have made a statistical analysis through the CHAID system (chi-square automatic interaction detection). The examined risk factors were age, gender, time of surgery, abdominal surgery, previous infection, immunodeficiency, preoperative stay, intrinsic risk of the surgery and preexisting pathology. Therefore, this index was applied in 59,352 operated patients in the period between 1975 and 1976. They previewed 73% of the infections.

In 1985, Haley and colleagues,[15] trying to simplify this methodology and analyzing the same data of the SENIC Project, reduced to a number of four the risk factors and studied them using a system of multiple regression. With this methodology, Haley and colleagues have previewed 69% of the postoperative infections. The four risk factors were contamination level (if the surgery was contaminated or infected), abdominal surgery, extended surgery (more than 2 hours), and the existence of more than three diagnoses or comorbidities in the patient.

In 1987, Christou and colleagues[16] also proposed a methodology of prognostic evaluation of the infection. They have analyzed in this proposal, through a logistic system of multiple regression, the contamination level of the surgery, serum albumin, age, cutaneous retarded sensibility test, and the time of surgery. The authors did not quantify the risk of the patient to have infection. The aim was to determine values that added together would show the chances of the patient to become infected after the surgical act. The final equation would be

$$\begin{aligned} P = 1 - \{1 + \exp[&-3.49 + 1.05 \text{ (albumine in g/L)}\\ &+ 0.17 \text{ (DTH score)} + 0.02 \text{ (age)}\\ &- 0.27 \text{ (surgery contamination)}\\ &+ 0.11 \text{ (time of surgery)}]\} \end{aligned}$$

where DTH score = logarithm expression of cutaneous reaction to hypersensibility test; surgery contamination = clean = 1; potential cont. = 2; cont. = 3; infected = 4; exp. = exponential; and P = risk of infection.

However, maybe the NISS system is the most used index of risk factors for infection, which was published in 1991 by Culver and colleagues.[17] In the NISS system, the time of surgery is used related to specific procedures, type of wounds, and ASA system of preoperative evaluation. In Table 36–1 we present the risk of infection according to the SENIC index, of Haley and colleagues, and the NISS.

The obese patient presents, in most varied analysis, a higher risk to develop infectious complications.[18-26] However, this kind of recognition has been based on empiric analysis and without a clear physiopathologic basis.[1] Experimental works in mice and rats have shown that, in obesity, there is retardation in the healing process, T cell lymphopenia, reduced macrophages and neutrophil activation, and chemotaxis and decrease in the expression of pro-inflammatory cytokines.[27-34] Clinical studies have also

confirmed this compromise in the inflammatory response and healing process.[27,33,34]

The inclusion of obesity as a risk factor in the development of infectious complications is related essentially to the existence of comorbidities, which usually comes with it. Among these comorbidities hyperglycemia and low oxygen tension in the tissues stand out. The chronic hyperglycemia, among many alterations, increases the surgical infection rates in a significant way.[1,35-40] Studies in intensive care unit patients have shown a great decrease in the bacteremia rates in those with rigorous control of blood sugar using insulin infusion.[35] The oxygen levels in tissues also influence in a significant way the incidence rate of the surgical site infection. It is believed that the bactericidal activity of neutrophils is dependent on superoxide radical production, which is dependent on the oxygen partial pressure in the tissues.[41,42]

A high surgical risk resulting from comorbidities requires special care and concern. Worried with this additional risk, Ferraz and colleagues,[43] in 2002, have compared the postoperative comorbidities and complications in the superobese with those of the operated severe obese patients, showing that the frequency in the first group is higher, formulating the score of Recife. This score quantifies the risk of the high severity of complications and death in the preoperative period.[43] The results of this present study indicate a 9.6% frequency of severe postoperative complications and 39.3% of mild postoperative complications in a superobese group of patients submitted to the Fobi-Capella gastric derivation surgery. The mortality rate was 3.6%. The main factors associated with the presence of mild complications were body mass index (BMI) over 55 kg/m^2, diabetes, and sleep apnea, while the factors associated with severe complications and death were BMI over 55 kg/m^2 and existence of coronary heart disease. In a multivariate analysis, the only factor that persisted and was associated with death in a significant way was BMI higher than 55 kg/m^2.

ANTIBIOTIC PROPHYLAXIS

Christou and colleagues, in a recent publication,[44] have considered that the incidence rate of surgical site infection in the surgical treatment for morbid obesity is high and the current recommendations of antibiotic prophylaxis are scant. In this type of patient, the surgical site infection tends to present significant morbidity.

Keighley,[45] in 1977, has postulated that prophylactic antibiotics should be prescribed in three occasions.

1. When the bacterial contamination risk is high (gastrointestinal, genitourinary, and respiratory surgeries among others).
2. When the contamination is not frequent, but the infection risks are high (amputation associated with vascular disorders, prosthesis and valve use, grafts).

Table 36–1.

Infectious Risk Distribution (According to the SENIC Project index, Haley & colleagues, and to NISS)

SENIC Project

Number of Factors	Clean	Pot. Contaminated	Contaminated	Infected
1	0.6	0.2	—	—
2	1.2	0.6	—	—
3	1.2	1.3	—	4.7
4	2.4	3.0	5.6	—
5	4.0	3.8	4.9	6.3
6	6.4	6.4	9.9	8.7
7	8.5	10.6	9.5	10.5
8	9.4	14.3	12.6	14.7
9	14.5	19.9	18.7	24.6
10	20.4	26.3	29.2	30.0
Haley and colleagues				
0	1.1	0.6	—	—
1	3.9	2.8	4.5	6.7
2	8.4	8.4	8.3	10.9
3	15.8	17.7	11.0	18.8
4	—	—	23.9	27.4
NISS SYSTEM				
0	1.0	2.1	—	—
1	2.3	4.0	3.4	3.1
2	5.4	9.5	6.8	8.1
3	—	—	13.2	12.8

3. When the contamination is not frequent but the host is immunosuppressed (transplants, chemo, and radiotherapy).

The use of prophylactic antibiotics in clean or potentially contaminated surgeries does not reduce the infection rate of surgical wounds.[46–49] In this kind of surgery, the benefits of antibiotic prophylaxis do not outweigh the risks, not being, therefore, a recommended application.[50–54] In order to execute the antibiotic prophylaxis in an effec-

tive way, it is necessary, among the minimal requirement, besides those recommended by Ferraz and Ferraz[12,13] (spectrum, pharmacokinetics, duration, toxicity), that it reaches maximum concentrations in the tissues at the incision time. Burke's work,[55] which has served as a foundation for these studies, however, was based on healthy and nonobese patients.

Under normal weight and conditions, the blood flow in the fat tissue is low and represents approximately 5% of cardiac output, while in the non-fat tissue this flow comes to

22%.[56] Therefore, it is important to reconsider antibiotic prophylaxis in morbid obesity. Information on the use of drugs and their distribution in obese patients and, particularly, in the morbidly obese is scarce. Very little is known about antibiotic pharmacokinetics in patients with BMI above 40 kg/m^2.[57]

Edmiston and colleagues[58] have emphasized the need of a better analysis of prophylaxis in morbid obesity, including the subgroups with BMI from 50 to 59 kg/m^2 and BMI over 60 kg/m^2. Evaluating the cefazolin concentration in its action place, it was observed that therapeutic levels were obtained in only 28.6% of the patients with BMI between 50 and 59 kg/m^2, and in only 10.2% of the patients with BMI equal or superior to 60 kg/m^2. A simple increase in the dose is not always sufficient to guarantee good prophylactic coverage. Forse et al.[59] have reduced the incidence rate of surgical site infection from 16.5% to 5.6%, enhancing the prophylactic cefazolin from 1 to 2 g. However, some prophylactic schemes must be reconsidered and even be replaced in the case of morbid obesity. The gastroplasty prophylaxis with cefazolin shows infection rates of the surgical site that varies from 5% to 20%.[44,58,59]

Ferraz and colleagues,[60] comparing patients submitted to gastric derivation with proximal Roux-en-Y, in which antimicrobial prophylaxis with ampicillin/sulbactam was used in a dose of 3 g (two doses), with those who received ceftriaxone in a dose of 1 g (single dose), did not observe a significant difference related with the incidence of infection in the surgical site. More information about drugs and doses in the prophylaxis of surgical site infection in severe obese patients is still missing. However, we must be aware that the increasing doses of known schemes, new drug utilization, and even modifications in the antimicrobial infusion technique may determine changes in the nosocomial microflora and in the appearance of resistant bacteria. Related with videosurgery, the choice of antibiotic, infusion technique, and antimicrobial duration do not differ from recommended basic rules concerning the use of prophylactic antibiotics in open surgery.[12,13]

POSTOPERATIVE INFECTION

Among the common infections of patients submitted to morbid obesity surgical treatment, we highlight the surgical site infection and the suture line leakage associated with intra-abdominal infections.

Surgical Site Infection

The infection rate in the surgical site in patients who were submitted to morbid obesity surgical treatment varies, in the literature, from 1% to 11%.[60–66] This large variation is related with high incidence of seroma in this type of patient, which mixes up and increases the incidence of this complication. In April 1999, the Centers for Disease Control published a consensus[67] about prevention of surgical site infection, which is still used by many people today. The incidence of abdominal wall infection is frequently higher in open surgeries.

Intra-Abdominal Infection

The management of the patient who has intra-abdominal infection must be aggressive, precise, and fast. The identification of intra-abdominal infection is merely clinical in 72% of the cases, a complementary confirmation with image exams being necessary in about 25%.[68] In the severe obese patients, the clinical appearance is nonspecific and the image examinations help us very little in the diagnosis. This way, we must suspect intra-abdominal infectious complication when the patient has tachypnea, tachycardia, fever and chills, and pleural effusion. The appropriate control of the infectious focus is the main factor that influences the reduction of mortality in this kind of patient.

The principles in the abdominal sepsis management are[69–71]

1. hemodynamic, immunological, and metabolic support;
2. antimicrobial therapy
3. infectious focus and basis disease control

Hemodynamic, Immunological, and Metabolic Support

Beyond the hydroelectrolytic and metabolic support, which the patient with abdominal sepsis must have, we could stratify the aims of management in this type of patient.[72]

Hemodynamic Support

Hemodynamic support to maximize oxygen support for tissues are

- hydroelectrolytic replacement
- inotropic agents
- vasoactive agents
- mechanical ventilation

Metabolic Support

Metabolic support aims essentially to reverse the catabolism state of the patient and the most effective measure is the control of the infectious focus. The nutritional support must be aggressive through enteral nutrition, preferably. The enteral nutrition presents a clear advantage in the inflammatory response modulation, decreasing TNF response.[73] The institution of enteral nutrition ameliorates, in a general way, the capacity of an individual to deal with and decrease the bacterial translocation, through reduction in catabolism, decreasing the cortisol serum level, and preventing gut mucosa atrophy.[74] But the translocation through the gastrointestinal barrier was not affected.[74] In case of an improper intestinal function, we must start parenteral nutrition. The nutritional therapy, besides preventing and treating deficiency of diet components, has been used to obtain similar responses to those of pharmacological agents, in a way to improve the immune response of the patients affecting some kinds of aggressive infections. A great variety of nutrients are associated with immunostimulator alterations in addition to their nutritional advantages.

Omega-3 fatty acids: The use of omega-3 fatty acids has aroused the attention of researchers, in the improvement of the patient immune response and also in the antirejection properties determined by this element.[75] The omega-3 fatty acid disjoins arachidonic acid, reducing the eicosanoid production. The use of this substance defines a certain immunosuppression degree, increasing the transplant's long life,[75] like anti-inflammatory action, with a significant decrease in the IL-1 and TNF synthesis, going back to normal levels 20 weeks after.[76] Clinically, a diet rich in fatty acids has been used in patients with inflammatory arthritis, psoriasis, and systemic lupus erythematosus, with the intention of reducing the severity of the cases.[77] The mortality of septic rats fed with omega-3 fatty acids was decreased.

Glutamine: Glutamine is a nonessential amino acid, and is considered as a primary fuel for lymphocytes, macrophages, and enterocytes. The use of solutions containing glutamine increases the nitrogenous balance of surgical and traumatized patients.[78] The mechanism through which glutamine contributes to this balance is by

- participating in protein synthesis of skeletal muscles;
- maintaining the structure and function of intestinal tract;
- improving glutathione levels inside the cell (an important cytosolic antioxidant);
- reducing the bacterial translocation rate; and
- improving the immune function.

Arginine: Is a partly essential amino acid which has important pharmacological properties. It is a source of nitrous and nitric oxides.[79] It is a powerful growth hormone stimulator of prolactin, pancreatic insulin, and glucagons; modulates protein metabolism; increases nitrogen retention; and increases collagen synthesis. Supplementary arginine decreases trauma effects over peripheral lymphocytic response.[80,81] Arginine also has important effects on organ rejection, increasing life span, and over malignant neoplasia, decreasing tumor size.[80,81]

The institution of balanced enteral nutrition has a fundamental role, as in maintaining and recuperation of the nutritional state of patients and also in inflammatory response modulation. Other elements have shown important properties on immune response modulation of the septic patient. Studies have demonstrated that the institution of balanced diets supplemented with arginine, nucleotides, and fish oil decrease patient's stay in the ICU as well as the infectious complications' incidence rates.[82]

Immunological Support

To prevent nosocomial infections, to eradicate existent infections, and to minimize to the maximum the metabolic response effects to infection, immunomodulation is the therapeutic intervention which aims to modify the damaged immune response.[83,84] The immunosuppressed patients, particularly those with basic diseases that do not suggest a reduction in immune defense, and patients with an overactive inflammatory response demand that we discover those patients who are sensitive to a detrimental organic response to the surgical-anesthetic experience. The surgery can be immunomodulating while controlling the infectious focus, but can be immunosuppressing while decreasing the reserve and resistance of the host immunological response.[85] In the literature, there are many efforts to modulate the surgical patient's immune response, but in practice only a few can still interfere in this response. Probably, they have not learned in an appropriate manner the number of each one of these countless variables that occur in sepsis and in systemic inflammatory response syndrome (SIRS). On the contrary, what has been obtained is how we interfere, in an inappropriate manner, in the healing of tissues by wrong use of antimicrobials and the incoherent utilization of invasive apparatus as well as using improper surgical techniques for infectious focus controlling.[86] Although until the last decade the decreasing mortality rate of the surgical patient was apparent, with larger use of this knowledge, the indication of a long road still to be traveled clearly exists. According to Baue et al.,[87] "When we reach the millennium, we recognize ourselves in the distance between our scientifical biologic process knowledge and the restricted capacity to treat our patients. Our science is strong. The molecular biology is powerful, but our therapeutic capacity is weaker and limited."

Antimicrobial Therapy

The obese patients, because of their physical composition, absorb, distribute, metabolize, and excrete drugs in a different way.[88-91] The relation between the size of the body, physiological functions, and pharmacokinetical variables on the obese population have been recently evaluated. Some physiological alterations, peculiar of the morbid obese, show potential consequences for drug kinetics. Among these alterations we can mention the following:

- Increased physical mass;
- increased total blood volume and cardiac debit;
- increased kidney clearance;
- increasing fat deposition on the liver; and
- serum levels of protein variations.

The antibiotic therapy in intra-abdominal infection, many times, starts in an empiric way and must cover a polymicrobial flora, essentially composed by gram-negative and anaerobic germs. The Gram stain is recommended and the culture will indicate the correct sensibility of pathogenic bacterias. The Surgical Infection Society[92] has presented some recommendations related to the choice of antibiotics in the intra-abdominal infection treatment, based on clinical rehearsals and the knowledge about pharmacokinetics and security profile of the antibiotics. The proposed schemes are presented in Table 36–2.

Table 36–2.

Antimicrobial Proposed Schemes for Intra-Abdominal Infection

Primary Peritonitis
  Cefotaxime
  Ciprofloxacin

Acquired Peritonitis in community, from mild to moderate
  Monotherapy
    Cefoxitin
    Cefotetan
    Cefmetazole
    Ampicillin-sulbactam
    Ticarcillin-clavulanic acid
    Ertapenem
  Antibiotic combination
    Aminoglycoside + Metronidazole

Severe peritonitis with bacterial resistance possibility
  Monotherapy
    Carbapenems
    Imipenem-cilastatin or meropenem
    Piperacillin-tazobactam
  Antibiotic Combinations
    Metronidazole + Third Generation Cephalosporins
      (or Cefepime)
    Clindamycin + Aztreonam
    Ciprofloxacin + metronidazole

Adapted, with permission, from Nathens AB, Rotstein, OD: Antimicrobial therapy for intra-abdominal infection. Am J Surg 172:1s–6s, 1996.

The specific treatment for *Candida* is recommended in immunosuppressed patients, who have peritonitis. The empiric addition of antimycotic therapy with fluconazole is recommended for patients who have postoperative intra-abdominal infection with high risk for *Candida* infection.[92] Particularly related to *Enterococcus*, the specific treatment is not recommended when it is for a polymicrobial infection of a peritonitis acquired in the community. When *Enterococcus* is identified in a remaining or recurrent process, it must be guaranteed an active treatment against this pathogen.[92]

After the infectious focus removal, the antibiotic therapy should be maintained until the patient presents[44]

- normal leucogram for more than 48 hours,
- no fever for more than 48 hours,
- no anorexia, and
- resettle conscious level.

The improper antibiotics use, especially in this kind of a patient, can determine infection by multiresistant pathogens and massive liberation of endotoxins. The endotoxin liberation determined by the antibiotic action is related with an increase in the mortality rate and must be considered in the choice of the therapeutic scheme.[93,94]

Vancomycin and aminoglycosides are one of the few antibiotics whose pharmacokinetics was extensively studied in the obese population. Despite the data not yet being definitive, primary recommendations can be made. Vancomycin doses should be calculated according to the total corporal weight (TCW). Aminoglycoside doses should be based on its distribution volume, using an FCDP of 0.4 approximately. The interval between the doses must be individualized, through dosaging of serum concentrations of these drugs.[95]

Allard and colleagues[96] have studied the ciprofloxacin distribution volume and drug degradation in the obese and observed that the maximum plasmatic concentration of ciprofloxacin is less in obese people than in nonobese after a 400 mg IV infusion, but the concentrations stay in the recommended therapeutic zone. These authors conclude that ciprofloxacin dose must be based on the TCW plus FCDP of 0.45. Few literature data can relate antimicrobial dose with morbid obesity. In Table 36–3, some suggestions of dosage optimization in the obese are presented.[57,59,96]

Table 36–3.

Antimicrobial Dosage Related to the Patient's Weight

Antibiotic	Dose Calculation Based on Weight
Beta-lactams	ICW + 0.30 (TCW – ICW)
Cefazolin	Double dose (2 g/qid)
Cefoxitin	Empiric – ICW
Ceftriaxone	ICW + 0.40 (TCW – ICW)
Cefepime	Empiric (2 g/bid)
Ceftazidime	Empiric – ICW
Ampicillin	Empiric – ICW
Imipenem	Empiric – ICW
Metronidazole	TCW
Gentamicin	ICW + 0.43 (TCW – ICW)
Amikacin	ICW + 0.38 (TCW – ICW)
Vancomycin	TCW
Ciprofloxacin	ICW + 0.45 (TCW – ICW)
Macrolides	ICW
Amphotericin B	TCW
Acyclovir	ICW

ICW, ideal corporal weight; TCW, total corporal weight.

Infectious Focus and Basis Disease Control

The intra-abdominal infection resulting from bariatric surgery can express itself in two manners: secondary peritonitis or intracavitary abscess. In the secondary peritonitis form, we recommend surgical treatment, objectifying:

1. elimination of the contaminant focus,
2. removal of secondary contamination sources,
3. drainage of established abscesses,
4. intense cavity washing, and
5. primary fascia closing.

In cases of secondary peritonitis, we do programmed relaparotomies every 48 hours until there are no infectious macroscopic signs in the abdomen. Our philosophy is now changing, as we do relaparotomies based on clinical/laboratorial indications.[1,97] The peritoniostomy constitutes an exception indication. It can bring damage to patient progress and needs to have its benefit clearly established. It is indicated in the impossibility of a primary closure of abdominal cavity and in fecal etiologies and diffuse peritonitis, with patient instability, secondary necrotic focus, tissue ischemia, and no focus control.

In the intra-abdominal abscess, the treatment is, invariably, drainage. The cavity abscess drainage can be done open or percutaneous. Analyzing the kind of drainage and correlating it with the APACHE II score, there was no difference between the drainage types in patients with low mortality risk. However, in severe patients, with high APACHE II scores, better results were obtained when the abscess was treated with open drainage.[98] Excellent results are associated with percutaneous drainage when some of the following are present[99]:

1. well-established unilocular liquid collection,
2. well-established drainage route, and
3. appropriate equipment and materials.

Surgical drainage would be indicated, which in turn leads to

1. percutaneous drainage fail,
2. multiples abscesses, and
3. abscesses associated with abdominal pathologies and fistulas.

But most important is effective drainage.

The antibiotic use in the intra-abdominal abscesses still is a polemic topic. Stable patients who have a single purulent collection, quite limited, precisely diagnosed by radiologic imaging method, can be submitted to surgical drainage, extra-serosa or by punch with or without ultrasonography or computerized tomography, with a single dose of the antibiotic administrated 30 or 60 minutes before the procedure. The antibiotic must cover anaerobic and gram-negative aerobic bacteria.[99] Except those cases, many patients with intra-abdominal abscess have an indication for antimicrobial use.

EVIDENCE BASED ANTIBIOTIC THERAPY

Evidence based medicine is a much explored field and it is necessary nowadays, especially if we consider the amount of available information and propagation speed of this information, which is not always authentic and based on controlled studies.

The antibiotic agent use in a systemic prophylactic way is a controversial question among surgeons, in greater part because of a lack of comprehension of the basic principles involved. The decision to use prophylactic antibiotic therapy, however, must be based on the weight of the evidence that has possible benefit in relation to the weight of evidence that has possible contrary effects. The improper use of prophylactic antibiotics increases the infection rate and adds to an unnecessary cost.[46–49] The wrong use of an antimicrobial determines, besides the immediate consequences of bad utilization in a specific patient, an important compromise for the whole nosocomial community, because it can determine or worsen the bacterial resistance effects.

In a general way, we can enumerate some evidence that must be followed when prophylactic antibiotic therapy is used.

1. Use it only in surgeries that probably have their infection rates reduced by the antibiotic administration;
2. use first line agents;
3. get antibiotic maximum serum levels on the exposure moment of the infecting agent (surgical moment);
4. restrict the prophylactic antibiotic use to the time of surgery. There is no evidence, in most of the surgeries, that the postoperative use reduces infection rates;
5. select an antimicrobial that is active against the majority of infecting agents of a certain surgery.

GUT DYSFUNCTION ON INFECTION GENESIS AND MAINTENANCE

The gastrointestinal tract takes part in an effective way not only on genesis, but also in sepsis perpetuation.[100–103] This perception has earned acceptance especially after the study published by Marshall, which is directly related with the bacterial translocation process.

In spite of the unquestionable occurrence, its clinical and pathological meanings are not properly explained yet, because clinical studies have not confirmed experimental finds. This does not mean there is no clinical importance of translocation. The correct reading is that, clinically, bacterial translocations have not had a defined role, despite probably existing. Bacterial translocation is directly related with bacterial adhesion capacity to the gut mucosa. This adhesion is avoided through mucous and IgA action.[104,105]

In trauma, humoral and cellular immunities are adversely compromised.[106] Sepsis and stress have a profound impact on B cell levels and, consequently, on IgA mucosa levels.[107–109] This impact is related to circulating glycocorticoid levels in trauma and sepsis situations. Glycocorticoids have a powerful immunosuppressive effect, acting on macrophages, inhibiting monocyte differentiation and B cell maturation.[106]

In Recife, Ferraz operated on 5 severe patients who had intra-abdominal sepsis and studied pieces of small intestine. Immunohistologic study by Coutinho and colleagues[110] in Oswaldo Cruz Institute, Recife, has revealed important alterations in the histological structure of small intestine, which could determine important alterations in the hemodynamics of patients. The authors have analyzed the alterations in small intestine mucosa and submucosa level, especially on IgA, IgM, J chain, HLA-DR, and plasmocytes level. The findings have encountered plasmocytes apoptosis which resulted in a decreased IgA and IgM expression that, certainly, favors bacterial adhesion to the intestinal mucosa and, consequently, bacterial translocation. The expressive increase of HLA-DR notifies the presence of a higher number of macrophages, necessary for the apoptotic cell phagocytosis. These findings plus small intestine pieces obtained in another 12 patients with similar clinical presentations from Aberdeen and Nottinghan Universities (England) have confirmed the alterations described in Recife and were an object of a multicentric publication that has defined these aspects in literature.[110] Meanwhile, not only mucous and IgA protect small intestine from bacterial and endotoxin passage through the intestinal lumen, but there are two other components that participate in an effective way on the mechanic protection of gastrointestinal tract, bacterial synergism and gastrointestinal motility.

In many sepsis cases, there is inappropriate antibiotic use, effectively eliminating the protector effect. The antimicrobial scheme utilization with large spectrum drugs favors bacterial selection and the colonization by multiresistant bacteria, like *Pseudomonas* and *Candida*.[12,13] The use of antibiotics by oral administration has caused a break on bacterial balance and a consequent proliferation and concomitant bacterial translocation.[111] Wells[112] has demonstrated the importance of anaerobic flora on the prevention of bacterial translocation.

This type of patient also shows significant alterations on intestinal motility, tending to paralytic ileus.[113] The paralytic ileus shows, in its physiopathology, multifactorial components that determine a hard control and complicate a therapeutic acting on its regression.[113] There is a gas and liquid accumulation and a bacteria proliferation that compromises normal intestinal functions. The main alteration on the myoelectric activity, evidenced on sepsis by peritonitis, is phase II absence. Phase III is preserved and phase I is also altered.[113] In this way, the protector effect of gastrointestinal motility is threatened.

Early enteral nutrition clearly benefits surgical patients and can be administrated in small volumes (10 mL/h), contending fundamental nutrients and, in turn, dispensing the traditional return of intestinal movements for its institution. This conduct can abbreviate the postoperative paralytic ileus,

decreasing the complication rate, as was very well demonstrated by Moore and Jones,[114] Moore and colleagues,[115] and Reissman and colleagues.[116] This relatively small volume of enteral feeding can establish the difference between a more effective postoperative recuperation, particularly in the severe surgical patient in whom enterocytic atrophy, reduction of systemic and intestinal induced by protein malnutrition that establish itself, initiates a whole sequence of events which is called intestinal dysfunction.

The presence of intestinal anastomoses, the fear of aspiration, and secondary nosocomial pneumonia have established a controversy in literature, which can only be lightened by random multicentric and well-controlled studies. However, precursory studies in patients submitted to this level of surgery suggest that early enteral alimentation is safe, well sustained, and reduces complication rates and improves prognosis. The intestinal dysfunction has a relevant role in genesis, continuity, and, eventually, in sepsis irreversibility of severe surgical patients, and the maintenance of an enteral alimentation, even in small quantities, acts in an efficient way on the enterocytes' atrophy prophylaxis and, this way, on the intestinal dysfunction prophylaxis.

IMMUNOMODULATION

We believe that the future of surgical infection treatment and sepsis is in immunotherapy utilization. The inhibition of neutrophil–endothelin interaction by the integrin or selectin blockade (CD 11 and CD 18) in inflammatory or infectious models has demonstrated conflicting results. On the other hand, the neutrophils' stimulation by administrating growth factors (G-CSF), which increases the PMNs number and activities, has demonstrated a rise in the long life of some experimental models, and there has also been an improvement in the symptoms of patients with pneumonia, with no alteration or decreasing mortality.

Clinical assays with cytokine antagonists have not shown benefits of this utilization. Studies with macrophage manipulation have resulted in the alteration of prognosis. The reduction in pulmonary macrophages has decreased the mortality and this reduction in liver and spleen has provocated a decrease on the MOF gravity.

In the eighties there were great expectations that the glucocorticoids could control the magnitude of inflammatory response. However, controlled studies have not demonstrated this expected action on sepsis and ARDS, and it was practically abandoned in clinic. Still, in 1998, two controlled studies—prospective, randomized, double-blind, and using placebo[117,118]—have demonstrated statistically significant reduction of morbidity and mortality and in turn have justified new studies, in progress, that aim to establish the glucocorticoid action before sepsis and inflammation.

The recombinant C protein utilization has been used in the treatment of severe sepsis patients who have high mortality risk. Its mechanism action promotes anti-thrombotics,

Table 36–4.

Experiment Type	Number of Experiments	Number of Patients	Mortality Placebo	Therapy
Antiendotoxin	4	2,010	35%	35%
Ab against IL-1	3	1,898	35%	31%
Antibradykinin	2	755	36%	39%
AntiPAF	2	870	50%	45%
AntiTNF	8	4,132	41%	40%
TN sol receiver	2	688	38%	40%
NSAI	3	514	40%	37%
Steroids	9	1,267	35%	39%
All studies	33	12,034	38%	38%

PAF, platelet activator factor; TNF, tumoral necrosis factor; NSAI, nonsteroidal anti-inflammatory.

anti-inflammatories, and profibrinolytic activities in the microcirculation, modulating the SIRS. Studies have shown that its use has caused a significant reduction in the mortality of patients with sepsis and acute organic dysfunction.[119]

The significant reductions of C protein levels in many patients with sepsis have raised the hypothesis regarding an excessive consumption of thrombomodulin by inflammatory cytokines.[119] However, rigorous controls of hemorrhagic phenomena must be followed during the recombinant C protein administration. While these studies are complete in themselves, it is really clear the importance of infectious focus control, like in the intra-abdominal infection and the efforts to avoid tissular hypoxia.[120,121] Luiz Alberto Toro and Alberto Garcia have synthesized in a table,[122,135] random, controlled experiments of immunotherapy in SIRS, sepsis, and septic shock (Table 36–4).

LATENT INFECTION

Viable bacteria can be present in wounds which have been healed for many years[123–125] and, in this way, represents a considerable factor for the development of a new infection episode. In 1989, Houck and colleagues[139] discovered a risk factor that was unsuspected before. The history of surgical site infection elevated the risk of a new infection in a significant way. A 41% surgical site infection rate is stated in patients with a history of infection and of 12% in patients without a history of infection, even after complete skin healing and total absence of cutaneous infection signs. Hesselink and colleagues[140] have also caught attention to this

fact; however, they have not shown statistically significant difference.

In 2003, Ferraz and Ferraz,[127,141] analyzing patients submitted to incisional hernioplasty, have observed that the global infection rate of surgical site was 6.7% (26/389). But this incidence was 27.6% (19/69) in the patients who had previous infection in the surgical site, while the wound infection rate of patients who did not have previous episodes of surgical site infection was 2.2% (7/320). In our study we observed a difference statistically significant between the infection rate in patients with a previous history of surgical wound infection (27.6% against 2.2%). These data take us to consider the possibility, also reminded by Houck and colleagues,[125] of existence of latent surgical site infection. The 80% coincidence of cultures (4/5), in our material, does not mean that the bacteria be the same. Only the bacterial DNA result could confirm this hypothesis. Houck and colleagues[125] have related a bacterial coincidence of 71.4% (5/7). In spite of the small number of cultures, this high percent of etiological agent's coincidence must not be unvalued.

The lifted hypothesis that a wound infection could determine the colonization by viable bacteria over years, and that new aggression or fall in defense mechanisms could favor the development of a new surgical site infection or even distant sites, still needs more evidence.

References

1. Chong AJ, Dellinger EP: Infectious Complications of Surgery in Morbidly Obese Patients. Available at: http://www.biomedcentral.com/1523–3820/5/387. Accessed December 27, 2005.

2. Mokdad AH, Serdula MK, Dietz WH: The spread of the obesity epidemic in the United States, 1991–1998. *JAMA* 282:1519–1522, 1999.

3. Flegal KM, Carroll MD, Ogden CL: Prevalence and trends in obesity among US adults, 1999–2000. *JAMA* 288:1723–1727, 2002.

4. Kluthe R, Schubert A: Obesity in Europe. *Ann Intern Med* 103:1037–1042, 1985.

5. Malheiros CA, Freitas Júnior WR: Obesidade no Brasil e no mundo. In: Garrido A Jr, Ferraz EM, Barroso FL, Marchesini JB, Szego T (eds.): *Cirurgia da Obesidade*. São Paulo, Atheneu, 2002; p. 19–23.

6. Baratieri R: Aspectos sociais e demográficos da obesidade. In: Silva RS, Kawahara NT (eds.): *Cuidados pré e pós-operatórios na cirurgia da obesidade*. AGE Editora, 2005. p. 39–45.

7. Balsiger BM, Kennedy FP, Abu-Lebdeh HS: Prospective evaluation of Roux-en-Y gastric bypass as primary operation for medically complicated obesity. *Mayo Clin Proc* 75:673–680, 2000.

8. Brolin RE: Bariatric surgery and long-term control of morbid obesity. *JAMA* 288:2793–2796, 2002.

9. Mason EE, Ito C: Gastric bypass in obesity. *Surg Clin North Am* 47:1345–1351, 1967.

10. Livingston EH: Obesity and its surgical management. *Am J Surg* 184:103–113, 2002.

11. Nichols RL: Postoperative infections in the age of drug-resistant gram-positive bacteria. *Am J Med* 104:11S–16S, 1998.

12. Ferraz EM, Ferraz AAB: Antibioticoprofilaxia. In: Ferraz EM (ed.): *Infecção em Cirurgia*. Rio de Janeiro, MEDSI, 1997; p. 345–352.

13. Ferraz AAB, Ferraz EM: Antibioticoprofilaxia em cirurgia. In: Colégio Brasileiro de Cirurgiões—Programa de atualização. Ano I, n 2, vol. 1. 2002. Pág.4–18.

14. Hooton TM, Haley RW, Culver DH, White JW, Morgan WM, Carroll RJ: The joint association of multiple risk factors with the occurrence of nosocomial infection. *Am J Med* 70:960, 1981.

15. Haley RW, Culver DH, Morgan WM, White JW, Emori TJ, Hooton TM: Identifying patients at high risk of surgical wound infection: A simple multivariate index of patient susceptibility and wound contamination. *Am J Epidemiol* 121:206, 1985.

16. Christou NV, Nohr CW, Meakins JL: Assessing operative site infection in surgical patients. *Arch Surg* 122:165, 1987.

17. Culver DH, Horan TC, Gaynes RP, et al.: Surgical wound infection rates by wound class, operative procedure, and patient risk index. National Nosocomial Infections Surveillance System. *Am J Med* 16;91(3B):152S–157S, 1991.

18. Choban PS, Heckler R, Burge JC, et al.: Increased incidence of nosocomial infections in obese surgical patients. *Am Surg* 61:1001–1005, 1995.

19. Birkmeyer NJ, Charlesworth DC, Hernandez, et al.: Obesity and risk of adverse outcomes associated with coronary artery bypass surgery. Northern New England Cardiovascular Disease Study Group. *Circulation* 97:1689–1694, 1998.

20. Engelman DT, Adams DH, Byrne JG, et al.: Impact of body mass index and albumin on morbidity and mortality after cardiac surgery. *J Thorac Cardiovasc Surg* 118:866–873, 1999.

21. Olsen MA, Mayfield J, Lauryssen A, et al.: Risk factors for surgical site infection in spinal surgery. *J Neurosurg* 98:149–155, 2003.

22. Knight RJ, Bodian C, Rodriguez-Laiz G, et al.: Risk factors for intra-abdominal infection after páncreas transplantation. *Am J Surg* 179:99–102, 2000.

23. Grady KL, White–Williams C, Naftel D, et al.: Are preoperative obesity and cachexia risk factors for post heart transplant morbidity and mortality: A multi-institutional study of preoperative weight-height indices. Cardiac Transplant Research Database (CTRD) Group. *J Heart Lung Transplant* 18:750–763, 1999.

24. Sawyer RG, Pellectier SJ, Pruett TL: Increased early morbidity and mortality with acceptable long-term function in severely obese patients undergoing liver transplantation. *Clin Transplant* 13:126–130, 1999.

25. Lauwers S, de Smet F: Surgical site infections. *Acta Clin Belg* 53:303–310, 1998.

26. Delgado–Rodriguez M, Medina-Cuadros M, Martinez-Gallego G, et al.: Usefulness of intrinsic surgical wound infection risk indices as predictors of post-operative pneumonia risk. *J Hosp Infect* 35:269–276, 1997.

27. Ozata M, Ozdemir IC, Licinio J: Human leptin deficiency caused by a missense mutation: Multiple endocrine defects, decreased sympathetic tone, and immune system dysfunction indicate new targets for leptin action, greater central than peripheral resistance to the effects of leptin, and spontaneous correction of leptin-mediated defects. *J Clin Endocrinol Metab* 84:3686–3695, 1999.

28. Tanaka S, Isoda F, Yamakawa T, et al.: T lymphopenia in genetically obese rats. *Clin Immunol Immunopathol* 86:219–225, 1998.

29. Loffreda S, Yang SQ, Lin HZ, et al.: Leptin regulates proinflammatory immune responses. *FASEB J* 12:57–65, 1998.

30. Fantuzzi G, Faggioni R: Leptin in the regulation of immunity, inflammation, and hematopoiesis. *J Leukoc Biol* 68:437–446, 2000.

31. Goodson WH 3rd, Hunt TK: Wound collagen accumulation in obese hyperglycemic mice. *Diabetes* 35:491–495, 1986.

32. Tsuboi R, Rifkin DB: Recombinant basic fibroblast growth factor stimulates wound healing in healing-impaired db/db mice. *J Exp Med* 172: 245–251, 1990.

33. Cottam DR, Schaefer PA, Fahmy D, et al.: The effect of obesity on neutrophil Fc receptors and adhesion molecules (CD 16, CD 11b, CD 62 L). *Obes Surg* 12:230–235, 2002.

34. Cottan DR, Schaefer PA, Shaftan GW, et al.: Effect of surgically-induced weight loss on leukocyte indicators of chronic inflammation in morbid obesity. *Obes Surg* 12:335–342, 2002.

35. van den Berghe G, Wouters P, Weekers F, et al.: Intensive insulin therapv in the critically ill patients. *N Engl J Med* 345:1359–1367, 2001.

36. Joshi N, Caputo GM, Weitekamp MR, et al.: Infections in patients with diabetes mellitus. *N Engl J Med* 341:1906–1912, 1999.

37. Malone DL, Genuit T, Tracy JK, et al.: Surgical site infections: Reanalysis of risk factors. *J Surg Res* 103:89–95, 2002.

38. Lathan R, Lancaster AD, Convington JF, et al.: The association of diabetes and glucose control with surgical-site infections among cardiothoracic surgery patients. *Infect Control Hosp Epidemiol* 22:607–612, 2001.

39. Golden SH, Peart-Virgilance C, Kao WH, et al.: Perioperative glycemic control and the risk of infectious complications in a cohort of adults with diabetes. *Diabetes Care* 22:1408–1414, 1999.

40. Pomposelli JJ, Baxter JK 3rd, Babineau TJ, et al.: Early postoperative glucose control predictsnosomial infection rate in diabetic patient. *JPEN J Parenter Enteral Nutr* 22:77–81, 1998.

41. Babion BM: Oxygen-dependent microbial killing by phagocytes (first of two parts). *N Engl J Med* 298:659–668, 1978.

42. Allen DB, Maguire JJ, Mahdavian M, et al.: Wound hypoxia and acidosis limit neutrophil bacterial killing mechanisms. *Arch Surg* 132:991–996, 1997.

43. Ferraz E, Arruda P, Ferraz A, Bacelar T, Albuquerque A: Severe obese pacients have a low incidence of operative mortality? The Recife score: A new morbidity and mortality grading scale. A preliminary Report. Paper presented at The VII World Congress of Bariatric Surgery, São Paulo, Brazil, 2002.

44. Christou NV, Jarand J, Sylvestre JL, McLean AP: Analysis of the incidence and risk factors for wound infections in open bariatric surgery. *Obes Surg* 14(1):16–22, 2004.

45. Keighley MRB: Prevention of wound sepsis in gastrointestinal surgery. *Br J Surg* 64:315–321, 1977.

46. Condon RE, Wittmann DH: The use of antibiotics in general surgery. *Curr Probl Surg* 12:807–907, 1991.

47. Ferraz EM, Bacelar TS, Aguiar JLA, et al.: Wound infection rates in clean surgery : A potentially misleading risk classification. *Infect Control Hosp Epidemiol* 13(8): 457–462, 1992.

48. Page CP, Bohnmem JMA, Fletcher R, et al.: Antimicrobial prophylaxis for surgical wound. *Curr Probl Surg* 128:79–88, 1993.

49. Daschner F, Kunin CM, Wittmann DH, Ferraz, EM, et al.: WHO Symposium: Use and abuse of antibiotics worldwide. *Infection* 17(1):46–57, 1989.

50. Baum ML, Anish DS, Chalmers TC: A survey of clinical trials of antibiotic prophylaxis in colon surgery: Evidence against further of no-treatment controls. *N Engl J Med* 305:795–799, 1981.

51. Ergina PL, Goold S, Meakins JL: Antibiotic prophylaxis for herniorrhaphy and breast surgery. *N Eng J Med* 322:1884, 1984.

52. Gross PA, Barret TL, Dellinger EP, et al.: Padrão de qualidade para profilaxia antimicrobiana em procedimentos cirúrgicos. *Infect Control Hosp Epidemiol* 15(3):182–188, 1994.

53. Hopkins CC: Antibiotic prophylaxis in clean surgery. Peripheral vascular surgery, noncardiovascular thoracic surgery, herniorrhaphy and mastectomy. *Rev Infect Dis* 13(Suppl 10):S869–S873, 1991.

54. Platt R, Zaleznik DF, Hopkins CC: Perioperative antibiotic prophylaxis for herniorrhaphy and breast surgery. *N Engl J Med* 322:253–260, 1990.

55. Burke JF: The effective period of preventive antibiotic action in experimental incisions and dermal lesions. *Surgery* 50:161–168, 1961.

56. Lesser GT, Deutsch S: Measurement of adipose tissue blood flow and perfusion in man by uptake of 85Kr. *J Appl Physiol* 23(5):621–630, 1967.

57. Ferraz AAB, Albuquerque AC: Farmacocinética no tratamento cirúrgico da Obesidade mórbida. In: Garrido A Jr, Ferraz EM, Barroso FL, Marchesini JB, Szego T (eds.): *Cirurgia da Obesidade*. São Paulo, Atheneu, 2002; p. 135–140.

58. Edmiston CE, Krepel C, Kelly H, et al.: Perioperative antibiotic prophylaxis in the gastric bypass patient: Do we achieve therapeutic levels? *Surgery* 136(4):738–747, 2004.

59. Forse RA, Karam B, MacLean LD, Christou NV: Antibiotic prophylaxis for surgery in morbidly obese patients. *Surgery* 106(4):750–756, 1989.

60. Ferraz AAB, Arruda PCL, Spencer Netto FAC, Albuquerque AC, Lima MHOLA, Ferraz EM: Estudo comparativo entre ampicilina/sulbactam e ceftriaxona na antibioticoprofilaxia de cirurgia bariátrica. *Rev Bras Med* 60(8):617–621, 2003.

61. Byrne TK: Complications of surgery for obesity. *Surg Clin North Am* 81:1181–1193, 2001, vii-viii.

62. Schauer PR, Ikramuddin S, Gourash W, et al.: Outcomes after laparoscopic Roux-en-Y gastric bypass for morbid obesity. *Ann Surg* 232:515–529, 2000.

63. Capella JF, Capella RF: The weight reduction operation of choice: Vertical banded gastroplasty or gastric bypass? *Am J Surg* 171:74–79, 1996.

64. Brolin RE, Kenler HA, Gorman JH, et al.: Long-limb gastric bypass in the superobese. A prospective randomized study. *Ann Surg* 215:387–395, 1992.

65. Demaria EJ, Sugerman HJ, Kellum JM, et al.: Results of 281 consecutive total laparoscopic Roux-en-Y gastric bypasses to treat morbid obesity. *Ann Surg* 235:640–645, 2002; discussion: 645–647.

66. Nguyen NT, Goldman C, Rosenquist CJ, et al.: Laparoscopic versus open gastric bypass: A randomized study of outcomes, quality of life, and costs. *Ann Surg* 234:279–289, 2001; discussion: 289–291.

67. Mangram AJ, Horan TC, Pearson ML, Silver LC, Jarvis WR: Guideline for prevention of surgical site infection, 1999. *Infect Control Hosp Epidemiol* 20(4):247–278, 1999.

68. Conor TJ, Garcha IS, Ramshaw BJ, et al.: Diagnostic laparoscopy for suspected appendicitis. *Am Surg* 61(2):187–189, 1995.

69. Christou NV, Barie PS, Dellinger EP, Waymack JP, Stone HH: Surgical infection society intra-abdominal infection study. Prospective evaluation of management techniques and outcome. *Arch Surg* 128(2):193–198, 1993.

70. Ferraz AAB, Ferraz EM: Abordagem cirúrgica da sepse abdominal. In: Petroianu A (ed.): *Terapêutica Cirúrgica*. Rio de Janeiro, Guanabara Koogan 2001; p. 640–645.

71. Wittmann DH: Tratamento cirúrgico das peritonites. In: Ferraz EM (ed.): *Infecção em cirurgia*. Rio de Janeiro, MEDSI, 1997; p. 387–420.

72. Marshall JC, Nathens AB: Multiple organ dysfunction syndrome. In: Wilmore DW, Cheung LY, Harken AH, Holcroft JW, Meakins JL, Soper NT (eds.): *ACS Surgery: Principles & Practice*. WEBMD Corporation, 2001; p. 1473–1494.

73. Fong Y, Lowry S: Cytokines and the cellular response to injury and infection. In: Meakins (ed.): *Surgical Infections*. New York, Scientific American, 1994; p. 65–86.

74. Faist E, Storck M, Hueltner L, et al.: Functional analysis of monocyte (MO) activity via synthesis patterns of interleukin 1, 6, 8 (IL-1, IL 6, IL-8) and neopterin (NPT) in surgical intensive care patients. *Surgery* 9:562–572, 1992.

75. Forse RA: Omega-3 PUFA. *J Intensive Care Med* 20(1):134, 1994.

76. Browder W, Williams D, Pretus H, et al.: Beneficial effects of enhanced macrophage function in the trauma patient. *Ann Surg* 211(5):605–613, 1999.

77. Bittiner SB, Tucker WF, Cartwright I, et al: Effects of manipulation of dietary fatty acids on clinical manifestation of rheumatoid arthritis. *Lancet* 1:184, 1988.

78. Wilmore DW: Role of glutamine. *J Intensive Care Med* 20(1):133, 1994.

79. Stuehr D, Gross S, Sakuma I, et al.: Activated murine macrophages secrete a metabolite of arginine with the bioactivity of endothelium derived relaxing factor and chemical reactivity of nitric oxide. *J Exp Med* 169:1011, 1989.

80. Barbul A: Arginine: Biochemistry, physiology and therapeutic implication. *JPEN* 10:227–238, 1986.

81. Barbul A, Sisto DA, Wasserkrug HL, Efron G: Arginine stimulates lymphocyte immune response in healthy humans. *Surgery* 90:244–251, 1981.

82. Alexander W: Can nutrition influence translocation? The effect of nutrition on translocation and host defense. *J Intensive Care Med* 20(1):134, 1994.

83. Horn JK: Origem da Sepse, In: Ferraz EM (ed.) *Infecção em Cirurgia*. Rio de Janeiro: MEDSI, 1997.

84. Faist E, Bawe AE: Imunoconseqüências do Trauma, do Choque e da Sepse: Mecanismos e abordagens contra-reguladoras. In: Ferraz EM (ed.): *Infecção em Cirurgia*. Rio de Janeiro: MEDSI, 1997.

85. Meakins JL: *Surgical Infections in Critical Care Medicine*. New York, Churchill Livingstone, 1985.

86. Condon RE: Infecções Cirúrgicas nos hospedeiros comprometidos. In: Ferraz EM (ed.): *Infecção em Cirurgia*. Rio de Janeiro: MEDSI, 1997.

87. Baue AE, Faist E, Fry DE: *Preface. Multiple Organ Failure, Pathophysiology, Prevention and Therapy*. New York, Springer-Verlag, 2000.

88. Cossu ML, Caccia S, Coppola M, et al.: Orally administered ranitidine plasma concentrations before and after bibliopancreatic diversion in morbidly obese patients, *Obes Surg* 9(1):36–39, 1999.

89. Macgregor AMC, Boggs L: Drug distribution in obesity and following bariatric surgery: A literature review. *Obes Surg* 6(1):17–27, 1996.

90. Dionne RE, Bauer LA, Gibson GA: Estimating creatinine clearence in morbidity obese patients. *Am J Hosp Pharm* 38:841–844, 1981.

91. Christoff PB, Conti DR, Naylor C, Procainamide disposition in obesity. *Drug Intell Clin Pharm* 17:516–522, 1983.

92. Nathens AB, Rotstein OD: Antimicrobial therapy for intra-abdominal infection. *Am J Surg* 172:1s–6s, 1996.

93. Mock CN, Jurkovich GJ, Dries DJ, Maier RV: Clinical significance of antibiotic endotoxin-releasing properties in trauma patients. *Arch Surg* 130(11):1234–1240, 1995.

94. Fry DE: Pathophysiology of peritonites. In: Fry DE (ed.): *Peritonites*. New York, Futura, 1993.

95. Bearden DT, Rodvold KA: Dosage adjustments for antibacterials in obese patients. *Clin Pharmacokinet* 38(5): 415–426, 2000.

96. Allard S, Kinzing M, Boivin G, Sorgel F, Lebel M: Intravenous ciprofloxacin disposition in obesity. *Clin Pharmacol Ther* 54:368–373, 1993.

97. Adeodato LCL, Pagnosin G, Ferraz EM: Relaparotomias programadas. In: Ferraz EM (ed.): *Infecção em cirurgia*. Rio de Janeiro, MEDSI, 1997; p. 441–468.

98. Levison MA, Zeigler D: Correlation of APACHE II score, drainage technique and outcome in postoperative intra-abdominal abscess. *Surg Gynecol Obstet* 172:89–94, 1991.

99. Ferraz EM, Ferraz AAB: Abscesso intra-abdominais. In: Coelho JCU (ed.): *Aparelho Digestivo: Clínica e Cirurgia*. Rio de Janeiro, Atheneu, 2005; p. 1929–1939.

100. Marshall JC, Christou NV, Horn R, Meakins JL: The microbiology of multiple organ failure. *Arch Surg* 123:309, 1988.

101. Bounous G: The intestinal factor in multiple organ failure and shock. *Surgery* 107:118, 1989.

102. Berg RD: Mechanisms confining indigenous bacteria to the gastrointestinal tract. *Am J Clin Nutr* 33:2472, 1980.

103. Alexander JW, Boyce ST, Babcock GF, et al.: The process of microbial translocation. *Ann Surg* 212:496, 1990.

104. Albanese CT, Cardona M, Smith SD, et al.: Role of intestinal mucus in transepithelial passage of bacteria across the intact ileum in vitro. *Surgery* 116:76, 1994.

105. Albanese CT, Smith SD, Watkins S, et al.: Effect of secretory IgA on transepithelial passage of bacteria across the intact ileum in vitro. *J Am Coll Surg* 179:679, 1994.

106. Cech AC, Shou J, Gallagher H, et al.: Glucocorticoid receptor blockade reverses postinjury macrophage suppression. *Arch Surg* 129(12):1227–1232, 1994.

107. Dhabhar FS, Miller AH, Mcewen BS, et al.: Effects of stress on immune cell distribution: Dynamics and hormonal mechanisms. *J Immunol* 154:5511, 1995.

108. Cox G: Glucocorticoid treatment inhibits apoptosis in human neutrophils: Separation of survival and activation outcomes. *J Immunol* 154:4719, 1995.

109. Arends MJ, Wyllie AH: Apoptosis: Mechanisms and roles in pathology. *Int Rev Exp Pathol* 32:223, 1991.

110. Coutinho HB, Robalinho TI, Coutinho VB, et al.: Intra-abdominal sepsis: An immunocytochemical study of the small intestine mucosa. *J Clin Pathol* 50(4):294–298, 1997.

111. Berg RD, Wommack E, Deitch EA: Immunosuppression and intestinal bacterial overgrowth synergistically promote bacterial translocation. *Arch Surg* 123:1359, 1988.

112. Wells CL, Maddaus MA, Reynolds CM, et al.: Role of anaerobic flora in the translocation of aerobic and facultatively anaerobic intestinal bacteria. *Infect Immun* 55:2689, 1987.

113. Frantzides CT, Mathias C, Ludwig KA, et al.: Small bowel myoelectric activity in peritonitis. *Am J Surg* 165:681, 1993.

114. Moore EE, Jones TN: Benefits of immediate jejunal feeding after major abdominal trauma: A prospective, randomized study. *J Trauma* 26:874–880, 1986.

115. Moore FA, Feliciano DV, Andrassy RJ, et al.: Early enteral feeding compared with parenteral reduce postoperative septic complications. *Ann Surg* 216:172–183, 1992.

116. Reissman P, Teoh TA, Cohen SM, et al.: Is early oral feeding safe after elective colorectal surgery? *Ann Surg* 222:73–77, 1995.

117. Dellinger RP, Carlet JM, Masur H, et al. Surviving sepsis campaign guidelines for management of severe sepsis and septic shock. *Crit Care Med* 32(3):858–873, 2004.

118. Rivers E, Nguyen B, Havstad S, et al. For The Early Goal-Directed Therapy Collaborative Group: Early goal-directed therapy in the treatment of severe sepsis and septic shock. *N Engl J Med* 345:1368–1377, 2001.

119. Van den Berghe G, Wouters P, Weekers F, et al.: Intensive insulin therapy in critically ill patients. *N Engl J Med* 345:1359–1367, 2001.

120. Van den Berghe G, Wilmer A, Hermans G et al.: Intensive insulin therapy in the medical ICU. *N Engl J Med* 354:449–461, 2006.

121. The Acute Respiratory Distress Syndrome Network (ARDSNET). Ventilation with low tidal volumes as compared with traditional tidal volumes for acute lung injury and the acute respiratory distress syndrome. *N Engl J Med* 342:1301–1308, 2000.

122. Annane D, Sébille V, Charpentier C, et al.: Effect of treatment with low doses of hydrocortisone and fludrocortisone on mortality in patients with septic shock. *JAMA* 288:862–871, 2002.

123. Bernard GR, Vincent J-L, Laterre P-F, et al.: The Recombinant Human Activated Protein C Worldwide Evaluation in Severe Sepsis (PROWESS) Study Group. Efficacy and safety of recombinant human activated protein C for severe sepsis. *N Engl J Med* 344:699–709, 2001.

124. Abraham E, Laterre P-F, Garg R, et al.: The administration of drotrecogin alfa (activated) in early stage severe sepsis (ADDRESS). Drotrecogin alfa (activated) for adults with severe sepsis and a low risk of death. *N Engl J Med* 353:1332–1341, 2005.

125. Warren B, Alain Eid, Pierre Singer, et al. For the KyberSept Trial Study Group: High-dose antithrombin III in severe sepsis: A randomized controlled trial. *JAMA* 286:1869–1878, 2001.

126. Abraham E, Wunderink R, Silverman H, et al.: Efficacy and safety of monoclonal antibody to human tumor necrosis factor alpha in patients with sepsis syndrome. A randomized, controlled, double-blind, multicenter clinical trial. TNF-alpha MAb Sepsis Study Group. *JAMA* 273:934–941, 1995.

127. Abraham E, Reinhart K, Opal S, et al.: Efficacy and safety of tifacogin (recombinant tissue factor pathway inhibitor) in severe sepsis: A randomized controlled trial. *JAMA* 290: 238–247, 2003.

128. Pieracci FM, Barie PS, Pomp A: Critical care of the bariatric patient. *Crit Care Med* 34(6):1796–1804, 2006.

37

Early Complications in Bariatric Surgery

Kenneth G. MacDonald, Jr, MD

▌ INTRODUCTION

This chapter will cover the diagnosis and management of early complications after bariatric surgery. While certain problems are more generic and may occur after any operation, others are specific to the particular procedure performed. In this chapter, I will concentrate on the problems after Roux gastric bypass, although some of the generic complications may also be discussed in other chapters.

The morbidly obese are challenging surgical patients; the technical aspects of any intra-abdominal procedure are more difficult than with normal weight individuals. Intravenous access, airway management, monitoring of the vital signs, and general logistics of transport and ambulation are all more problematic. Diagnosis and management of complications is hampered by difficulty with physical examination and radiologic diagnostics.

It is difficult to compare complication rates between open and laparoscopic bariatric procedures, as the more current reports on laparoscopic series can be compared only to historical control groups. Experience, instrumentation, surgical techniques, diagnostic and therapeutic radiology, and critical care have evolved considerably in the last decade, no doubt improving outcomes in this group of patients. Concurrent groups cannot be compared, as open bariatric operations are now generally performed on the highest risk patients, either because of higher body mass index (BMI), past operations, or some other complicating factor. There is little doubt that abdominal wall complications, such as wound infections and incisional hernias, have declined significantly with the laparoscopic procedures. Mortality rate and length of hospitalization are also reduced from earlier experience, although the same is true of most major operative procedures.

Finally, the complication and mortality rates of many operations, ranging in complexity from laparoscopic inguinal hernia repair to Whipple pancreaticoduodenectomy and coronary artery bypass, have been shown to decrease with increased numbers of operations performed by individual surgeons and institutions. A similar association has been documented with Roux gastric bypass. Nguyen and others demonstrated significantly reduced hospital stay, overall complications, and cost in high-volume hospitals (>100 cases/year) compared to that in low-volume hospitals (<50 cases/year).[1] The observed mortality, particularly in patients older than 55 years, was also lower in the high-volume centers. Courcoulas and colleagues have reported significantly reduced adverse outcomes and mortality with high-volume surgeons compared to low-volume (<10 cases/year) surgeons.[2]

COMPLICATIONS

Leaks

A leak is perhaps the most feared single complication after gastric bypass, occurring with a reported incidence of 0%–5.6%.[3,4] Leaks are one of the most common causes of mortality and a source of serious morbidity. While most occur at the gastrojejunostomy, the staple-line closures of the gastric pouch or the distal stomach and the jejunojejunostomy anastomosis are other potential sites. Potential causes include technical factors, stapler malfunction, and tissue ischemia. Ischemia may occur from division of blood supply, dissection injury, or tension. However, the etiology of a leak cannot be defined frequently, even with reoperation.

Diagnosis

Most leaks present in the first week after surgery, most commonly on postoperative days 1 through 3. Those with a more delayed presentation generally are more contained and have a better prognosis. Physical examination is notoriously misleading; significant tenderness and peritonitis are often absent. Tachycardia, with a heart rate greater than 120 per minute, is the most common early finding. In fact, persistent unexplained tachycardia must be presumed to represent a leak until proven otherwise. Fever is very nonspecific and may be absent. Patients usually do not look well, with a flushed and anxious appearance, although they may not have a specific complaint other than an inability to "get comfortable." Anxiety and a "feeling of doom" are not uncommon. Tachypnea and confusion may occur. Oliguria, hypoxemia, and hypotension are late findings that occur with progressive development of sepsis. Leukocytosis and/or left shift is usually present, but not required for diagnosis. Later abnormalities in the laboratory values may include increased creatinine, rise in bilirubin, decreased serum bicarbonate, and hypoalbuminemia.

A Gastrografin swallow may reveal a leak at the gastrojejunostomy, but false negative examinations do occur. Further, this study does nothing to evaluate leaks from the distal stomach or the jejunojejunostomy. A left pleural effusion is frequently noted if a chest x-ray or abdominal series is performed during evaluation. Computed tomography of the abdomen will usually show a fluid collection or perhaps free intraperitoneal air, but the patient's size and weight may limit the value of this examination or prevent it entirely by exceeding the limits of the scanner.

Management

The key to management of a leak is early diagnosis and return to the operating room for exploration. Delay results in increased morbidity and mortality. While the procedure may be performed laparoscopically, exposure and visualization may require conversion to an open operation. In addition, the thickened, inflamed tissue and the dilated bowel increase the difficulty of manipulation with laparoscopic instruments.

The source of the leak should be identified and repair should be attempted, using adjacent bowel or omentum to buttress the repair if at all possible. Injection of air or methylene blue via endoscope or tube may aid in identification of a leak from the pouch or gastrojejunostomy if not readily apparent. Wide drainage of the area of the leak is essential, as it should be assumed that any surgical repair will break down. Closed suction or sump drains are recommended. As collections frequently occur in the left subdiaphragmatic space, the splenic hilum, and the lesser sac, the drainage should include these areas. Placement of a gastrostomy tube in the distal stomach should be considered to allow postoperative decompression and provide access for enteral nutrition, which should begin as soon as the patient's condition permits. A nasogastric tube placed through the gastrojejunostomy may help to maintain patency of the anastomosis or prevent stenosis.

Postoperative management should include broad-spectrum antibiotic coverage, including an antifungal agent. Thromboembolism prophylaxis is crucial. Aggressive fluid resuscitation is important to try to minimize the incidence of acute renal failure. Anticipate a difficult course with high probability of pulmonary problems, which could require prolonged mechanical ventilation. Use of appropriate beds and nursing care to avoid prolonged pressure on any part of the body is essential to prevent decubitus ulcers or nerve compression syndromes. The operative drains should be left in place until the patient's nutritional parameters are close to normal levels and a tract has formed around the drains, usually at least 3 weeks. It is not unusual for drains to erode into adjacent bowel or stomach, or to prevent complete closure of a leak. Once a stable fistulous tract has formed, the drains can be removed, allowing the tracts to drain as needed and subsequently close without problem.

Occasionally, a contained leak will present several days or even weeks after operation as a discrete abscess. In retrospect, these patients often had unexplained fever, tachycardia, or leukocytosis in the immediate postoperative period. The presentation may be subtle, with complaints of intermittent fever or nausea. Abdominal pain may occur, but is frequently absent. The more frequent laboratory abnormalities include leukocytosis, left shift, and hypoalbuminemia.

Fortunately, these cases are adequately managed by percutaneous drainage in radiology with a course of antibiotics. Bowel rest and parenteral nutrition may be required, depending on overall status of the patient and whether or not an ongoing leak is demonstrated by contrast studies.

Venous Thromboembolism

Pulmonary embolism is another common cause of mortality after gastric bypass. The morbidly obese are at higher risk for development of deep venous thrombosis, and they have little cardiopulmonary reserve if a pulmonary embolus occurs. The incidence of symptomatic pulmonary emboli after bariatric surgery is generally reported as 1%–2%,[3,5] although many are likely not diagnosed and the actual incidence in these patients is probably much higher. The estimated mortality of pulmonary emboli in this population has been reported to be 20%–30%.[6] The importance of pulmonary embolus in overall mortality from gastric bypass was emphasized by a small autopsy study, which reported PE as a cause in 3 of 10 gastric bypass deaths, while 80% of this group were found to have microscopic evidence of pulmonary emboli.[7] In comparison, a large review of 6,833 autopsies performed on patients who died while hospitalized in England confirmed pulmonary emboli as the cause of death in 5.2% of adult cases.[8]

Diagnosis

As with many complications after bariatric surgery, a high index of suspicion must be maintained to assure timely diagnosis and treatment of pulmonary emboli. The most common presentation includes tachycardia and hypoxia, often combined with hypocarbia due to hyperventilation. Patients may exhibit similar anxiety, dyspnea, and feelings of doom as do patients with a leak. In fact, differentiating between these two complications is not an uncommon dilemma. Abrupt onset of symptoms would seem to favor a pulmonary embolus, but this observation is generally not helpful in making a diagnosis. Sudden cardiovascular collapse with pulseless electrical activity does strongly suggest pulmonary embolus, although this condition is rarely remediable.

Contrast studies are usually not helpful, as a negative examination does not rule out intraperitoneal sepsis. Nuclear medicine ventilation–perfusion studies offer only probabilities, expend considerable time, perhaps delaying treatment, and again do not evaluate the abdomen. The traditional gold standard examination for diagnosis of pulmonary embolism, pulmonary angiography, is not possible in many morbidly obese patients because of weight limitations. For patients who are sufficiently stable and of appropriate weight for computed tomography, a CT of the chest and abdomen is the most productive examination. The negative predictive value of a normal helical chest CT is greater than 99%.[9] Quantitative D-dimer assays also are reported to have a high negative predictive value, but they currently appear to be most useful in ruling out embolism in combination with a low clinical probability.[10]

Management

Management of a patient with suspected pulmonary embolus depends on the clinical probability of the complication and the results of the diagnostic procedures performed. In a patient with high clinical suspicion for PE or leak with a normal CT examination of the chest and the abdomen, or in a patient whose weight precludes CT scanning, prompt abdominal exploration should be performed. If no evidence of leak or intra-abdominal sepsis is found, then anticoagulation is indicated. This sequence is recommended as anticoagulation is best initiated after abdominal exploration and because many patients with suspected pulmonary emboli are ultimately found to have leaks. In patients with low or moderate clinical suspicion of PE or leak, additional supportive testing may be performed, such as ventilation–perfusion scanning, compression ultrasonography, and quantitative D-dimer assay.

Because of the high risk of venous thromboembolism in the morbidly obese, any discussion of treatment should include prophylaxis. Perioperative subcutaneous heparin administration and use of sequential compression devices on the legs or pumps on the feet is considered standard. However, fixed or weight-based dosing may not be optimal, leading to either inadequate prophylaxis or to bleeding.[11] Additional measures, including early ambulation and limiting the amount of time in reverse Trendelenburg position in the operating room, should be employed.

Although of yet unproven benefit, preoperative placement of inferior vena cava filters is increasingly considered in morbidly obese patients at increased risk for occurrence of pulmonary embolism. Risk factors include high BMI (greater than 50 kg/m²), marked truncal obesity, history of venous stasis disease, presence of a hereditary hypercoagulable condition (such as Factor V Leiden mutation; lupus anticoagulant; and Antithrombin III, protein C, or protein S deficiencies), personal history of prior deep venous thrombosis or pulmonary embolus, and immobility.[12,13] Patients with pulmonary artery hypertension should also be considered for filter placement because of the increased risk of mortality with pulmonary embolism. Options for filter placement have increased with introduction of retrievable filters as well as use of intravascular ultrasound for accurate localization.

Bowel Obstruction/Acute Gastric Distension

Early postoperative bowel obstruction after gastric bypass has many potential causes, including internal hernia (Peterson's, mesocolic, and mesenteric), kinking or luminal narrowing at the jejunojejunostomy, incarcerated abdominal wall hernia, twisted alimentary limb, and the "Roux-en-Y" and the more generic and traditional adhesive obstruction. Other uncommon causes include scarring around the alimentary limb at the level of the transverse mesocolon and jejunojejunal intussusception, both antiperistaltic (retrograde) and isoperistaltic.[14] Altered motility of the Roux limb has been documented by manometric evaluation of one patient after suffering both an antiperistaltic followed by an isoperistaltic intussusception, suggesting the etiology of this complication.[15]

Early obstructions have significant potential for serious complications, such as leakage from a proximal anastomosis or staple-line, acute distal gastric distension, aspiration, and sepsis. Acute distension of the distal stomach can occasionally occur even in absence of distal obstruction, most often as a consequence of sepsis from another source. Regardless of the etiology, ischemia and necrosis of the gastric wall, usually involving the fundus, can result. Internal hernias are dangerous, as most result in closed-loop obstruction with a propensity for ischemic necrosis.

The incidence of postoperative small bowel obstruction after laparoscopic gastric bypass ranges from 1% to 7%.[16,17] The incidence of early and late small bowel obstruction is generally felt to be higher after laparoscopic than after open gastric bypass,[18] although some report no difference in obstruction between the two techniques.[19] An explanation for an increase in obstruction after the laparoscopic approach is an increased mobility of the small bowel due to decreased tethering by adhesions, increasing potential for internal hernias. The incidence of internal hernias after laparoscopic gastric bypass has been reported to decrease with antecolic versus retrocolic passage of the Roux limb because of elimination of the mesocolic window.[20,21]

Diagnosis

Early postoperative small bowel obstruction often presents with refractory nausea and vomiting and with intolerance of oral liquids. Abdominal pain may not be a significant symptom in the early postoperative period and physical examination is usually unrevealing. Plain abdominal films may show dilation of the bypassed distal stomach. Significant small bowel distension or air-fluid levels may not be present, as many of these obstructions, particularly those caused by internal hernias, involve proximal bowel. Contrast swallow studies may demonstrate dilation of the alimentary limb, but are not generally helpful other than to rule out proximal obstruction at the gastrojejunostomy. Computed tomography of the abdomen is helpful, both for diagnosis and for localization of the point of obstruction. Identification of the cause of obstruction is occasionally possible; twisting or whirling of the mesenteric vessels may be seen with internal hernia and the appearance of intussusception is quite characteristic.

Late presentation of internal hernias deserves special mention. Recurrent periumbilical pain should always be presumed to be internal hernia until proven otherwise. While barium swallow and CT scan may demonstrate obstruction, negative studies do not rule out hernia. The bowel may move in and out, causing intermittent obstruction before incarceration or volvulus finally occurs.

Management

Because of the risk of serious morbidity and mortality with small bowel obstruction after gastric bypass, early operation is advised in most cases. Unlike traditional obstructions after other types of abdominal surgery, nasogastric tubes are rarely effective for decompression of the proximal bowel and do nothing for distension of the bypassed stomach. Additionally, placement of such tubes in the early postoperative period is essentially contraindicated due to the risk of perforation or disruption of the proximal pouch or gastrojejunostomy.

While management of obstructions is frequently possible laparoscopically, identification of the anatomy with incarcerated internal hernias may be difficult and visualization may be hampered by the bowel distension. Risk of perforation of the thin, distended bowel with laparoscopic manipulation is also significant. For these reasons, there should be a low threshold for conversion to an open procedure.

Surgical management of the obstruction depends on the etiology. Internal hernias are reduced and the bowel carefully placed in the proper orientation. Compromised bowel is resected. The internal defect is closed with permanent suture. Obstructions at the jejunojejunostomy frequently require revision of the anastomosis. When only the alimentary limb is obstructed proximal to the anastomosis, an anastomosis may be created between the limb and a segment of bowel distal to the jejunojejunostomy. As with most cases of intussusception in adults, resection of the involved bowel is usually required.

Measures to avoid potential causes of postoperative bowel obstruction should be taken at the time of the original operation. The mesocolic, Peterson's, and mesenteric defects should be closed with permanent suture. Antiobstruction sutures are placed at the jejunojejunostomy to prevent kinking. The fascia in the larger trocar sites (at least 12 mm and 15 mm) is closed with suture. Existing umbilical or incisional hernias should be repaired due to the apparent increased incidence of incarceration in the early postoperative period or perhaps due to increased intra-abdominal pressures from distended bowel or tissue edema. Exceptions occasionally can be made for very large hernias which would require use of prosthetic patches or mesh or for hernias filled with incarcerated omental or preperitoneal fat.

References

1. Nguyen NT, Paya M, Stevens CM, et al.: The relationship between hospital volume and outcome in bariatric surgery at academic medical centers. *Ann Surg* 240(4):586–593, 2004.
2. Courcoulas A, Schuchert M, Gatti G, et al.: The relationship of surgeon and hospital volume to outcome after gastric bypass surgery in Pennsylvania: A 3 year summary. *Surgery* 134(4):613–621, 2002.
3. Schauer PR, Ikramuddin S, Gourash W, et al.: Outcomes after laparoscopic Roux-en-Y gastric bypass for morbid obesity. *Ann Surg* 232:515–529, 2000.
4. Fernandez AZ Jr, DeMaria EJ, Tichansky DS, et al.: Experience with over 3000 open and laparoscopic bariatric procedures: Multivariate analysis of factors related to leak and resultant mortality. *Surg Endosc* 18:193–197, 2004.
5. Livingston EH: Procedure, incidence and complication rates of bariatric surgery in the United States. *Am J Surg* 188:105–110, 2004.
6. Brolin RE: Complications of surgery for severe obesity. *Probl Gen Surg* 17:55–61, 2000.
7. Melinek J, Livingston E, Cortina G, et al.: Autopsy findings following gastric bypass surgery for morbid obesity. *Arch Pathol Lab Med* 126:1091–1095, 2002.

8. Alikhan R, Peters F, Wilmott R, et al.: Fatal pulmonary embolism in hospitalized patients: A necropsy review. *J Clin Pathol* 52:1254–1257, 2004.

9. Michiels JJ, Gadisseur A, van der Planken M, et al.: Screening for deep venous thrombosis and pulmonary embolism in outpatients with suspected DVT or PE by the sequential use of clinical score: A sensitive quantitative D-dimer test and noninvasive diagnostic tools. *Semin Vasc Med* 5:351–364, 2005.

10. deGroot MR, van Marwijk Kooy M, Pouwels JG, et al.: The use of a rapid D-dimer blood test in the diagnostic work-up for pulmonary embolism: A management study. *Thromb Haemost* 83:180–181, 2000.

11. Shepherd MF, Rosborough TK, Schwartz L: Heparin thromboprophylaxis in gastric bypass surgery. *Obes Surg* 13:249–253, 2003.

12. Keeling WB, Haines K, Stone PA, et al.: Current indications for preoperative inferior vena cava filter insertion in patients undergoing surgery for morbid obesity. *Obes Surg* 15:1009–1012, 2005.

13. Atluri P, Raper SE: Factor V Leiden and postoperative deep venous thrombosis in patients undergoing open roux-en-y gastric bypass surgery. *Obes Surg* 15:561–564, 2005.

14. Goverman J, Greenwald M, Gellman L, et al.: Antiperistaltic (retrograde) intussusception after roux-en-Y gastric bypass. *Am Surg* 70:67–70, 2004.

15. Hocking MF, McCoy DM, Vogel SB, et al.: Antiperistaltic and isoperistaltic intussusception associated with abnormal motility after roux-en-Y gastric bypass: A case report. *Surgery* 110:109–112, 1991.

16. Hwang RF, Swartz DE, Felix EL: Causes of small bowel obstruction after laparoscopic gastric bypass. *Surg Endosc* 18:1631–1635, 2004.

17. Papasavas PK, Caushaj PF, McCormick JT, et al.: Laparoscopic management of complications following laparoscopic roux-en-y gastric bypass for morbid obesity. *Surg Endosc* 17:610–614, 2003.

18. Podnos YD, Jimenez JC, Wilson SE, et al.: Complications after laparoscopic gastric bypass: A review of 3464 cases. *Arch Surg* 138:957–961, 2003.

19. Smith SC, Edwards CB, Goodman GN, et al.: Open vs laparoscopic roux-en-Y gastric bypass: Comparison of operative morbidity and mortality. *Obes Surg* 14:73–76, 2004.

20. Cho M, Carrodeguas L, Pinto D, et al.: Diagnosis and management of partial small bowel obstruction after laparoscopic antecolic antegastric roux-en-Y gastric bypass for morbid obesity. *J Am Coll Surg* 202:262–268, 2006.

21. Champion JK, Williams M: Small bowel obstruction and internal hernias after laparoscopic roux-en-Y gastric bypass. *Obes Surg* 13:596–600, 2003.

38

Late Complications: Ulcers, Stenosis, and Fistula

Scott A. Shikora, MD • Leonardo Claros, MD • Julie J. Kim, MD • Michael E. Tarnoff, MD

INTRODUCTION

Since its inception in the 1950s, bariatric surgery has evolved into a field that offers safe and effective operations, which result in meaningful and sustainable weight loss. However, even with successful weight loss, patients may still develop complications long after the surgical procedure was performed. With early recognition and appropriate management, these problems are generally nonlethal and minor. However, left untreated, they may result in devastating complications. It is therefore critical that all health care professionals responsible for bariatric patients recognize the signs and symptoms, know the proper diagnostic maneuvers, and institute the correct treatment in a timely fashion.

This chapter will cover three of the more commonly seen complications: ulcers, stenosis, and fistula. Since these issues are less commonly seen after laparoscopic adjustable gastric banding (LAGB) or vertical banded gastroplasty (VBG), the chapter will focus mainly on procedures that involve an anastomosis such as the Roux-en-Y gastric bypass (RYGBP),

biliopancreatic diversion (BPD), and the biliopancreatic diversion with duodenal switch (BPDDS).

Ulcers

Generally speaking, ulcers after bariatric surgery will be either anastomotic (marginal ulcers) or peptic. Peptic ulcers occur in the distal gastric antrum or duodenum as they would occur in people who have not had bariatric surgery. After LAGB or VBG, the incidence of peptic ulcer disease is similar to that of nonbariatric patients. However, after GBP it is thought to be much lower in incidence. Printen et al. reported an incidence of 0.26% in over 3000 gastric bypasses.[1]

Marginal ulceration represents a mucosal erosion on the intestinal side of the anastomosis with the gastric pouch (Figure 38–1). In humans, the intestinal mucosa is normally not exposed to gastric acid, which gets neutralized by the alkaline biliopancreatic secretions. Unlike the stomach, which is resistant to acid, the intestinal mucosa has no natural barriers and easily ulcerates. Marginal ulceration has been reported to

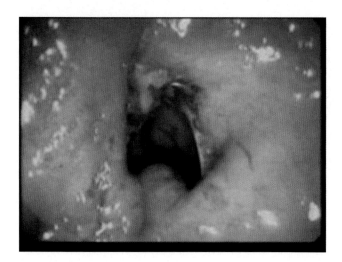

Figure 38–1. Endoscopic view of a marginal ulcer at the gastro-jejunal anastomosis of a gastric bypass.

occur in 5–15% and 3–5% of patients who undergo undivided and divided RYGBP, respectively.[2–5]

The majority of stomal ulcers that occur in the undivided RYGBP operation occur in conjunction with a disrupted vertical staple line (gastrogastric fistula).[4] The incidence of stomal ulcers is higher when a gastrogastric fistula is present because the gastric acid from the excluded fundus is able to come in contact with the intestinal mucosa. Gastrogastric fistula can occur after both divided and undivided RYGBPs. However, it occurs more commonly in the undivided procedure where the staple line dehiscence rate is as high as 29%.[6–8] In divided RYGBPs without gastrogastric fistula, the etiology of marginal ulceration remains unclear. Acid output by parietal cells in the standard 30-cc gastric pouch is minimal but not usually absent.[2,9,10] Large pouches may likely contain more acid-producing parietal cells thus increasing the incidence of ulceration.[4,9] Some studies have also suggested that the injudicious use of nonsteroidal antiinflammatory agents,[11] *Helicobacter pylori*,[12] tobacco smoking, ischemia, and Roux limb tension are also possible etiologic factors.[4]

Marginal ulceration can also occur with the biliopancreatic procedures (BPD). The incidence has been reported to range from 2.8% to 10.6%.[13,14] The gastric pouch of the BPD is typically 200 cc in capacity and contains gastric tissue rich in parietal cells. It is surprising that the incidence is not in fact, even higher. With the BPDDS, the duodenum and its ability to neutralize acid are left intact, and not surprisingly, the incidence is significantly lower than that after the classic BPD where the ileum is anastomosed directly to a large acid-producing gastric pouch. The incidence has been reported to range from 0% to 1.6%.[15,16]

Marginal ulcers can present at any time after surgery but seem to be more common within the first few months.[17] The anastomotic technique may or may not influence the likelihood of ulceration. Capella et al. demonstrated in a large retrospective review of their practice that the incidence of ulceration was 6.8% with a stapled anastomosis, 1.6% for a two-layer hand-sewn anastomosis where the outer layer was silk, and 0% for a two-layer hand-sewn anastomosis where the inner layer was constructed with absorbable sutures.[6] However, since these were consecutive series in their practice, the results must be considered with caution. In contrast, Gonzalez et al. found no difference in ulcer rates between circular stapled, linear stapled, and hand-sewn anastomoses.[18] Patients with marginal ulcers will usually present with upper epigastric pain and burning. The pain may radiate to the back. Substernal chest pain can also occur. Nausea, vomiting, and food intolerance are often commonly seen with ulcers. While massive upper GI (UGI) bleeding is uncommon, iron deficiency anemia is more commonly associated with chronic or recurrent ulcers. Not all gastrogastric fistulas will result in ulceration. Some patients who have developed a gastrogastric fistula present only with increased appetite and weight gain. There are also patients with gastrogastric fistula who remain asymptomatic.

The evaluation of a patient who presents with symptoms suggestive of ulceration is very straightforward. A barium swallow radiograph is simple, noninvasive, and often the first diagnostic test ordered. However, while it may delineate large deep ulcers and demonstrate gastrogastric fistulas, it might miss more shallow ulcerations. Upper endoscopy, while more invasive, is a superior test to diagnose ulceration. It is much more specific for identifying ulcers. If an ulcer is found, the treatment includes removal of irritants such as tobacco or nonsteroidal antiinflammatory drugs (NSAIDs) and the prescription of either a histamine-receptor antagonist or proton-pump inhibitor. Unless the ulcer is due to ischemia or a gastrogastric fistula, medical therapy will usually succeed.[3,19]

Ulcers that are ischemic in origin or secondary to a gastrogastric fistula will often be resistant to medical therapy and generally require surgery. To decrease the incidence of marginal ulceration, many programs maintain their patients on histamine-receptor antagonists for a period of time after surgery.

Stenosis

In addition to small pouch size, a narrow anastomotic diameter is believed to be a key component in maintaining durable weight loss after RYGBP and VBG. Most authors agree that creation of a gastrojejunostomy with an internal diameter not exceeding 1.5 cm provides optimal results, though recent analysis has called this theory into question.[20] With these narrow anastomoses, patients must eat slowly and chew very well or food will not be able to pass through the anastomosis. However, should the outlet narrow from inflammation, ulceration, swelling, ischemia with scarring, etc., food will not be able to pass leading to frequent and often progressive vomiting. This is called an anastomotic stricture or stenosis. Anastomotic (gastrojejunostomy) stenosis occurs in 1–15% of patients who undergo RYGBP and typically occurs within 2 years of the procedure.[21] However, most seem to occur within the first 4–8 weeks after surgery.[22] In our series of over 750 retrocolic, retrogastric anastomoses created with the 25-mm circular stapler, the incidence of outlet stenosis has been 0.8%.[5] The incidence is reported to be about 1% with the BPDDS.[23]

It is controversial whether anastomotic technique, i.e., circular versus linear versus hand sewn, retrocolic versus antecolic, truly alters the incidence of stenosis. Some studies have suggested that circular stapled anastomoses may result in higher stricture rates than hand sewn or linear stapled. In a small, nonrandomized retrospective review, Gonzalez et al.[18] found a significantly higher stricture rate with the 21-mm circular stapler than the hand-sewn and linear stapled anastomosis (31% vs 3% vs 0%, respectively; $p < 0.01$). However, the 31% with the circular seems quite high and although not stated, the circular technique was probably the first one used in their operative experience. In contrast, in another small retrospective review, Abdel-Galil et al.[24] found a higher stricture rate with hand sewn over circular or linear 33.3% versus 16.6% versus 10%, respectively.

There may be a trend toward a higher stricture rate with antecolic Roux limbs compared with retrocolic presumably secondary to tension or blood supply. Additionally, stapler diameter may influence the incidence of stenosis. Nguyen et al.[22] compared the stenosis rate with both the 21-mm and 25-mm circular staplers for creation of the gastrojejunostomy. The stricture rate was significantly higher with the 21-mm stapler than the 25-mm stapler (26.8% vs 8.8%, respectively; $p < 0.01$).

Patients who develop anastomotic stenosis develop progressive vomiting first for solids and eventually liquids. The history of such complaints is vital to recognition of this complication. Constant and progressive symptoms are characteristic of stenosis, while episodic or transient vomiting is more likely from dietary indiscretion. Although generally not life threatening, unrecognized and prolonged vomiting resulting from anastomotic stenosis can cause dehydration, and if chronic, protein-calorie malnutrition, and vitamin or thiamine deficiency.

Anastomotic strictures can usually be diagnosed by history alone. UGI fluoroscopy can also be helpful in demonstrating narrowing of the gastrojejunal anastomosis and delayed emptying of the gastic pouch. However, should the suspicion of a stricture be high enough, upper endoscopy is superior because it not only can establish the diagnosis but treat it as well. Inability to pass a 9-mm endoscope through the anastomotic outlet is considered by many to be diagnostic of anastomotic stricture.[25] Balloon dilatation with a through the scope balloon is highly effective in reestablishing an adequate lumen and resolving the patient's symptoms (Figure 38–2a and b). A stepwise approach is usually performed, dilating 3–5 mm above the size of the lumen at the first endoscopy and then using subsequent endoscopy to dilate to a final lumen of 12 mm.[26] The majority or strictures are successfully corrected with endoscopic balloon dilatation with one dilatation.[22,25,27]

Outlet stenosis is also common after VBG.[28] In one study, Hocking et al. found the incidence to be 14%.[29] Stenosis

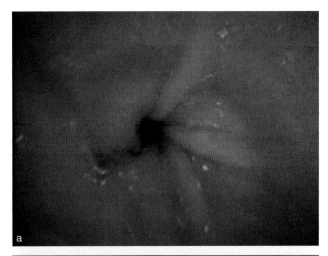

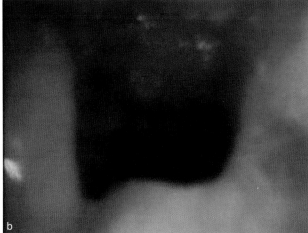

Figure 38–2. Endoscopic view of an anastomotic stricture before and after balloon dilatation.

is often due to a fibrotic reaction around the band compressing the lumen. It may occur as a result of band or ring erosion into the lumen which incites an inflammatory response and fibrosis. It can also be seen with band or ring angulation leading to kinking of the outlet. Since the band or ring is a fixed structure, endoscopic dilatation is often unsuccessful leaving revisional surgery as the only treatment option.

Gastrogastric Fistula

Gastrogastric fistulas are abnormal luminal communications between the gastric pouch and the excluded gastric fundus. Compartmentalizing the stomach to restrict food intake creates the potential for developing a fistula between gastric segments, a complication usually followed by weight gain and/or marginal ulceration. The incidence reported in the literature is extremely wide, ranging from as low as 0% in some series up to 49% in other ones, highlighting the number of factors that may influence their formation.[6,7] The etiology of gastrogastric fistula is partly due to the type of gastric bypass procedure performed. At one time, a partitioned gastric bypass, where the stomach was stapled with a noncutting linear stapler that segmented rather than divided the stomach, was very popular. The earlier descriptions of partitioned RYGBP used a single application of two- or four-row staples to create a 15–30-cc gastric pouch. However, with this technique, a high rate of staple line dehiscence was seen.[2,6] Jones reported a low incidence with a double application of a four-row stapler.[30] Sugerman et al. demonstrated that three superimposed staple lines (four rows each) significantly reduced the incidence (1%) of this troubling complication.[21] In our series of nearly 800 open, partitioned GBP procedures using two overlapping applications of a four-row stapler, we have seen this complication in 4% of patients.

Studies by MacLean et al.[2] and others demonstrated that when the gastric pouch was physically separated from the pouch by using a linear cutting stapler, the incidence of gastrogastric fistula was significantly less than when the stomach was stapled in continuity (3% vs 29%). These data led many surgeons to abandon gastric partitioning in favor of gastric division. Furthermore, the introduction of laparoscopic gastric bypass dramatically increased the prevalence of the divided gastric bypass. Numerous studies have subsequently reported low fistula rate with this technique. For example, Carrodeguas et al. reported an incidence of 1.2% of gastrogastric fistulas in a large series of 1292 consecutive patients who underwent a laparoscopic RYGBP procedure at their institution.[31] In our own series of 750 consecutive laparoscopic RYGBPs, the incidence was 0.4%.[5]

For the divided gastric bypass, there are several potential causes of gastrogastric fistula formation. It is thought that for fistulization to occur, a digestive process involving the gastric acid and pepsin must take place.[6] Digestion of tissue probably begins in the excluded stomach since a small, well-constructed pouch with an intact staple line has little or no acid. Studies by MacLean et al.[2] as well as Siilin et al.[9] demonstrated that gastric pouches had almost undetectable quantities of acid but also that invariably the proximal gastric pouch contained acid-producing parietal cells. Therefore in order to reduce acid production and, hence, the risk of potential stomal ulcers and fistula formation, the pouch has to be made as small as possible. A break in gastric mucosa appears necessary for acid and pepsin to begin digestion of the stomach wall. Staples and other foreign material have a tendency to migrate toward the lumen of the bowel, disrupting the continuity of the mucosa and theoretically allowing the escape of gastric juices from inside the gastric lumen. This migration phenomenon is seen frequently with an upper endoscopy. There is also a well-documented association between gastrogastric fistulas and marginal ulceration in the bariatric population. Studies have reported rates as high as 53.3% of marginal ulceration when associated with fistulas.[31]

Carrodeguas et al.[31] have divided the etiologic reasons for the development of gastrogastric fistulas into six categories:

1. *Iatrogenic*: The most common cause is an error in judgment and inadvertent failure to divide the stomach completely while constructing the proximal pouch. This could be due to difficulty visualizing the angle of His and the gas-

troesophageal junction because of various reasons such as an enlarged liver, spleen, multiple adhesions, or a large omental fat pad.
2. *Leaks*: This would also include small, contained, subclinical leaks where the pouch leak spontaneously drains into the gastric fundus.
3. *Mechanical and device related*: Infrequent, but possible is the fact that the stapler, despite properly firing, would fail to divide the stomach.
4. *Gastric tissue migration*: It is possible that the gastric wall mucosal tissue has the capability to migrate back and reattach to the gastric remnant in the absence of an inflammatory process.
5. *Marginal ulceration and perforation*: Marginal ulceration if not treated can erode through the wall of the anastomosis and lead to a communication between the gastric pouch and the gastric remnant.
6. *Foreign body erosion*: Much more common in those procedures that had a ring of some sort of material in order to prevent dilatation of the gastrojejunal anastomosis or pouch.

While the likelihood of preventing the formation of gastrogastric fistula is remote, there have been multiple attempts with an assortment of technical modifications to decrease the incidence. The use of sealants, oversewing the staple lines, and the use of buttressing material have been advocated.[32–36] In addition, jejunal and/or omental interposition have also been shown to decrease the likelihood of this complication.[6,37]

Diagnosing gastrogastric fistula is not a complicated endeavor. Close and careful patient observation during follow-up visits for any deviation from a normal and expected postoperative course should raise a red flag. Nonspecific but yet suggestive symptoms of gastrogastric fistulas include nausea, vomiting, development of marginal ulcerations, chronic upper abdominal pain, bleeding, and failure to lose weight or weight regain after initial weight loss. Diagnosis of a gastrogastric fistula is best made by UGI fluoroscopy with water-soluble contrast (Figure 38–3). Esophagoduodenoscopy can be useful for characterizing the size and location of the fistula. It may also diagnose concomitant marginal ulcers.

The treatment of gastrogastric fistula has traditionally been surgical. Revisional surgery to resect the gastrogastric fistula is extremely challenging and is associated with a high incidence of recurrence.[30] In addition, it cannot always be completed laparoscopically. However, not all fistulas require treatment. Many may be found incidentally. Small fistulas may not lead to weight gain or marginal ulceration and therefore only require observation. Uncomplicated marginal ulcers secondary to gastrogastric fistula should first be treated like any other marginal ulcers. Removal of any irritants such as NSAIDs, alcohol, and tobacco is essential. Histamine-receptor antagonists or proton-pump inhibitors may be effective. Should nonoperative treatment fail, surgery should be considered to prevent the complications of hemorrhage, perforation, dehydration, malnutrition, or significant weight regain.

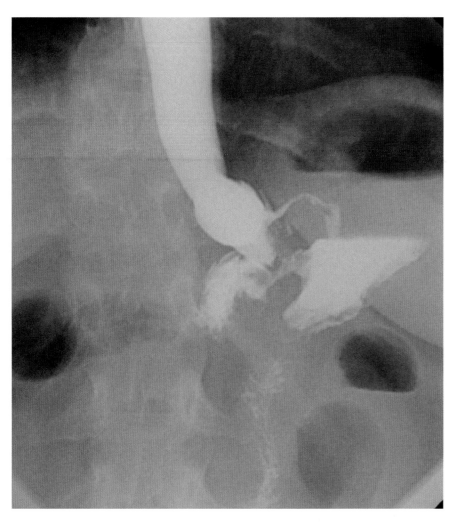

Figure 38–3. Upper GI contrast x-ray demonstrating a gastrogastric fistula. The contrast can be seen in the excluded fundus.

There is currently significant interest in developing safer, nonsurgical treatments. Endoscopic techniques involving injection of fibrin sealants and/or clips are being explored. At our institution, we have found that this therapy promotes the healing of fistula approximately half of the time and is most successful for long narrow fistulas. Recently, endoscopic suturing and stapling techniques are being developed and used to treat fistulas. However, it is early to make any conclusions. Further research and validation is pending and warranted.

CONCLUSIONS

Since its inception approximately 50 years ago, bariatric surgery has matured into a safe and effective frontline treatment for morbid obesity. In fact, it is currently the only treatment option that will usually provide meaningful and sustainable weight loss, which results in dramatic improvements in health and well-being. However, complications such as anastomotic stenosis, marginal ulceration, and gastrogastric fistula may occur. It is important for all clinicians involved with bariatric patients to understand, recognize, and be able to properly treat these patients when these complications occur to ensure their long-term success.

References

1. Printen KJ, LeFave J, Alden J: Bleeding from the bypassed stomach following gastric bypass. *Surg Gynecol Obstet* 156:65–66, 1983.
2. MacLean LD, Rhode BM, Nohr C, et al.: Stomal ulcer after gastric bypass. *J Am Coll Surg* 185:342–348, 1997.
3. Sanyal AJ, Sugerman HJ, Kellum JM, et al.: Stomal complications after gastric bypass. Incidence and outcome of therapy. *Am J Gastroenterology* 87:1165–1169, 1992.
4. Sapala JA, Wood MH, Scapala MA, et al.: Marginal ulcer after gastric bypass. A prospective 3 year study of 173 patients. *Obes Surg* 5:509–516, 1998.
5. Shikora SA, Kim JJ, Tarnoff ME, et al.: Laparoscopic roux-en-Y gastric bypass. Results of learning curve of a high-volume academic program. *Arch Surg* 140:362–367, 2005.
6. Capella JF, and Capella RF: Gastro-Gastric Fistulas and marginal ulcers in gastric bypass procedures for weight reduction. *Obes Surg* 9:22–27, 1999.
7. Cucchi SG, Pories WJ, MacDonald KG, et al.: Gastrogastric fistulas: a complication of divided gastric bypass surgery. *Ann Surg* 221:387–391, 1995.
8. MacLean LD, Rhode BM, Sampalis J, et al.: Results of the surgical treatment of obesity. *Am J Surg* 165:155–159, 1993.

9. Siilin H, Wanders A, Gustavsson S, et al.: The proximal gastric pouch invariably contains acid-producing parietal cells in Roux-en-Y gastric bypass. *Obes Surg* 15:771–777, 2005.

10. Smith CD, Herkes SB, Behrns KE, et al.: Gastric acid secretion and vitamin B12 absorption after vertical roux-en-Y gastric bypass for morbid obesity. *Ann Surg* 218:91–96, 1993.

11. Wallace JL: Pathogenesis of NSAID-induced gastroduodenal mucosal injury. *Best Pract Res Clin Gastroenterol* 15:691–703, 2001.

12. Schirmer B, Erenoglu C, Miller A: Flexible endoscopy in the management of patients undergoing roux-en-Y gastric bypass. *Obes Surg* 12:634–638, 2002.

13. Scopinaro N, Gianetta E, Adami GF, et al.: Biliopancreatic diversion for obesity at eighteen years. *Surgery* 119:261–268, 1996.

14. Totte E, Hendrickx L, van Hee R: Biliopancreatic diversion for treatment of morbid obesity: Experience in 180 consecutive cases. *Obes Surg* 9:161–165, 1999.

15. Baltasar A, Bou R, Bengochea M, et al.: Duodenal switch: An effective therapy for morbid obesity-intermediate results. *Obes Surg* 11:54–58, 2001.

16. Hess DS and Hess DW: Biliopancreatic diversion with a duodenal switch. *Obes Surg* 8:267–282, 1998.

17. Pope GD, Goodney PP, Burchard KW, et al.: Peptic ulcer/stricture after gastric bypass: a comparison of technique and acid suppression variables. *Obes Surg* 12:30–33, 2002.

18. Gonzalez R, Lin E, Venkatesh KR, et al.: Gastrojejunostomy during laparoscopic gastric bypass. Analysis of 3 techniques. *Arch Surg* 138:181–184, 2003.

19. Schauer PR, Ikramuddin S, Gourash WF, et al.: Outcomes after laparoscopic roux-en-y gastric bypass for morbid obesity. *Ann Surg* 232:515–529, 2000.

20. Wittgrove AC and Clark GW: Laparoscopic gastric bypass, Roux-en-y 500 patients: Technique and results with 3–60 month follow-up. *Obes Surg* 10:233–239, 2000.

21. Sugerman HJ and DeMaria ES: Gastric surgery for morbid obesity. In: *Mangot's Abdominal Operations*, 10th edn. Stamford, Appleton and Lange, 1997; p. 982–991.

22. Nguyen NT, Stevens CM, Wolfe BM: Incidence and outcome of anastomotic stricture after laparoscopic gastric bypass. *J Gastrointest Surg* 8:997–1003, 2003.

23. Rabkin RA, Rabkin JM, Metcalf B, et al.: Laparoscopic technique for performing duodenal switch with gastric reduction. *Obes Surg* 13:263–268, 2003.

24. Abdel-Galil E and Sabry AA: Laparoscopic Roux-en-Y gastric bypass-Evaluation of three different techniques. *Obes Surg* 12:639–642, 2002.

25. Rossi TR, Dynda DI, Estes NC, et al.: Stricture dilation after laparoscopic Roux-en-Y gastric bypass. *Am J Surg* 189:357–360, 2005.

26. Bell RL, Reinhardt KE, Flowers JL: Surgeon-performed endoscopic dilatation of symptomatic gastrojejunal anastomotic strictures following laparoscopic Roux-en-Y gastric bypass. *Obes Surg* 13:728–733, 2003.

27. Barba CA, Butensky MS, Lorenzo M, et al.: Endoscopic dilation of gastroesophageal anastomosis stricture after gastric bypass. *Surg Endosc* 17:416–420, 2003.

28. Sataloff DM, Lieber CP, Seinige UL: Strictures following gastric stapling for morbid obesity. Results of endoscopic dilatation. *Am Surg* 56:167–174, 1990.

29. Hocking MP, Bennett RS, Rout WR, et al.: Pouch outlet obstruction following vertical ring gastroplasty for morbid obesity. *Am J Surg* 160:496–500, 1990.

30. Jones KB: The double application of the TA-90B four row stapler and pouch formation: Eight rows are safe and effective in Roux-en-Y gastric bypass. *Obes Surg* 4:262–268, 1994.

31. Carrodeguas L, Szomstein S, Soto F, et al.: Management of gastrogastric fistulas after divided Roux-en-Y gastric bypass surgery for morbid obesity: Analysis of 1292 consecutive patients and review of literature. *SOARD* 1:467–474, 2005.

32. Baker RS, Foote J, Kemmeter P, et al.: The science of stapling and leaks. *Obes Surg* 14:1290–1298, 2004.

33. Liu CD, Glantz GJ, Livingston EH: Fibrin glue as a sealant for high-risk anastomosis in surgery for morbid obesity. *Obes Surg* 13:45–48, 2003.

34. Sapala JA, Wood HH, Schuhknecht MP, et al.: Anastomotic leak prophylaxis using vapor-heated fibrin sealant: report on 738 gastric bypass patients. *Obes Surg* 14:35–42, 2004.

35. Shikora SA: The use of staple-line reinforcement during laparoscopic gastric bypass. *Obes Surg* 14:1313–1320, 2004.

36. Shikora SA, Kim JJ, Tarnoff ME: Reinforcing gastric staple-lines with bovine pericardial strips may decrease the likelihood of gastric leak after laparoscopic Roux-en-Y gastric bypass. *Obes Surg* 13:37–44, 2003.

37. Zorrilla PG, Salinas RJ, Salinas-Martinez AM. Vertical banded gastroplasty-gastric bypass with and without the interposition of jejunum: Preliminary report. *Obes Surg* 9:29–32, 1999.

39

Nutritional Consequences and Management

Ampadi Thampi, KMD, FRCS • Robert N. L. Corprew Jr. • Michael Barker, MD • Walter J. Pories, MD, FACS

Bariatric surgery is misnamed. Weight control is only one of the objectives of the surgery. The others, such as the control of diabetes, sleep apnea, asthma, and gastroesophageal reflux disease, are in the long run much more important. Metabolic surgery would be a far more appropriate name for the discipline. No matter which of the common procedures is done—the vertical banded gastroplasty, adjustable gastric banding, gastric tube, Roux-en-Y gastric bypass (RYGB), or biliopancreatic diversion—the goal of all of these operations is to induce controlled malnutrition.

All of the procedures induce malnutrition by a reduction in volume as well as a change in the type of food. The gastroplasty and the bands not only reduce the gastric reservoir to the size of a golf ball but also limit the choice of foods to those that do not require a lot of chewing, such as water soluble starches and fats. Beef and those foods that form lumps like white bread may be difficult to pass. The malabsorptive procedures, in addition, exclude various sections of the foregut, dumping undigested food into the small bowel that can induce dumping, thus forcing the avoidance of foods rich in sugar.

Since most vitamins and minerals are absorbed in the upper small intestines, namely the duodenum and jejunum,[1] it should not be surprising that some patients may develop malabsorptive syndromes, some induced by variations in the operations, by differences in patient response, by starvation by strictures of the gastroenterostomy, by bowel obstructions caused by adhesions, internal hernias, or kinking of the enteroenterostomy, or by the failure of the patient to comply with the instructions to take nutritional supplements on a regular basis. While most nutritional problems are minor and readily managed by doubling vitamin and mineral supplements for a month, some patients develop serious deficiencies that can lead to life-threatening complications and permanent disabilities.

An example of a complication is demonstrated by the case of a 46-year-old woman, a composite of several such patients seen in our clinics who had undergone an intestinal or gastric bypass. Note that the onset can often be subtle and confusing.

A 46-year-old white woman, 5′2″ tall who weighed 308 lb with a BMI of 48.4, underwent a gastric bypass to treat her morbid obesity as well as her diabetes, GERD, and sleep apnea. Her early postoperative course was marked by frequent emesis due to a stricture that required dilatation on three occasions. Three months after gastric bypass surgery, she presented with tingling and numbness of her lower extremities. She was reassured by her referring physician that these "kinds of symptoms" are not infrequent after bariatric surgery. Even though she was seen by a number of other specialists, her symptoms continued to worsen. When she developed diplopia and gait difficulty, she was referred to a neurologist.

Neurological examination revealed horizontal nystagmus with intact extraocular movements, bilateral lower-extremity weakness, and diminished light touch, pinprick, and temperature sensations in both lower limbs and in her right hand. She had an ataxic gait with intact coordination and normal bladder and bowel functions. Deep tendon reflexes were symmetrically diminished with flexor plantars. Physical examination was otherwise unremarkable.

Laboratory examination revealed an elevated sedimentation rate of 54 mm/h (reference range, 0–20 mm/h) with a diminished vitamin B1 (thiamine) level of 25 ng/mL (reference range, 87–280 ng/mL). Serum erythrocyte transketolase activity was unavailable at our laboratory. Serum vitamin B12 level was not low at 1188 pg/mL (reference range, 200–600 pg/mL).

Magnetic resonance imaging (MRI) scan of the brain showed increased T2 signal in the head of the right caudate nucleus and adjacent putamen, with a similar ill-defined focus in the left frontal horn. Results of MRI of the spine were normal. These changes are consistent with Wernicke encephalopathy.[2] Only after all of these studies had been completed, the original bariatric surgeon was consulted. She was placed on a carefully controlled program of nutritional replacement with some but not full recovery of function.

In addition to Wernicke's encephalopathy, bariatric procedures may also induce other malabsorption deficiency disorders such as anemia, pernicious anemia, osteomalacia, osteoporosis, marasmus, kwashiorkor, pellagra, beriberi, and rarely ocular blindness. Note that patients may differ sharply in their response to malnutrition. Even though they may

Table 39–1.

Various Sites of Absorption of Nutrients in the Body

Stomach	Monosaccharides, alcohol
Proximal duodenum	Vitamins A, B, folic acid, iron, disaccharides Distal duodenum Disaccharides and dipeptides
Entire duodenum and proximal jejunum	Glucose, galactose, vitamin C, amino acids, glycerol and fatty acids, folic acid, biotin, copper, zinc, potassium, pantothenic acid Vitamins D, E, K, B1, B2, B3, B6, calcium, magnesium, and phosphorus
Jejunum	Glucose, galactose, vitamin C, amino acids, glycerol and fatty acids, folic acid, biotin, copper, zinc, potassium, pantothenic acid
Ileum	Entire Sodium, chloride Proximal Disaccharides, potassium Distal Vitamin B12 and intrinsic factor
Colon	Water, biotin

have undergone similar procedures, they may develop sharply different malnutrition syndromes. Understanding the potential nutritional consequences of bariatric operations will aid in decreasing the mortality and morbidity following surgery. This chapter highlights the effects of malnutrition and the preventive measures especially in the setting of postsurgical bariatric patients.

THE NORMAL PHYSIOLOGY OF DIGESTION AND ABSORPTION

Carbohydrate Digestion and Absorption

Carbohydrates consist of polysaccharides, disaccharides, and in the simplest form monosaccharides. The major dietary carbohydrates are the disaccharides sucrose (table sugar), lactose (milk sugar), and the polysaccharide starch, which is the glucose polymer storage form of carbohydrates in plants. Most starch consumed is present as amyopectin (α-1, 4 linked chains with α-1, 6-linked branches) as opposed to amylase (long, unbranched chains with glucose units linked α-1, 4). Glycogen, the animal storage form of carbohydrate found mostly in long glucose chains, is ingested in much lesser amounts. Although most diets contain significant quantities of the carbohydrate cellulose, humans cannot cleave the β-1, 4 bonds rendering cellulose indigestible.

The enzyme α-amylase found in salivary and pancreatic secretions cleaves the α-1, 4 linkages between glucose residues. During mastication, salivary α-amylase (ptyalin) mixes with food, which begins the process of digestion. However, only a small percentage of starch is hydrolyzed by ptyalin due to the brief period food spends in the mouth and rapid drop of pH in the stomach, which inhibits the enzyme. The optimal pH of this enzyme is 6.7, and it is obtained when bicarbonate secreted by the pancreas raises the pH in the duodenum. Additionally, α-amylase is secreted by the pancreas during this time. As a result, the starch is nearly completely hydrolyzed to the glucose, disaccharide maltose, trisaccharide maltotriose, and α-dextrin (glucose polymers containing α-1, 6 linkages) before it has passed beyond the duodenum and upper jejunum.

The small intestine surface area is increased through projections of villi lined by enterocytes. Each enterocyte contains a microvilli forming brush border, with tips projecting into a glycocalyx containing the oligosaccharidases that further digest the starch and other dietary carbohydrates. Maltase, α-dextrinase, and sucrase cleave the oligosaccharides to molecules of glucose. Lactase splits lactose to a molecule of galactose and glucose. Sucrase splits sucrose into a molecule fructose and glucose. While trehalase splits trehalose (α-1,1 dimer of glucose) to two molecules of glucose. Thus, these newly formed monosaccharides are ready for absorption by the small intestine.

Monosaccharides are the predominant form of carbohydrate that is absorbed across the mucosal membrane of the intestine. Absorption of monosaccharides takes place in the upper, mid, and lower small intestine. Glucose composes 80% of absorbable monosaccharide with galactose and fructose compiling the remaining 20%. Glucose enters intestinal epithelial cells by active transport using sodium glucose cotransport system (SGLT) in the apical membrane. This increases the intracellular glucose concentration above the blood glucose concentration, and glucose moves passively into the blood via carrier mechanisms (GLUT2) in the basolateral membrane. The sodium ions that enter the cell with the glucose molecules on SGLT are pumped out by Na/K ATPase located in the basolateral membrane.[3] Fructose is absorbed through facilitated diffusion using a different membrane transporter, GLUT5 into the cell and GLUT2 outside into the interstium, while galactose uses the same transporters as glucose.[4,5]

Protein Digestion and Absorption

Protein digestion starts in the stomach with pepsin, which is secreted as a proenzyme, pepsinogen, and activated by acid in the stomach. But most of the digestion takes place in the small intestine. Majority of proteases is secreted as proenzymes. In the duodenum, enteropeptidase converts trypsinogen to trypsin, which then converts other proenzymes to active enzymes. Pancreatic proteases are classified as endopeptidases (trypsin, chymotrypsin, and elastase) and exopeptidases (carboxypeptidase A and B) depending on the specificity of action. The final products of protein digestion are amino acids and small peptides.

Amino acids are absorbed via secondary active transport system in to the enterocytes. Like glucose, the uptake of amino acids is dependent on sodium concentration gradient across the brush border membrane. Proteins are also absorbed as dipeptides and tripeptides, and their uptake is more efficient than amino acid uptake. Complex peptides are broken down by peptidases located in the enterocytes before being absorbed. Malnourished patients are given di- and tripeptides instead of amino acids due to their better absorption and taste. In adults, negligible amounts of proteins are absorbed undigested.

Most of amino acid absorption takes place in the duodenum and jejunum and is completed at the ileum; none is absorbed in the colon. The major source of protein to the body is dietary in origin. There are also proteins derived from endogenous sources like pancreatic (20–30 g/day), biliary (10 g/day), and intestinal secretions and the cells shed from the intestinal villi (50 g/day).[6]

Lipid Digestion and Absorption

The major source of dietary lipids is triglycerides. Other lipids in human diet are cholesterol and phospholipids. Fats are acted upon by lingual lipase, which is secreted by the Ebner's glands of the tongue, and gastric lipase secreted by the stomach. The gastric lipase contributes very little to fat digestion. The main location of fat digestion is within the small intestine. Arrival of fat into the duodenum causes the release of the gut hormone, cholecystokinin (CCK), which slows gastric motility and emptying, stimulates pancreatic enzymes release, and causes contraction of the gallbladder with subsequent release of lecithin and bile salts. The churning of fat in the stomach and the small intestines plus the addition of bile salts in the duodenum causes the emulsification of fat into tiny droplets. The enzyme pancreatic lipase then hydrolyzes the 1- and 3-bonds on the triglycerides leaving a 2-monoglyceride. Colipase, which is activated by trypsin, and bile salt activated lipase are also released by the pancreas but play a lesser role in fat digestion. Cholesteryl ester hydrolase cleaves the ester from the dietary cholesterol ester forming cholesterol and a free fatty acid. In addition, pancreatic phospholipase A2 hydrolyzes one of the fatty acids from a phospholipid leaving lysophospholipid and a free fatty acid.

The bile salt micelle is composed of 2-monoglyceride, free fatty acids, cholesterol, and lysophospholipids obtained from lipid digestion in the lumen of the duodenum, jejunum, and to a lesser extent the ileum. Bile salts transfer the lipids to mucosal surface where they enter the cells. Unlike carbohydrates and proteins, lipids are believed to enter enterocytes by passive diffusion.

Once inside the enterocyte, monoglyceride is acylated back to triglyceride which occurs within the smooth endoplasmic reticulum. This is the major source of triglycerides, while short- and long-chain fatty acids supply only a minute amount of the triglyceride. Short-chain fatty acids, less than 10–12 carbon atoms, are relatively hydrophilic and able to pass through the enterocyte unchanged into the portal circulation. Longer-chain fatty acids, those greater than 10–12 carbon atoms, are hydrophobic and must be reesterified to triglycerides. A portion of the cholesterol absorbed into the enterocyte is also esterified. In forming the chylomicron, which will transport the lipids through the lymphatic system, the triglycerides and cholesterol esters are coated with a layer of protein, cholesterol, and phospholipids.[7–11]

Vitamin and Mineral Absorption

The absorption of vitamins and minerals occurs mainly in the upper small intestines. The absorption of the fat-soluble vitamins such as vitamins A, D, E, and K decreases with decrease in absorption of fat. This may occur due to lack of pancreatic enzymes or the absence of bile within the intestine. Vitamin B12 absorption takes place in the ileum. Vitamins and mineral transport across the mucosa is generally largely dependent on valency. Monovalent ions have a much greater maximal absorption than a bivalent ion.

Mineral levels are frequently below normal in the morbidly obese prior to surgery, especially in terms of calcium and iron. The sufficiency of the trace elements, including zinc, copper, and chromium, is less clear although zinc deficiencies have been reported by some and not others. The disagreements in the micronutrient studies may well be due to the difficulties in the collection, preservation, and analyses of these elements. Problems with absorption of vitamins and minerals can lead to serious morbidities and possibly mortality.

DEFICIENCIES, THEIR PREVENTION, AND MANAGEMENT

Protein Deficiency

Bariatric surgery is a metabolic surgery designed to produce malnutrition. Energy deficit occurs due to low food intake, food intolerance, and nutrient malabsorption. We aim to achieve malnutrition to lose weight but without complications. Protein deficiency can occur after any bariatric operation. The ratio of fat mass to fat-free mass loss is about 4:1 in restrictive operations like RYGB.[12] It is probably even more severe after biliopancreatic diversion (BPD). The literature is not clear. Some report severe protein-calorie malnutrition[13] although low incidences have been described by others.[14,15]

Protein deficiencies manifest themselves initially with fatigue and loss of muscle strength, especially with greater than expected weight loss as in patients who have strictures of the gastrojejunal anastomosis. Progression of protein deficiency is predictable with continuing weight loss with the additional development of hair loss, poor wound healing, wasting, emaciation, kwashiorkor, and marasmus.

Protein deficiencies should be addressed promptly with supplementation. Although normal protein requirement for the average individual is 1 g/kg body wt/day, this formula does not work for the morbidly obese with weights of 200 kg or more. Most bariatric surgeons aim for 60–90 g per day for their postoperative patients, but, in fact, there is little evidence for this guideline. Protein deficiency can be assessed by checking serum albumin levels at regular intervals, but it is not a reliable measure. We have seen virtual normal albumin levels in patients who were severely malnourished that fall to extremely low values when additional nutrition is provided. It almost appears that the patients lack the enzymes to utilize the albumen, building albumen stores that cannot be used.

Our usual approach is to proceed promptly by supplementing these patients with one or two cans of a liquid, high protein, high vitamin preparation such as Ensure Plus if they are able to tolerate an oral diet. This approach rarely fails but may take weeks to restore patients to euproteinemia. If the patients are unable to eat or drink, however, total parenteral nutrition should be started promptly with an emphasis on slow rather than fast correction. In our experience, badly malnourished patients should be corrected slowly; they are unable to manage sudden large loads of nutrients when they are first seen.

Carbohydrate Deficiency

Carbohydrate deficiency, manifested as episodic hypoglycemia, is probably quite common. Many patients admit to having episodes of feeling "shaky and light-headed" during the day, usually about 2 hours or so after meals. When our series of gastric bypasses was about 1000 cases over 16 years, we found 47 patients in our practice who developed documented glucose levels in the 30–40 d/mL range. The hypoglycemia appeared to be independent of age, gender, race, original weight, and degree of weight loss and could appear as late as 14 years after the operation. Fortunately, all of our patients were managed well with candy taken at the first "aura" of hypoglycemia, i.e., weakness, shaking, sweatiness, etc. All cleared within a year of the appearance of symptoms. A recent report of nesidoblastosis requiring pancreatic resection suggests that refractory cases exist possibly due to the development of secondary tumors.[16,17]

Fatty Acid Deficiency

Linoleic acid and linolenic acid are not synthesized in humans and hence are classified as essential fatty acids. Deficiency of clinically essential fatty acid has been recorded with deficiency of linoleic acid. This occurs in extreme malnutrition. The deficiency results in a clinical syndrome characterized by scaly skin rash, poor wound healing, increased susceptibility to infections, growth retardation, and sparse hair growth. Treatment with one of the high-caloric liquid preparations such as Ensure Plus or, in severe cases, with total parenteral nutrition should provide restoration of normal values. Intravenous fat preparations are not needed.

Vitamin B12 Deficiency

Vitamin B12 deficiency may be seen as early as 1 year and as late as 9 years after gastric bypass surgery. Most patients have substantial stores of vitamin B12, at about 2000 μg, prior to surgery. The daily requirement of vitamin B12 is around 2 μg.

Vitamin B12 absorption is significantly altered following RYGB. In the stomach, pepsin and hydrochloric acid cleave vitamin B12 from food, primarily meats. The free vitamin B12 binds to R-binder protein seen in saliva and proximal alimentary tract. Inside duodenum, degradation of R-binder proteins occurs by pancreatic peptidases and proteases releasing vitamin B12 to form a complex with intrinsic factor (IF), a carrier protein produced in the stomach. The vitamin B12–IF complex gets absorbed in the terminal ileum. Some of the vitamin B12 is also absorbed from the large bowel, taking advantage of the B12 produced by the colonic flora. Mechanisms of vitamin B12 deficiency include achlorhydria preventing cleavage of vitamin from food, decreased intake of meat and milk, and inadequate secretion of intrinsic factor from the stomach after surgery.

In patients after RYGB, the prevalence of vitamin B12 deficiency is estimated to be around 12–33%.[18] Significant vitamin B12 deficiency can lead to megaloblastic anemia, thrombocytopenia, leukopenia, and glossitis, all of which are reversible with supplementation. If deficiency persists, demyelination can occur, leading to irreversible loss of peripheral sensation.[19] Although incidence of symptomatic vitamin B12 deficiency is low, there is a general consensus that most gastric bypass patients cannot maintain adequate vitamin B12 levels without supplementation. The best route of supplementation is controversial. Supplementation with 300–500 μg/d orally or as 1000 μg/month intramuscular shots is sufficient to prevent deficiency disorder. Other available forms of supplementation include sublingual 350 μg/d and nasal spray 500 μg weekly.

There is a case reported of an exclusively breastfed infant with vitamin B12 deficiency, born of an asymptomatic mother who had gastric bypass surgery.[20] In addition, we have had one post-gastric-bypass surgery patient who died of pernicious anemia after stringent refusal to take any form of vitamin B12, reasoning that the supplement was satanic and not in accord with her religion.

Folate Deficiency

Folate deficiency is much less common than vitamin B12 deficiency. Folate absorption is facilitated by hydrochloric acid in the stomach and primarily occurs in the upper part of small intestine. Vitamin B12 acts as a coenzyme for the conversion of methyl THF to tetrahydrofolate; therefore, a deficiency in vitamin B12 may subsequently cause folate deficiency. Despite these two mechanisms for folate deficiency, decreased folate consumption from dietary sources is thought to be the predominant cause of deficiency. It can also present with megaloblastic anemia, thrombocytopenia, leukopenia, and glossitis. Serum deficiencies are quite common and symptoms are rare and easily corrected with supplementation; 1 mg a day should correct the deficiency. Folate deficiency is a serious threat to women getting pregnant after gastric bypass, as it can lead to increased risk of neural tube defects in the baby. Although folate absorption occurs in the proximal small bowel, it can take place along the entire small bowel with adaptation after surgery.

Vitamin B1

A well-known risk associated with obesity surgery in patients who have intense and persistent vomiting is the development of vitamin deficiency in a short time, especially thiamine. Mild deficiency causes anorexia, irritability, apathy, and generalized weakness. Major deficiency leads to beriberi and a variety of neurological manifestations such as polyneuropathies Wernicke's encephalopathy (WE)[21] and Wernicke-Korsakoff psychosis.

Thiamine was the first vitamin B to be identified and therefore also referred to as vitamin B1. Thiamine deficiency is also seen in alcoholism, hyperemesis gravidarum, prolonged fasting, prolonged parenteral nutrition, and dialysis and acquired immunodeficiency syndrome.

Thiamine pyrophosphate, a coenzyme form of thiamine, is required for the branched-chain amino acid metabolism and carbohydrate metabolism. It has also been postulated that thiamine plays a role in peripheral nerve conduction, although the exact chemical reaction underlying this function is unknown.

Thiamine is absorbed from proximal jejunum by active transport and passive diffusion.[22] Once absorbed, it circulates bound to plasma proteins (mainly albumin) and erythrocytes. Storage sites include muscle, heart, liver, kidney, and brain, muscle being the principal storage site. Total body storage is mainly in the form of thiamine pyrophosphate, which amounts to approximately 30 mg, with a biological half-life ranging between 9 and 18 days.

Mild deficiency leads to anorexia, irritability, apathy, and generalized weakness. Prolonged deficiency causes beriberi. It can be wet beriberi with cardiovascular involvement presenting with enlarged heart, tachycardia, high output cardiac failure, edema, and peripheral neuritis or dry beriberi presenting with symmetrical peripheral neuropathy of the motor and sensory systems with diminished reflexes. The neuropathy markedly affects legs, and patients have difficulty rising from squatting position. The pathological event is axonal degeneration. Dry beriberi is usually seen in the setting of energy deprivation and inactivity, two conditions commonly seen after bariatric surgery.

Chronic vitamin B1 deficiency can involve CNS known as Wernicke's encephalopathy, consisting of horizontal nystagmus, ophthalmoplegia, cerebellar ataxia, and mental impairment. Additional memory loss and confabulatory psychosis make it Wernicke-Korsakoff syndrome.

Diagnosis of WE is mainly clinical. It is associated with neuronal loss and vascular damage about the third and fourth ventricles, vermix and periaqueductal gray matter. Patients can be tested for functional enzymatic assay of transketolase activity before and after the addition of TPP. A stimulation of more than 25% is considered abnormal. Thiamine or TPP levels can be measured by high-performance liquid chromatography to detect deficiency. Urinary thiamine <27 μg/g of creatinine per day is abnormal.

Treatment. Acute thiamine deficiency is treated with parenteral thiamine 100 mg/d for 7 days followed by 10 mg/d orally until complete recovery.[23] Prophylaxis is given to all bariatric patients in the form of multivitamin supplementation. There is no routine test to check the levels of thiamine in the postoperative follow-up period. But it is important to start intensive vitamin B1 therapy at the earliest suspicion of deficiency. Anaphylaxis has been reported with high doses, but no adverse effects have been recorded.

Vitamin A

Gastric bypass procedures can cause vitamin A deficiency leading to serious ocular complications, including xerophthalmia, nyctalopia, and ultimate blindness.[24] The increasing incidence of obesity and gastric bypass procedures warrants patient and physician education regarding strict adherence to vitamin supplementation. Education is imperative to avoid detrimental ophthalmic complications resulting from hypovitaminosis A and to prevent a potential epidemic of iatrogenic xerophthalmia and blindness. Fat-soluble vitamin deficiencies are known complications of this BPD,[25] with incidence rates reported as high as 6%.

Two curious aspects of bariatric surgery are the great variation in the deficiency syndromes and that severe consequences can occur even after the least intrusive surgical procedure. A recent case report[26] provides a sobering example: a 36-year-old morbidly obese female with BMI 60.6 kg/m^2 underwent laparoscopic adjustable gastric banding, followed 2 years later by BPD in an attempt to control her weight. Following BPD, she failed to attend outpatient appointments and was poorly compliant with daily multivitamins and monitoring of serum vitamin and mineral levels. She developed symptomatic vitamin A deficiency, with vitamin A levels <0.1 μmol/L, and night blindness, as well as deficiencies of vitamins D, E, and K, zinc, and selenium.

Iron

Iron deficiency is one of the most frequent deficiencies after obesity surgery. The incidence is about 14–16% in RYBG and 21–26% after BPD.[27] The etiology of iron deficiency is multifactorial. Iron deficiency after gastric bypass results from both malabsorption and maldigestion of dietary iron. Iron is absorbed in the ferrous form only. Dietary iron (ferric) is reduced to ferrous form by the acid in the stomach. Restrictive surgeries cause less production of acid in the stomach and hence less absorption. Moreover, with the exclusion of duodenum and proximal jejunum, the main areas of iron absorption are bypassed. Postoperative changes in eating habits and food preferences may also contribute to development of iron deficiency anemia.

Women during the child-bearing age after gastric bypass are at high risk for developing iron deficiency anemia. Iron stores in menstruating women are estimated at approximately 300 mg, which is about one third of the stores of adult males.

The regulation of body iron stores is effected by control of intestinal mucosal absorption. The daily requirements are 30–35 mg. Normal diet provides about 15–30 mg. Body iron loss for men is 1.0–1.5 μg/d, but it is 2–3 μg/d for women. Iron is stored as ferritin, and measurement of serum ferritin is the most useful indirect estimate of body iron stores. Levels decline with storage iron depletion. Iron deficiency presents with low hemoglobin, microcytic hypochromic anemia, low serum iron, low serum ferritin, and high total iron-binding capacity.

Most multivitamin and mineral supplements contain sufficient amount of iron to prevent deficiency. However, iron deficiency and anemia sometimes persist even in patients taking multivitamins. As a preventive measure, all menstruating women are prescribed ferrous sulfate 325 mg every day. Patients diagnosed with anemia are treated with ferrous sulfate 325 mg three times a day along with vitamin C. Sometimes parenteral iron therapy is necessary to correct anemia. Iron therapy is associated with constipation as a common side effect.

Calcium

Moderate weight loss has been reported to reduce bone mineral density.[28–30] Drastic weight loss following bariatric procedures results in increased risk of low bone mass[31] and metabolic bone disease.[32] This results from calcium and vitamin D malabsorption and from secondary hyperparathyroidism. The latter results from insufficient calcium intake, low calcium absorption (due to decreased gastric acidity, reduced surface of absorption, and from increased production of calcium-binding substances in the plasma), and low serum calcium levels.

Calcium is absorbed in duodenum and proximal jejunum by an active process mediated by vitamin D. Elevation of PTH and reduction of vitamin D have been reported in obese patients.[33] Obesity associated vitamin D3 deficiency is likely due to decreased bioavailability of vitamin D3 from cutaneous and dietary sources because of its deposition in body fat compartments.[34]

Calcium deficiency leads to osteoporosis. Osteoporosis has been difficult to diagnose during its early stages. Secondary hyperparathyroidism occurs when there is inadequate absorption of calcium and can be detected by the elevated PTH levels. Serum calcium may be normal due to efficiency of the parathyroid glands.

Routine monitoring of vitamin D and Ca intake is necessary for all bariatric surgery patients. Recommended screening tests include Serum Ca, Serum C-telopeptide, 25-OH D, and PTH. A rise in C-telopeptidase is the first sign of calcium deficiency and would indicate the need to increase treatment with calcium and vitamin D.

Recommendation to prevent osteoporosis after bariatric surgery includes ingestion of 1200–1500 mg of calcium and 800 IU of vitamin D per day.[35] If the patient has extreme malabsorption, higher doses are needed to prevent secondary hyperparathyroidism. The efficacy of calcium absorption varies inversely with the calcium intake. At low doses (<500 mg), calcium absorption is by active transport. At higher doses, calcium is absorbed by diffusion. Calcium is absorbed in most parts of the intestine, but mainly in duodenum and proximal jejunum where pH is lower. In a low-acid environment as seen in achlorhydria and gastric bypass, absorption of calcium carbonate is poor.[26] A recent study reported that absorption of amino acid chelated calcium is twice that of calcium carbonate.[36]

A cross-sectional survey was conducted by Ybarra et al. on 144 patients of whom 80 had not undergone bariatric surgery, while 64 had bariatric surgery at a mean of 36 months previously.[37] Eighty percent of the patients presented with low vitamin D levels and mild secondary hyperparathyroidism. Hypovitaminosis D with secondary hyperparathyroidism due to low calcidiol bioavailability should be added to the crowded list of sequelae of morbid obesity. While further studies are warranted, it seems advisable to support vitamin D supplementation in the morbidly obese population.

Zinc

Zinc deficiency has been recorded in patients following gastric bypass surgery. Zinc is required for protein synthesis and is a component of more than 100 enzymes, among which are DNA polymerase, RNA polymerase, and transfer RNA synthetase. Zinc deficiency has a profound effect in rapidly proliferating tissues. Deficiency is associated with poor wound healing, diarrhea, dermatitis, alopecia, glossitis, corneal clouding loss of dark adaptation, and behavioral changes. Acrodermatitis enteropathica is a rare, recessively inherited disease in which intestinal absorption of zinc is delayed.

Multivitamin therapy containing zinc will help to prevent deficiency disorders.

Acute zinc toxicity develops if more than 200 mg of zinc is taken in a single day. It is manifested by abdominal pain, nausea, vomiting, and diarrhea.

Cu and Zn compete for intestinal absorption and hence long-term ingestion of >25 mg of Zn can lead to Cu deficiency. No accurate laboratory test is available to check Zn deficiency. Plasma, hair, and red blood cell zinc levels are often misleading.

CLINICAL APPLICATIONS

Nutritional deficiencies are expected following obesity surgery and supplementing them is the best way of prevention. At East Carolina University, our Obesity Surgery Program has a standardized vitamin and mineral supplementation protocol that includes daily oral supplementation of two chewable multivitamins (Flintstones complete or Bugs

Bunny with Vitamins and Minerals are recommended), 250 μg of vitamin B12, and calcium citrate 1000 mg. Menstruating females are advised to take ferrous sulfate elixir 325 mg every day by mouth. Iron and calcium supplements are advised to be taken at least 3 hours apart, as both compete for absorption in the body.

In addition to spending significant time with patients before and after the surgery with discussions of the importance of vitamin and mineral supplementation, we follow limited nutritional parameters at regular intervals but depend greatly on the interview, the degree of weight loss, and the quality of daily function to pick up any emerging deficiencies. There is no overall reliable laboratory test for malnutrition. Standard gastric bypass laboratories done in our department include CBC with differential, serum albumin, and vitamin B12 levels. These are done at 2 weeks, 4 weeks, 3, 6, 9, and 12 months, and thereafter annually. The patient's multiple comorbidities are addressed separately.

Iron deficiency anemia is treated with ferrous sulfate 325 mg three times a day. Parenteral iron therapy may be necessary in selected patients, but the indications are very rare for this degree of intervention. Refractory and severe anemia may require blood transfusion. Thiamine and folate deficiencies are suspected in patients who present after repeated vomiting. They should be treated with parenteral thiamine and folate before starting fluid replacement. Acute thiamine deficiency is treated with parenteral thiamine 100 mg/d for 7 days followed by 10 mg/d orally until there is complete recovery. Vitamin B12 deficiency has to be corrected by supplementing 300–500 μg/d orally or as 1000–2000 μg/month intramuscular shots. Protein deficiencies are identified and corrected by dietary modification and protein supplementation. Total parenteral nutrition may be necessary for patients with extreme degree of malnutrition.

CONCLUSIONS

Bariatric surgery is a great medical advance but it is not without risk. The inducement of rapid massive weight loss in patients who are already ill with comorbidities and chronic malnutrition can lead to severe and permanent consequences from deficiencies of carbohydrates, proteins, fatty acids, macroelements, trace elements, and vitamins. Those who care for bariatric surgical patients must be aware of these complications that vary sharply between patients and are all too often subtle and difficult to treat.

References

1. Ponsky TA, Brody F, Pucci E: Alterations in gastrointestinal physiology after Roux-en-Y gastric bypass. *J Am Coll Surg* 201(1):125–131, 2005.
2. Nautiyal A, Singh S, Alaimo DJ: Wernicke encephalopathy—an emerging trend after bariatric surgery. *Am J Med* 117(10):804–805, 2004.
3. Rhoades RA, Tanner GA: *Medical Physiology*, 2nd edn, Chapter 2. Philadelphia, PA, Lippincott Williams and Wilkins, 2002; p. 29–31.

4. Gartner L, Hiatt J: *Color Atlas of Histology*, 3rd edn. Philadelphia, PA, Lippincott Williams and Wilkins, 2000.

5. Johnson L: *Gastrointestinal Physiology*, 6th edn. St. Louis, Mosby, 2001.

6. Rhoades RA, Tanner GA: *Medical Physiology*, 2nd edn, Chapter 2. Philadelphia, PA, Lippincott Williams and Wilkins, 2002; p. 503–505.

7. Guyton A, Hall J: *Textbook of Medical Physiology*, 9th edn. Philadelphia, PA, W.B. Sauders Company, 1996.

8. Ganong W: *Review of Medical Physiology*, 22nd edn. Lange Medical Books/McGraw-Hill, 2003.

9. Costanzo L: *Physiology*, 3rd edn. Philadelphia, PA, Lippincott Williams and Wilkins, 2003.

10. Marks D: *Biochemistry*, 3rd edn. Philadelphia, PA, Lippincott Williams and Wilkins, 1999.

11. Goldberg S: *Clinical Physiology Made Ridiculously Simple*. Medmaster Inc., 2002.

12. Faintuch J, Matsuda M, Cruz ME, et al.: Severe protein-calorie malnutrition after bariatric procedures. *Obes Surg* 14(2):175–181, 2004.

13. Sugerman HJ: Bariatric surgery for severe obesity. *J Assoc Acad Minor Phys* 12:129–136, 2001.

14. Totte E, Hendrickx L, van Hee R: Biliopancreatic diversion for treatment of morbid obesity: Experience in 180 consecutive cases. *Obes Surg* 9:161–165, 1999.

15. Scorpinaro N, Adami GF, Marinari GM, et al.: Biliopancreatic diversion. *World J Surg* 22:936–946, 1998.

16. Kaiser AM, Carpender T, Trautmann ME, et al.: Hyperinsulinemic hypoglycemia with nesidioblastosis after gastric bypass surgety. *N Engl J Med* 353(20): 2192–2194, 2005.

17. Service GJ, Thompson GB, Andrews JC, et al.: Hyperinsulenimic hypoglycemia with nesidioblastosis after gastric bypass surgery. *N Engl J Med* 21;353(3):249–254, 2005.

18. Brolin RE, Leung M: Survey of vitamin and mineral supplementation after gastric bypass and biliopancreatic diversion for morbid obesity. *Obes Surg* 9:150–154, 1999.

19. Brolin RE, Gorman JH, Gorman RC, et al.: Are Vitamin B12 and folate deficiency clinically important after roux-en-y gastric bypass? *J Gastrointest Surg* 2:436–442, 1998.

20. Grange DK, Finlay JL: Nutritional vitamin B12 deficiency ina breast-fed infant following maternal gastric bypass. *Pediatr Hematol Oncol* 11:311–318, 1994.

21. Loh Y, Watson W, Verma A, et al.: Acute Wernicke's encephalopathy following bariatric surgery:clinical course and MRI correlation. *Obes Surg* 14:129–132, 2004.

22. Mhan LK, Escott-Stump S: *Vitamins. Krause's Food Nutrition abd Diet Therapy*, 11th edn. Philadelphia, PA, Saunders, 2004; p. 93–95.

23. Russell RM: *Principles of Internal Medicine*, 15th ed, Vol. 1. p. 461–462.

24. Lee WB, Hamilton SM, Harris JP: Ocular complications of hypovitaminosis a after bariatric surgery. *Ophthalmology* 112(6):1031–1034, 2005.

25. Hatizifotis M, Dolan K, Newbury L, et al.: Symptomatic vitamin A deficiency following biliopancreatic diversion. *Obes Surg* 13(4):655–657, 2003.

26. Recker RR: Calcium absorption and achlorhydria. *N Rng J Med* 313:70–33, 1985.

27. Brolin RE, Leung M: Survey of vitamin and mineral supplementation after gastric bypass and biliopancreatic diversion for morbid obesity. *Obes Surg* 9:150–154, 1999.

28. Luciana JE, Kadre: Paulo Roberto savassi-Rocha calcium metabolism in pre and postmenopausal morbidly obese women at baseline and after laparoscopic Roux-en-y gastric bypass. *Obes Surg* 14:1062–1066, 2003.

29. Shapes S: Weight loss and the skeleton. In: Burckhardt P, Heaney R, Dawson Hughes B, et al. (eds). *Nutritional Aspects of Osteoporosis*. New york, Springler-Verlag, 2001.

30. Guney E, Kisakol G, Ozgen G, et al.: Effect of weight loss on bone metabolism:comparison of vertical banded gastroplasty and medical intervention. *Obes Surg* 13:383–388, 2003.

31. Bano G, Rodin DA, Pazianas M, et al.: Reduced bone mineral density after surgical treatment for obesity. *Int J Obes* 23:361–365, 1999.

32. Crowley l, Seay J, Mullin G: Late effects of gastric bypass for obesity. *Am J Gastroenterol* 79:850–860, 1984.

33. Bell N, Epstain S, Green A, et al.: Evidence of alteratinof the vitamin D endocrine system in obese subjects. *J Clin Invest* 76:370–373, 1985.

34. Wortsman J, Matsuoka LY, Chen TC, et al.: Decreased bioavailability of vitamin D in obesity. *Am J Clin Nutr* 72:690–693, 2000.

35. American association of Clinical Endocrinologist Medical guidelines for clinical practice for the prevention and management of postmenopausal osteoporosis. *Endocr pract* 7:293–312, 2001.

36. Heaney RP, Recker RR, Weaver CM: Absorbability of calcium sources: the limited role of solubility. *Calcif Tissue Int* 46:300–304, 1990.

37. Ybarra J, Sanchez-Hernandez J, Gich I, et al.: Unchanged hypovitaminosis D and secondary hyperparathyroidism in morbid obesity after bariatric surgery. *Obes Surg* 15(3):330–335, 2005.

40

Weight Recidivism

José Carlos Pareja, MD, PhD • Daniela Magro, PhD

It is common knowledge among bariatric surgeons that, sometime after surgery, patients tend to present with higher weight than the least measured in the period between 18 and 24 months after the procedure, the interval in which weight loss plateau is reached. Weight regain occurs usually between 2 and 5 years after gastric bypass, in a significant percentage of the patient population depending on patient compliance and the attention given by the bariatric medical staff and support groups.

In a seminar of the American Society for Bariatric Surgery and the Academy of Alimentary Disorders, Carol Signore[1] asked surgeons and colleagues from support groups (psychologists, nutritionists) about the extent of weight regain in operated patients and if they considered support groups important to improve weight loss. Many of the attending professionals agreed that the number of patients regaining weight was certainly increasing along with the follow-up time. A consensus was reached and patients having gastric bypass were divided into groups regarding weight regain:

GROUP 1—about 25% of patients lose 80%–100% of their excess weight, regardless of medical or support groups' aid.

GROUP 2—25% of patients do not lose enough weight, or display weight regains, even with medical and support group care.

GROUP 3—about 50% of patients might achieve good results, but this is primarily dependent of the efficacy of medical staff and the attention of support groups. For these patients, the ability of the multi-professional team

to keep patients involved in support group programs is vital. Should these data be confirmed, it is possible that, in long-term analysis (5–10 years after surgery), almost half of the patients could experience suboptimal results.

According to the professionals attending the seminar, many patients do not take advantage of the help from these groups, without which they may not reach the expected goals.

There are few published works to date on patient's long-term follow-up, but most surgeons are aware that weight regain is really taking place. Long-term weight-loss maintenance after bariatric surgery depends, among other things, on change in alimentary habits, being essential to identify those patients who present with *binge eating disorder (BED)* before the procedure so that these patients can receive more adequate treatment in the postoperatory period. BED, as stated by Saunders,[2] was present in 33.3% of the cases studied by her. These data are similar to those found by Spitzer,[3] from which BED prevalence was 30% in patients who submitted to medical treatment for weight loss. Hsu et al.[4] found 38% of BED in preoperative bariatric surgery patients.

It is important to consider other eating disorders that do not fulfill BED's criteria, but may cause problems to the patients postoperatively. A high incidence of depression is associated with severe *binge eating (BE)* in the postoperative period, showing that the patient's psychological state is related to BE regardless of weight.

Nonetheless, one paper notes that BED individuals have weight loss similar to non-BED at 1-year follow-up.[5] Other authors, following patients from 13 to 15 years after surgery, found that 49% of the subjects had BED preoperatively, compared to only 6.4% postoperatively.[6] Some studies demonstrate that preoperative BED patients experience less weight loss, or regain weight after surgery.

A review article stated that gastric bypass patients lost 60%–70% of excess weight, but 30% regained some weight at 18–24 months postoperatively. However, the studies on which it was based did not quantify the mean increase in weight per unit time.[7] Given that, we still lack sufficient evidence to define the importance of previous eating habits after bariatric surgery. Some questions are yet to be answered, such as: Does BED influence postoperative weight loss? What is the real impact of bariatric surgery on BED patients? Is it of utmost importance to start BED treatment preoperatively, or is it useless? To obtain these answers, long-term follow-up studies are necessary.[2]

Psychotherapists say that complete cure of eating compulsion habits is difficult and often temporary. Many subjects manage to temporarily avoid alimentary compulsions, and then return to the old eating habits they had before surgery.

If support groups are effective, the group 3 patients may become 70%–80% of the operated patients, instead of only 50%. The need for support groups, with meetings with psychologists, psychiatrists, nutritionists, and surgeons, is a widely accepted reality; these meetings should occur twice a month, for at least 2 years. Nevertheless, the author has observed that patients give up the meetings, for different reasons: lack of time, economic issues, and individual problems. After some time, the heavier noncompliant patients get back to support groups, depressed by weight increase.

In a seminar carried out in Utah in the mid-nineties, an experienced bariatric surgeon, Charles B. Edwards,[8] commented

> Why do some of the patients submitted to gastric bypass lose weight effectively and keep this state for many years, while others display good initial results and gain weight later?
>
> If we could clarify this matter, we would know in advance how each patient should respond to surgery.
>
> Our experience shows that the patients followed the recommendations given by the medical staff in the beginning. However, after some years (2 to 5), they returned to old habits, forgetting the eating modifications previously learned. Why does it happen? Why do some of the patients adapt to new habits and succeed and some don't? Why do some of them see themselves as the only reason for their long-term weight loss, while others believe only surgery could make them thinner?
>
> It is likely that the patients who give up trying and regain weight share some characteristics and, on the other hand, the subjects who permanently succeed must have many things in common too.
>
> If we could identify what the successful patients have in common, we could set guidelines and solid orientations for all patients. The way of knowing it could be at the postoperative visits and support groups meetings, by means of investigation of the parameters and habits that lead these patients to sustained weight loss.

A study was then designed to identify successful patient habits, and was presented by Cook and Edwards,[8] in 1998, at the American Society for Bariatric Surgery Annual Meeting in Orlando, FL. This study was later published in *Obesity Surgery*, in February 1999.

A hundred gastric bypass patients studied between 1979 and 1995 answered a questionnaire about personal habits such as eating, sleeping, drinking liquids and alcohol, and physical activities. They experienced a mean excess weight loss of 74%. In this study of very successful patients, six long-lasting good habits were identified as determinant of weight reduction maintenance.

1. Concerning eating, the subjects had three balanced meals and two snacks a day. Food ingestion consisted of three portions of protein, three portions of vegetables, one portion of fruit, and two portions of carbohydrate per day. Two portions of sweets per week were allowed.
2. As for daily ingestion of liquids, they drank plenty of water (about 1.2–1.8 L/day) and few carbonated drinks: About 55% of them avoided soft drinks, 55% drank no juices or sweet drinks, 53% drank no caffeine containing liquids (colas, tea, or coffee), and 74% did not consume alcoholic beverages.
3. Up to 92% took vitamin preparations, 68% took calcium supplements, and 39% took iron pills.
4. They slept an average of 7 hours a night and 76% of them felt well and energetic for daily work.
5. Most did regular physical exercise: About 77% practiced some significant physical activity for 40 minutes, 4 times a week, as they believed that exercise was essential for their weight loss.
6. Regarding personal responsibility, the patients agreed that the task of losing weight was their own: over 69% weighed weekly. They understood that surgery was an instrument to help them achieve their goal, not a panacea.

Table 40–1.

Follow-up of Operated Patients, Relative to Time After Surgery

Time After Surgery (Months)	Number of Operated Patients	Number of Patients Followed	% Follow-Up
12	782	580	74.1
24	575	313	54.4
36	415	265	63.8
48	216	143	66.2
60	86	40	46.5

Table 40–2.

Comparative BMI Analysis Patients

Interval in Months (Number of Patients)	Mean 1	Mean 2	Mean Difference	P
12–18 (272)	29.1 ± 4.8	28.0 ± 4.6	1.06 ± 2.0	0.00*
18–24 (174)	28.3 ± 5.1	27.9 ± 4.8	0.29 ± 2.1	0.06
18–36 (168)	28.9 ± 5.4	28.8 ± 5.2	0.11 ± 2.8	0.59
18–48 (107)	29.1 ± 5.4	29.9 ± 5.8	−0.84 ± 3.3	0.01*
18–60 (40)	30.9 ± 6.7	30.8 ± 5.7	0.15 ± 3.6	0.79

Among the nonsuccessful individuals, the absence of one or more of these characteristics was frequent. The most common flaw was lack of exercises, followed by eating errors, such as snacking several times a day and drinking soda. Still, up to 97% of patients were happy with their surgery. Long-term weight increase was a median 5.5 kg in the successful group and 25.5 kg in the nonsuccessful one.

Gastric bypass and biliopancreatic diversion procedures result in about 70% or more excess weight loss 18 months after surgery. In the 2–5-year post-bypass interval, the majority of patients succeed in keeping excess weight loss between 50% and 70%. In a famous publication that followed 600 patients for 14 years, Pories[9] found an excess weight loss higher than 50% in most subjects, associated with effective resolution of comorbidities, such as diabetes, arterial hypertension, and sleep apnea.

Total weight loss failure relative to preoperative weight is rare. In spite of that, when considering the lowest postoperative weight, regain may take place in varying degrees with the different techniques. Many studies[10–12] have noticed 5–6-year failure—excess weight loss lower than 50% after gastric bypass—of 5%–7%. There are few publications with more than 10-year follow-up in the United States, where private practice medicine is strong, but long-term follow-up is hampered by costs, the same happening to a lesser extent in Brazil. In smaller countries, with socialized medicine, there is better patient follow-up. Biron,[13] in a Canadian study of over 900 BPD–duodenal switch patients followed for 7–14 years (mean = 10), managed to achieve 97% follow-up. He found excess weight loss failure at 5 years in 10% of the operated morbidly obese patients (considered as return to BMI > 35 kg/m^2) and 20% in the superobese group (return to BMI > 40 kg/m^2). In a 10-year period, failure indexes doubled in both groups. This work did not present weight regain comparative analysis for each year. A few studies have found, in 5–6-year follow-up, 5%–10% mean weight regain from the lowest preoperative weight between 24 and 60 months after gastric bypass. Follow-up, however, was not always higher than 50%–60%.

We conducted, in the Obesity Surgery Centre of Campinas, São Paulo, Brazil, a longitudinal study to assess weight regain in patients between 18 and 60 months after gastric bypass. All 782 subjects from both genders had a gastric bypass with sylastic ring, the Fobi pouch technique. The following interval was between June 1998 and June 2003. Patients were studied from 18 to 60 months post-operatively. The

Table 40–3.

Weight Recidivism Characteristics

	Follow-Up in Months (Number of Patients)			
	18 × 24 (174)	18 × 36 (168)	18 × 48 (107)	18 × 60 (40)
Patients who regained	80	87	68	21
% of weight increase	45.9	51.8	63.6	52.5
Mean gain (kg)	2.63 ± 3.12	7.14 ± 7.99	9.8 ± 7.20	8.8 ± 6.61
% of mean gain (kg)	3.6	6.5	8.9	8.0

Table 40–4.

Distribution of Operated Patients According to Gender

Month interval	Female		Male	
	N	%	N	%
18–24	138	46.37	36	44.44
18–36	116	51.72	44	40.90
18–48	76	65.78	31	54.84
18–60	29	51.72	11	54.54

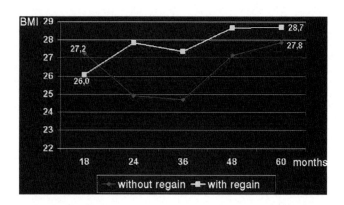

Figure 40–3. Evolution of weight increase in patients with preop BMI between 40 and 45 kg/m^2.

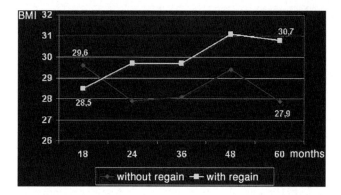

Figure 40–4. Evolution of weight increase in patients with preop BMI between 45 and 50 kg/m^2.

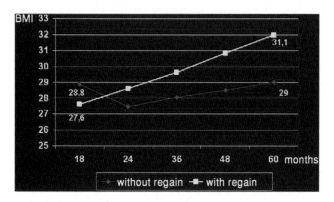

Figure 40–1. Evolution of BMI in patients with and without weight regain.

variables assessed were percentage of excess weight loss, lost weight, change in BMI, and percentage of regained weight. The *Metropolitan life tables of height and weight*[14] were used as a reference. In order to identify the starting point of weight regain and how it changes during the follow-up, a comparative analysis was carried out, with evaluation of postoperative patients in the following date pairs: 1–18 and 24 months postop; 2–18 and 36 months postop; 3–18 and 48 months postop; and 4–18 and 60 months postop. Although the usual

follow-up is 75% at 5 years, this index could not be sustained due to an exclusion criterion, which did not consider patients who were checked 4 months before or after the previously set dates, even though they were normally included in the study.

Table 40–1 shows the number of patients operated, the number actually evaluated, and the follow-up index over time. BMI comparative analysis for each time interval is tracked in Table 40–2. Weight loss remained steady for 18 months after the procedure ($p < 0.0001$). From 24 months postop on, weight loss varied, and subjects from 18–48-month group had the highest percentage of weight gain

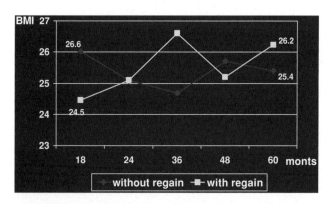

Figure 40–2. Evolution of weight increase in patients with preop BMI < 40 kg/m^2.

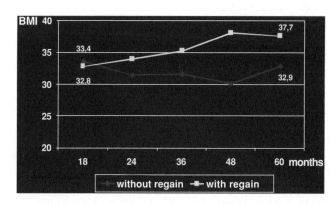

Figure 40–5. Evolution of weight increase in patients with preop BMI > 50 kg/m^2.

Table 40–5.

Distribution of Surgical Failure Percentage, Between Morbidly Obese and Superobese Subjects, According to Excess Weight Loss and BMI

Time After Surgery (months)	Total Operated Patients	Total Followed Patients	% of Follow-Up	Number of Patients (MO) (SO)	Percentage of Failure (EWL < 50%)	Failure (BMI $\geq$ 35 kg/m^2) Morbidly Obese (%)	Failure (BMI $\geq$ 40 kg/m^2) Superobese (%)
18 MO	462	354	76.6	277	21 of 277 7.6	3.9	—
18 SO				77	8 of 77 10.4	—	11.7
24 MO	575	313	54.4	241	13 of 241 5.4	5.4	—
24 SO				72	6 of 72 8.3	—	4.2
36 MO	415	265	63.8	191	13 of 191 6.8	4.7	—
36 SO				74	10 of 74 13.5	—	14.9
48 MO	216	143	66.2	90	10 of 90 11.11	6.7	—
48 SO				53	10 of 53 18.8	—	13.2
60 MO	86	40	46.5	14	2 of 14 14.3	0	—
60 SO				26	2 of 26 7.7	—	11.5

MO, morbidly obese; SO, superobese.

($p < 0.01$). Table 40–3 displays weight regain percentage, mean weight increase, and percentage of weight regained from the lowest postop weight. After 60 months, mean weight increase was 8.8 kg, and the percentage of weight gained from the lowest weight reached was 8%, though the highest percentage occurred by 48-month follow-up. Males represented 1/3 of the total, but there was no difference in weight regain between genders, as shown in Table 40–4. There was no significant BMI difference at 60 months between the patients who did or did not present with weight recidivism (Figure 40–1). The same happened when considering stratified groups with initial BMI $\leq$ 40 kg/m^2 (Figure 40–2), with BMI between 40 and 45 kg/m^2 (Figure 40–3), and with BMI between 45 and 50 kg/m^2 (Figure 40–4). The superobese group (BMI $\geq$ 50 kg/m^2), despite similar excess weight loss at 18 months, regained more at 60 months, and the BMI difference was significant—32.9 kg/m^2 for those who did not have regain, compared to 37.7 kg/m^2 for those who did (Figure 40–5).

We were able to conclude that patients lose weight until the 18th postoperative month. From that time on, 46%–60% of them regain weight all the way to 60 months. In this study, weight regain was higher among the superobese. Table 40–5 data confirm that failure in the superobese group is worse when evaluating both excess weight loss and BMI. While failure in the morbidly obese varied from 7.6% at 18 months to 14.3% at 60 months, in the superobese group the change was from 10.4% at 18 months to 18.8% at 48 months. Thus, superobese individuals should be more closely monitored relative to clinical, nutritional, and psychological concerns.

Therefore, the truth about weight recidivism is that many patients do not receive necessary postoperative follow-up care from the groups who operated them in the first place, thereby not reaching sufficient loss of weight. It is essential for us to precisely determine the extent of this subjective problem. Further studies with better 5–10-year follow-up indexes are needed. Support groups and psychological follow-up must always be available to the patients, as we continually empha-size their importance. A major concern is the fact that, if the professionals involved in obesity treatment do not work together with the patients from the outset, with the intent to solve the weight regain problem and control the eating compulsion, surgical treatment can be compromised.

References

1. Signore C: *Beyond Change, "Information Regarding Obesity Surgery."* Bloomfield Hills, MI, JKS Associates, 2004.
2. Saunders R: Binge eating in gastric bypass patients before surgery. *Obes Surg* 9(1):72–76, 1999.
3. Spitzer RR, Devleu M, Waish BT, et al.: Binge eating disorder: A multisite field trial of the diagnostic criteria. *Int J Eat Disord* (11):191–203, 1992.
4. Hsu LK, Betancourt S, Sullivan SP: Eating disturbances before and after vertical banded gastroplasty: a pilot study. *Int J Eat Disord* 19(1):23–34, 1996.
5. Malone M, Alger-Mayer S. Binge status and quality of life after gastric bypass surgery: A one-year study. *Obes Res* 12(3):473–481, 2004.
6. Mitchell JE, Lancaster KL, Burgard MA, et al.: Long-term follow-up of patients' status after gastric bypass. *Obes Surg* 11(4):464–468, 2001.
7. Hsu LK, Benotti PN, Dwyer J, et al.: Nonsurgical factors that influence the outcome of bariatric surgery: A review. *Psychosom Med* 60(3):338–346, 1998. Review.
8. Cook CM, Edwards C: Success habits of long-term gastric bypass patients. *Obes Surg* 9(1):80–82, 1999.
9. Pories WJ, Macdonald KG, Morgan EJ, et al.: Surgical treatment of obesity and its effects on diabetes: 10yr follow-up. *Am J Clin Nutr* 55:5825–5855, 1992.
10. Fobi MA, Lee H, Igwe D Jr, et al.: Revision of failed gastric bypass to distal Roux-en-Y gastric bypass: A review of 65 cases. *Obes Surg* 11(2):190–195, 2001.
11. Capella JF, Capella RF: The weight reduction operation of choice: Vertical banded gastroplasty or gastric bypass? *Am J Surg* 171(1):74–79, 1996.
12. Brolin RE, Kenler HA, Gorman JH, Cody RP: Long-limb gastric bypass in the superobese. A prospective randomized study. *Ann Surg* 215(4):387–395, 1992.
13. Biron S, Hould FS, Lebel S, et al.: Twenty years of biliopancreatic diversion: What is the goal of the surgery? *Obes Surg* 14(2):160–164, 2004.
14. Harrison GG: Height-weight tables. *Ann Intern Med* 103:489–494, 1985.

41

Radiographic Evaluation and Treatment

Ester Labrunie, MD, PhD • Edson Marchiori, MD, PhD • Cid Pitombo, MD, PhD

 ROLE OF IMAGING STUDIES AFTER BARIATRIC SURGERY

Imaging methods play an important role in the evaluation of patients undergoing bariatric surgery; the objective of these methods is to provide precise and early diagnosis of complications. This helps to minimize clinical repercussions by allowing quick, appropriate treatment of complications.[7,18]

Whenever possible, the surgical team should accompany examinations and provide specific details of the procedure employed and any clinical suspicions of each patient. Special care should be taken, together with the surgical team, in respect to the administration of oral contrast, always considering the normal precautions related to venous contrast contraindications (severe allergy, alterations in the renal function, etc.).

Radiological aspects vary depending on the surgical technique utilized (Please see Chapter 14). Knowledge of anatomical–radiological and functional changes is essential in the investigation of possible complications. It is important that the surgeon and radiologist work together as a team for correct image interpretation. Specific, relevant perioperative data may guide the radiological study and minimize false positive or negative reports.

The patient's body weight may be a limiting factor in performing imaging and in the quality of the images obtained, as well as in attaining quality fluoroscopic images. Conventional radiology and computed tomography (CT) equipments have maximum weight limits established by manufacturers, which frequently make the study of superobese patients difficult or even impossible. Additionally, the abdominal diameter may be a limiting factor when performing the examination, specifically with small ring gantry CT devices or the equipment used in conventional upper gastrointestinal studies.

In these patients, the GI series may be performed with the patient in the standing position. The study can also be done in angiography suites, as this equipment often has higher weight limits. Radiology suites with digital acquisition in general allow post-processing adjustments that improve the quality of the images, giving better and quicker final technical results, frequently preventing repeating radiographs.

With CT, details such as removing the mattress from the examination table can improve the quality of the images and reduce artifacts. Other important factors include the utilization of higher kilovolt (kV) and milliampere (mA) settings for image acquisition and the use of softer filters in their reconstruction.

Pulmonary complications frequently occur in patients submitted to bariatric surgery, independent of the technique utilized. Pneumonia and pleural effusions are relatively common, with pulmonary embolism being the most severe complication with the highest mortality rate. Its radiological aspects are similar to those in the nonobese population suffering from pneumonia and will not be described in this chapter.

Ultrasonography is utilized mainly in the preoperative period, to evaluate cholelithiasis and steatosis. Restrictions in the assessment of obese patients are inherent to the ultrasound method. Sound wave penetration is greatly attenuated by the fat layers, making good image acquisition difficult. The presence of dressings, incisions, and drains can also adversely affect the acquisition of quality images. Therefore, it is a method that is little used in the postoperative period with these patients, even though there are cases where its use is essential. Critically ill patients who are unable to be moved to the radiology department or those who exceed the equipment's weight limits may be submitted to ultrasonographic examinations. Pleural effusions are visible and sometimes free liquid and intestinal loop distension can be visualized. The presence of pneumoperitoneum may make the examination impossible. Ultrasonographic evaluation of the wound in the postoperative period may identify fluid collections, such as seromas, hematomas, and abscesses, with the occasional need to correlate these with the patient's clinical status for an etiological diagnosis. Sometimes wound hernias are also identified, especially when they involve an intestinal loop.

Conventional radiography and CT examinations use ionizing radiation; therefore, specific precautions should be taken to protect both the physician and the patient. In general, CT scans are reserved for patients with suspected complications or to evaluate the extent of complications and to follow them up. When investigating late complications, the possibility of pregnancy should always be ruled out before performing the examination, as with all patients submitted to x-ray examinations. Imaging examinations can be very useful to guide invasive procedures in the treatment of specific postoperative complications, notably those involving the aspiration and percutaneous drainage of fluid collections as well as gastrostomies.

This chapter describes the main radiological aspects in different surgical techniques, highlighting possible postoperative abdominal complications. Additional cases may be seen on the accompanying DVD. The reader may analyze the images and make their own diagnosis before reading the results.

GASTRIC BAND

Normal Study

Imaging methods allow evaluation of the band position and its relation to the subcutaneous tissue and also the size of the stomach and the gastric pouch above the band (Figure 41–1(a)). Postoperative band adjustment should be performed with upper GI series guidance.[12,24] Oral administration of a small quantity of contrast helps to evaluate band restriction on the food flow, and thus may guide band volume adjustment[7] (Figure 41–1(b)).

The different types of bands have already been discussed (please see Chapters 14 and 16). Band radiopacity depends on the manufacturer and the materials used. Among the most commonly used bands in Brazil are the LAP-BAND (Inamed Health, formerly BioEnterics Corporation, Santa Barbara, CA) and the Swedish Adjustable Gastric Band (SAGB, Obtech Medical AG, Switzerland). The first is totally radiopaque, with the reservoir sewn to the abdominal fascia on the left flank. It is usually adjusted through the injection of saline solution into the reservoir. The latter type, the SAGB, has little radiopacity. Its reservoir is generally fixed to the sternum and it has metallic components that guarantee its radiopacity. A contrast solution should be used when adjusting this Swiss band, thereby permitting its visualization.

Aseptic technique, including sterile gloves, mask, and adequate disinfection of the skin puncture site and the injection of sterile solution, must always be used when adjusting the band in order to prevent infection. This should be performed guided by fluoroscopy, which also helps to localize the reservoir membrane. Some teams adjust the band in their own offices without radiological guidance, which may result in a greater incidence of infection as well as damage to the system (perforation of the tube that connects to the reservoir, hematomas, seromas, infection around the system, etc.). The examinations are normally quick and the dose of radiation during fluoroscopy is not significant for the patient or for the physician, even with repeated examinations, as long as routine protection is used (protective lead aprons, thyroid protectors, etc.).

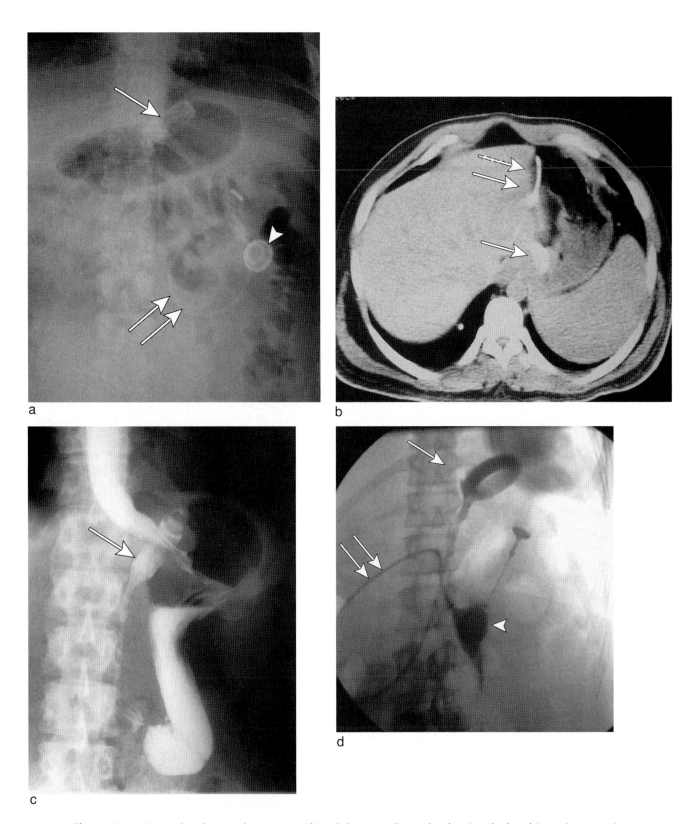

Figure 41–1. Gastric band, normal aspect. (a) Plain abdomen radiography showing the band (arrow), connective tube (two arrows), and the port access (arrowhead). (b) Abdomen CT of band (arrow) near to the esophagogastric junction and connective tube (two arrows). (c) Contrasted examination, normal aspect: band (arrow) located near to the esophagogastric junction. (d) Verification of band integrity (arrow) and connective tube (two arrows) by guided puncture of the cutaneous reservoir (arrowhead) and contrast injection.

The injection of a diluted iodinated contrast under fluoroscopy may be useful in evaluating band integrity. In cases of rupture, leakage of contrast into the cavity occurs. Fluoroscopy can also help to puncture the cutaneous ring, notably in cases where there is postoperative rotation or displacement (Figure 41–1(c)). CT plays a limited role in the postoperative period of these patients; it may be useful in cases where complications are suspected. As illustrated in Figure 41–1(d), the band is seen as a hyperdense ring encircling the proximal stomach. The connecting tube and its access port are easily identified.

Postoperative Complications

Possible complications related to the band are[7] displacement, erosion of the gastric wall, and gastric necrosis. Also, gastrointestinal complications have been related to the technique, including gastroesophageal perforation, esophagitis, gastric leaks, bleeding, hepatic hematoma, fluid collections, and abscesses.[3,7] Stoma narrowing can cause gastric pouch dilation and impaction of ingested foods. Complications related to the insufflation tube are perforation, rotation, and inversion of the port device in the subcutaneous tissue, with possible local infections and hematomas.

A plain abdominal radiograph may be useful to visualize the band. Sometimes this is enough to diagnose complications such as band slippage. In these cases, the ring is frequently horizontally oriented. The distended upper gastric pouch commonly presents fluid-air levels, which can be seen to the left and posterior to the ring.[7] Conventional radiological studies with the administration of oral contrast also allow the evaluation of band slippage, gastric pouch enlargement, as well as other complications, some viewed specifically on dynamic examinations under fluoroscopy.

In normal examinations, contrast passes through the narrow orifice of the ring, without change in the dynamics of emptying. With band stenosis, a delay in the passage of the contrast between the small upper gastric pouch and lower stomach can be visualized. Alterations secondary to stenosis are gastroesophageal reflux, esophageal dilation, esophageal peristaltic waves, as well as delays in the food flow. In some cases, impacted and retained food is present inside the distal esophagus, giving the appearance of a foreign body (Figure 41–2(a) and (b)). In cases of severe gastroesophageal reflux, there may be some nocturnal aspiration. Chest radiography and CT may be necessary to evaluate these pulmonary complications. In severe cases with perforation and gastric necrosis, thickening of the gastric wall and pneumatosis in cases of ischemia can sometimes be seen with CT.[7]

Dilation of the upper gastric pouch may not be related to displacement of the ring, but to the slippage of the gastric fundus through the band with a consequent increase in the size of the upper pouch. In these cases, the patient commonly presents with weight gain (Figures 41–2(c) and 41–2(d)). In some cases, there may be narrowing of the stoma and upper gastric pouch dilation secondary to the formation of perigastric fibrous tissue due to overdistention of the ring or a small

ring.[7] In the radiographic study, overdistention of the pouch, with the ring in the normal position, and delay in emptying the stoma are observed. Some patients present with upper pouch dilation because they do not change their eating habits, thereby causing chronic overdistention. In these cases, there is no stenosis of the stoma, only concentric pouch dilation.[9] CT multiplanar reconstruction may show band slippage and migration. It can also assess infection of the port device with the formation of abscesses and other complications such as band and connecting tube perforation.

Transmural band penetration is a late complication caused by the progressive penetration of the band through the gastric wall to the mucous membrane. In general, it is a chronic blocked perforation and signs of pneumoperitoneum or contrast extravasation are very rare. The most common aspect is the presence of orally administered contrast medium surrounding the band portion in contact with the gastric lumen.[21]

ROUX-EN-Y GASTRIC BYPASS SURGERY

Normal Study

Evaluation by routine GI series in the postoperative period prior to introducing oral diet is recommended by some authors[7,23,25] and criticized by others.[9,14,24] The GI series can evaluate the integrity and patency of the gastrojejunal anastomosis and help rule out possible leaks or contrast extravasations. The examination can significantly change the course of treatment and indicate surgical reintervention.[25]

Upper GI series should be performed obtaining early images during and after swallowing a small amount of non- or slightly diluted iodinated contrast to assess the esophagogastrojejunal flow. The gastric ingestion capacity is reduced with gastroplasty; therefore, the examination should be done in the early postoperative period with only about 30–50 mL of contrast. Administration of greater amounts of contrast media is only possible after the radiological documentation of good distal contrast progression. In the late postoperative period, greater amounts of contrast are possible, as long as they are administered slowly.

In general, the left anterior oblique position will best demonstrate the anastomosis; however, complementary views can and should be utilized when necessary. Whenever possible the study should include studies in the decubitus position, in order to better study the row of staples up to the proximal esophageal–gastric junction. Studies with barium contrast should only be performed after excluding the possibility of leaks or contrast extravasation, but may be necessary in some cases. Delayed radiographic images should be obtained to evaluate the progression of the contrast and the jejunojejunal anastomosis.

The Higa and Fobi-Capella surgical techniques (please see Chapter 14) present with some distinct radiological aspects that identify the technique that the surgeon employed (Figures 41–3(a) and 41–4(a)). Plain radiography should be performed before the administration of oral contrast to

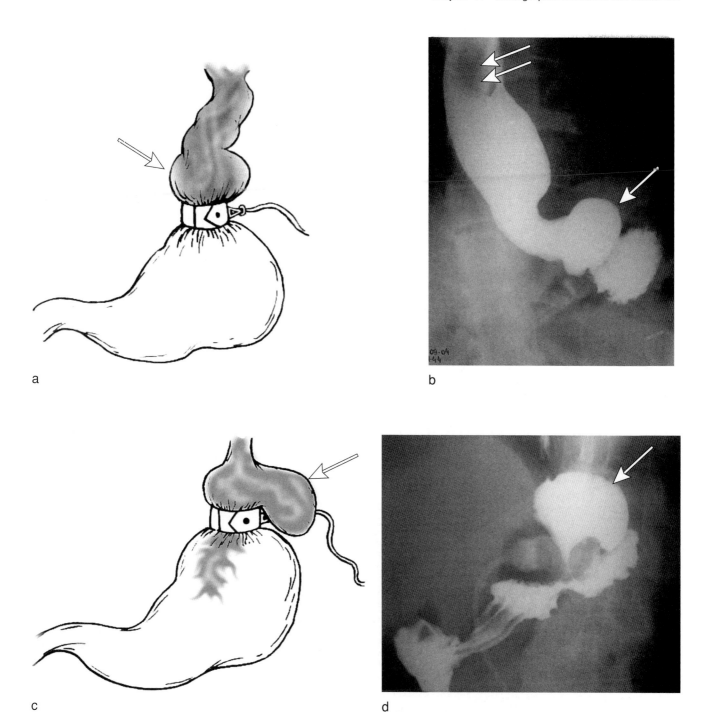

Figure 41–2. Gastric band complications. (a) and (b) Band stenosis with dilation of the gastric pouch (arrow) and the esophagus. Note food remnants causing filling defects in the stomach (two arrows). (c) and (d) Dilation of the upper gastric pouch (arrow).

visualize the superior staple-line and the location of cavity drains, when present (Figure 41–3(b)). In the Fobi-Capella technique, a band around the gastric pouch can also be seen when it is made of Silastic, a radiopaque material; but when it is made of Marlex netting, the band cannot be visualized. Some teams also attach the excluded gastric stomach to the wall, marking the region with a radiopaque ring, which allows its identification and serves as a guide for possible percutaneous gastrostomies in cases of postoperative gastric overdistention (Figure 41–4(b)).

In GI series, the small gastric pouch, the gastrojejunal anastomosis, and the alimentary limb can be identified. Evaluating flow progress from the esophagus to the loops of the small intestine below the enteroenteric anastomosis is essential. In the Higa technique, the gastric pouch is very small and the closed limb of Roux-en-Y loop, in general, is short and can have a shepherd's crook-like appearance (Figure 41–3(c) and (d)). In the Fobi-Capella surgery, on the other hand, the closed afferent loop is larger, longer, and vertical; it is also possible to see the restriction ring around the gastric

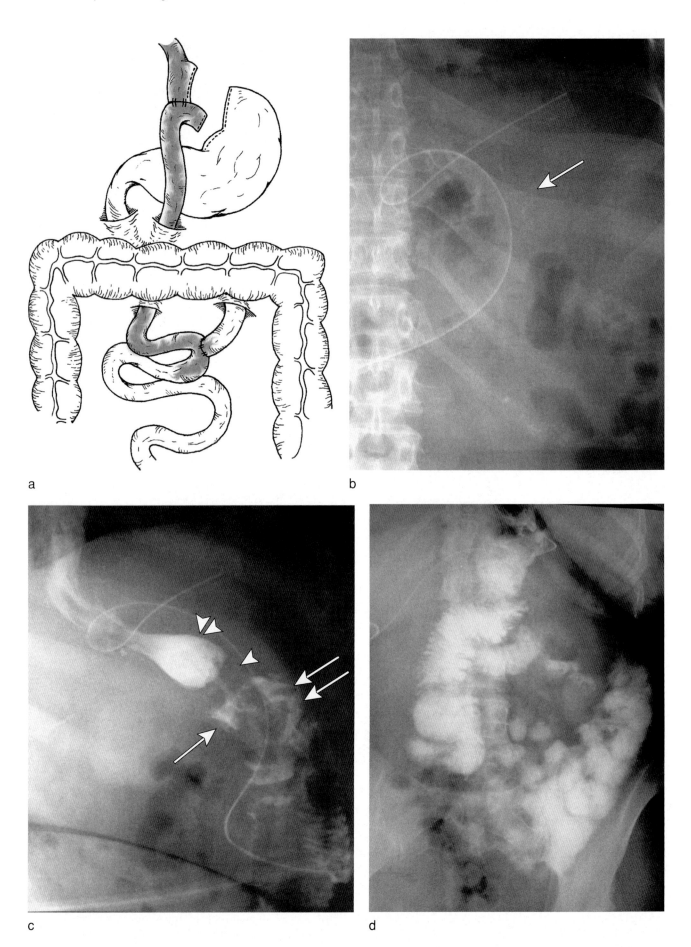

a

b

c

d

Figure 41–3. *(Continued)*

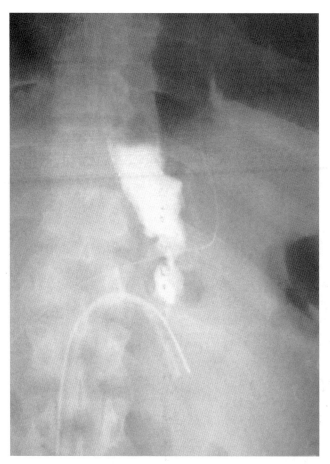

e

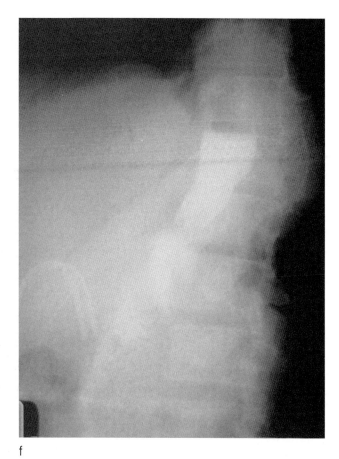

f

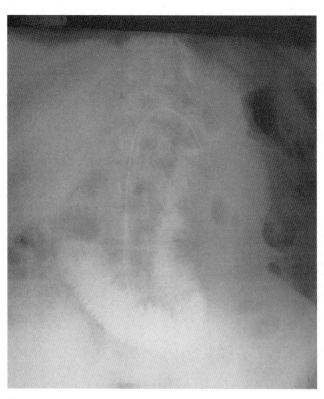

g

Figure 41–3 Normal aspects of the contrasted examination of the Higa surgery in two patients with uneventful clinical evolution. (a) Diagram of the technique. (b–d) The first patient: (b) Plain radiograph showing the surgical drain and dense threads of the gastric and gastrojejunal anastomosis staple-line (arrow); (c) small gastric pouch (two arrowheads), gastrojejunal anastomosis (arrowhead), and Roux-en-Y loop (two arrows). Note the reflux of the contrast to the closed loop (arrow); (d) opacification of the alimentary limb and the normal-sized common channel providing normal patency to the jejunojejunal anastomosis. (e)–(g) The second patient: (e) Relative delay in the passage through the gastrojejunal anastomosis with fluid-air level in the esophagus (arrow); (f) integrity gastrojejunal anastomosis (arrow); (g) slight ectasia of the alimentary limb (two arrows).

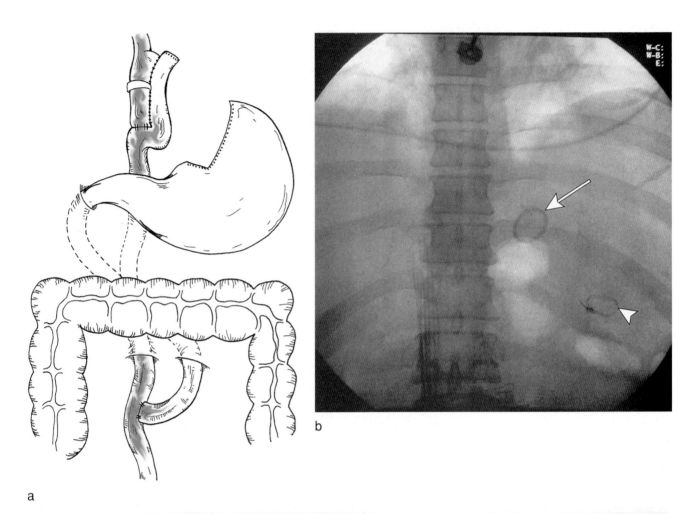

a

b

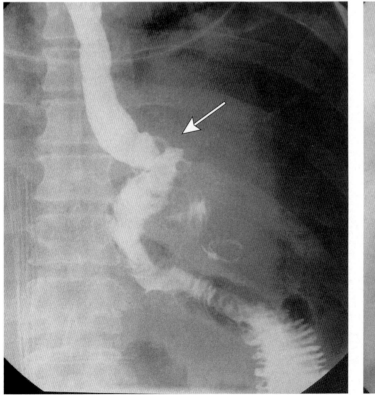

c

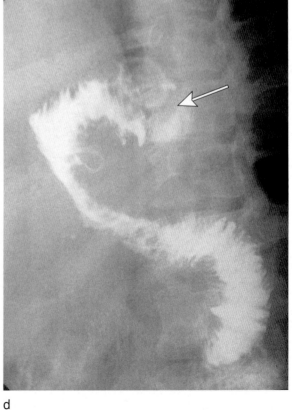

d

Figure 41–4. *(Continued)*

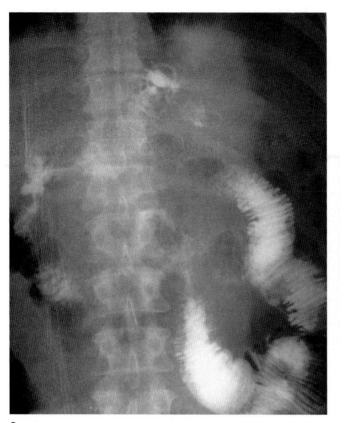

e

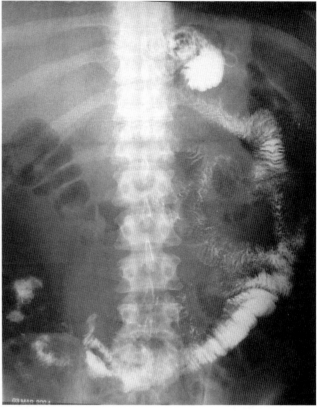

f

Figure 41–4. Normal aspects of the Capella surgery. (a) Diagram of the technique. (b) Plain radiography demonstrating the restrictive band (arrow) and the anchoring of the excluded stomach (arrowhead). (c) Passage of contrast through the integral gastrojejunal anastomosis (arrow). (d) Contrast reflux to the loop (arrow). (e) Postoperative examination in D1 showing edema and slight ectasia of the small intestinal loops. Also note the contrast to the duodenum and the stomach after coughing. (f) Control 10 days after demonstrating normal-sized loops. There was no gastric opacification, showing absence of gastrogastric leaks.

reservoir, cranial to the gastrojejunal anastomosis. The afferent limb of the Roux-en-Y loop is normally slightly longer in this technique and it is laterally attached to the gastric pouch (Figures 41–4(c) and (d)). Contrast reflux to this closed intestinal loop segment is common and should not be mistaken for a leak. The gastroenteroanastomosis in general is wider in Fobi-Capella than in Higa technique, as the ring placed on the gastric pouch has a restrictive function.

In the first postoperative days, a certain amount of dysmotility and a relative delay in the esophagogastrojejunal contrast flow is common, and should not be mistaken for anastomotic stenosis (Figure 41–3(e) and (f)). Similarly, the Roux-en-Y loop may be slightly dilated and distended in the early postoperative period due to the surgical manipulation and/or edema at the lower anastomosis (Figures 41–3(g), 41–4(e)–(f), and 41–5). Contrast reflux to the closed segment of the Roux-en-Y loop should not be mistaken for a leak or contrast extravasations (Figures 41–4(c) and (d)). Also, contrast reflux through the enteroenteric anastomosis to the duodenal arch and excluded stomach may occur, which is generally better seen by CT (Figure 41–4(e) and (f)). A gastrogastric leak should be differentiated, as will be discussed later in this chapter. A later imaging examination may be necessary to rule out a leak.

Computed tomography is usually reserved for patients with suspicion of a postoperative complication and for its follow-up. In the Higa technique, the alimentary limb is located anteriorly to the bypassed stomach and its transmesocolic passage is viewed anteriorly to the transverse colon. The gastric row of staples and the gastrojejunal anastomosis are easily identified with CT, specifically before intake of oral contrast, as is the suturing of the enteroenteric anastomosis. In the Fobi-Capella technique, the alimentary limb is seen between the small gastric pouch and the excluded stomach and its route is generally retrogastric retrocolic.

The excluded stomach generally contains fluids in the early postoperative period and can also present a fluid-air level. It is important to remember this aspect so as not to mistake it for a subphrenic fluid collection. In the late postoperative period, the stomach in general presents collapsed.

Postoperative Complications

Imaging examinations are extremely useful in the diagnosis and follow-up of complications and can also guide percutaneous treatment using interventional radiology. Whenever possible, CT should be performed with the oral and intravenous administration of iodinated contrast.

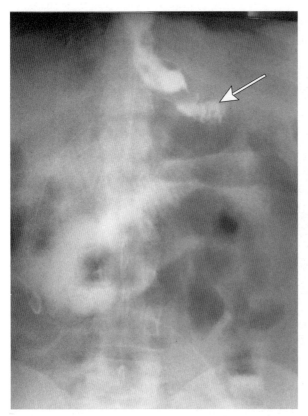
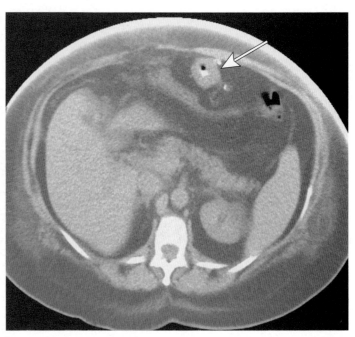

a

b

Figure 41–5. Control in D1 after the Higa surgery showing relative edema and distention of the alimentary limb. The start of the diet was delayed for 24 hours, with regression of the edema and a good clinical evolution. (a) Upper GI series showing major contrast leaks to the left subphrenic space (arrow) due to suture dehiscence. (b) Upper GI series showing a small contrast leak removed by the drain (arrow) and not depicted in CT (not shown).

In some patients, a nasoenteric tube is placed below the gastroenteric anastomosis during the surgical procedure itself. In other patients it can be done postoperative through endoscopy. Iodine contrast can be administered through this tube for the opacification of intestinal loops. However, whenever possible, the patient should be asked to swallow a small amount of contrast during the acquisition of images to evaluate the integrity of the gastrojejunal anastomosis.

In cases in which oral administration of contrast is contraindicated, patients with gastrostomy or jejunostomy may benefit from the administration of contrast through the ostomy, identifying the biliopancreatic loops. In these cases, contrary to oral administration, the noncontrasted intestinal portion is the alimentary limb. Here we will describe aspects that may be observed in several postoperative complications.

ANASTOMOTIC LEAKS

This is a dreaded complication that can result in sepsis and is potentially lethal.[9,61] Leaks are more common within the first 10 postoperative days[9] (please see Chapter 17). They mainly occur at the gastrojejunal anastomosis, but can also occur at the jejunojejunal anastomosis, excluding stomach, esophagus, and hypopharynx.[9,16,21,48]

Upper GI series and CT are indicated for the evaluation of these leaks as they are reliable imaging methods and complementary to diagnosis. CT should be performed whenever there is a clinical suspicion of leaks not identified by conventional contrast examinations and also during their follow-up, in order to evaluate secondary complications.

Major leaks or dehiscence are easily identified by upper GI series (Figure 41–6(a)). Small contrast leaks can be difficult to see in contrasted examinations during the early postoperative period. Opacification of a surgical drain may be the only radiological sign, which is better observed at GI series (Figure 41–6(b)). With CT, these minor leaks may not be diagnosed, as most drains are spontaneously hyperdense in images, and therefore do not allow the identification of any contrast medium within.

Sometimes the leak is not identified by contrast extravasations. Other aspects are found, such as the appearance of an increase in extraluminal gas in the perigastric region after the administration of oral contrast without any leak of oral contrast itself (Figure 41–7(a)–(d)).

Abdominal fluid collections can occur due to leaks and are better identified in CT studies. They are more common

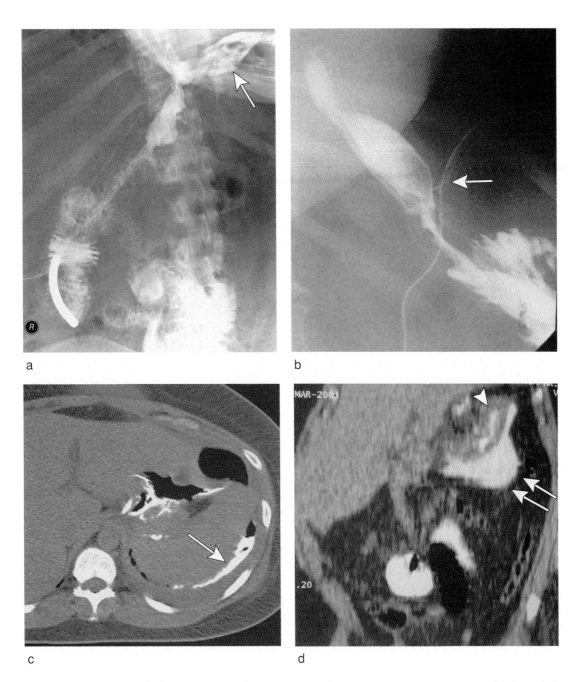

Figure 41–6. Anastomotic leaks in 4 patients. (a) Upper GI series shows extensive contrast extravasation (arrow), due to suture dehiscence. (b) Small contrast extravasation oriented to abdominal drain (arrow), not visualized in CT (not shown). (c) CT shows perisplenic oral contrast (arrows), with air-fluid level. (d) Coronal reformatted CT image shows extraluminal oral contrast along the gastric long curvature (double arrows). Note oral contrast in excluded stomach, due to gastro-gastric fistula (arrowhead).

in the upper left quadrant of the abdomen, mainly in the perisplenic region[7] and can evolve to abscesses; peripheral impregnation by the contrast medium can be observed combined with the presence of gas bubbles (Figure 41–8(a)). It is possible in some cases to identify the presence of oral contrast within the fluid collection. In other instances, extraluminal contrast is not observed and so the fluid collection may or may not be related to the anastomotic leak.[16]

The percutaneous punction and draining of fluid collections guided by imaging methods is a procedure that can frequently avoid further surgical intervention[7,26] (Figure 41–8(b)).

Stoma Obstruction

Stoma obstructions occur more frequently in laparoscopic surgeries; it is the most common late complication of this surgical technique.[20] Diagnosis, confirmation, and treatment by dilatation are usually made by digestive endoscopy.[7,15,22]

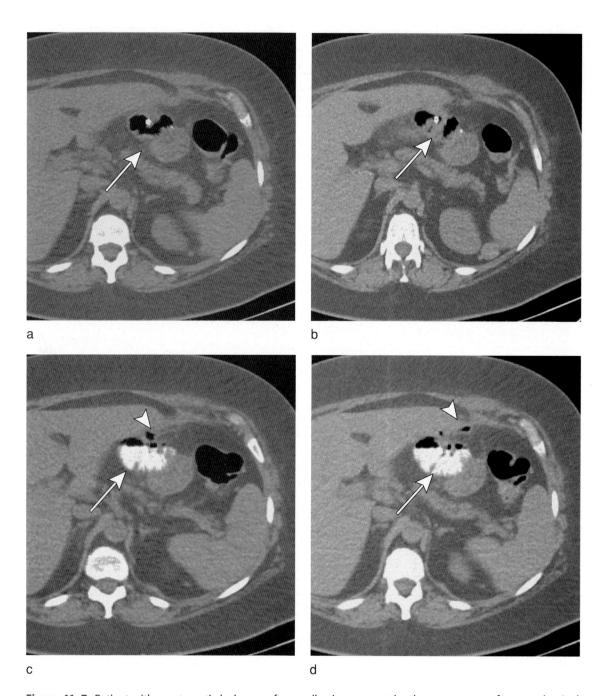

a

b

c

d

Figure 41–7. Patient with anastomotic leak seen after swallowing contrast by the appearance of an extraluminal gaseous bubble. (a) and (b) CT without contrast at the gastrojejunal anastomosis (arrows). (c) and (d) CT after the oral administration of contrast. Contrasted Roux-en-Y loop (arrows) and the appearance of extraluminal gaseous bubbles (arrowheads).

In upper GI series, the following aspects have been described[22]: Stenosis at the anastomosis (diameter less than 8–10 mm); accentuated angulation of the gastric pouch; complete stoma obstruction and significant delay in the passage of contrast through the gastric pouch. Upper GI series also allow the diagnosis of other anomalies that might make the endoscopic procedure difficult or impair its success, such as the presence of diverticulum and esophageal dysmotility. It also assists in verifying the integrity of the gastric staple row and presence of stoma ulcers.[22]

Complications from endoscopic surgery are rare and include perforation, bleeding, and cardiorespiratory complications.[22] A plain radiological examination may be useful in the diagnosis of perforation evidenced by pneumoperitoneum.

Intestinal Obstruction

Small bowel obstruction occurs in patients submitted both to open surgery or to laparoscopy. In laparoscopic surgery, there is less surgical trauma, with less formation of adhesions,

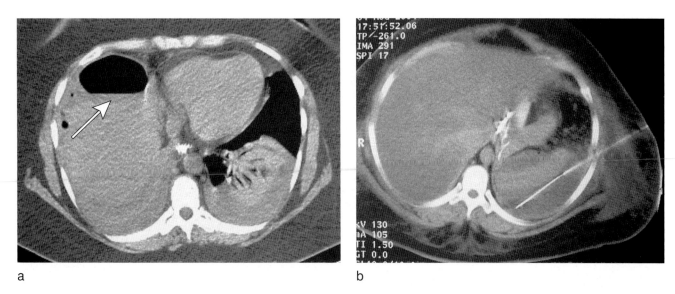

Figure 41–8. Fluid collections in patients with leaks. (a) Right subphrenic collection with fluid-air level (arrow) treated by surgical intervention. (b) Perisplenic collection treated by percutaneous drainage.

contrary to laparotomies. Internal hernias are more commonly described in video surgery. Improved techniques, such as closure of surgically created orifices in the mesenteric and mesocolon and anchoring of the Roux-en-Y loop, have significantly reduced their incidence.

The causes of obstruction in general are related to internal hernias,[7,16] adhesions,[1] or stenosis of the enteroenteric anastomosis.[2,17,20] They also occur secondary to incarcerated hernias of the abdominal wall, formation of bezoar in the gastric pouch, and intussusceptions at the site of entreroenterotomy.[7]

Ultrasonography plays a limited role in these patients; it may be useful when other imaging examinations are un-

available. The presence of free fluids and distention of the intestinal loop due to fluid can be seen by ultrasonography, with this latter condition constituting an important finding in the late postoperative period. In these cases, intestinal obstruction should be suspected.

Abdominal radiography and/or a study of the flow of food with oral contrast administration may assist in the diagnosis, demonstrating jejunal distention and delay in the passage of the contrast.[17] Radiological signs of small intestinal obstructions, independent of whether caused by hernias or adhesions are diameter of the loop greater than 2.5 cm and an abrupt change in the caliber with the distal loop collapsed[6,19] (Figure 41–9(a)–(b)).

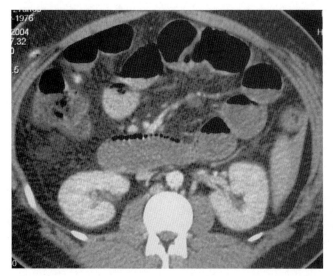
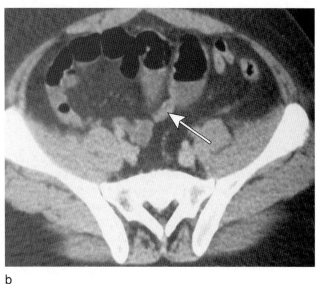

Figure 41–9. Intestinal obstruction due to adhesion in the early postoperative period of the Higa surgery by laparoscopy. (a) Dilated jejunal loops with fluid-air level. (b) Abrupt transition of loop diameter at the site of the adhesion (arrow). During surgery, adhesion and volvulus of the small intestine were evidenced as well as a gastrojejunal anastomotic leak.

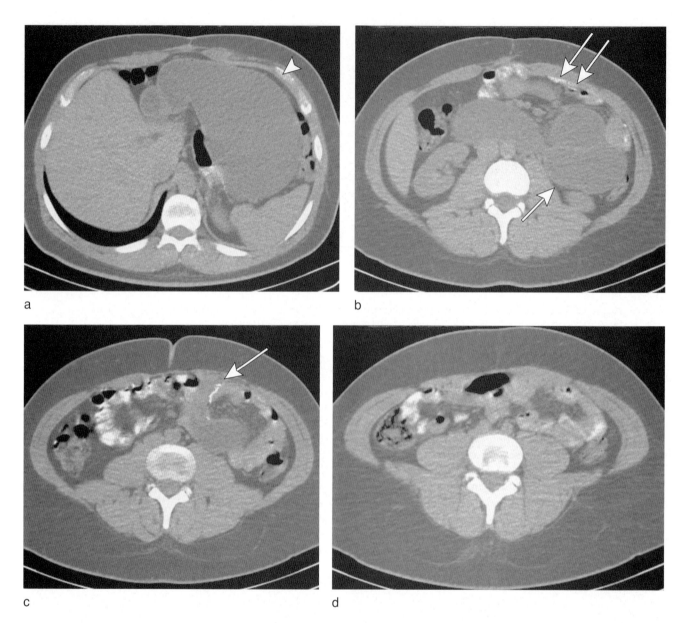

Figure 41–10. Patient submitted to the Higa surgery 3 years ago. The patient presented with intestinal obstruction secondary to a bridle with adhesion and volvulus of the jejunojejunal anastomosis at the surgical instrumentation site. (a) Hyperdistended excluded stomach (arrowhead). (b) Hyperdistended biliopancreatic loop (arrow) and normal diameter alimentary limb (two arrows). (c) Transition of diameter of loop at the suture of the lower anastomosis which is anteriorly displaced and in contiguity to the abdominal wall (arrow). (d) Common loop with normal diameter.

Intestinal obstructions lead to distention upstream of the loop—distention of either the food or biliopancreatic tracts or both (Figure 41–10(a)–(b)). There is a consequent increase in the tension at the gastrojejunal anastomosis, which may cause dehiscence of this suture, with a consequent leak and its complications—this is the cause of death of some patients.[16]

Internal hernias described in bariatric surgery occur due to three defects or potential spaces created during surgery: In the mesentery of the enteroenteric anastomosis, in the transverse mesocolon, and in the Petersen defect or hernia.[11,17] The herniated intestine may be the Roux-en-Y loop itself together with a variable length of the small intestine.[9]

Internal hernias are difficult to diagnose preoperatively; however, they have high morbidity and mortality rates. Herniation can also be intermittent, which further hampers diagnosis.[9]

Upper GI x-ray series and CT to investigate internal hernias are a challenge for the radiologists. A negative examination does not necessarily exclude its diagnosis. Delay in the diagnosis and treatment may lead to severe complications secondary to ischemia of the intestinal segment. CT can suggest the diagnosis in the majority of the cases when analyzed by experienced specialists. If herniation is intermittent, it can only be diagnosed by imaging methods if they are performed during the phase in which the patient is symptomatic.[17]

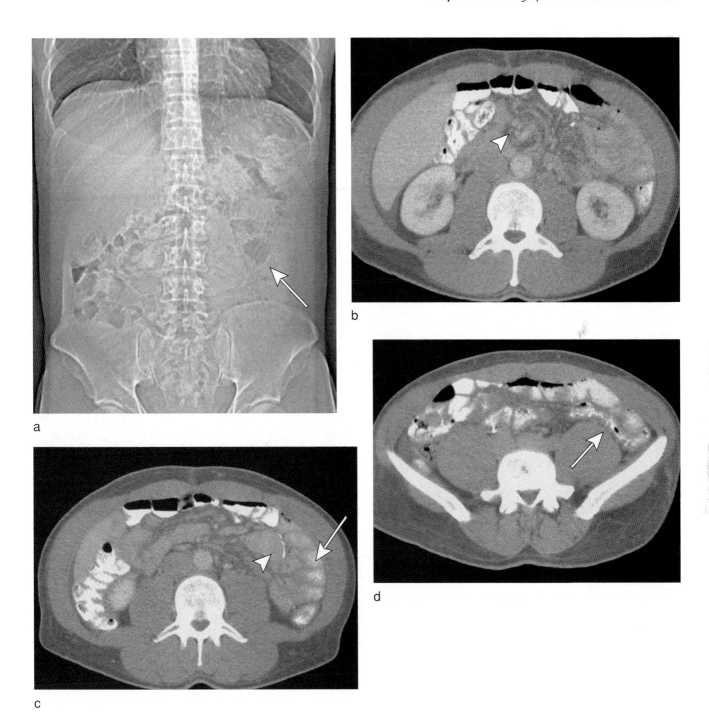

Figure 41–11. Petersen hernia 3 years after the Higa surgery. (a) CT scout view showing distended small intestinal loops on left flank (arrow). (b) Stretching and engorgement of mesenteric vessels (arrowhead). (c) Edema of the small intestinal loops (arrow) at the jejunojejunal anastomosis (arrowhead). (d) Parietal thickening of distal jejunal loops (arrow).

Conventional GI series may identify loops of the small intestine clustered in the left upper quadrant, with delay in the flow of contrast medium.[7,8] The appearance of the internal hernia with CT depends on its location.[9] A clustering of dilated small bowel segments associated with stretched, displaced, crowded, and engorged mesenteric vessels and displacement of other bowel segments is generally present.[5,6,7] In transmesocolic hernias, the distended loops are clustered posteriorly to the excluded stomach, exerting a compressive effect.[7] In mesenteric defects, the distended loops of the small intestine are found adjacent to the abdominal wall, without being covered by omentum and medially displacing to the transverse colon.[6,7,8] They can frequently present with complications such as volvulus of the small intestine[5,6] and intestinal ischemia.[6] Petersen's hernias may be very difficult to diagnose and may not be evident with CT. They do not have a characteristic location, nor a defined hernial sac around the loops.[4,7] Frequently, the only signs are crowding and engorgement of mesenteric vessels, and signs of small bowel obstruction[4] (Figure 41–11(a)–(d)).

There are also reports of proximal small bowel obstruction secondary to bleeding and the formation of intraluminal blood clots[2] and obstruction due to superior mesenteric syndrome after significant weight loss in the postoperative period.[13]

ABDOMINAL WALL COMPLICATIONS

Surgical wound complications are an important cause of morbidity in obese patients, independent of the type of surgical procedure employed. They occur both in open surgeries and in laparoscopy, but are more frequent in the first.[17]

Seromas occur in up to 40% of cases.[18] Wound infections are more frequent in open surgery than in videolaparoscopy.[17] When the wound infection occurs after laparoscopy, it is normally less severe and easier to treat, with little or no predisposition for evisceration.[20] Patients with a wound seroma and ongoing fever should be submitted to CT to search for intracavitary fluid collections[18] or other complications. The presence of gas within a fluid collection may suggest infection and/or association with a leak (Figure 41–12(a)–(c)).

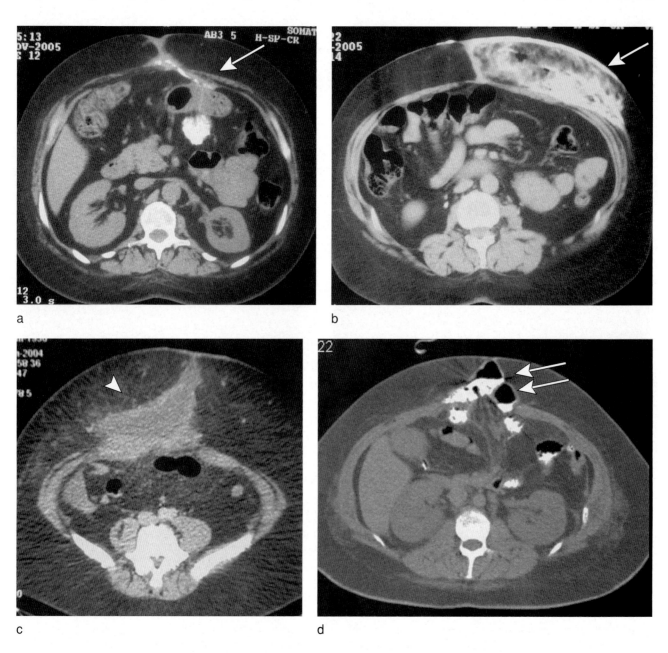

Figure 41–12. Complications of the abdominal wall. (a) and (b) Postoperative period of the Capella surgery with an increase in the volume of the abdominal wall. CT with oral contrast. (a) Contrast leak at the gastrojejunal anastomosis with extravasation to the wound (arrow). (b) Leakage of oral contrast infiltrating the subcutaneous cellular tissue (arrow). (c) Fluid collection in the wall during the postoperative period, with peripheral impregnation by venous contrast (arrowhead). (d) Postoperative herniation of the intestinal loops at surgical wound site (two arrows) of laparoscopic Higa technique surgery.

Obese patients have a greater risk of evolving incisional hernias,[17] although their incidence is significantly less after laparoscopic surgeries[7,15,26] (Figure 41–12(d)). The size of the hernia is related to the size of the incision.[20] This is the most common late complication in laparotomies.[15,16] Incisional hernias in laparoscopic surgeries can occur at the insertion site of the surgical instrument; because of the small caliber of the instruments, the diameter of the hernia orifice is smaller in videolaparoscopy and delay in diagnosis may lead to intestinal loop compromise.[26]

INTRACAVITARY BLEEDING

Hemorrhage in the postoperative period is more frequent in videolaparoscopy surgery than in open surgeries.[16,20] It may originate from the staple-line in the gastric remnant, from the gastrojejunostomy or from the jejunostomy.[20] Bleeding can occur to the peritoneal cavity and be exteriorized through surgical drains, or it can occur to the gastrointestinal tract.[1,16] In the majority of cases, conservative treatment is sufficient, but occasionally surgical reinterventions are required.[1] Externalization by the upper gastrointestinal tract can also be secondary to bleeding of the gastric remnant and duodenum. In these cases endoscopic diagnosis is very difficult or even impossible.[15] Bleeding of the lower gastrointestinal tract in general is due to bleeding at the enteroenteric anastomosis.[16] CT is indicated in the evaluation of these patients. The presence of hyperdense fluid collections (hematomas) and/or free fluid in the peritoneal cavity may be evidenced (Figure 41–13(a)–(c)). A small amount of free liquid in the peritoneal cavity may be a common aspect in the postoperative period, and may not be related to bleeding or infection.[80]

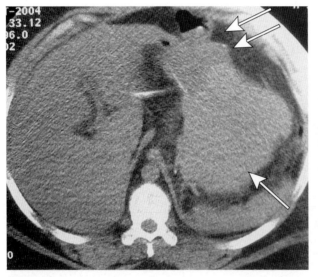

a

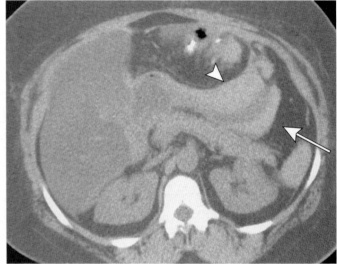

b

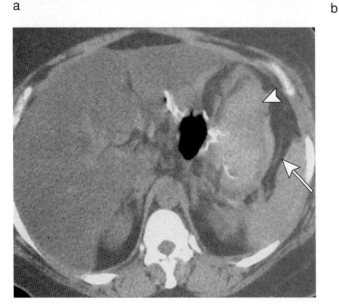

c

Figure 41–13 Postoperative bleeding. (a) Hematic collection (arrow) posterior to excluded stomach, which is anteriorly pulled (two arrows). (b) and (c) Bleeding inside of (arrowheads) and posteriorly to (arrows) excluded stomach.

ACUTE GASTRIC DISTENTION

The gastric remnant may contain a small or moderate amount of fluid, principally in the early postoperative period, due to physiologic alterations, but without clinical symptoms and patient evolution is event free. Acute gastric over distension may put the staple line under tension. In these cases, the surgical team should be immediately contacted because of the possibility of perforation of the gastric remnant or the gastrojejunal anastomosis, which could cause fistula and dehiscence in this region.[18,26]

Dilation of the afferent loop and the gastric remnant is more common in superobese, diabetic, and elderly patients, secondary to gastroparesis, but overall it has a low incidence,[15,18] occurring more in laparotomy surgeries than in videolaparoscopy.[7] It can also be secondary to volvulus of the gastric remnant,[7] edema, or obstruction of the enteroentero anastomosis.[15,18,26]

Conventional radiologic studies can demonstrate gastric distention, by identifying the fluid-air level in the left hypochondrium. However, when the dilation is due to fluid without gas, visualization is hampered in radiography. CT allows a better visualization of the entire segment (dysfunctional stomach, duodenum, biliopancreatic loop), as well as the enteroentero anastomosis (Figure 41–10(a)–(d)). Gastric decompression can be successfully achieved by aspiration and/or percutaneous drainage guided by fluoroscopy or CT. Surgery is the indicated treatment in case of loop obstruction.

GASTROGASTRIC FISTULA

Gastrogastric fistulas can occur in the early or late postoperative period but do not present the same morbidity and mortality rates as free leaks to the peritoneal cavity.[10] This complication should be suspected when there is unsatisfactory weight loss in the postoperative period or when there is opacification of the excluded stomach at CT but no or very little opacification of the duodenum.[26]

Upper GI series can demonstrate the fistula (Figure 41–14(a) and (b)). When there is oral contrast to the left of the gastrojejunal anastomosis, opacification of the excluded stomach should be suspected, and must be differentiated from intracavitary leakage. Diagnosis can be accomplished by complementary incidences at right posterior oblique projection, mobilizing the contrast of the gastric fundus and opacifying the antroduodenal region. The quantity

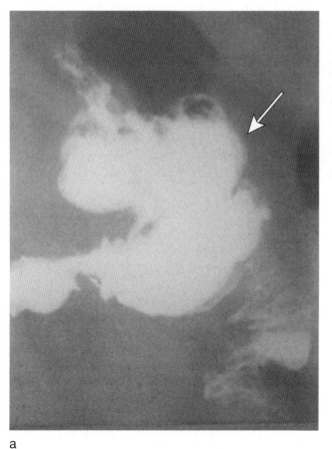

a

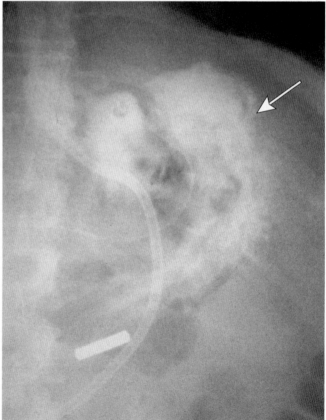

b

Figure 41–14. Opacification of the excluded stomach (arrows) by gastrogastric fistula in two patients. (a) Late postoperative period of patient with unsatisfactory weight loss. (b) Follow-up of a patient with prior anastomotic leak shows a gastrogastric fistula (conservative treatment).

of contrast that passes to the excluded stomach seems to be related to the severity of the leak.[26]

The presence of contrast in the excluded stomach may also be due to reflux through the jejunojejunal anastomosis into the biliopancreatic loop. It occurs late during the upper GI series, and frequent retrograde opacification of the duodenum can also be identified[10] (Figure 41–4(e) and (f)).

SPLENIC AND HEPATIC LACERATIONS

These occur more frequently in laparotomy surgery. In video-laparoscopy, there is better access and visualization of the operative field by the pneumoperitoneum, reducing the risk of injury.[20] Splenic lesions can be observed at CT as sub-capsular fluid collections.[28] Other times, splenectomy is performed during the surgical procedure. There are also reports of splenic infarcts, which may be single, multiple, or may even compromise the entire organ.[28]

Hepatic infarcts have already been observed in the left lobe secondary to surgical manipulation. As with splenic infarcts, they present as hypodense areas at CT. They can evolve to abscesses.[28]

GASTRIC STOMA ULCERATION

The detection of gastric stoma ulceration by upper GI series is difficult.[18] Ulceration can occur in the early or late postoperative period and may be the cause of anastomotic stenosis or even digestive tract hemorrhage.[17] Diagnosis is normally made by digestive endoscopy. The leak is, in the majority of cases, situated in the jejunal portion of the anastomosis.

SCOPINARO AND DUODENAL SWITCH

Normal Study

In both cases there is little restriction to ingestion and a great malabsorptive component (Figure 41–15(a) and (b)). They involve partial gastrectomy that allows the ingestion of a greater volume (around 200–400 mL), associated to a large intestinal diversion greatly reducing the intestinal absorptive area.

In the surgery described by Scopinaro, horizontal gastrectomy is performed with a broad gastroileal anastomosis; an alimentary limb of around 250 cm and short common absorptive loop, initially described as being of 50 cm (please

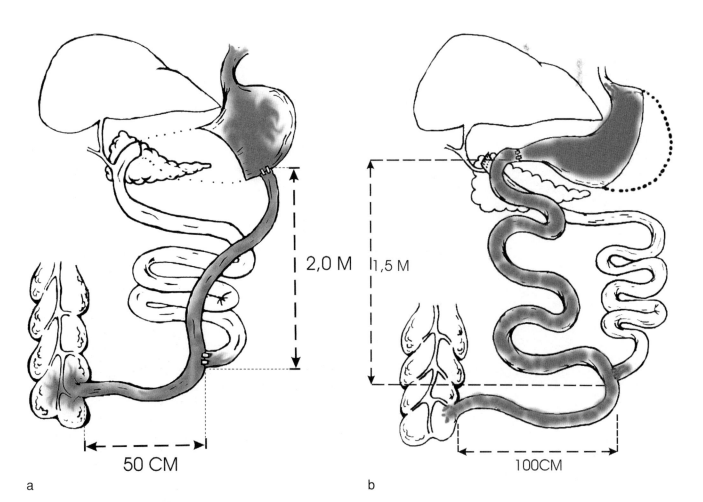

a   b

Figure 41–15. Diagrams of (a) the Scopinaro and (b) duodenal switch surgeries.

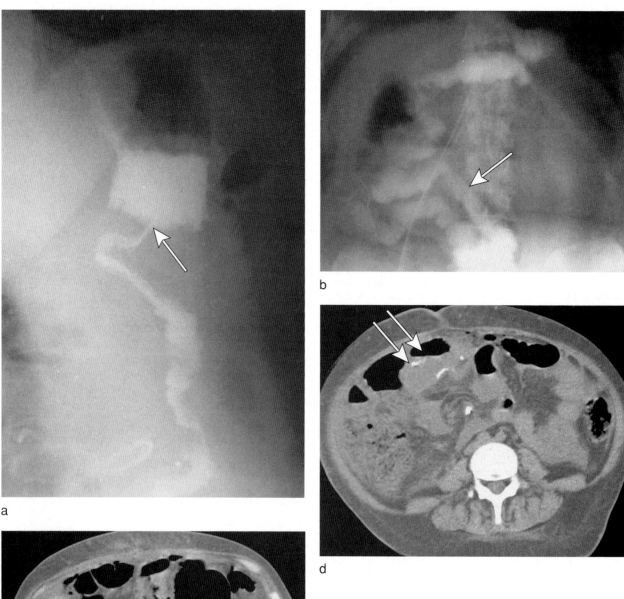

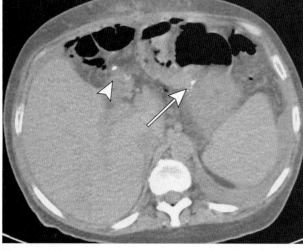

Figure 41–16 Scopinaro surgery—normal appearance. (a) Upper GI series of the gastroenteric anastomosis (arrow). (b) Upper GI series showing the short alimentary limb located predominantly to the right of the abdomen (arrow). (c) CT showing the dense threads of the sutures at the gastroenteric anastomosis (arrow) and of the closure of the duodenum (arrowhead). (d) Enteroenteric anastomosis, located to the right of the midline (two arrows).

see Chapters 10 and 14). Technical modifications have been proposed, mainly in the late postoperative period with the inclusion of a longer absorptive loop in order to reduce malabsorption in patients who present with protein–calorie insufficiency.

The duodenal switch surgery, modified in 1990 by Dr. Marceau in Canada (please see Chapters 10 and 14), consists

of a gastrectomy along the greater curvature together with a gastric tube constructed based on the lesser curvature. The duodenum is sectioned 2 cm below the pylorus, which remains on the alimentary limb. The upper anastomosis is with a Roux-en-Y ileal loop (duodenoileal anastomosis). The distal anastomosis is jejunal–ileal with a common absorptive loop of around 100 cm. The larger common loop reduces

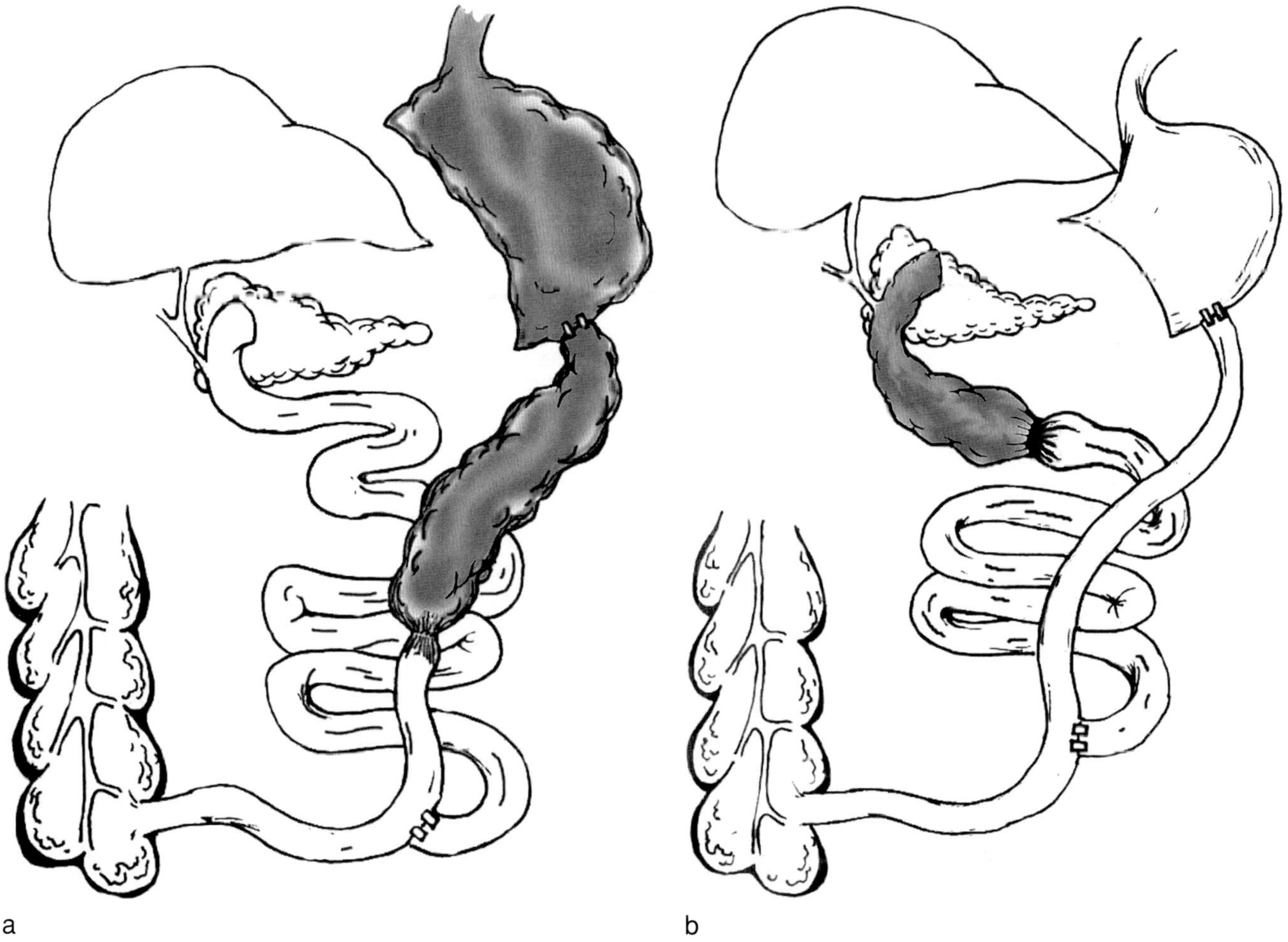

Figure 41–17. Diagram of intestinal obstruction in Scopinaro surgery. (a) Obstruction of the alimentary limb. (b) Obstruction of the biliopancreatic loop. This segment can only be adequately studied by computed tomography.

the diarrheic evacuations. A reduction in the number of epithelial cells, associated with the preservation of the pylorus, reduces the incidence of stoma ulcers and the effect of dumping. Cholecystectomy and appendectomy are frequently performed in the same operation as a prophylactic measure in both techniques.

In the radiological examination, a larger gastric chamber is seen and there are no gastric segments excluded in the abdominal cavity. The horizontal gastrectomy with gastroileal anastomosis, according to Scopinaro, is easily studied by upper GI series (Figure 41–16(a)). The pylorus is preserved in the duodenal switch. The orally contrasted segment is shorter. In CT, dense suture threads of the partial gastric resection and the closure of the duodenum are frequently seen. The enteroenteric anastomosis is more distal, often located to the right of the fossa iliac in Scopinaro's technique (Figure 41–16(b)–(d)).

Postoperative Complications

The complications described in this type of surgery include leaks, surgical wound complications and wound dehiscence, bleeding, splenic lacerations, and the adhesions. Stenosis of the gastroenteric and enteroenteric anastomoses, food impaction above the anastomosis, or stenosis can also occur. Anastomotic ulcers are less common in the duodenal switch technique than the Scopinaro technique.

Conventional GI series allows evaluation of the anatomical surgical changes, as well as identification of leaks, stenosis of the gastroenteroanastomosis, gastric tunneling in the duodenal switch procedure, and obstruction of the afferent loop or of the common channel.

In these patients, the excluded segment of the alimentary tract (biliopancreatic loop) is very long. In the late postoperative period, there is generally no more gas in this segment, which impairs its visualization by conventional radiological technique. In case of distention of this segment, whether by stenosis, obstruction, or adynamic, ileum can only be adequately evaluated by CT (Figure 41–17(a) and (b)). Delay in performing this examination and consequently late diagnosis of obstruction can lead to the compromise of this intestinal segment and place the life of the patient at risk.

References

1. Amir M, Samuel S, Nathan Z, Raul R: Management of acute bleeding after laparoscopic Roux-en-Y gastric bypass. *Obes Surg* 13:842–847, 2003.

2. Awais O, Raftopoulos I, Luketich JD, Courcoulas A: Acute, complete proximal small bowel obstruction after laparoscopic gastric bypass due to intraluminal blood clot formation. *Surg Obes Relat Dis* 1:418–422, 2005.

3. Biertho L, Steffen R, Riclin T, et al.: Laparoscopic gastric bypass versus laparoscopic adjustable gastric banding: A comparative study of 1200 cases. *Laparosc Proc Morbid Obes* 197(4):536–545, 2003.

4. Blachar A, Federle MP: Gastrointestinal complications of laparoscopic Roux-en-Y gastric bypass surgery in patients who are morbidly obese: Findings on radiography and CT. *AJR* 179:1437–1442, 2002.

5. Blachar A, Federle MP, Brancatelli G, Peterson MS, Oliver JH III, Li W: Radiologist performance in the diagnosis of internal hernia by using specific CT findings with emphasis on transmesenteric hernia. *Radiology* 221:422–428, 2001.

6. Blachar A, Federle MP, Dodson SF: Internal hernia: Clinical and imaging findings in 17 patients with emphasis on CT criteria. *Radiology* 218:68–74, 2001.

7. Blachar A, Federle MP, Pealer KM, Abeid SA, Graif M: Radiographic manifestations of normal postoperative anatomy and gastrointestinal complications of bariatric surgery, with emphasis on CT imaging findings. *Semin Ultrasound CT MR* 25(3):239–251, 2004.

8. Blachar A, Federle MP, Pealer KM, Ikramuddin S, Schauer PR: Gastrointestinal complications of laparoscopic Roux-en-Y gastric bypass surgery: Clinical and imaging findings. *Radiology* 223:625–632, 2002.

9. Camerini G, Pretolesi F, Mariani GM, et al.: Radiology of patients with vertical banded gastroplasty. *Obes Surg* 12:57–61, 2002.

10. Carucci LR, Turner MA: Radiologic evaluation following Roux-en-Y gastric bypass surgery for morbid obesity. *Eur J Radiol* 53:353–365, 2005.

11. DeMaria EJ, Sugerman HJ, Kellum JM, Meador JG, Wolfe LG: Results of 281 consecutive total laparoscopic Roux-en-Y gastric bypasses to treat morbid obesity. *Ann Surg* 235:640–647, 2002.

12. Frigg A, Zynamon A, Lang C, Tondelli P: Radiologic and endoscopic evaluation for laparoscopic adjustable gastric banding: Preoperative and follow-up. *Obes Surg* 11:594–599, 2001.

13. Goiten D, Gagné DJ, Papasavas PK, et al.: Superior mesenteric artery syndrome after laparoscopic roux-en-Y gastric bypass for morbid obesity. *Obes Surg* 14:1008–1011, 2004.

14. Higa KD, Ho T, Boone KB: Laparoscopic Roux-en-Y gastric bypass: Technique and 3-year follow-up. *Laparoendosc Adv Surg Tech A* 11(6):377–382, 2001.

15. Kirby DF: The management of obesity for the primary care physician. In: *American College of Gastroenterology 68th Annual Scientific Meeting: Primary Care Focus.* Baltimore, MD, em 10–15 outubro de 2003. Available at: www.medscape.com/viewarticle/463770. Accessed October 31, 2003.

16. Luján JA, Frutos MD, Hernández Q, et al.: Laparoscopic versus open gastric bypass in the treatment of morbid obesity: A randomized prospective study. *Ann Surg* 239(4):433–437, 2004.

17. Martin LF: *Obesity Surgery*, McGraw-Hill, 2004, pp. 259–274. Chapter 14.

18. Merkle EM, Hallowell PT, Crouse C, Nakamoto DA, Stellato TA: Roux-en-Y gastric bypass for clinically severe obesiy: Normal appearance and spectrum of complications at imaging. *Radiology* 234:674–683, 2005.

19. Passa V, Karavias D, Grillias D, Birbas A: Computed tomography of left paraduodenal hérnia. *J Comput Assist Tomogr* 10:542–543, 1986.

20. Podnos YD, Jimenez JC, Wilson SE, Stenvers CM, Nguyen NT: Complications after laparoscopic gastric bypass—a review of 3464 cases. *Arch Surg* 138:957–961, 2003.

21. Pomerri F, De Marchi F, Barbiero G, Di Maggio A, Zavarella C: Radiology for laparoscopic adjustable gastric banding: A simplified follow-up examination method. *Obes Surg* (13):901–908, 2003.

22. Sataloff DM, Lieber CP, Seinige UL: Strictures following gastric stapling for morbid obesity: Results of endoscopic dilatation. *Am Surg* 56:167–174, 1990.

23. Serafini F, Anderson W, Ghassemi P, Poklepovic J, Murr MM: The utility of contrast studies and drains in the management of patients after Roux-en-Y gastric bypass. *Obes Surg* 12:34–38, 2002.

24. Singh R, Fisher BL: Sensitivity and specificity of postoperative upper GI series following gastric bypass. *Obes Surg* (13):73–75, 2003.

25. Toppino M, Cesarani F, Com A, et al.: The role of early radiological studies after gastric bariatric surgery. *Obes Surg* (11):447–454, 2001.

26. Yu J, Turner MA, Cho S-R, et al.: Normal anatomy and complications after gastric bypass surgery: Helical CT findings. *Radiology* 231:753–760, 2004.

27. Zacharoulis D, Roy-Chadhury SH, Dobbins B, et al.: Laparoscopic adjustable gastric banding: Surgical and radiological approach. *Obes Surg* (12):280–284, 2002.

42

Radiographic Evaluation and Treatment: Intervention

Ester Labrunie, MD, PhD • Edson Marchiori, MD, PhD • Cid Pitombo, MD, PhD, TCBC

I. ANASTOMOTIC LEAKS AND FLUID COLLECTIONS

II. PERCUTANEOUS GASTROSTOMY

III. GASTRIC OUTLET OBSTRUCTION

Interventional radiology plays an important role in the treatment of patients with postoperative complications, decreasing morbidity, and mortality in many cases.

ANASTOMOTIC LEAKS AND FLUID COLLECTIONS

Abdominal abscesses can be treated by percutaneous drainage guided by computed tomography (CT) or ultrasound. It is an efficacious treatment, as long as adequate technique and patient selection are carefully performed.[3,6] In obese patients, CT is usually better in visualizing the lesion and surrounding anatomy. The cutaneous entry site should be meticulously planned. In general, the shortest distance to the lesion should be traversed, obviously avoiding structures such as bowel, spleen, lung, and blood vessels. Coagulopathies, if present, should be corrected, and written informed consent should be obtained prior to the procedure.

Patients with leaks presenting insidious or minimal clinical findings usually can be treated nonoperatively, with antibiotics, maintenance of surgical drains (when present),

with holding oral intake, and administration of total parenteral nutrition.[3] CT should be performed on these patients. It can determine if there is any abdominal collection. Any suspicious fluid collection detected by CT should be promptly submitted to percutaneous aspiration and drainage.[1,2,7] Catheter drainage may obviate surgery in many cases.

Patients with leaks, who exhibit hemodynamic instability, should undergo operative treatment. Inflammatory changes around the gastrojejunostomy and excluded stomach may significantly hamper the surgical access and treatment.[3,4] These patients can also beneficiate from percutaneous drainage of fluid collections.

Fluid collections occur most frequently in the left upper abdomen, especially in the perisplenic area,[6] but can also occur elsewhere in the abdomen and pelvis. Fluid collections may evolve into abscesses, and are not always related to anastomotic leaks.

Diagnostic puncture and aspiration guided by CT or ultrasound may be useful in distinguishing abscesses from other fluid collections. Hematomas usually present as high attenuation collections (60–80 HU). They are usually treated conservatively, or may be submitted to surgical drainage in

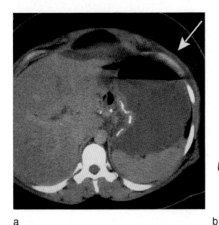

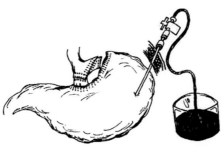

a   b

Figure 42–1. Excluded stomach overdistention. (a) CT in early post-op period shows significant distention of excluded stomach, with air-fluid level (arrow). (b) Diagram of percutaneous gastrostomy.

case of large collections. They may become infected, and percutaneous puncture may be performed for diagnosis. Percutaneous drainage of hematomas is controversial, usually requiring longer drainage, bigger catheter size, and more catheter replacements due to drain obstruction.[7]

PERCUTANEOUS GASTROSTOMY

Acute postoperative distention of the excluded stomach may occur after gastric bypass surgery, usually due to adynamic ileus, edema, and obstruction at jejunojejunal anastomosis or small bowel obstruction. Marked distention of the excluded limb should be promptly diagnosed and treated, because excessive tension on the staple-line may result in free leak (Figure 42-1a).

The excluded segment of the gastrointestinal tract is not readily available for either mechanical, radiological, or endoscopic evaluation. CT scans must be obtained to evaluate gastric distention, as it may not be evident in conventional radiological studies. Decompressive gastrostomy is indicated, and it can be performed by surgery, endoscopy, or percutaneously. Percutaneous gastrostomy (Figure 42-1b) has proved to be safe and effective, with similar or fewer complications than percutaneous endoscopic gastrostomy.[8] Patients with bowel obstruction should be ultimately submitted to surgery. Decompressive gastrostomy in these patients may provide short-term relief of symptoms, but with a higher risk for acute leak and peritonitis around the gastrostomy tube.[8]

Some surgeons routinely place a radiopaque marker around the gastrostomy site at the excluded stomach, which enables easy radiological localization of the bypassed stomach, and thus easier percutaneous access. Others place surgical gastrostomy tubes during the primary gastric bypass surgery. These procedures may add operative risk, and the gastrostomy is needed in only 2% of the patients.[8] Percutaneous fine-needle decompression of gastric acute distention may also be performed.[5] It can be a temporarily successful procedure; however, if distention recurs emergent surgery may be necessary.

GASTRIC OUTLET OBSTRUCTION

Gastric bypass surgery and vertical banded gastroplasty may present late progressive stenosis of the gastric outlet, with symptoms of obstruction. This complication is usually treated by endoscopically guided balloon dilatation, which has proved to be an effective procedure. Balloon dilatation can also be performed guided by fluoroscopy.[9] A guide wire is placed beyond the stenosis through fluoroscopic guidance and the ballon is advanced over a guide wire.

Possible complications are laceration and perforation of the stoma. This complication seems to be more frequent when performed without introduction of a guide wire, and without fluoroscopic guidance, for the end tip of the balloon may lacerate the gut.[9]

References

1. Civardi G, Fornari F, Cavanna L, Sbolli G, Di Stasi M, Buscarini L: Ultrasonically guided percutaneous drainage of abdominal fluid collections: A long-term study of its therapeutic efficacy. *Abdom Imaging* 15:245–250, 1990.
2. Gerzof SG, Robbins AH, Birkett DH, Johnson WC, Pugatch RD, Vincent ME: Percutaneous catheter drainage of abdominal abscesses guided by ultrasound and computed tomography. *AJR* 133:1–8, 1979.
3. Gonzalez R, Nelson LG, Gallagher SF, Murr MM: Anastomotic leaks after laparoscopic gastric bypass. *Obes Surg* 14:1299–1307, 2004.
4. Yu J, Turner MA, Cho S-R, et al.: Normal anatomy and complications after gastric bypass surgery: Helical CT findings. *Radiology* 231:753–760, 2004.
5. Merkle EM, Hallowell PT, Crouse C, Nakamoto DA, Stellato TA: Roux-en-Y gastric bypass for clinically severe obesiy: Normal appearance and spectrum of complications at imaging. *Radiology* 234:674–683, 2005.
6. Blachar A, Federle MP, Pealer KM, Abeid SA, Graif M: Radiographic manifestations of normal postoperative anatomy and gastrointestinal complications of bariatric surgery, with emphasis on CT imaging findings. *Semin Ultrasound CT MR* 25(3):239–251, 2004.
7. Garcia-Vila J, Saiz-Paches V, Domenech-Iglesias MA, et al.: Infected intraabdominal hematomas: Percutaneous drainage. *Abdom Imaging* 18(4):313–317, 1993.
8. Nosher JL, Bodner LJ, Girgis WS, Brolin R, Siegel RL, Gribbin C: Percutaneous gastrostomy for treating dilatation of the bypassed stomach after bariatric surgery for morbid obesity. *AJR* 183:1431–1435, 2004.
9. Marshal JS, Srivastava A, Gupta SK, et al.: Roux-en-Y gastric bypass leak complications. *Arch Surg* 138:520–523, 2003.

43

Endoscopic Evaluation and Treatment

Paulo Sakai, MD • Fauze Maluf Filho, MD • Marcelo Lima, MD • Kendi Yamazaki, MD

INTRODUCTION

Obesity is an emerging global health problem, which threatens to negatively impact gains in longevity. In 1991, the National Institutes of Health consensus development panel recommended bariatric surgery for patients with grade 3 obesity (BMI > 40 kg/m^2) or with grade 2 (BMI 35–40 kg/m^2) with coexisting comorbidities. The endoscopic treatment, mainly through the intragastric balloon placement, has been also an attractive procedure since it can be easily deployed and is reversible. Currently available balloons can usually induce short-term weight loss, but are not more effective than a diet and are ineffective for sustained weight loss. New endoscopic techniques are being developed aiming at minimally invasive treatments and as a primary intervention for obesity.[1,2] The development of Endoscopic suturing devices and the concept of "NOTES—natural orifice transluminal Endoscopic surgery" are creating expectations regarding the possibility of endoscopically created restrictive gastroplasty and gastrojejunal anastomosis. Currently these procedures are being tested in animal models and it will take some time before confirmation of its efficacy.

Bariatric surgery has emerged as the treatment of choice for the patients with morbid obesity. The widespread use of bariatric surgery is justified by its safety and good results, associated with the impact that these procedures have through media.

Multidisciplinary teams composed of surgeons, clinicians, endocrinologists, psychologists, and nutritionists prepare patients for surgery in order to decrease the frequency of postoperative complications. Endoscopists should be a part of that team because endoscopic evaluation may be necessary to investigate and treat various surgical complications. With this in mind, the primary aim of this study is to review some endoscopic procedures during the pre- and postoperative period of these patients.

The most commonly employed surgical options include Roux-en-Y gastric bypass (RYGBP) procedure with or without silicone ring (SR) and adjustable gastric banding (Lap-Band).

EQUIPMENT AND SEDATION

For most patients with RYGBP, a standard gastroscope can be used to evaluate the esophagus, gastric pouch, gastrojejunal anastomosis, and proximal portion of the Roux limb. A pediatric colonoscope or enteroscope may be required to examine the jejunojejunal anastomosis. More recently, the equipment named Double Balloon Enteroscope (Fujinon Corporation, Saitama, Japan) may be used to examine the biliopancreatic limb and the bypassed stomach.

The Endoscopy Unit should have appropriate bariatric hospital beds as well as the availability of facilities for general anesthesia. Morbid obesity is associated by marked respiratory comorbidities such as obstructive sleep apnea, restrictive lung disease, and occasionally pulmonary hypertension. During anesthesia, patients with morbid obesity may develop large alveolar-to-arterial oxygen gradients that may require higher inspiratory oxygen to maintain adequate oxygenization. The use of supplemental oxygen may improve this situation, but it must be emphasized that this may mask alveolar hypoventilation. In fact, the sampling rates of commonly used pulse oximeters may affect the detection of hypoxemia. The type and the sedation dose should be individualized. The careful association of fentanyl and midazolam gives an adequate short time and safe sedation which can be reversible with antagonists naloxone and flumazenil, respectively. In obese patients with respiratory insufficiency or other limitations, the anesthesiologist assistance is a must. An important aspect is that in obese patients the upper gastrointestinal (GI) endoscopy is feasible utilizing topical anesthesia without sedation and seated in a special wheelchair, using the standard or ultrathin endoscope for nasogastroscopy.

PREOPERATIVE ENDOSCOPIC EVALUATION

The upper GI endoscopic examination is a part of the preoperative evaluation for patients who will be undergoing bariatric surgery. It is mostly desirable in the treatment of GI diseases such as gastroesophageal reflux disease or peptic ulcers before surgery and in some cases, the presence of upper GI tumors or other lesions seen during the endoscopic evaluation, causing changes in the surgical approach. This happens in 5%–10% of the patients.[3] For example, atrophic gastritis is a risk factor for the development of gastric adenocarcinoma. On the other hand, it is known that *Helicobacter pylori* may cause histological changes such as chronic gastritis, atrophy, and intestinal metaplasia, which suggests that the diagnosis and treatment for *H. pylori* be instituted on a routine basis as part of the usual measures that precede the bariatric surgery.[4] Some surgeons believe that after treating this infection the incidence of marginal ulcer diminishes. In the same way, endoscopic findings like the stromal tumors (GIST, gastrointestinal stromal tumors) and the leiomyomas indicate further investigation with endoscopic ultrasound and sometimes biopsies or even complete endoscopic resection of these lesions.[5]

POSTOPERATIVE ENDOSCOPIC EVALUATION

Endoscopic evaluation may be necessary to investigate and treat various surgical complications. The complications may be early such as bleeding and anastomotic leaks and late such as luminal stenosis, primary surgical failure, and gallstones. Other complications are more specific to the particular type of procedure, e.g., gastric erosions and acid reflux are seen following gastric banding procedure. When called upon to evaluate the postoperative bariatric patient, GI endoscopists will be confronted with an altered anatomy, so whenever possible, it is important to discuss the bariatric surgery technique with the patient's surgeon so that preparation may be done with adequate equipment and accessories for each situation.[6] Sometimes drawings or diagrams of the bariatric surgery technique used are more valuable than any transcribed text. And it is very useful to review all available postoperative abdominal imaging studies and examinations. When the patient is at the beginning of the "losing weight curve," sedation should be carefully managed, as previously recommended, in the preoperative period.

During the postoperative period, GI endoscopy control is done every year, even in asymptomatic patients and every time there is a suspicion of any complication in the process of evaluation of the failure to lose weight or even in the investigation of the cause of regaining weight. Specific symptoms like abdominal pain were not predictive in any particular endoscopic finding, especially when these symptoms occurred 6 months after surgery.[7] Some authors describe marginal ulcers in almost 16% of the operated patients, which does not correspond to our experience.[8] Maybe the variation of the surgical technique might explain that difference, which some authors advocate as the incidence where this complication is reduced when the anastomosis is done in two layers with absorbable line suture.

FOOD IMPACTION IN THE GASTRIC POUCH

After the RYGBP procedure, some patients continue to persist in inappropriate eating habits thereby causing the most common postoperative complication in this kind of surgery, which is the impaction of food in the gastric pouch, usually

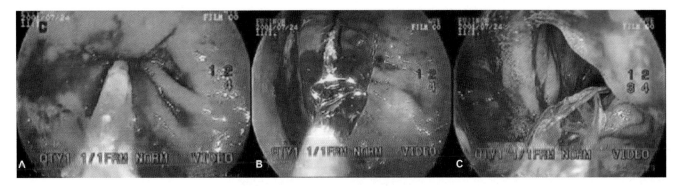

Figure 43–1. (A) Deflated balloon placed at the gastrojejunal stoma stenosis, (B) balloon's dilation, and (C) post-dilation appearance.

above the gastric SR or the gastrojejunal bypass. The most common symptoms in this situation are nausea, vomiting, and persistent sudden salivation after a meal. The endoscopic findings vary from small fragments or even larger fragments obstructing the gastric pouch above the gastric ring constricted area, or, if not, at the gastrojejunal anastomosis.

Stomal stenosis or the excessive calibration of the anastomotic banding is rarely associated with food impaction. The endoscopic treatment consists of suction of the smaller fragments and removal of the bigger ones by using a polypectomy snare, Dormia basket, and even the plastic cap that can be used to apprehend compacted boluses of food with the help of close suction vacuum. After "cleaning" the gastric pouch, the SR constriction and the gastrojejunal anastomosis should be evaluated for stenosis.

STOMAL ULCERS AND STENOSIS

Anastomotic ulcers, also referred to as stomal or marginal ulcers, are a well-recognized complication of bariatric surgery that often present as retrosternal or epigastric pain. Symptoms typically develop in the first 3 months following surgery; however, ulceration may occur at any time. The exact etiology is unclear; however, many factors are thought to be associated with their development including *H. pylori*, gastrogastric fistula, increased acid exposure, mucosal ischemia, pouch size, pouch orientation, and NSAIDs. When stomal ulcerations are not associated with significant staple-line, failure management consists of PPI therapy and elimination of ulcerogenic medications.

After diagnosing stomal stenosis, one should have in mind that the bypass is a terminal-lateral gastrojejunal anastomosis and the passage of balloons or Savary bougie offers potential risk for jejunal perforation. Most times the anastomotic stenosis is suspected at the end of the first week postoperatively when liquid diet is given to the patient. The endoscopic aspect is like an inflammatory stenosis, with intense edema, redness, flat ulcers, and frequently with various suture materials at the gastrojejunal anastomosis. It is important to remove foreign bodies before dilation, because even the metallic suture material coming out of the lumen could perforate the balloon. The removal of the suture method

is important to reduce the inflammatory reaction. The esophageal or pyloric balloon used has 12 mm of diameter with 5.5 cm of length, which is passed through the scope (TTS) to the jejunal loop (Figure 43–1). Abrupt dilation at the jejunal loop should be avoided because of the perforation risk. Sometimes it is not possible to make the passage through the anastomosis and an alternative measure is to use dilation balloons with a guide-wire with hydrophilic tip, passing it under fluoroscopic control. In some difficult cases, the use of pediatric endoscope and fluoroscopy may be necessary. In 42 patients who underwent this kind of technique, the resolution of the stenosis with a 12-mm dilation of the anastomosis with a total of three sessions per patient was possible in all cases. In two patients, intralesional steroid injection was also done, in stenosis that occurred on the third postoperative week with an ischemic component factor. Good results have been seen with this technique in more than 90% of the cases, which was described by other authors[9] (Figure 43–1).

CONSTRICTION OF THE GASTRIC SILICONE RING

Some surgeons have placed an SR in some patients at the distal portion and around the gastric pouch and when it gets too tight, obstruction symptoms may occur. To inexperienced endoscopists, it is not an easy task to distinguish this situation with a stomal stenosis because some bariatric surgeons place the gastric ring near the anastomosis. In a practical way, it is possible to distinguish both situations. The dilation of the gastric ring constriction is not effective. Since the gastric ring is made of silicone, dilation will be compressing the gastric pouch wall against a fixed structure, which is nonexpandable and will cause edema to the gastric wall. If the weight loss is higher than planned and the food impaction symptoms like nausea and vomiting are frequent, the possibility of surgical removal of the gastric ring should be considered.

GASTRIC SILICONE RING EROSION

Another complication is the erosion of the gastric pouch wall with the spontaneous extrusion of the band and in this case

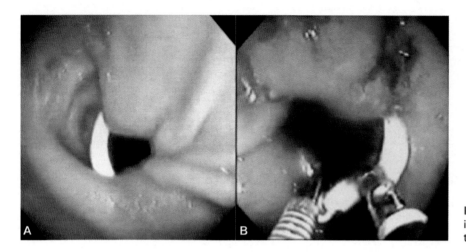

Figure 43–2. (A) Silicone ring migration into the gastric pouch. (B) Silicone ring cut to be removed.

dyspeptic symptoms or a self-limited episode of GI bleeding might happen (Figure 43–2). The removal of this band is indicated by many surgeons because it has lost its function. The most effective way of removing the band is by using a double channel endoscope and through one of the channels pass a grasping forceps to catch and stabilize the plastic ring. Using the scissors passed through the other one the ring is cut. The best cutting device is a scissor with a hook shape. If double channel endoscope is not available, a plastic "cap" may be adapted to the tip of the endoscope, so the scissor may do the cutting movements with the plastic ring fixed against the "cap." In 27 patients, the double channel technique was used in 22 and "cap" technique in 5. This result has been repeated in other studies.[10]

GASTRIC SILICONE RING MIGRATION

The ring can migrate to the gastrojejunal anastomosis causing stenosis of the jejunal segment. This kind of complication is very rare and happens late, after the procedure. The clinical symptoms are similar to a distal esophageal obstruction. The endoscopic findings reveal intense esophagitis, reflux, stasis in the esophagus and the gastric pouch, and the absence of the ring constriction associated to an excessively large stoma below them. And finally, one may identify the jejunal mucosa converging to the point of obstruction, which looks like a pinwheel shape. In this situation, the endoscopist can only pass a feeding tube beyond the point of obstruction and advise the patient for a new surgical procedure.

FISTULA

Gastrocutaneous fistula, near the stapled His angle, is one of the most frequent complications, ranging toward 8% in different studies.[11] It is a morbid condition and very difficult to treat and sometimes needing repeated surgical procedures with low odds of success. The classic treatment of ruptured stapled line and peritonitis is early surgical reintervention with debridement of the fistula region, cleaning, local exposition, and resuture. The removal of the plastic ring is mandatory when dehiscence occurs above it. The drainage and gastrostomy of the excluded stomach completes the reoperation.[12]

For some surgeons the drainage of the stapled vertical line and gastrostomy have been routinely part of the RYGBP, so when there is an anastomosis rupture, clinical and conservative treatment of the fistula may be considered a valid option.

Working toward a minimum invasive therapy, GI endoscopy has been using different methods to treat postoperative fistulas.[13–20] In the literature, there are case reports using endoscopic clips, fibrin glue, and recently Surgisis® SIS (Wilson Cook, WS, NC).[21] Surgisis® is an acellular matrix used as a prosthetic material for abdominal hernia correction and chronic cutaneous ulcers and other applications. This material, a product of swine small bowel submucosa, is a support for proliferation of inflammatory cells and fibroblasts (Figure 43–3). Our experience counts with 19 patients treated endoscopically with that material placed inside the fistula. Of the 19 patients, 14 had the fistula closed by this method (73.7%). Only 1 needed one session (7.1%), 11 needed two applications (78.6%), and 2 patients had to have a third session (14.2%) to obliterate the fistula. In five cases, the treatment has failed after the third week (three sessions) but in all of them size reduction of the fistula was noticed.

In some cases, with large fistulas almost 20 mm in diameter and no internal drainage and the use of self-expandable plastic stent allowed the patient to discharge with a diet oral intake (Figure 43–4). Baptista et al. describe the closure of this kind of fistula in 8 patients treated with a covered self-expandable metallic stent and mention that there is some difficulty removing it afterward.[10]

The use of endoscopic therapy with adhesives or healing agents benefits small fistulas with low volume leakage. On the other hand, removable self-expandable stent may have an important role in larger fistulas with a high volume leakage.

The endoscopic evaluation is needed when the expected weight loss is not achieved. Two endoscopic diagnoses are

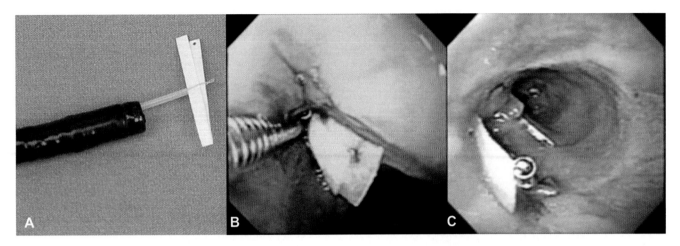

Figure 43–3. (A) Small soft ribbon of Surgisis®, (B) stuffing the fistula, and (C) fixed by a hemoclip.

possible in this situation. First of all, a gastric pouch fistula to the excluded stomach. In this situation, barium contrast radiograph helps to confirm the diagnostic suspicion. A surgical technique modification like the interposition of jejunal segment and complete exclusion of the stomach in this kind of situation is uncommon. On the other hand, the spontaneous rupture of the gastric ring or excessive enlargement of the stoma may cause a gain of the lost weight. Some studies propose injection of a substance at the anastomosis, creating a stenotic "chemical ring," where one can reduce it to about 40% of the anastomosis calibration.[22] Probably, in the future, devices for endoscopic suture will be available to suture the enlarged stoma.

Biliary Stone

Following the RYGBP procedure, late complications such as fatty liver and gallstones may occur with varying incidence. Biliary acute pancreatitis is one of the severe complications and ERCP may be necessary. An ERCP, in the setting of RYGBP, can be performed in an antegrade fashion utilizing a percutaneous gastrostomy. In a retrograde fashion, the ERCP can be performed utilizing the pediatric colonoscope or double balloon enteroscope.

Endoscopic Evaluation of the Bypassed Stomach

There is no formal indication for endoscopic evaluation for the excluded stomach. The conventional enteroscopy evaluated the excluded stomach in 33 (65%) patients submitted to gastric "bypass." In 32 patients, there was bile at the defunctionalized stomach and antral gastritis. Atrophy and intestinal metaplasia were identified in 4 (12%). The intensity of the gastritis had no time relation between the intervals from the operation to the examination. That interval varies from 3 to 24 months.[23]

A new model of enteroscope called double balloon enteroscope has been gaining favor. It consists of an overtube where the enteroscope slides through and uses the double balloon system, avoiding the formation of jejunal loops. It is a technique that offers an easy possibility to examine the bypass stomach, in order to assess changes in the gastric mucosa mainly after long-term follow-up (Figure 43–5). Atrophic

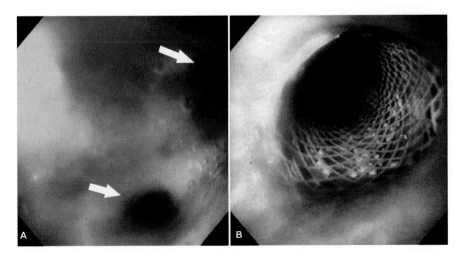

Figure 43–4. (A) Gastric pouch double fistula orifice and (B) self-expandable plastic stent placement.

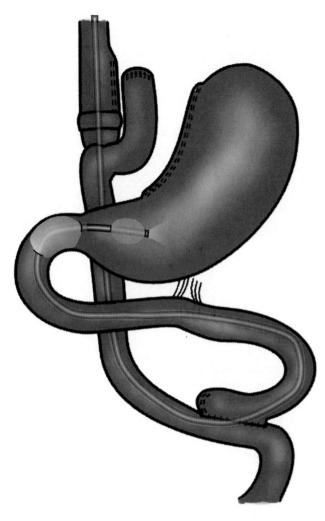

Figure 43–5. Illustration of the double balloon enteroscope approaching the bypassed stomach.

gastritis pattern with intestinal metaplasia, erosive hemorrhagic gastritis, and *H. pylori* infection have been described.[24]

ADJUSTABLE GASTRIC BAND EROSION

One of the complications that happens in patients after laparoscopic adjustable gastric banding is erosion and intrusion of the gastric band into the lumen. This complication occurs in 8% of the operated patients and its laparoscopic treatment has a 10% rate of complications.[25]

This increases the interest of removing the band by endoscopy. Using the YAG laser may be an alternative but it is not easily available. A method very similar to biliary stone lithotripsy was developed to cut the band by endoscopy. It consists of cutting the band with a guide wire made of steel which slides the metallic sheath accessory of the lithotripsy toward the band. The endoscopist grabs one of the extremities of the band with a polypectomy snare, removing it through the patient's mouth (Figure 43–6). It may be a time-consuming technique and demands general anesthesia and the presence of the surgeon. The risk of pneumoperitoneum is a fact and it may be revealed by a simple radiological imaging after the procedure. If pneumoperitoneum occurs, and the patient is asymptomatic, antibiotic therapy and no oral intake might be the treatment of choice[26] (Figure 43–6).

CONCLUSIONS

Endoscopy has an important role before and after surgical treatment of obesity. Sometimes the endoscopic findings of asymptomatic lesions may change the previously proposed

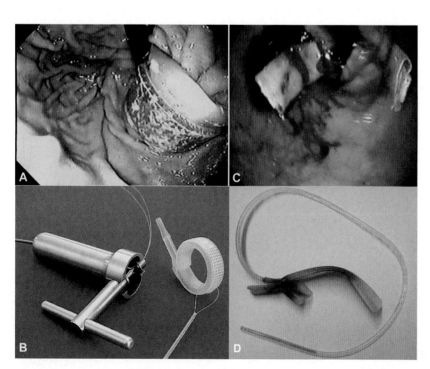

Figure 43–6. (A) Adjustable gastric band migrated into the stomach, (B) accessory to cut the band, (C) the cut band "in vivo," and (D) removed after cutting it.

treatment. In the postoperative period, endoscopy can identify complications and there is a possibility of treatment for them. The further development of endoscopic accessories such as suturing devices and flexible staplers will likely improve endoscopic outcomes and result in a reduced need for surgical revisions. The role of endoscopy as a primary intervention for obesity is yet to be determined.

References

1. Hu B, Chung SCS, Sun LCL, Kawashima K: Transoral obesity surgery: Endolumial gastroplasty with an endoscopic stuture device. *Endoscopy* 37:411–414, 2005.
2. Kelleher B, Yurek M, Swain P: Creation of a gastric partition using an endoscopic stapler. *Gastrointest Endosc* 5:AB236, 2006.
3. Schirmer B, Eronoglu C, Miller A: Flexible endoscopy in the management of patients undergoing Roux-em-Y gastric bypass. *Obes Surg* 12:634–638, 2002.
4. Cordeiro F, Ferraz E: *H. pylori* and gastroplasty in the treatment of morbid obesity. *Am J Gastroenterol* 96:605–606, 2001.
5. Sanchez BR, Morton JM, Curet MJ, Alami R, Safadi BY: Incidental finding of gastrointestinal stromal tumors (GISTs) during laparoscopic gastric bypass. *Obes Surg* 15:1384–1388, 2005.
6. Stellato TA, Crouse C, Hallowell PT: Bariatric surgery: Creating new challenges for the endoscopist. *Gastrointest Endosc* 57:86–94, 2003.
7. Huang CS, Forse AR, Jcobson BC, Farraye FA: Endoscopic findings and their clinical correlations in patients with symptoms after gastric bypass surgery. *Gastrointest Endosc* 58:859–866, 2003.
8. Capella JF, Capella RF: Staple disruption and marginal ulceration in gastric bypass procedures for weight reduction. *Obes Surg* 6:44–49, 1996.
9. Capella JF, Capella RF: Gastro-gastric fistulas and marginal ulcers in gastric bypass procedures for weight reduction. *Obes Surg* 9:22–27, 1999.
10. Baptista A, Raijman I, Bonilla Y, et al.: Endoscopic management of complications after bariatric surgery. *Gastrointest Endosc* 61:5:AB160, 2005.
11. Murr M, Balsinger B, Kennedy F, Mai J, Sarr M: Malabsorptive procedures for severe obesity: Comparison of pancreaticobiliary bypass and very very long limb Roux-en-Y gastric bypass. *J Gastrointest Surg* 3:607–612, 1999.
12. Barroso FL, Alonso ADS, Leite MA: Complicações cirúrgicas intra operatórias e do pós operatório recente, Cirurgia da Obesidade, Ed. Atheneu, 2001.
13. Thurairajah P, Hawthorne AB: Endoscopic clipping of a nonhealing gastrocutaneous fistula following gastrostomy removal. *Endoscopy* 36:834, 2004.
14. Familiari P, Macri A, Consolo P, et al.: Endoscopic clipping of a colocutaneous fistula following necrotizing pancreatitis: Case report. *Dig Liver Dis* 35:907–910, 2003.
15. Papavramidis ST, Eleftheriadis EE, Papavramidis TS, Kotzampassi KE, Gamvros OG: Endoscopic management of gastrocutaneos fistula after bariatric surgery by using a fibrin sealant. *Gastrointest Endosc* 59:296–300, 2004.
16. Rabago LR, Ventosa N, Castro JL, Marco J, Herrera N, Gea F: Endoscopic treatment of postoperative fistulas resistant to conservative management using biological fibrin glue. *Endoscopy* 34:632–638, 2002.
17. Papavramidis ST, Eleftheriadis EE, Apostolidis DN, Kotzampassi KE: Endoscopic fibrin sealing of high-output non-healing gastrocutaneous fistulas after vertical gastroplasty in morbidly obese patients. *Obes Surg* 11:766–769, 2001.
18. Dunn CJ, Goa KL: Fibrin sealant: A review of its use in surgery and endoscopy. *Drugs* 58:863–886, 1999.
19. Cellier C, Landi B, Faye A, et al.: Upper gastrointestinal tract fistulae: Endoscopic obliteration with fibrin sealant. *Gastrointest Endosc* 44:731–733, 1996.
20. Shand A, Pendlebury J, Reading S, Papachrysostomou M, Ghosh S: Endoscopic fibrin sealant injection: A novel method of closing a refractory gastrocutaneous fistula. *Gastrointest Endosc* 46:357–358, 1997.
21. Maluf-Filho F, Moura F, Sakai P, et al.: Endoscopic treatment of esophagogastric fistulae with an acellular matrix. *Gastrointest Endosc* 59:AB151, 2004.
22. Catalano MF, George S, Tomas M, Geenen JE, Chua T: Weight gain following bariatric surgery secondary to staple line disruption and stomal dilation: Endotherapy using sodium morrhuate to induce stomal stenosis prevents need for surgical revision. *Gastrointest Endosc* 59:AB149, 2004.
23. Sinar DR, Flickinger EG, Park HK, Sloss RR: Retrogrande endoscopy of the bypassed stomach segment after gastric bypass surgery: Unexpected lesions. *South Med J* 78:255–258, 1985.
24. Sakai P, Kuga R, Safatle-Ribeiro A, et al.: Is it feasible to reach the bypassed stomach after Roux-en-Y gastric bypass for morbid obesity? The use of the double-balloon enteroscope. *Endoscopy* 37:566–569, 2005.
25. Keidar A, Szold A, Carmon E, Blanc A, Abu-Abeid S: Band slippage after laparoscopic adjustable gastric banding: Etiology and treatment. *Surg Endosc* 19:262–267, 2005.
26. Sakai P, Hondo FY, Artifon ELA, Kuga R, Ishioka S: Symptomatic pneumoperitoneum after endoscopic removal of adjustable gastric band. *Obes Surg* 15:893–896, 2005.

New Technology

44

Gastric Pacing

Angelo Loss, MD • Marcel Milcent, MD • Georgia Bartholdi, MD

▮ INTRODUCTION

The human kind becomes heavier every day and this excess weight is progressively increasing.[1] More than 58% of the United States adult population is presently overweight (BMI > 25 kg/m^2).[2] In addition, 4.7% (14–16 million) of American people are morbidly obese (BMI > 40 kg/m^2).[3] The consequence of this pandemic is the increase in comorbidities[4,5] and premature death[6,7] in this group. These individuals suffer from a wide variety of obesity-related diseases and integrate the second largest group of avoidable deaths, coming after smokers (>300,000 annually).[3] The cost of this obese population reaches approximately US$70 billion a year.[8] Overweight/obesity prevalence worldwide is esti-mated around 1.7 billion people,[9] what leads to more than 2.5 million deaths a year.[10]

Many ways of treatment are available for obesity, with variable efficacy: diets, appetite suppressor drugs, and surgery.[2] For the patients considered morbidly obese (BMI > 40 kg/m^2), the US National Institutes of Health concluded that obesity surgery is the most adequate therapeutic option.[11] Several studies have shown dramatic improvement in obesity-related comorbidities in patients submitted to diverse surgical treatments (restrictive, malabsorptive, or combined) after weight loss.[12] Throughout the last 50 years, with the development of adequate techniques and instruments, surgical treatment has evolved into a safe and efficient treatment. In addition, the emerging of minimally invasive surgery such as laparoscopy has increased the safety and popularity of these procedures. Nevertheless, in spite of all technical and technological advances, every procedure may lead to short-term postoperatory complications and long-term nutritional and gastrointestinal consequences.[13]

Less than 1% of the obese patients that fulfill the criteria for surgical treatment actually have access to it, however. While many potential candidates have their operations denied by health insurance companies, lack of knowledge about the efficacy of the specific method and other reasons, a great number of individuals will avoid surgery because of the fear of the possible complications and long-term consequences of the procedures performed to date.[12]

The implantable gastric stimulation (IGS), usually referred as the gastric pacemaker, comes as a new concept for the treatment of severe obesity. Unlike other ways of bariatric surgery, it involves minimal manipulation of the normal gastrointestinal tract anatomy, and is feasible by laparoscopy. These features minimize the risks of postoperatory complications and the development of late nutritional and gastrointestinal disturbances; it is even a possibility for the patients not eligible for invasive procedures for presenting with BMI < 35 kg/m^2.[13]

PHYSIOLOGIC BASIS OF THE IMPLANTABLE GASTRIC STIMULATOR

Gastric Motility and Emptying

Motility is one of the major functions and characteristics of the gastrointestinal tract, without which the progression of food, its digestion, and absorption would be impaired. In order to perform this task adequately, the stomach needs to generate coordinated contractions (peristalsis) to propel nutrients to regions of maximum absorption in a regular rate. Thus, coordinated gastric contractions are necessary to gastric emptying. These contractions are born from a gastric native electric activity.[13]

The pattern of gastric electric activity is different in fasting and postprandial periods.[14] In the postprandial phase, the human stomach contracts in the maximum frequency of three cycles per minute (cpm). This contractile wave originates proximally and propagates forward, toward the pylorus. In healthy humans, 50% or more of the ingested food leaves the stomach after 2 hours and 95% or more is propelled within 4 hours after ingestion.[15] When empty, the pattern of gastric motility alters. The fasting phase follows a cycle of periodic fluctuations divided in three phases: Phase I—no contraction, 40–60 minutes; phase II—intermittent contractions, 20–40 minutes; and phase III—regular and rhythmic contractions, 2–10 minutes.

Stomach Myoelectrical Activity

Gastric contractile action is regulated by its myoelectric activity, which normally compounds two components: slow waves and spike potentials. Slow waves occur in regular intervals,

whether there is gastric contraction or not; they originate in the proximal stomach and propagate distally to the pylorus; they also determine the maximum frequency, speed of propagation, and direction of gastric contraction. When a spike potential happens over a slow wave a vigorous gastric contraction takes place.[13]

Gastric arrhythmias represent anomalies in the myoelectric activity. Like cardiac arrhythmias, they include abnormal rapid contractions (tachygastrias) and abnormal slow contractions (bradygastrias).[12] Recently, the prevalence and origin of gastric arrhythmias have been investigated.[16] It was noted that the majority of bradygastrias initiated in the proximal stomach and propagated through the gastric wall to the antrum. Consequently, the bradygastrias were assumed to be caused by a decrease in the generation of waves by the gastric topic pacemaker. On the other hand, tachygastrias originated in the distal antrum and propagated partially or entirely through the gastric wall to the proximal stomach. During these tachygastrias, waves generated by the topic pacemaker were still present. Therefore, it was not unusual to have the proximal stomach under influence of the normal slow waves and the distal organ dominated by tachygastria. Moreover, the prevalence of arrhythmias was higher in the distal antrum and lower in the proximal stomach.

Gastric Emptying and Obesity

Gastric emptying has an important role in the regulation of the ingestion of food. Several studies have demonstrated that gastric distention acts as a satiety-signaling mechanism, inhibiting continuation of ingestion,[17] and that the rapid gastric emptying could be associated with excess feeding and obesity, especially in animals with hypothalamic lesions.[18] In a study carried out by Wright, in a group of 77 individuals (46 obese and 31 nonobese) of similar age, sex, and race, the obese ones presented with much faster gastric emptying than did the nonobese.[19] Despite the fact that the cause of this alteration remains obscure, Carlson proposed a relation between the gastrointestinal tract and the hypothalamus regulating food ingestion in his classical 1913 work at the University of Chicago.[20] It has also been observed that some peptides such as cholecystokinin (CCK) and corticotrophin releasing factor (CRF) inhibit hunger and gastric emptying.[21] More recently, it has been demonstrated that ob/ob rats (genetic model for obesity) display accelerated gastric emptying when compared to nonobese ones.[22] A peptide similar to CRF, Urocortin, would be capable of diminishing food ingestion and weight gain as well as gastric emptying in ob/ob rats. This suggested that gastric emptying might contribute to hyperphagia and obesity in those animals, rendering new insights in the treatment of obesity.

Gastric Stimulation

Gastric stimulation involves application of an electric current to the stomach wall in order to alter its emptying. Its use would only be possible if this artificially generated current overwhelmed the gastric physiologic slow waves. This has indeed been proven possible in humans.[23] The electric stimulus in the stomach can be guided to caudal (anterograde or aboral) or cephalic (retrograde or orad) directions. Studies of anterograde stimulation have assessed its effects on gastric myoelectric activity, gastric motility, gastric emptying, and gastrointestinal symptoms. They have shown that the interference in gastric slow waves is possible with the use of artificial generators, but it depends on some features like intensity and frequency of the electric stimulus. In addition, anterograde stimuli could interfere with the slow waves through electrodes located over the serosa or inside gastric lumen.[24–31]

Retrograde stimuli could be beneficial in patients with accelerated gastric emptying, such as those with dumping syndrome and morbid obesity. The original concept was that retrograde stimulation might retard gastric emptying, which would be useful in the treatment of obesity given that slowed gastric emptying is associated with early satiety and diminished food intake. This has been true in non-obese individuals, whether assessed indirectly by symptoms induced by it,[32] or by direct measurement of gastric emptying and food intake.[33]

To provide these electric currents, an electric impulse generator should be connected to the distal stomach region, along the lesser curvature, which would result in electric waves that would propagate from the antrum to the fundus. Consequently, a gastric arrhythmia would be induced and the physiologic emptying—dependent on the slow waves—would be compromised. The degree of impairment of the gastric emptying would be determined by the intensity of the electric stimuli.

DEVELOPMENT AND EVOLUTION OF IGS

Whether gastric emptying could be slowed by electric stimuli or not, this possibility proved to be safe and feasible for the treatment of morbid obese patients.

An Italian surgeon, Valério Cigaina, first developed the idea of gastric electric stimulation for weight loss in the late eighties. By that time, the accepted theory was that exogenous electric impulses could be used to alter gastric electromotor activity in obese patients, resulting in weight loss.[34] In 1992, Cigaina et al.[35,36] demonstrated that the retrograde electric stimulus was feasible, safe, and was associated with weight loss in porcine. Studies in humans followed in 1995.[37] A stimulator with platinum electrodes was implanted by laparoscopy in four women with BMI > 40 kg/m², in the anterior gastric wall; they were followed for 40 months. All were allowed to eat freely. At the end, one had lost 32 kg, one had lost 62 kg, while the other two had not lost weight; in the latter two, rupture of the wire connecting the generator and the electrodes was noted. It did become a fact that chronic gastric stimulation in humans was safe, for no collateral effects had been observed.

Another study came out in 1998, with 10 morbid obese patients.[35] No deaths or other medical problems were observed during the study, both early and late. There was no rupturing of wires or electric component flaws. After 51 months of electric stimulation, 23% excess weight loss (EWL) was reached, and apparently sustained. However, battery exhaustion lead to weight regain, and its replacement resulted in novel weight loss.

SURGICAL TECHNIQUE

After Cigaina's proposal of an implantable electric stimulator for the treatment of morbid obesity, the device was developed in collaboration with Transneuronix Inc. (Arlington, NJ). Two of the components are permanently implanted in the patient. One is the conducting wire, which contains two platinum–iridium electrode plates. The other is the electric current provider, the implantable pulse generator (IPG). A computer, used for data retrieval and the generator programming, controls the device. Communication between the IPG and the computer is noninvasive and transcutaneous, established by radiofrequency waves (wand).[38]

The installation procedure of the IGS is carried out in a minimally invasive manner, by laparoscopy, using regular laparoscopic instruments and the four components (wire, IPG, program, and wand), supplied by Transneuronix. Candidates for the IGS are informed of the risks and benefits of the operation with an informed consent. Prophylactic antibiotics and heparin are used. Patients under general anesthesia are put in 20° reverse Trendelenburg, lithotomy position. A minimum of three trocars are inserted. One middle line, supraumbilical trocar is used for the optic system. One right superior quadrant port is used for insertion of a grasper. The conducting wire and electrodes will pass through the left subcostal 10-mm port, in the anterior axillary line. If necessary, a fourth trocar is used for the liver retractor and its position will depend on the surgeon's preference.

The region where the electrodes will be implanted is identified. The ideal position is yet to be determined. A useful reference for the site is the junction of the lesser curvature with neurovascular plexus fat. Other easily identifiable reference is the *pes anserinus*, the region where the vagus nerve motor branch (Latarget's nerve) crosses the serosa of the stomach. The points of entrance and exit of a 3-cm muscular tunnel are marked with the electrocautery. Rulers or other distance-measuring instruments can be used. The conducting wire is then cautiously inserted in the abdominal cavity, as problems with the equipment will require reintervention for replacement of wires or electrodes. The wire is inserted in the muscular tunnel; gastric counter-traction is important at this time. The tunnel of appropriate size guarantees that both electrodes stay inside the muscular wall. Endoscopic control is performed after the electrodes' positioning to make sure that there is no perforation into the lumen. Should the electrodes be seen inside the stomach, they are to be removed and reinserted in another tunnel made nearby. Repair of the penetrating point is not necessary, with no risk of fistulae. Once adequately implanted, the wire is attached to the outer gastric wall via nonabsorbable seromuscular stay-stitches. After fixation, the proximal end of the cable is withdrawn from the peritoneal cavity through the left subcostal port.

A subcutaneous site for the generator is prepared. It should be located under the fat in the anterior abdominal wall. The skin incision should not be over the generator. The generator's posterior side will be in contact with the rectus anterior sheet and will be fixed by two stitches. Upon completion of the generator implantation, electrocautery should not be used anymore, as it might cause damage to the generator's electronic parts. The proximal tip of the wire is cleaned with sterile water (never saline) and then connected to the generator. Misconnections may be associated with short circuits or insufficient impedance. The wand is covered with sterile plastic and the system is checked with the computer. Once the parameters are accepted the generator is positioned and fixed. The abdominal cavity is refilled with gas and the team confirms the correct position of the wires and electrodes after manipulation. Any excess of conducting wire is left in the cavity, forming a delicate curve. The pneumoperitoneum is exsufflated and the trocars removed. Wounds are closed.

INTERNATIONAL EXPERIENCE WITH IGS FOR WEIGHT LOSS

European Multicentric Study

In a multicentric study conducted in Europe, morbidly obese patients were submitted to IGS implantation in seven different centers (Italy,[39] France,[40] Germany, Sweden, Greece, Austria, and Belgium), 15 individuals each. The study profiles differed according to the center, but no complications were observed in any patient. Mean EWL exceeded 40% in a 2-year follow-up. More recently, a second multicentric study is being carried out, the laparoscopic obesity stimulation survey (LOSS). Like the aforementioned study, no complication was noted. Mean EWL was more than 20% in a 12-month follow-up and about 25% 2 years after the implementation. Baroscreen-selected[41] patients achieved a 31.4% EWL, versus 15% in the group not selected by this screening.[42]

United States O-01 Trial

The first study conducted in the United States was multicentric, double-blinded, randomized, and controlled. A total of 103 morbid obese patients were followed; in 100 of them, the procedure was laparoscopic, being open in 3. After the first month, patients were randomized in groups where the generator would be turned on or not. After 7 months, the inactive generator's group had them turned on too. Patients were followed monthly for 2 years. No dietary or behavioral counseling was offered. There were no deaths or complications related to the implant in the study. Although there were not any collateral effects from the procedure, 17 of the first 41 cases had migration of electrodes and conducting wires from the proper position.[43] This led to a technical modification and more adequate fixation of the wire to avoid dislodgements. This affected weight loss results in this group anyway. Curiously, during the first 6 months many patients admitted to have recklessly ingested food to identify if their respective generators were functional or not. Despite this bias, in the first-year follow-up 20% of the patients had lost 5% of total weight, with mean EWL of 11%.

DIGEST

Given the lessons learned from the European and American trials, a new study was launched in the United States with intent to improve IGS results. The Dual-Lead Implantable Gastric Electrical Stimulation Trial (DIGEST) involved 30 patients in two centers. In this trial, binge eaters were excluded, patients were advised to alimentary and behavioral changes, the system was composed of two wires (four electrodes) that could be programmed altogether or separate, and finally, programming was individual for each patient, which had not happened previously. A mean 15% EWL was observed in 38-week follow-up. In one of the centers, a mean EWL of 30.4% was noted in 9.5 months. In this group, 80% of the patients had lost weight and 60% had lost more than 10% excess weight. The great differences between these two groups reflected the differences in patient selection and corroborated the importance of this issue.

World experience with IGS has then proved that, like all surgical procedures for the treatment of obesity, no technique is equally effective for all patients, as shown by an international retrospective survey conducted in over 250 countries. Motivational aspects were important in the assessment of good results. Well-motivated patients displayed more satisfactory results. In both American studies, care about this selection issue would have excluded 75% of the patients who received the IGS implant. However, the remaining 25% would have obtained excellent results.

DISCUSSION

IGS displays some advantages when compared with other treatments for morbid obesity. There is no limiting of food intake or higher rates of esophageal reflux as in restrictive procedures such as vertical banded gastroplasty or gastric banding. Furthermore, there is no reason to believe that IGS could cause metabolic deficiencies due to malabsorption.

The exact mechanism of IGS action is yet to be defined. Although previously attributed to retarded gastric emptying, this was not ascertained in humans. Other causes were considered as an indirect effect through gastrointestinal hormone secretion and neural signaling generated by the IGS. Cigaina found alterations in the release of the hormones CCK and somatostatin[44] and lower basal levels of glucagon-like peptide and leptin as results of gastric electric stimulation. Other works with gastrointestinal hormones such a ghrelin are being conducted, and motilin may also play a role.[45] Xing suggested that gastric electric stimulation would lead to an expansion of the gastric fundus, hence causing satiety, like in a postprandial state.[46] Ouyang showed that gastric stimulation alters gastric slow waves,[47] while Chen discovered changes in the antrum contraction pattern.[48] Nutritional and psychological counseling revealed to be of utmost importance for the good results ascribed to IGS, as well as with other bariatric procedures. Motivated patients with good acceptance of habit modification had better results of sustained weight loss and satiety from meals.

Some issues are to be considered, though. The population of patients that would benefit most from the method still needs to be defined. Obesity is a very heterogeneous pathology. The development of patient-selection tools to identify the ones prone to respond adequately to the treatment would be the first step. Initial assessments showed good results with IGS use in patients with BMI between 35 and 40 kg/m^2, not repeated with patients with BMI > 60 kg/m^2. Perhaps IGS would be more effective in patients between 30 and 40 kg/m^2. Approximately 50 million Americans are in this BMI range; they are usually not considered for surgical treatment, and yet do not respond to other forms of therapy. IGS would be an attractive way of treating these individuals, as well as obese teenagers, for weight loss maintenance after other therapies.[12]

CONCLUSION

Weight loss caused by IGS is lower than the observed with other forms of surgical treatment, but higher when compared with nonsurgical modalities such as diet of medication. On the other hand, IGS has a much lower potential of surgical or metabolic complications than do other operative procedures. Thus, it might be beneficial to strata of the obese population not eligible to bariatric surgery by the present criteria. Some subsets of this population should be evaluated and compared by sex, body fat distribution (android X gynecoid), influence of preexisting comorbidities, and obesity degree. It is even possible that IGS plays a prophylactic role, preventing obese individuals to reach morbid weight levels and the development of related comorbidities.[2] Answers to these questions are to come from the ongoing studies and from the experience gained from the method application.

> We get the impression that this is the beginning of a long, exciting, challenging and potentially very rewarding investigative journey.
>
> —Dr. Mitiku Belachew

References

1. Kuczmarski RJ, Flegal KM, Campbell SM, et al.: Increasing prevalence of overweight among US adults. The National Health and Nutritional Surveys 1960 to 1991. *JAMA* 272:205–211, 1994.

2. Belachew M, Greenstein RJ: Implantable gastric stimulation (IGS) as therapy for human morbid obesity: Report from the 2001 IFSO symposium in Crete. *Obes Surg* 12, 3S–5S, 2002.

3. Mokdad AH, Ford ES, Bowman BA, et al.: Prevalence of obesity diabetes, and obesity-related health risk factors, 2001. *JAMA* 289:76–79, 2003.

4. Pi-Sunier FX: Medical hazards of obesity. *Ann Intern Med* 119:655–665, 1993.

5. Foster WS, Burton BT, Van Itallie TB: Health implications of obesity: NIH consensus development conference. *Ann Intern Med* 103(Suppl 2):981–1077, 1985.

6. Calle EE, Thun MJ, Ptrelli JM, et al.: Body-mass index and mortality in a prospective cohort of US adults. *N Engl J Med* 341:1097–1105, 1999.

7. McGinnis JM, Foege WH: Actual causes of death in the United States. *JAMA* 270:2207–2212, 1993.

8. Colditz GA: Economic costs of obesity and inactivity. *Med Sports* 31:S663–S667, 1999.

9. Rigby N: Call for obesity review as overweight numbers reach 1.7 billion. Online 2003. http://www.iotf.org/media/iotfmar17.htm

10. World Health Report 2002.

11. Gastrointestinal Surgery for Severe Obesity: National Institutes of Health Consensus Development Conference Statement. *Am J Clin Nutr* 55:615S–619S, 1992.

12. Shikora SA: Laparoscopic Gastric Pacing, in Inabnet WB, Demaria EJ, Ikramuddin S (eds.): *Laparoscopic Bariatric Surgery*, 1st ed. Philadelphia, LWW, 2004; p. 285.

13. Shikora SA, Chen J, Cigaina V: *Gastric Pacing*, in Martin LF (ed.): Obesity Surgery, 1st ed. New York, McGraw-Hill, 2003; p. 243.

14. Hasler WL: The physiology of gastric motility and gastric emptying. In: Yamada T, Alpers DH, Owyang C, Powell DW, Silverstein FE (eds.): *Textbook of Gastroenterology*. 2nd edn. Philadelphia, PA, Lippincott Williams & Wilkins, 1995; pp. 181–206.

15. Tougas G, Eaker EY, Abell TL, et al.: Assessment of gastric emptying using a low fat meal: Establishment of international control values. *Am J Gastroenterol* 95:1456–1462, 2000.

16. Quian LW, Pasricha PJ, Chen JDZ: Origins and patterns of spontaneous and drug-induced canine gastric myoelectrical dysrrythmia. *Dig Dis Sci* 48:508–515, 2003.

17. Philips RJ, Powley TL: Gastric volume rather then nutrient content inhibits food intake. *Am J Physiol* 271:R766–R779, 1996.

18. Duggan JP, Booth DA: Obesity, overeating and rapid gastric emptying in rats with ventromedial hypothalamic lesions. *Science* 231:609–611, 1986.

19. Wright RA, Krinsky S, Fleeman C, et al.: Gastric emptying and obesity. *Gastroenterology* 84:747–751, 1983.

20. Carlson AJ: *The Control of Hunger in Health and Disease*. Chicago, IL, University of Chicago Press, 1916.

21. Moran TH, McHugh PR: Cholecystokinin suppresses food intake by inhibiting gastric emptying. *Am J Phisiol* 242:R491–R497, 1982.

22. Asakawa A, Inui A, Ueno N, et al.: Urocortine reduces food intake and gastric emptying in lean and ob/ob MMice. *Gastroenterology* 116:1287–1292, 1999.

23. Miedema BW, Sarr MG, Kelly KA: Pacing the human stomach. *Surgery* 111:143–150, 1992.

24. Lin ZY, McCallum RW, Schirmer BD, et al.: Effects of pacing parameters in the entrainment of gastric slow waves in patients with gastroparesis. *Am J Physiol Gastrointest Liver Physiol* 274:G186–G191, 1998.

25. Eagon JC, Kelly KA: Effects of gastric pacing on canine gastric motility and emptying. *Am J Physiol* 265:G767–G774, 1993.

26. Hocking MP, Vogel SB, Sninsky CA: Human gastric myoelectrical activity and gastric following gastric surgery and with pacing. *Gastroenterology* 103:1811–1816, 1992.

27. Lin XM, Peters LJ, Hayes J, et al.: Entrainment of segmental small intestinal slow waves with electrical stimulation in dogs. *Dig Dis Sci* 45:652–656, 2000.

28. McCallum RW, Chen JDZ, Lin ZY, et al.: Gastric pacing improves emptying and symptoms in patients with gastroparesis. *Gastroenterology* 114:456–461, 1998.

29. Qian LW, Lin XM, Chen JDZ: Normalization of atropine-induced postprandial dysrhythmia with gastric pacing. *Am J Physiol Gastrointest Liver Phisyol* 276:G387–G392, 1999.

30. Abo M, Liang J, Qian LW, et al.: Normalization of distention-induced intestinal dysrhythmia with intestinal pacing in dogs. *Dig Dis Sci* 45:129–135, 2000.

31. Bellahsene BE, Lind CD, Schlimer BD, et al: Acceleration of gastric emptying with electrical stimulation in canine model of gastroparesis. *Am J Physiol* 262:G826–G834, 1992.

32. Yao S, Ke M, Wang Z, et al.: Visceral response to acute retrograde gastric electrical stimulation in healthy human. *World J Gastroenterol* 11(29):4541–4546, 2005.

33. Yao S, Ke M, Wang Z, et al.: Retrograde gastric pacing reduces food intake and delays gastric emptying in humans: a potential therapy for obesity: *Dig Dis Sci* 50(9):1569–1575, 2005.

34. Shikora SA: Implantable gastric stimulation for the treatment of severe obesity. *Obes Surg* 14:545–548, 2004.

35. Cigaina V: Gastric pacing as therapy for morbid obesity: Preliminary results. *Obes Surg* 12:12S–16S, 2002.

36. Cigaina VV, Saggioro A, Rigo VV et al.: Long-term effects of gastric pacing to reduce feed intake in swine. *Obes Surg* 6:250–253, 1996.

37. Cigaina V, Rigo V, Greenstein RJ: Gastric myo-electrical pacing as therapy for morbid obesity: Preliminary results [abstract]. *Obes Surg* 9:333–334, 1999. Abstract 33A.

38. Miller KA: Implantable electrical gastric stimulation to treat morbid obesity in the human: Operative technique. *Obes Surg* 12:17S–20S, 2002.

39. Favretti F, De Luca M, Segato G, et al.: Treatment of morbid obesity with the transcend implantable gastric stimulator: A prospective survey. *Obes Surg* 14:666–670, 2004.

40. D'Argent J: Gastric electrical stimulation as therapy of morbid obesity: Preliminary results from the french study. *Obes Surg*, 12, 21S–25S, 2002.

41. Shikora SA, Mande – Griffin R: Barroscreen: Using machine learning to improve patient selection for implantable gastric stimulation. *SCARD* 1(3):242–249, 2005.

42. Miller K, Hoeller E, Aigner F: The implantable gastric stimulator for obesity. An update of the European experience in the LOSS (laparoscopic obesity stimulation survey) study. *Treat Endocrinol* 5(1):53–58, 2006.

43. Shikora SA, Knox TA, Bailen L, et al.: Successful use of endoscopic ultrasounds (EU) to verify lead placement for implantable gastric stimulators (IGS). *Obes Surg* 11:403, 2001.

44. Cigaina V, Hirschberg A: Gastric pacing and neuroendocrine response: A preliminary report [abstract]. *Obes Surg* 10:334, 2000. Abstract 89.

45. Yang M, Fang D, Li Q, et al: Effects of gastric pacing on gastric emptying and plasma motilin. *World J Gastroenterol* 10(3):419–423, 2004.

46. Xing JH, Brody F, Brodsky J, et al.: Gastric electrical stimulation at proximal stomach induces gastric relaxation in dogs. *Neurogastroenterol Motil* 15:15–23, 2003.

47. Ouyang H, Yin J, Chen JD: Therapeutic potential of gastric electrical stimulation for obesity and its possible mechanisms: A preliminary canine study. *Dig Dis Sci* 48:698–705, 2003.

48. Chen JD, Qian L, Ouyang H, et al.: Gastric electrical stimulation with short pulses reduces vomiting but not dysrhythmias in dogs. *Gastroenterology* 124:401–409, 2003.

45

Intragastric Balloon

José A. Sallet, MD • João C. Marchesini, MD • Pablo Miguel, MD • Paulo C. Sallet, MD

INTRODUCTION

The incessant increase of obesity in the world and the natural evolution of science aiming at solving our patients' problems and based on two fundaments—safety and lesser trauma, minimizing risks in the treatment of this disease—were decisive factors to make us seek a new alternative technique, the intragastric balloon. We took into consideration the in- numerous patients with morbid obesity, the high rates of increase in weight with its associated diseases, the threats to their lives, and, in the case of surgery, the anguish caused to the patients themselves, doctors, and family members. In many cases, these patients would postpone surgeries, exposing themselves to an even greater risk: the excess weight itself with the limitations it imposes and its severe consequences; the interference in their quality of life and life expectancy.

The objective of this chapter is to report this method among our colleagues involved in the treatment of obesity, to establish multidisciplinary teams for both clinical and surgical treatment, as well as to inform the lay public and potential candidates about this technique. It is important to stress the selection criteria used to indicate this method of treatment to the patients. The target population consists of massively obese patients with severe associated illnesses (sleep apnea, DM, systemic arterial hypertension, etc.) in the preoperative period for bariatric, cardiovascular, orthopedic, abdominal surgery, or surgery in general. Another indication would be overweight individuals or patients with grade I obesity, who fail in well-oriented clinical treatment and suffer from or run the risk of developing associated diseases. It could also be a temporary option for morbid obesity patients who do not accept surgery or are not in good clinical condition for surgery. In this latter case, the procedure can in fact be repeated.

We would like to emphasize that the technical placement of the balloon is simple and can be performed by most endoscopists. What is essential for achieving good results is the preparation of a multidisciplinary team consisting of clinician, psychiatrist, psychologist, dietitian, and a physical activity professional.

As to correct and appropriate preparation of patients, the indications and limitations of the method should be made clear, thus avoiding unrealistic expectations. Likewise, it is important that patients comply with the treatment as a whole, understanding that the method "facilitates" following a hypocaloric diet and oriented physical activity.

BACKGROUND TO THE DEVELOPMENT OF THE BIB AND THE EVOLUTION OF ITS TECHNICAL CHARACTERISTICS

The concept of the balloon was developed through observation of the effects naturally caused by bezoar (formation of large food bolus impairing gastric emptying) in weight loss. The presence of bezoar leads to weight loss and its removal results in recovering initial weight. The SIB (later BIB) was developed incorporating the positive aspect of weight loss induced by bezoar and adapting to its physiology and anatomy.

The BIB was designed to be placed closed or deflated in the stomach and later expanded through injection of saline solution, thus acting as an artificial bezoar. Upon expansion, the BIB acquires a spherical shape. A valve permits the external catheter to be removed on closure of the valve. The BIB was designed to float freely in the stomach. Its shape allows adjusting volume for each patient during placement and during the course of treatment.

The design of the first SIB aimed at incorporating qualities that were considered fundamental for good performance of the intragastric balloon. These attributes were improved following a series of studies carried out by the SIB/BIB project and included the following features: Development of a thin external layer of silicone to avoid formation of protuberances on inflation, thus preventing irritation of the gastric mucosa,

erosions, or ulcers; this increases flexibility and enables more delicate handling, making it easier to place or remove the balloon with direct endoscopic visualization; the balloon may be inflated with air or liquid; it is made of a soft and very elastic biologically inert material, which may be safely used in vivo for a prolonged period; and it also permits radiological control in radiopaque areas.

The SIB system used in the first clinical study consisted of an elongated spherical balloon with a placement and retubing catheter, with the balloon being positioned, deflated, in the stomach via the esophagus. Afterward, the gastroscope was passed through the esophagus, beside the catheter, to allow direct observation of the balloon and its correct positioning in the stomach. Once in place in the intragastric space, the SIB was inflated with saline solution, up to a maximum volume of 700 mL. This would rupture the protective cover of the inserting catheter, and then the set comprising catheter/protective sheath was withdrawn through the mouth, via the esophagus.

After the SIB-001 1987–1988 intragastric balloon, the clinical studies were completed and results pointed to the need to improve the SIB prototype before initiating a new clinical study. Because of some cases of early deflation and in order to improve performance and durability of the SIB, some changes were made to its physical properties: Thickness of the balloon was increased and possible variations in thickness were controlled by various government inspections and the method of manufacturing the valve was altered to eliminate possible damage. The valve was redesigned and became more elongated and marks were added to its surface to help visualization and recognition of its exact position. The inserting catheter was simplified, using a PVC model that made it easier to introduce the balloon into the stomach.

In May 1989, permission was obtained from the Food and Drug Administration (FDA), U.S., to initiate the protocol study of the new SIB model, denominated SIB-002 A. Other improvements were made in BIB manufacture to get to the current shape; this brings the benefits of technical improvements associated with the fundamental characteristics of the original form. The BIB system consists essentially of the balloon itself, placement catheter, and the fill tube. The balloon is protected by a delicate silicone sheath which facilitates its oral insertion and progression. The sheath opens when the balloon is inflated. The radiopaque marks orient positioning the balloon and reentubing the valve.

EVOLUTION AND RESULTS OF CLINICAL INVESTIGATION IN THE UNITED STATES

In December 1986, the FDA protocol research division authorized INAMED Corporation to initiate a clinical study using the SIB (SIB-001 Protocol). Two investigation settings were approved: St. Francis Hospital, in Illinois, having Dr. Gau as the main investigator, and the University of Arizona, in Tucson, AZ, with Dr. Shneiderman as the main investigator. The study by Dr. Gau lasted 6 months and by

Dr. Schneiderman, 3 months, since some balloons could move with more prolonged use (over 3 months).

A total of 26 patients were selected for this study. Two patients were unable to receive the SIB due to contraindications in the selective endoscopic examination. Another two patients had the balloon removed on day 8 because of the intolerance to the balloon. The remaining 22 patients were divided into two groups. In Dr. Gau's group, 9 patients were morbidly obese (BMI > 40 kg/m^2) and in Dr. Schneiderman's group, 7 patients presented this characteristic.

Considering an average weight loss of 20%, Dr. Gau's patients lost 12% more weight than those of Dr. Schneiderman. This difference was probably due to the longer use of the balloon by Dr. Gau's patients. There were no deaths, neither were there any adverse reactions. No intestinal obstruction occurred and none of the balloons had to be removed surgically. Two patients had to be admitted to hospital; one patient developed a gastric ulcer, which was resolved after the removal of his second balloon; the other presented with intense vomiting and required intravenous rehydration. A third patient developed an ulcer in week 4 and did not respond to ranitidine; the ulcer healed after removal of the SIB. Three patients did not agree to adequate clinical control, resulting in less weight loss in comparison with the rest of the group. Another three patients gained weight again after spontaneous deflation of the SIB.

This study demonstrated that, in spite of the importance of dietetic control and the need to modify patients' lifestyle, weight loss was directly related to the use of the SIB. All the patients submitted to this study had poor results regarding weight loss in numerous other clinical treatments with diets, modification of living habits, and exercises. This fact made clear the importance of the SIB, promoting greater compliance of patients to clinical treatment and resulting in more adequate weight loss. The final results of these studies were submitted to the FDA by Dr. Schneiderman in October 1988 and by Dr. Gau, in March 1989.

EUROPEAN CLINICAL STUDY WITH THE SIB-002/SIB-002 A

After the end of the first clinical study, a new protocol proposing a second clinical study with the SIB-002 was submitted to FDA. In May 1989, after several modifications and additions, the FDA approved the SIB-002, which was denominated SIB-002 A. At the beginning of 1992, after refining the manufacture of the SIB, the FDA authorized INAMED to initiate a protocol study using the SIB-002 A in Holland. The study coordinator was Professor Lisbeth Mathus-Vliegen, who trained with Dr. Gau before beginning the study in Holland.

Professor Mathus-Vliegen carried out this study over a 2-year period. The results of the study were published in the "Annual Report for the IDE-1996" and, in 1997, in two reprints during the 8th European Congress of Obesity, held in Dublin, Ireland. This study involved 43 patients: 7 male and 36 female, mean age of 41.4 years. These individuals participated in the study for 2 years, including 1 year with active use of the balloon and 1-year follow-up without the balloon.

During the first 12 months, these patients received three balloons (one balloon every 4 months). The treatment program consisted of hypocaloric diet, psychological support, group meetings, and physical exercises. Out of 43 patients, 3 were excluded from study for not tolerating the balloon, 1 patient did not agree with placement of the balloon, and another spontaneously dropped out the protocol before insertion of the balloon. Out of the 38 patients who continued in the protocol, 5 (13%) did not lose sufficient weight and were excluded from the second phase of the study, 12 patients suffered from mild esophagitis, and 6 had severe esophagitis, with both groups recovering after the appropriate clinical treatment. Two patients experienced a transitory intolerance to the balloon and were submitted to another endoscopy to replace the valve and reduce the volume of the balloon by 100 mL, resulting in improved clinical symptoms. There were three cases of gastric erosion: one balloon deflated in the stomach and was removed endoscopically, while two other balloons moved spontaneously through the digestive tract. Cultures were randomly performed in the balloon liquid from 15 patients, and 3 had positive results. The average weight loss of these 15 patients during the first year of study (with the balloon) was 26.3 kg. However, the weight loss was partially maintained after withdrawal of the balloon; the average weight loss during 1-year follow-up was 14.7 kg.

Professor Mathus-Vliegen concluded that a multidisciplinary treatment obtained with moderate dietary restriction and the use of the intragastric balloon results in an average weight loss of 25 kg. Nevertheless, in spite of the maintenance of the multidisciplinary treatment, the withdrawal of the balloon resulted in partial weight gain in the patients studied.

BRAZILIAN MULTICENTRIC STUDY OF THE NEW INTRAGASTRIC BALLOON

First Stage of the results

Methods

Subjects: In the period from November 2000 to March 2006, more than 1000 patients were treated with BIB.

This study analyzes the results in the first stage of this technique used in Brazil in the period from November 2000 to February 2004; after the Brazilian Health Ministry's approval of BIB protocol, 483 overweight and obese patients recruited in six Brazilian private clinics were treated with the intragastric balloon (BIB). Demographic and clinical data from the 323 patients who completed a 6-month follow-up after BIB placement are provided in Table 45–1. The remainder 160 patients had not completed a 6-month follow-up yet. All patients were informed about the study and gave written consent.

Table 45–1.			

Demographic and Clinical Data at Baseline in 323 Obese Patients Submitted to the Intragastric Balloon for a Mean 6-Month Follow-Up

Demographic and Clinical Data	Men ($n = 127$) (39.3%)	Women ($n = 196$) (60.7%)	Subjects Total # ($n = 323$)
Age (years)	38.0 ± 12.9	37.2 ± 12.1	37.5 ± 12.4
Weight (kg)	134.1 ± 36.5	94.1 ± 21.0	110.1 ± 34.4
Weight excess (kg)[a]	56.2 ± 34.4	27.4 ± 19.5	38.7 ± 29.9
BMI (kg/m^2)	42.8 ± 10.6	35.2 ± 7.2	38.2 ± 9.4
Comorbidities	94 (74.0%)	62 (31.6%)	156 (48.3%)
Systemic hypertension	67 (52.8%)	35 (17.9%)	102 (31.6%)
Arthropathies	24 (18.9%)	47 (24.0%)	71 (22.0%)
Hyperlipoproteinemia	27 (21.3%)	16 (8.2%)	43 (13.3%)
Sleep apnea	26 (20.5%)	9 (4.6%)	35 (10.8%)
Diabetes mellitus	22 (17.3%)	13 (6.6%)	35 (10.8%)
Cardiovascular diseases	19 (15.0%)	12 (6.1%)	31 (9.6%)

Values are referred to as mean ± standard deviation.
[a] *Excess weight was calculated on the basis of kilograms exceeding a body mass index of 25 kg/m^2.*

Results

Six-month follow-up: Patients showed a global weight reduction from baseline BMI of 38.2 ± 9.4 kg/m^2 to 6-month BMI of 32.9 ± 8.3 kg/m^2 (paired samples t-test $= 28.0$, $p < 0.000$). Compared to baseline values, subjects showed highly significant reductions in weight (-15.2 ± 10.5 kg), BMI (-5.3 ± 3.4 kg/m^2), percent excess weight loss (%EWL $= 48.3 \pm 23.3\%$), and percent loss of total weight (%LTW $= 13.6 \pm 7.3\%$). Results distributed in gender and BMI differences are presented in Table 45–2 and Figure 45–1.

With regard to weight loss results, we have considered a generally accepted criterion in clinical treatments: the method failed if %EWL was lower than 20%. According to this criterion, 275 subjects (85.1%) succeeded and a global failure was observed in 48 subjects (14.9%). With reference to gender, in men the method succeeded in 99 cases (78.0%) and in women it succeeded in 176 cases (89.8%). Indeed, despite the fact that women showed lower baseline BMI compared to men (which should render women prone to higher %EWL), analysis of variance taking %EWL as dependent variable and baseline BMI as covariant showed a trend to better results in women (F $= 3.5$, $p = 0.06$). Age showed no significant correlation with %EWL or BMI reduction. However, 21 adolescents (age ≤ 18 years) changed from a pretreatment BMI of 36.5 ± 8.4 kg/m^2 to a 6-month BMI of 31.5 ± 9.1 kg/m^2 (BMI reduction $= -5.0 \pm 3.6$ kg/m^2), with a mean %EWL of $57.4 \pm 37.0\%$. The 5 adolescents who completed a 1-year follow-up maintained a mean %EWL of $46.5 \pm 30.4\%$—a result statistically not different from their 6-month %EWL of $49.2 \pm 27.3\%$ (t-test $= 0.35$, $p = 0.74$).

Massively obese patients (baseline BMI > 50 kg/m^2) under preoperative preparation ($n = 32$) showed mean weight loss of 26.1 kg (range: 3.6–77.0 kg), mean %EWL of 23.5% (range: 3.0–54%), and mean BMI reduction of 8.5 kg/m^2 (range: 1.3–24.9 kg/m^2). Considering surgical risk, most patients (16 patients with %EWL $> 20\%$, 66% of cases) showed a significant improvement from American Society of Anesthiology (ASA) III-IV before placement of the balloon to ASA II, with easier control of comorbidities, particularly hypertension, diabetes mellitus, and sleep apnea. These results enabled safer surgical procedures. Patients with BMI < 35 kg/m^2 ($n = 148$) showed a %EWL of $63.4 \pm 28.6\%$, both men and women showing a rate of success of 94%.

Estimation of global benefits: From the 323 subjects taken for the study, 76 were followed with the Bariatric Analysis and Reporting Outcome System (BAROS), a specific questionnaire for bariatric surgery involving %EWL, clinical improvement, procedure's complications, and quality of life.[2] Total BAROS was designated as insufficient by 4 (5.3%), acceptable by 7 (9.2%), good by 43 (56.6%), very good by 18 (23.7%), and excellent by 4 (5.3%) subjects. Clinical comorbidities were regarded as unchanged in 7 (9.2%), improved in 31 (40.8%), and one of them solved with others improved in 38 (50%) cases. Most of these subjects described a global improvement in the quality of life subscale (mean of 1.6 ± 0.8).

The most prevalent side effects were nausea and vomiting (129 cases, 39.9%). Epigastric pain affected 65 patients (20.1%). There was dehydration requiring intravenous saline infusion in 15 patients (4.6%), and 11 patients (3.4%) had early intolerance leading to prosthesis removal.

Table 45–2.

Results Regarding Weight Loss, Percent Excess Weight Loss, and BMI Reduction in 323 Patients Distributed Along BMI Categories and Sexual Gender Treated with the Intragastric Balloon at 6-Month Follow-Up

BMI Category (Baseline) (kg/m²)	N	Weight Loss (kg)	Percent Excess Weight Loss (%)	BMI reduction (kg/m²)
Men	127 (39.3%)	18.7 ± 13.4	38.8 ± 24.5	5.9 ± 4.2
25–30	4 (3.1%)	8.0 ± 4.5	69.4 ± 35.4	2.9 ± 1.4
30–35	30 (23.6%)	14.9 ± 10.9	54.4 ± 26.9	4.6 ± 3.1
35–40	29 (22.8%)	15.1 ± 11.7	38.3 ± 24.5	4.7 ± 3.6
40–50	37 (29.1%)	20.4 ± 10.9	34.5 ± 17.7	6.5 ± 3.4
>50	27 (21.3%)	26.0 ± 17.9	23.2 ± 12.9	8.2 ± 5.8
Women	196 (60.7%)	12.9 ± 7.2	54.4 ± 28.7	4.8 ± 2.6
25–30	33 (16.8%)	8.2 ± 4.6	77.5 ± 30.8	3.0 ± 1.7
30–35	81 (41.3%)	12.4 ± 5.5	61.2 ± 26.4	4.7 ± 2.1
35–40	58 (29.6%)	12.7 ± 6.8	39.4 ± 21.7	4.8 ± 2.5
40–50	19 (9.7%)	20.5 ± 8.7	38.9 ± 15.9	7.4 ± 3.0
>50	5 (2.6%)	26.4 ± 5.2	25.2 ± 3.4	9.9 ± 2.1
Total	323 (100%)	15.2 ± 10.5	48.3 ± 28.1	5.3 ± 3.4
25–30	37 (11.5%)	8.1 ± 4.5	76.7 ± 30.9	3.0 ± 1.7
30–35	111 (34.4%)	13.1 ± 7.4	59.4 ± 26.6	4.7 ± 2.4
35–40	87 (26.9%)	13.5 ± 8.7	39.0 ± 22.6	4.7 ± 2.9
40–50	56 (17.3%)	20.4 ± 10.1	36.0 ± 17.1	6.8 ± 3.3
>50	32 (9.9%)	26.1 ± 16.5	23.5 ± 11.9	8.5 ± 5.4

Results are reported as mean ± standard deviation.

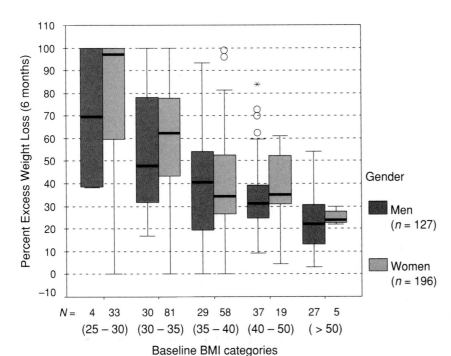

Figure 45–1. Boxplot showing percent excess weight loss in 323 patients treated with the intragastric balloon (BIB) at 6-month follow-up.

Table 45–3.

Results Regarding Weight Loss in 85 Patients Treated with the Intragastric Balloon after 1-Year Follow-Up

Subjects	Baseline BMI (kg/m^2)	6-month BMI Reduction	6-month %EWL	1-year BMI Reduction	1-year %EWL
Men ($n = 42$)	41.9 ± 8.9	6.8 ± 3.4	47.7 ± 25.3	6.5 ± 4.4	43.3 ± 25.9
Women ($n = 43$)	34.4 ± 4.1	6.0 ± 2.4	66.8 ± 24.2	5.3 ± 2.9	58.4 ± 29.8
Total ($n = 85$)	38.1 ± 7.8	6.4 ± 3.0	57.4 ± 26.4	5.9 ± 3.7	50.9 ± 28.8

Minor complications were clinically controlled: reflux esophagitis in 40 patients (12.4%) and symptomatic gastric stasis in 28 patients (8.7%) due to transient obstruction of the pyloric antrum by the balloon. Major complications were balloon impaction (2 cases, 0.6%) in the antrum with gastric hyperdistension, requiring removal of gastric content under general anesthesia. There was one case (0.3%) of spontaneous deflation of the balloon and migration to the digestive tract, causing intestinal obstruction after 5 months of BIB placement. This patient was submitted to conservative treatment in the first 24 hours without satisfactory result. Therefore, we decided to perform a minilaparotomy and the prosthesis was located at 40 cm from the ileocecal valve. We induced its movement up to the right colon, with simultaneous removal by colonoscopy, avoiding further complications. The spontaneous balloon deflation was related to the patient spontaneously discontinuing his daily dose of omeprazole, which probably caused damage to the prosthesis by the persistent action of gastric acid.

One-year follow-up: Patients who completed 1 year after BIB placement (6 months after BIB removal) were contacted by mail or telephone call and invited for a reinforcement visit in their respective clinics. Table 45–3 shows results regarding 85 patients who have returned for a visit (34% of the 250 patients who completed 1 year after BIB placement). Overall, these patients have maintained a substantial weight reduction, even if their 1-year %EWL ($50.9 \pm 28.8\%$) was significantly lower than their 6-month %EWL ($57.4 \pm 26.4\%$) (t-test = 2.9, $p = 0.004$). However, 17 patients who were followed 2 years after BIB placement (11% of the 158 patients who completed 2 years after BIB placement) showed 2-year %EWL ($56.9 \pm 36.5\%$) not significantly different from their 6-month %EWL ($66.1 \pm 28.0\%$) (t-test = 1.4, $p = 0.19$) (Table 45–4).

THE INTRAGASTRIC BALLOON PROTOCOL

Indications

1. Patients with a BMI > 35 kg/m^2, who are resistant to clinical treatment or present contraindications to surgical treatment, or who do not accept surgical treatment and present obesity-associated diseases.

2. Patients with a BMI < 35 kg/m^2, presenting with secondary diseases associated with obesity or resistant to regular clinical treatment for obesity for a period longer than 3 years, contraindication to drugs used in clinical treatment or susceptible to secondary diseases concomitant to treatment with medication (secondary hypothyroidism, drug-dependent psychiatric disorders).

3. Preparation and selection of patients with extreme obesity (BMI > 50 kg/m^2) for gastric restrictive surgery (BIB test). Reduction of anesthetic risk (bariatric surgery, general surgery, orthopedic surgery, cardiovascular surgery, paroxysmal nocturnal dyspnea, sleep apnea, etc.).

4. Reduction of surgical risk (extreme BMI with associated diseases).

5. Reduction of clinical risk of severe chronic diseases or those that cause disability.

Contraindications

Absolute
- previous gastric surgery
- alcohol or drug dependence
- active gastric or duodenal ulcer
- chronic use of anticoagulants
- collagen diseases
- inflammatory bowel diseases (Crohn's, ulcerative colitis)
- hiatal hernia >5 cm
- hepatic cirrhosis
- chronic renal failure
- pregnancy
- AIDS

Relative
- potential upper gastrointestinal bleeding conditions (excluding those related to portal hypertension)
- grade III esophagitis
- Barrett's esophagus
- chronic use of NSAIDs and anticoagulant agents

Pre-procedure Routine

Routine laboratory tests
- full blood count
- glycemia

Table 45–4.

PubMed—MEDLINE Indexed Studies on Obese Patients Treated with the BioEnterics Intragastric Balloon (BIB)

Reference	Sample	Method	BL Weight	BL BMI	Weight loss	%EWL	BMI Reduction	Side Effects	Complications	Comments
1. Galloro et al. (1999)[11]	13 (6:7)	BIB	134.4	47.6	10.1	18.3	4.1	–	Peptic ulcer (1); candidiasis (1)	
2. Vandenplas et al. (1999)[a,19]	5 adolescents	BIB	198.6	BMI% (148–293%)	3 m–11.2 6 m–+10.2	–	–	–	–	BMI reduced at 3 months and increased at 6 months
3. Weiner et al. (1999)[12]	14 (7:7)	BIB	194.7	60.2	18.1	±16	±5.6	–	Early removal (2); BIB dysfunction (1)	BIB preoperative for LAGB
4. Doldi et al. (2000)[a,14]	132 (36:96)	BIB diet 1000 kcal/day	115.4	41.0	14.4	–	5.2	Vomiting leading to removal in 9 cases (7%)	Early removal (9); spontaneous deflation (1); gastric ulcer (2)	(*) Preliminary report of Doldi et al. (2002). Better results in males
5. Hodson et al. (2001)[a,15]	10 (1:9)	BIB diet 800 kcal/day	–	39	18.6	40	–	Vomiting (1)	BIB rupture (1)	Patients with 1 balloon had %EWL of 19%; patients with 2 balloons had %EWL of 54%
6. Loffredo et al. (2001)[16]	64 (23:54)	BIB BIB-test	128.0	46.6	14.3	23.5	5.3	–	Gastric ulcer (2); spontaneous deflation (15); candidiasis (4)	Good results with BIB predict good outcome with gastric banding
7. Totte et al. (2001)[17]	126 (5:121)	BIB diet 800 kcal/day	Weight excess = 35.3 kg	37.7	15.7	50.8	5.7	(69 eligible) Vomiting (41)	Early removal (3); reflux esophagitis (11)	Final evaluation in 69 patients (bias). Satisfaction correlated poorly with %EWL
8. Evans et al. (2001)[18]	63 (10:59)	BIB	124.5	46.3	15	18.7	5.6	Vomiting (31)	Early removal (4); displacement (18); obstruction (3) (laparotomy)	
9. Doldi et al. (2002)[14]	281 (73:208)	BIB diet 1000 kcal/day	117.4	41.8	13.9	18.1	4.8	–	Early removal (17); deflation (5); gastric ulcer + erosion (4)	BIB + diet produced higher WL than diet alone
10. Sallet et al. (2004)[9]	323 (127:196)	BIB diet 1000 kcal/day	110.1 ± 34.4	38.2 ± 9.4	15.2 ± 10.5	48.3 ± 23.3	5.3 ± 3.4	Vomiting (129); Epigastric pain (65)	Early intolerance (11); reflux esophagitis (40); gastric stasis (28); impaction (2); deflation (1)	Best indications: preoperative in superobese, teenagers, and BMI < 35 kg/m²
Mean of studies[b]	884 Females (72%) Male (28%)	BIB + Diet (800–1000 kcal/day)	117.5 kg	40.9 kg/m²	14.7 kg	34.2 %	5.2 kg/m²	Side effects: Vomiting: 202/465 (43%); epigastric pain: 65/323 (20%)	Complications: Early intolerance (removal): 37/807 (4.6%); reflux esophagitis: 51/449 (11%); spontaneous deflation: 23/692 (3.3%); intestinal obstruction: 4/884 (0.5%)	

[a] Not included in the analysis due to lacking or repeated data.
[b] Means weighted for the size of the studies.

- parasitological examination of feces
- Na$^+$
- K$^+$
- creatinine
- coagulogram
- albumin
- cholesterol—total and fractions
- triglycerides
ECG
- with heart evaluation, if necessary
- chest x-ray
- spirometry, in case of associated respiratory disease
- upper abdomen ultrasound
- psychological assessment
- esophagogastroduodenoscopy with test for *Helicobacter pylori* (30 days before placement of BIB)
- in the presence of *H. pylori* or diseases such as gastritis or ulcer, proceed with treatment.

Procedure (Please see the DVD)

1. The BIB placement procedure should be carried out on outpatient basis or in a day hospital regimen, and the patient is admitted in the morning.
2. Placement should be performed under deep sedation or superficial general anesthesia, at the anesthesiologist's discretion, with heart monitoring and oximetry.
3. Introduction of the deflated balloon through the mouth and positioning in the stomach cavity, under endoscopic control.
4. Injection of 500 mL (400–700 mL) of 0.9% isotonic saline solution with 10 mL methylene blue, under endoscopic control.
5. After inflation of the balloon, carry out maneuver to close the balloon valve.
6. Cephalic traction of inflation probe, slowly, until the balloon is freed within the stomach, withdrawing the probe and the outer wrapping of the balloon via the esophagus.
7. Checking on correct positioning of the balloon under endoscopic control.
8. Patient is discharged 2 hours after placement of the balloon and, if necessary, receives home care. The balloon is kept in an average for 4 months (maximum 6 months).

Follow-Up

- Continuous use of omeprazole 40 mg/day while the balloon is in place.
- In case of intolerance after 7 days, the removal of the balloon should be considered.
- Follow-up visits for medical control: weeks 1, 2, and 4; after that a minimum of once-a-month checking after placement, up to removal of the balloon.
- Abdominal ultrasound in the third month to evaluate balloon volume.

- Control of feces and urine color.
- Follow-up by dietitian, psychiatrist, or psychologist and physical instructor.

Removal of the Intragastric Balloon

1. The removal of the balloon should be done preferentially under deep sedation or general anesthesia, at the anesthesiologist discretion, with cardiorespiratory assessment.
2. After the patient has been sedated, the digestive endoscopy is initiated and the balloon is positioned in the fundus.
3. Perform a "U"-turn maneuver with the endoscope tip and proceed with puncturing of the BIB with a sclerosis needle, which should penetrate into the balloon 10 cm. Remove the needle and initiate suction of the liquid measuring the volume aspirated. The balloon should be completely empty in order to be removed.
4. After it is completely empty, the balloon should be grabbed with the two-pronged wire grasper at the opposite end of the valve.
5. The balloon should be extracted slowly and gradually; it should always be kept together with the tip of the endoscope.
6. After removal, the patient should be kept under observation for 30 minutes, and then discharged.

Complications

- Deflation of the balloon and natural expulsion—0.25% to 1%.
- meteorism—8%
- nausea and persistent pain (>2 weeks after placement)—3%
- ulcer from decubitus—1%
- peptic ulcer—1%
- spontaneous deflation of BIB, evolving with intestinal obstruction and need for surgical treatment—0.13% to 0,25%
- Gastric perforation—0.05%

Day Hospital Anesthetics Protocol for Placement and Removal of the Intragastric Balloon

- Preanesthetic evaluation
- Drugs used during the procedure
  - Fentanyl 1.0–1.5 μg/kg IV
  - propofol 0.015–0.035 mg/kg/min IV in infusion pump or microdrops
  - ondansetron 8 mg IV
  - dexamethasone 2.5 mg IV
  - Buscopan 20 mg IV
- Anesthetic procedure—Conscious sedation, maintaining natural and assisted breathing, with oxygen 100% 5 L/min through nasal catheter (98% of our patients), or under general anesthesia (only 2% of our patients).

- Postanesthetic recovery—The patient remains in the recovery room until discharge, in accordance with the criteria set by resolution 1363/93 of the Federal Medical Council.
- Monitoring—During the whole procedure, the patient will be monitored by cardioscopy, oximetry, and noninvasive measurement of blood pressure by means of automated equipment. Monitoring continues in the recovery room until discharge.
- Postdischarge orientation—Antiemetic medication, PO, ondansetron (4 times a day) for 72 hours, omeprazole 40 mg, oral via, until the sixth month (during all the time in which the BIB is in the stomach); buscopan, 4 times a day, during 3 days, and in the event of uncontrollable nausea and vomiting, prescribe IV therapy. The first-line antiemetic agent is ondansetron 32 mg/day, divided into three doses (every 8 hours).

NUTRITIONAL ORIENTATION

The objective of this orientation is to make the body adapt to the new condition brought about by the presence of the intragastric balloon.

First three days after BIB placement. During the first 2–3 days after placement of the BIB, a semiliquid diet is recommended, that is, thin semisolid foods, such as thin soups prepared in blender, porridges made from corn flour or oats, soft gelatin, water, juices, milk, thin mashed potatoes, bean broth, and blended papaya or banana. At this stage it is important to

- have 3–4 meals a day (breakfast, lunch, afternoon snack, and dinner);
- take small mouthfuls, holding the head in an upward position;
- make sure that there is an interval of at least 1 hour between meals;
- avoid excessive consumption of condiments like pepper, oil, and salt;
- drink 1–1.5 L of liquids per day (water, tea, juices);
- avoid coffee (use decaffeinated coffee), chocolate, cold foods like ice cream, sweets in general, soft drinks and other fizzy drinks, fat foods in general, and snacks.

After the fourth day. Begin transition to solid diet, e.g.,
Breakfast: milk or yogurt, 150 mL; savory biscuit, 1.
Lunch: noodles, two tablespoons; shredded chicken, two tablespoons; cooked vegetables, carrot, pumpkin).
Afternoon snack: 4 tablespoons papaya or banana.
Dinner: mashed potatoes, 1 tablespoon; stewed fish, 3 tablespoons; cooked vegetables, broccoli, zucchini, beetroot.

Note: During this phase, the transition should take place gradually over the following 4 days. If there is vomiting, return to the semiliquid diet for three successive meals.

DIETARY REEDUCATION FIFTEEN DAYS AFTER PLACEMENT OF THE BIB

It is particularly important that the prescribed dietary indications be strictly followed rigorously during the adaptation period.

Orientations

- During the first month light food is indicated.
- Eat very slowly! Rest the cutlery on the plate between mouthfuls.
- Upon beginning to eat solid food, it is absolutely essential to ingest only small quantities in each mouthful, chewing food very well!
- Do not drink liquids during the meal, but drink approximately 10 glasses of water throughout the day. Always wait for 1 hour after eating before you drink. Avoid fizzy water.
- Do not drink coffee, chocolate drinks, and soft drinks (even diet ones).
- Divide food intake into three main meals and, if necessary, two mid-day snacks.
- Control the amount of oil used in preparation of food to a maximum of 4 teaspoons.
- Have meat, fish, or chicken once a day. Consume plenty of greens and fruits in all meals, varying them as much as possible, depending on what is in season.
- Do not lie down soon after meals.
- Do not eat between meals.
- Do not eat while watching television, studying, or working.
- Do not eat foods that are rich in fat, such as fried snacks (pasties, savories, etc.); cold cuts (salami, frankfurters, ham, etc.); sweets (especially those containing cream, condensed milk, or whipped cream), chocolate, ice creams, fat meats (sausage, cuts of beef with fat, bacon, leg of pork, etc.), and mayonnaise-based sauces or dressings.
- Use only sweeteners to sweeten liquids. These may be aspartame (Zero Cal, Finn, or Equal®), cyclamate/saccharine (Tal e Qual), or sucralose (Splenda).
- Prefer white meat (poultry and fish), always grilled, baked, or cooked.
- Use only skimmed dairy products: milk (Molico), cottage cheese, ricotta, and light Minas type cheese (Danúbio), light yogurts).
- Choose whole grain or diet breads.
- Instead of sweets, choose diet gelatins or fresh fruits for dessert.
- Season salads with vinegar, salt, mustard, or soy sauce. Do not use oils, olive oil, or mayonnaise-based dressings.
- In case of vomiting, return to a light diet for three consecutive meals.

- Keep a food diary: write down everything that you are actually consuming (quantity and quality), in particular specify gastrointestinal symptoms (nausea, difficulty in swallowing, regurgitation, vomiting, and diarrhea).

ORIENTATION FOR PHYSICAL ACTIVITY

After the appropriate cardiorespiratory and physical conditioning assessment (carried out during the preparation for placement of the intragastric balloon), the patient is oriented to proceed with daily aerobic physical activities (walking, swimming, hydrogymnastics, etc.), for a minimum of 40 min/day and combined with weight lifting under the physical instructor's orientations.

PSYCHOLOGICAL SUPPORT

The frequency of psychological support after placement of the intragastric balloon should be determined based on the individual needs of each specific patient, minimum once a month.

References

1. Sallet JA, Marchesini JB, Miguel P, et al.: Brazilian multicentric study of the Intragastric Balloon. *Obes Surg* 14(7):991–998, 2004.
2. Galloro G, De Palma GD, Catanzano C, et al.: Preliminary endoscopic technical report of a new silicone intragastric balloon in the treatment of morbid obesity. *Obes Surg* 9(1):68–71, 1999.
3. Weiner R, Gutberlet H, Bockhorn H: Preparation of extremely obese patients for laparoscopic gastric banding by gastric-balloon therapy. *Obes Surg* 9(3):261–264, 1999.
4. Doldi SB, Micheletto G, Perrini MN, et al.: Treatment of morbid obesity with intragastric balloon in association with diet. *Obes Surg* 12(4):583–587, 2002.
5. Hodson RM, Zacharoulis D, Goutzamani E, et al.: Management of obesity with the new intragastric balloon. *Obes Surg* 11(3):327–329, 2001.
6. Loffredo A, Cappuccio M, DeLuca M, et al.: Three experience with the new intragastric balloon, and a preoperative test for success with restrictive surgery. *Obes Surg* 11(3):330–333, 2001.
7. Totte E, Hendrickx L, Pauwels M, et al.: Weight reduction by means of intragastric device: Experience with the bioenterics intragastric balloon. *Obes Surg* 11(4):519–523, 2001.
8. Evans JD, Scott MH: Intragastric balloon in the treatment of patients with morbid obesity. *Br J Surg* 88(9):1245–1248, 2001.
9. Vandenplas Y, Bollen P, De Langhe K, et al.: Intragastric balloons in adolescents with morbid obesity. *Eur J Gastroenterol Hepatol* 11(3):243–245, 1999.

46

Hand-Assisted Laparoscopic Duodenal Switch

Robert A. Rabkin, MD, FACS

I. INTRODUCTION AND OVERVIEW

II. THE OPERATION—STEP BY STEP

III. DISCUSSION

IV. CONCLUSION

INTRODUCTION AND OVERVIEW

Gastric reduction/duodenal switch procedure is the most physiologically sound of current commonly performed weight loss operations. It is a combined procedure that relies on both moderate restriction and controlled absorption. The restrictive component arises from a vertical gastrectomy, wherein the easily expendible greater curvature of the stomach is removed leaving a 2–3-cm wide gastric tube along the lesser curvature of the stomach. This preserves the gastric antrum, which retains the gastric resevoir capabilities to macerate protein rich food, and protects the normal emptying mechanism of the stomach. It also preserves contact between food and the most proximal portion of the duodenum, a segment which neutralizes gastric acid and produces important intestinal hormones. To reduce absorption, the most distal 250 cm of ileum is employed to conduct the foodstream and the channel common to food and biliopancreatic juices.

Like most intra-abdominal operations, exposure for gastric reduction/duodenal switch procedure can be established using a traditional extended midline incision or via minimally invasive laparoscopic techniques. Safety must

always be the highest priority. A secondary consideration is the maintenance as much as possible of the same materials and calibrations regardless of type of exposure. That being said, there are advantages and disadvantages to each technique and accordingly times where one technique may be preferable. In this chapter we will discuss the hand-assisted laparoscopic approach. We will discuss the procedure step by step and describe other techniques which we have used but subsequently discarded and why.

THE OPERATION—STEP BY STEP

The midline is incised 18 cm below the xyphoid and the incision extended 7-cm caudad. This distance most often coincides with the level of the umbilicus, and therefore works well to minimize cosmetic concerns. Additionally this facilitates the repair of umbilical hernias which are not infrequent.

Exploration of the abdomen is performed in the usual manner. Using a large Richardson retractor, the cecum can be grasped with a Babcock clamp and the appendix identified. If present, at this point early in the procedure the mesoappendix only is transected using the Ligasure device. To minimize the potential for contamination, the appendix itself will be transected only at the conclusion of the procedure.

The terminal ileum is now identified. By grasping the ileum in serial fashion with two large Babcock clamps under moderate tension (to achieve "maximum stretch"), the ileum is measured and marked at 100 cm from the ileocecal valve with two sutures, of which the more proximal is cut short. This identifies not only the 100-cm distance from the ileocecal valve, but also marks the direction of the bowel. This distance may be diminished or extended, by referencing it to 10% of the total bowel length[1]; however, we utilize the 100-cm length as described by Marceau et al.[2]

Measuring of the bowel is continued proximally for an additional 150 cm. It is again marked with doubled strands of suture to distinguish this area from the previously marked 100-cm site. According to Hess and Hess, a dividing point marking at 30% of the total bowel length may be used.[1] The remainder of the small bowel is measured and total length is recorded. The small bowel is transected between the sutures at the more proximal mark using the linear stapler. We use the 3.5-mm staple length cartridges throughout the entire procedure for simplicity but one could use the 2.5-mm staple length cartridges for the small bowel.

The mesentery at this location is divided for a distance of 6 cm to achieve length adequate to reach proximal duodenum. The line of division is made with the Ligasure device oriented perpendicular to the long axis of the bowel to avoid devascularizing the respective ends. The distal part of the transected small bowel is cleared of mesentery for a 3–4 cm distance with *Metzenbaum* scissors. We do not use cautery in this area and accept a small amount of oozing in order to avoid the potential for electrical injury. After this preparation, the bowel is then sutured to an 8-cm rubber tube. (This tubing will be used later as a handle to identify this bowel and to bring it up to the duodenum.)

The proximal end of transected small bowel (biliopancreatic limb) is then brought inferolaterally and juxtaposed to the small bowel 100 cm from the ileocecal valve. It is then anastomosed to the small bowel at this location. The mesenteric defect is now closed. The hand port is then placed in the midline incision. One 10-mm port is then placed with the guidance of the surgeon's left hand about 2 fingerbreadths lateral to the hand port on the patient's right side. A 12-mm port is placed about 4 fingerbreadths lateral to this port and a second 12-mm port is placed about 4 fingerbreadths lateral to the hand port in the left abdomen.

CO_2 insufflation is established at 15-cm water pressure. Two insufflators are used—one on each 12-mm port site, leaving the camera port (immediately to the right of the hand port) available to vent smoke as needed. A small stab incision is made at the xyphoid and through this the right lobe of the liver is sampled using a biopsy needle. The needle exit site is cauterized for hemostasis.

Divide adhesions as necessary. Using a fascial closure device, doubled #2-0 nylon ties are placed at the xyphoid incision around the round ligament and held up with a Kelly

clamp. This maneuver will retract the liver and the ligament from the operative field. Suture the 8-cm rubber tubing at the greater curvature aspect of the pylorus and using this mark the greater curvature of the stomach at 7-cm proximal to the pylorus with a clip.

Dissect the lateral aspect of the duodenum from just proximal to where the pancreas becomes adherent to the duodenum toward the pylorus. Grab the base of the gallbladder and retract laterally using the hook cautery. Grasp the duodenum with the Dorsey instrument and retract it lateral and cephalad to facilitate dissection of the medial aspect of the duodenum from the pancreas and retroperitoneum. Once a window is developed between the retroperitoneum and the duodenum, transect duodenum with the linear stapler as far distally as possible. Note that it is important to dissect directly on the duodenum to avoid excessive bleeding.

At that time you can proceed to the cholecystectomy when present. The greater curvature of the stomach is now cleared of all vessels starting from the marking clip previously placed 6-cm proximal to the pylorus to the angle of His using the Ligasure instrument. At this point the anesthesiologist will pass a #58F bougie into the stomach. Vertical gastrectomy is now performed using serial firings of the 60 mm × 3.5 mm linear stapler starting at about 6 cm from the pylorus and continuing toward the angle of His. A helpful landmark to follow is the line along which the lesser curvature vessels disappear into the serosa, staying a comfortable distance from the bougie and this will correspond to the area where the vessels on the anterior aspect of the stomach disappear into the serosa. Deliver the greater curvature of the stomach.

After bluntly making a hole in the transverse colon mesentery overlying the duodenum, the ileum may be brought up retrocolic, using the rubber tubing as a handle, to the duodenum. The bowel is now checked from the cecum through the distal anastomosis and up to the area of the duodenum making sure there are no twists in the bowel from placing it through the retrocolic tunnel.

Perform the duodenal–ileal anastomosis using a triangulation technique with the linear blue stapler as follows (Figure 46–1(a)). Cut a small hole in the mesenteric border of the ileum which was earlier cleared of mesentery. Cut a small hole on either side of the duodenum adjacent to the corners of the staple-line. Holding the corner of the staple-line of the duodenum with a Maryland grasper will facilitate this. Place and fire the 45 mm × 3.5 mm linear stapler after placing cartridge into the ileum and anvil into the duodenum. The stapler should be positioned immediately past the lateral hole in the duodenum to allow the proper amount of posterior wall to be stapled but not make too large a defect in the small bowel when it fires.

Three sutures (black, white, and purple) are used to approximate the hole in the medial aspect of the anastomosis making sure the black suture is across the posterior staple-line. Retract the #58F bougie back to the gastroesophageal junction and advance the inner #32 tube through the pylorus and into the ileum. Holding traction on the three sutures, place a second 45 mm × 3.5 mm linear stapler across the

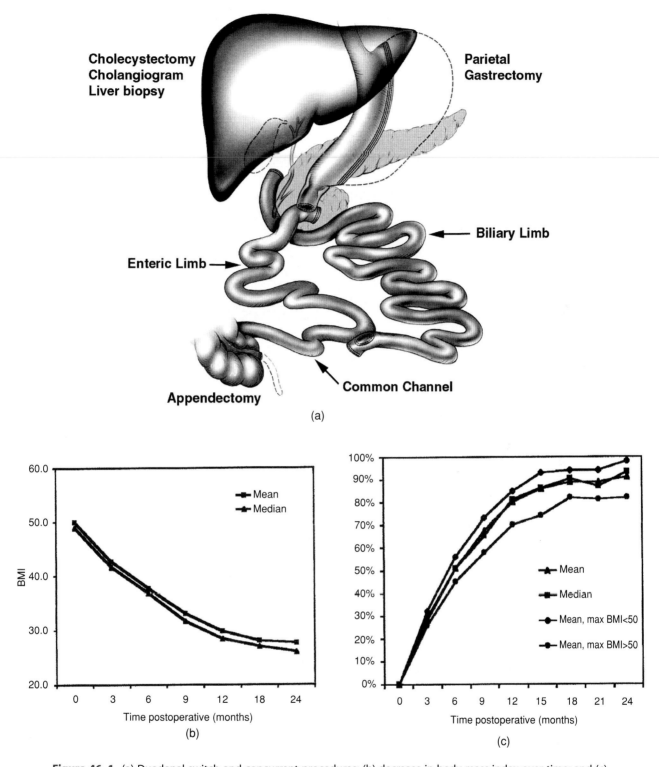

Figure 46–1. (a) Duodenal switch and concurrent procedures; (b) decrease in body mass index over time; and (c) percent excess weight loss over time.

anteromedial defect. The crotch of the instrument must incorporate the black suture that is across the initial posterior staple-line to ensure that the entire hole closes. After firing this second staple-line, place a single holding suture across the posterior staple-line lateral to the hole in the duodenum. Fire a third 45 mm × 3.5 mm linear stapler across the remaining defect. Remove the small piece of distal ileum with

a small part of the distal duodenum. When complete, the anastamosis should give an end-to-end appearance stapled circumferentially.

Note: We have constructed the proximal anastomosis in a retrocolic fashion using at various times the circular stapler and the Valtrac anastomosing ring. Neither of the latter techniques proved as reliable or as versatile and on occasion, because of the size or angulation, the small bowel was noted to tear, particularly when attempting antecolic proximal anastamosis. The circular stapler technique yields fewer strictures when a #25 diameter anvil is used, and we have found that this is the easiest and most consistent technique; however, the #25 anvil does not always pass readily through the pylorus, necessitating purse string placement on those occasions.

Withdraw the #32 inner tube back into the proximal duodenum and pull the #58F bougie back to the gastroesophageal junction to occlude the gastroesophageal junction. Clamp the ileum just distal to the anastomosis and infuse into the stomach, by gravity, methylene blue colored saline solution to check for the leaks as well as to calibrate the size of the stomach.

Transect the appendix from the cecum with a linear stapling instrument. The midline fascia is closed with #1 PDS and the skin is closed with 3-0 and 4-0 subcuticular Biosyn. All patients undergo a water-soluble contrast upper gastrointestinal x-ray series on the first postoperative day, after which a clear liquid diet is started.[3]

DISCUSSION

Although initially more time consuming than open laparotomy, laparoscopic hand-assisted technique now yields operating times comparable to open technique. Compared to using conventional ports alone, the surgical port count is reduced from 6 or 7 down to 4. The extracorporeal portion of the technique allows measurement of the small bowel to the same degree of accuracy provided by a long midline incision. In addition, meticulous closure of the small bowel mesenteric defect can be performed. During the intracorporeal portion, the pylorus is more readily located and confirmed and as well the diameter of the gastric remnant can be calibrated by palpation. Any anastomotic concerns and areas of bleeding can be corrected and reinforced more quickly, even in the superobese, in whom a retrocolic proximal anastomosis is particularly important to avoid constricting the colon. Over 95% of the patients qualify for the laparoscopic-assisted approach. The procedure is scalable: The heaviest woman in our series had a BMI of 118 kg/m^2 and the heaviest man weighed 338 kg. The current contraindications to the laparoscopic approach are the following two: History of multiple prior operations with associated dense adhesions and medical concerns related to anesthesia.

Our approach has yielded acceptable morbidity (10%) compared to the open DS series.[4–6] The range of complications is similar to that reported in open DS series. We have had 2 operative mortalities in 1,150 laparoscopic DS patients in our series to date. Most procedures are completed in less than 3 hours, including routine cholecystectomy and appendectomy. Liver biopsy is obtained routinely for baseline and because of the known high incidence of steatosis and pre-existing liver pathology in the obese population. When present, the appendix and the gallbladder are removed concurrently. Their removal has no known direct effect on weight loss; however, a significant incidence of cholecystitis is documented as associated with rapid weight loss. The incidence of appendicitis is low but abdominal pain is not uncommon. Both cholecystectomy and appendectomy therefore can simplify postoperative management (Figure 46–1).

Our technique of constructing the proximal anastomosis initially required a purse string suture to secure the EEA anvil within the open end of the duodenum and then doing an end-to-side duodenoenterostomy. On an intermediate basis, we used a transoral insertion of the anvil with no purse string. By eliminating the EEA stapler altogether in the thin-walled duodenum, we believe we have reduced the potential for leaks and strictures. Obstructions occurred early in our series because of the antecolic positioning of the proximal anastamosis, now abandoned in favor of retrocolic.

CONCLUSION

Both conventional laparoscopic and hand-assisted techniques are technically feasible and have an acceptable morbidity. A steep learning curve is generally acknowledged and prior laparoscopic and bariatric surgical experience is essential. Advantages of the laparoscopic hand-assisted approach include decreased pain, improved pulmonary function in the early postoperative period, reduced hospital stay, and improved cosmetic result due to the use of shorter incisions. Those candidates that may be excluded include patients with a history of extensive prior surgery or very large patients with a high medical risk who may not tolerate a potentially prolonged operation and the attendant pneumoperitoneum. In conclusion, our technique has evolved to the hand-assisted approach because of the reduced operating time and its applicability to nearly all patients regardless of size. Longer-term data reflecting weight loss and comorbidities do not differ from that of the open technique patients as the sutures, staples, measurement techniques, and all other aspects are identical between the two techniques apart from the use of the handport. Our current protocol is to approach nearly all patients laparoscopically.

References

1. Hess D, Hess D: Biliopancreatic diversion with duodenal switch. *Obes Surg* 8:267–282, 1998.
2. Marceau P, Biron S, Simard S, et al.: Biliopancreatic diversion with a new type of gastrectomy. *Obes Surg* 3(1):29–35, 1993.
3. Rabkin R, Rabkin J, Metcalf B, et al.: Laparoscopic technique for performing duodenal switch with gastric reduction. *Obes Surg* 13:263–268, 2003.
4. Rabkin RA: Distal gastric bypass/duodenal switch, Roux-en-Y gastric bypass and biliopancreatic diversion in a community practice. *Obes Surg* 8(1):53–59, 1998.
5. Marceau P, Hould FS, Simard S: Biliopancreatic diversion with duodenal switch. *World J Surg* 22(9):947–954, 1998.
6. Baltasar A, Bou R, Bengochea M: Duodenal switch: An effective therapy for morbid obesity-intermediate results. *Obes Surg* 11:54–58, 2001.

Special Topics in Bariatric Surgery

47

Cost and Economic Impact of Bariatric Surgery

Eldo E. Frezza, MD, MBA, FACS

PRACTICE OF BARIATRIC SURGERY

Operative Costs of Bariatric Surgery

Introduction

Obesity is a worldwide epidemic. In the United States alone, not only are the majority of adult Americans overweight, but approximately 30% of its citizens are affected by morbid obesity. The resultant increase in bariatric surgical procedures mandates examination of operative costs of this surgery. Our group analyzed, for the US Southwest region, the cost of the two most common procedures, laparoscopic Roux-en-Y gastric bypass (LRYGBP) and laparoscopic adjustable gastric band (LAGB). Operative cost categories included the following costs:

1. Anesthesia professional costs, defined as charges rendered by an anesthesiologist or certified registered nurse anesthetist according to the guidelines of the American Society of Anesthesiologists (ASA).
2. Operating room costs, defined as nonprofessional anesthesia and operating room utilization fees.
3. Instrument costs, which included two subcategories, disposable items and reusable items.
4. Hospital costs.

Results

Anesthesia Professional Costs

The relative value guide booklet issued by the ASA recognizes LRYGBP and LAGB as one and the same. A unit is a $70 charge. For each case, an initial 10-unit charge is rendered. After the first scalpel cut occurs, every 15 minutes yields a 1-unit charge; thus, each hour of surgery costs 4 units. An LAGB that takes an average of 2.5 hours is charged 20 units or $1400; the LRYGBP that takes an average of 3 hours incurs a $1540 charge. In addition, more units are added to the case depending on the complexity of the patient's management, which is at the discretion of the anesthesiologist. Anesthesia time ends when the patient is signed out to the nursing team in the postanesthesia recovery room.[1]

Operating Room Costs, Reimbursement of Bariatric Costs

Operating Room Costs

LRYGBP. An LRYGBP that takes 3 hours is charged as follows. OR fees for anesthesia equipment is $454 per hour. LRYGBP is a complexity level 4 laparoscopic procedure, the room utilization fee of which is $4485 for the first hour and $767 for each additional half hour. The OR room cost is $3 \times \$454 + 1 \times \$4485 + 4 \times \$767 = \$8915$.

LAGB. Like LRYGBP, LAGB is also charged on hourly basis. If the LAGB takes 2.5 hours, the total OR fees would be $2.5 \times \$454 + 1 \times \$4485 + 3 \times \$767 = \$7921$.

Tables 47–1 to 47–3 delineate actual instrument costs. The aforementioned examples are instructive, but Table 47–4 should be specifically referenced, as it reflects average actual OR charges and anesthesia charges for the two procedures.

Disposable instrument costs for LAGB, as a fraction of total operative costs, are twice those of LRYGBP. Because the greatest potential price reductions occur due to technological innovation and competition among vendors in this area, cost containment efforts in regard to LAGB should focus upon disposable instrument costs.[1]

Table 47–1.

Reusable Instruments Costs, to Be Used in Both Operations

A. Reusable items*	
1	Harmonic scalpel machine: $19,969.50
2	Omni retractor: $11,000
3	Storz camera: $15,000
4	Storz 45° 5-mm lens: $5000
5	Bariatric tray: $11,000

LRYGBP and LAGB have different costs.
* This equipment cost does not apply to each operation and is incorporated in overall cost to the operating room.

Table 47–2.

Laparoscopic Roux-en-Y Gastric Bypass Disposable Equipment

1	Endo clip applier: $105.97
2	Endo 150-mm pneumoperitoneum needle (Veress): $19.18
3	Extension flexible linear cutter/stapler: $298.31
4	Angled Harmonic scalpel: $358.31
5	Autosuture endostitch: $215.27
6	Endolinear cutter/stapler 45 mm: $281.60
7	Surgiwand suction/irrigation: $97.53
8	Reload EndoGIA 45 mm (white): $90.69
9	Reload EndoGIA 45 mm (blue): $90.69
10	Surgidac (Endostitch reload) #2–0: $41.45
11	Surgidac (Endostitch reload) #0: $41.45
12	5 mm trocar: $48.17 × 3 = $144.51
13	12 mm trocar $58.01
14	10 mm trocar: $58.01

Disposable items total cost: $1900.98 (each aforementioned price applies to a single item which is often used more than once, for instance the Surgidac and EndoGIA reloads).

Reimbursement Following Bariatric Surgery

Insurance Payments

Angus[2] uncovered fascinating dichotomies in insurance payments for gastric bypass procedures. Private sector surgeons received $3178; public sector surgeons received $1004. In contrast, private hospitals received $7541 while public hospitals received $16,235. Open Roux-en-Y gastric bypass was reimbursed $8158; LRYGBP was reimbursed $6425.

Reimbursement to Surgeons, Office Collections

The difference in reimbursement for open versus laparoscopic gastric bypass did not reflect a greater instrument cost for the latter procedure. Open gastric bypass requires a TA90B stapler and a GIA 60 linear stapler. The laparoscopic technique, as established by Wittgrove,[3] requires seven nonreusable trocars, multiple EndoGIA II staplers, and an EEA stapler. Indeed, Angus[2] found that the difference in disposable equipment charges meant that LRYGBP had a $1000 higher direct cost than did open gastric bypass. Note that Angus' reimbursement calculation differs from ours because ours only calculated the direct costs of the operating room, including anesthesia and instruments.[1]

Table 47–3.

Laparoscopic Adjustable Gastric Band Disposable Equipment

1	Endo clip applier $105.79
2	Endo pneumoperitoneum needle 150 mm: $19.18
3	Autosuture Endostitch: $215.27
4	Surgidac #0: $41.45
5	Surgidac #2-0: $41.45
6	5 mm trocar: $48.17 × 3 = $144.51
7	12 mm trocar $58.01
8	10 mm trocar: $58.01
9	15 mm trocar: $126.25
10	Vanguard 10 laparoscopic band: $3195 (permanent)
11	Angled harmonic scalpel: $358.31

Disposable items total cost (each of the aforementioned prices apply to a single item which will be used more than once, for instance the Surgidac): $4363.32 (note this includes the band cost).

Table 47–4.

Surgical Office Versus CPT Codes

	Laparoscopic Gastric Bypass		Laparoscopic Gastric Banding	
	Cost ($)	%	Cost ($)	%
Anesthesia costs	1,540	13	1,400	14
Operating room charges	8,320	71	5,577	55
Disposable instrument costs	1,901	16	3,195	32
Total	11,761	100	10,141	100

Angus'[2] most important finding was that public insurance, such as Medicare and Medicaid, rewards physicians poorly for their efforts. Such reimbursement has the unfortunate consequence of discouraging care for those who need it most: lower income individuals correlate with a much greater risk of morbid obesity.[4,5] In contrast, public hospitals receive reimbursements far more than private hospitals for bariatric procedures. In addition, the difference between reimbursements for open and laparoscopic gastric bypass has the potentially deleterious effect of encouraging open procedures, even though LRYGBP is safer and requires a shorter hospital stay.

Because the surgeon, and not the hospital, performs the procedure, indigent people are less likely to receive the surgery. Reimbursements to surgeons in this circumstance do not cover expenses. Moreover, because the treatment of obesity-related illnesses increases health-care costs, the resultant lack of surgery ultimately costs the public sector more money.[6,7]

Bariatric Practice Office Reimbursement

Introduction

Office Policy, CPT Codes

Because office fees paid at the front desk, also called "window collections," generate less revenue than do surgical procedures, it receives insufficient attention from surgeons. In fact, co-payments can be high: Some patients pay over $300 for a presurgical weight management evaluation.[2,7]

To ensure window collections generate as much revenue as possible, patients must learn to pay before actually being seen by the physician. This important information should be provided by a note sent before the visit, as well as by a large poster in the waiting room. The fee should be received from self-pay patients before they even enter the office. Stress is laid upon this point because many people who do not undergo surgery are reluctant to pay for the cost of the evaluation, even though it is a very legitimate fee.

Figures 47–1 to 47–3 illustrate this argument. Figure 47–1 shows how office revenue is generated through insurance and procedural charges and "window collection" of co-payments. Figure 47–2 displays the large discrepancy between the amounts charged and the fees collected for the office visit in most bariatric practices. Figure 47–3 shows a policy of office charges being paid prior to the actual evaluation brings collections to almost 100% within 2 months (Figure 47–3).

How Do You Adjust Office Policy?

Because a bariatric practice is expensive to operate, every effort must be made to collect what is due. Obtaining co-payment before an evaluation will bring office window collections to 99% of the charges. This change in policy usually covers the cost of one-half to one full-time employee; the

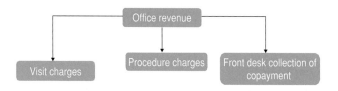

Figure 47–1. How an office obtains revenue.

- Big discrepancy
- High charges
- Low collection

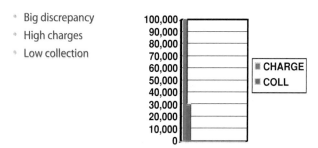

Figure 47–2. Front desk charging and collecting in the bariatric office.

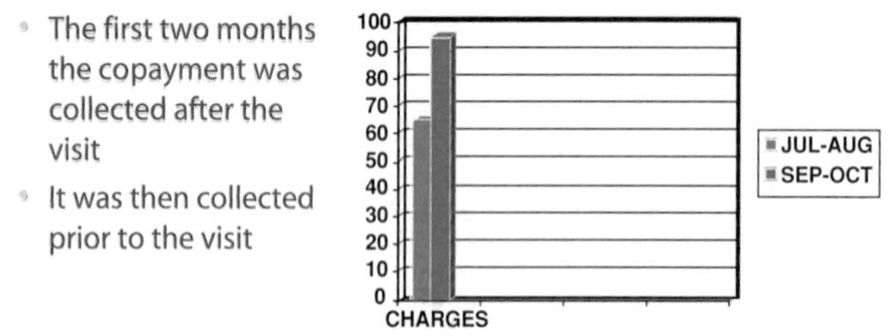

- The first two months the copayment was collected after the visit
- It was then collected prior to the visit

Figure 47–3. Four months adjustment in our front desk office charges.

office staff should be apprised of this so that they will be motivated to implement this policy.

All Visits Merit High-Complexity CPT Codes

All bariatric surgery consultations are of high complexity and should be charged as such. The morbidly obese usually have multiple disorders, each of which must be evaluated and taken into account. Almost always the visit requires more than an hour. Durations of interactions with the physician, the nutritionist, and the coordinator should be recorded in the patient's chart. Always use CPT codes such as 99275 and 99274. For each half hour spent beyond one hour, apply a 99355 CPT charge.[6,7]

Health-Care Costs, Expenses, and Commentary

What About Presurgery Collections?

Most of the bariatric surgeries are scheduled weeks in advance, which means that some patients can cancel a few days before surgery for a variety of reasons. If patients pay a deposit when the operation is scheduled, cancellation is less likely. The deposit should be returned if the patient cancels ten or more days prior to the surgery. The justification is that late cancellation denies another patient his or her operation. Because the deposit is credited to the final bill, it does not add to the expense of the surgery. Making patients pay deposits will permit a tight schedule and decrease losses from unwarranted cancellations.

Conclusion

Since the expenses to operate a bariatric practice are quite high, any physician should perform an accurate and detailed

office analysis of window collections in order to have a profitable practice. These profits will allow for needed personnel to be hired, avoid loss of income and time due to unwarranted cancellations, and, most importantly, permit the running of an efficient and profitable bariatric practice.

Local and State Health-Care Economy for Bariatric Surgery

Health-Care Expenditures for Bariatric Surgery

In addition to the increased risk for mortality and morbidity, obesity consumes a large portion of health-care expenditures through both direct and indirect costs related to the management of obesity and its sequelae.[8–13] Obesity has been shown to be associated with a 36% independent increase in inpatient and outpatient spending and a 77% increase in medication use.[14] Weight loss in the morbidly obese is anticipated to yield health and economic benefits.[15]

Direct Cost of Obesity, Medication Costs of Obesity

Sampalis[16] compared direct health-care costs related to hospitalization for two cohorts of obese patients, one that underwent bariatric surgery and one that did not. Universal health insurance in the nation where the study was performed, e.g., Canada, enabled excellent follow-up. Evaluation of hospital and provincial insurance administrative databases contrasted direct health-care costs among morbidly obese patients treated with bariatric surgery to those of matched controls that were not treated surgically.

In the first year, total costs for hospitalizations in the surgery cohort were higher by over C$8 million for patients when compared to the controls. This difference was reversed in subsequent years, reaching a maximum during the fifth year when the costs for the control cohort were more than C$4 million higher on the average when compared to the bariatric cohort. After 5 years, the total cost per 1,000 patients for hospitalizations in the control cohort was 29% higher when compared to that of the bariatric patients. For 3.5 years, the initial average cost was higher for the bariatric cohort. But, in the next 1.5 years, the cost was lower in patients who underwent surgery. Thus, after 3.5 years, the initial investment for the weight reduction surgery and related hospital care was compensated for by a reduction in total costs.

Sampalis' conclusion[16] shows there is a net reduction of C$5.7 million for health-related complications per 1,000 patients treated within 5 years after surgery.

The direct cost of obesity is between 2% and 5% of most developed countries' health-care expenditures.[17] Ten years ago, the cost of obesity in the United States was estimated to be US$99 billion, of which US$52 billion represented direct health costs; this comprised 5.7% of total health costs.[18] When one includes the direct cost of physical inactivity, the estimated cost of obesity is 9.4% of the US health-care spending.[19] Direct medical costs attributable to obesity are 2.4% of Canada's total direct medical costs.[20] The chief expense lies in the cost of managing comorbidities associated

Table 47–5.

Surgical Office Versus CPT Codes

	Office Visits—New PL		Consultations		Prolonged Physician Service
99201	Prob. focus/straight	99241	Prob. focus/straight	99354	First hour (In addition to E&M code)
99202	Exp. prob. focus/straight	99242	Exp. prob. focus/straight forward	99355	Additional 30 min
99203	Detailed/low complexity	99243	Detailed/low complexity		
99204	Comprehensive/Mod. Complexity	99244	Comprehensive/moderate complexity		
99205	Comprehensive/High Complexity	99245	Comprehensive/high complexity		
	Established Patients				
99211	Minimal/nurse only		**Confirmatory Consultation**		
99212	Prob. focus/straight	99271	Problem focused		
99213	Expanded/low complexity	99272	Expanded/straight forward		
99214	Detailed mod. complexity	99273	Detailed/low complexity		
99215	Comprehensive/high complexity	99274	Comprehensive/moderate complexity		
104038	Preop N/C	99275	Comprehensive/high complexity		
99024	Postop N/C				

with obesity.[21,22] Obesity accounts for 85% of the cost of type 2 diabetes and 45% of the cost of hypertension.[23] Nonsurgical interventions for weight loss in severely obese patients are usually ineffective.[24–28]

Demographics of Bariatric Patients, Occupations of Obese Patients

Narbro[29] compared pharmaceutical costs for 510 obese individuals who underwent weight reduction surgery with 455 randomly selected obese individuals who did not undergo weight reduction surgery over a 6-year period. The surgery lowered the costs of diabetes and cardiovascular medications and increased the costs for other medications, including gastrointestinal, anemia, and vitamin deficiency medications. Overall, medication costs were similar for the two groups. Potteiger[30] found a 77.3% reduction in the total cost of diabetic and antihypertensive medications with surgically induced weight loss, particularly Roux-en-Y gastric bypass.

Flum[31] reported that the bariatric surgery patients have a higher readmission rate, but that average total cost and average accumulated cost show a cost ratio between controls and bariatric of 1.29, indicating a definite decrease in cost for pa-

tients who undergo bariatric surgery. Despite increased rehospitalization, the economic evidence, especially with the adoption of the laparoscopic approach, strongly favors bariatric surgery over the long term.

Patient Base of Bariatric Surgery

Introduction

What is the patient base of bariatric surgery and what type of background do these individuals have? Obesity and its associated illnesses[32] have lowered productivity[33] and wages.[34,35] Because treatment of obesity-related ailments increases health-care costs, many have considered governmental interventions to ameliorate this condition.[36] Surgical cure exists, but financing for bariatric surgery is not often included in health insurance plans, and the expense is often beyond the means of the uninsured.

We evaluated bariatric surgery demographics at a large university hospital and compared them with the broader region's population statistics. The data should permit the development of an economic model capable of evaluating the costs and benefits of obesity surgery to society.

Costs of Obesity, Impact on Local and State Economy

Description of Sample

The age, race, education level, employment status, occupation, and bariatric surgical choice of 150 patients was collected and compared with the state of New Mexico. Of the patients reviewed, 87.5% (130/150) were female, 62% (93/150) were Caucasian, 28% (42/150) were Hispanic, 4.5% (7/150) were African American, and 0.5% (1/150) were Native American. Half (75/150) had a high school degree, 20% (30/150) had a Bachelor's degree, 6% (9/150) had an Associate's degree, 13 (19/150) had a Master's degree, 1% (2/150) had a PhD, 0.5% (1/150) were physicians, 0.5% (1/150) were veterinary assistants, and 1.5% (3/150) had an education up to the eleventh grade. Of this sample, 82% (123/150) were employed, 10% (15/150) were homemakers, 32% (48/150) were nurses, secretaries, or managers, 4.5% (7/150) were supervisors in companies, 3% (5/150) were students, 4% (6/150) were teachers, and 2.5% (4/150) were in customer service. The remainder had a wide array of occupations. In terms of age, 13% (8/150) were 40 years or older, 4.5% (7/150) were 30–39 years old, and 7% were 20–29 years old. Our results showed that morbid obesity affects all "classes" of the population. Bariatric surgery was particularly sought out by women with high school diplomas and higher degrees.

Statistical Analysis of Surgery Choice

In the future, we will need to use a series of appropriate parametric and nonparametric tests (e.g., t-statistics, χ^2-statistics, etc.) to compare the patient sample to the population at large. From this information, an economic choice model can be derived to predict individuals who will opt to have this surgery. Identifying a set of predictor variables may be important for the efficient allocation of scarce health-care state and federal resources.

The Impact of Obesity on the Local and State Economy

A number of attempts have been made to quantify the economic costs of obesity and/or the economic or societal benefits associated with treatment and prevention.[8,37,38]

The costs are usually broken down into three cost categories: direct, indirect, and personal.[37] Much debate exists as to the appropriate cost–benefit measurement and, moreover, on whether or not economic methodology should be focused on evaluation of policy under the constraint of scarce resources instead of on the traditional role of costing.[38]

State Losses from Obesity, Illness and Obesity

The economic evaluation of solutions pays particular attention to direct costs of obesity that accrue to a community, as health-care resources must be diverted from one activity to another in order to deal with obesity-related illnesses. In terms of personal costs, some studies show that persons deemed overweight or obese have lower wages, though other studies have not found this to be true.[10,11] Besides the "wage penalty" (in the jargon of economists) assessed for being obese, society suffers productivity losses from illnesses associated with obesity[9]; this is an indirect cost of obesity.

Currently underway is a study in our division that will estimate the economic impact of obesity on a specific local economy in terms of lost business output, lost employment, and lost income. The study uses information gathered on bariatric patients at a large university hospital. The region of analysis, dictated by patient residence and employment location, includes the state of New Mexico. Our goal is to quantify the state's loss in jobs, income, and output attributable to obesity-related illnesses.

Absenteeism and Obesity, Job Cost Loss

Obesity is hypothesized to increase absenteeism. The associated lost productivity would yield lost output, jobs, and income through a mechanism known as the economic multiplier. Economic Impact Analysis studies the direct benefits and costs of an event (or, in our case, the existence of obesity) as it affects local, regional, or national economies (Economic Analysis Primer, USDOT, FHWA 2003). Economic impacts arise from payroll spending, business/organizational operating expenses, and construction projects; these factors in turn generate jobs and income through a process known as the "multiplier effect."

MATERIALS AND METHODS

Input–output (I–O) analysis, which estimates margins and regional purchase coefficients (RPC), was used to model the regional economy. Margins refer to the prices of purchases made by final consumers (or households) of goods and services. RPC measures the percent of spending from local suppliers. Collected patient data used in conjunction with IMPLAN model data sufficed to estimate a complete set of economic accounts for local areas,[39] which are converted to an industry-by-industry formulation of I–O accounts and then into a set of multipliers.

From each data set were derived final demands, value added, output, and employment. Actual local employment by industry was used to partly validate the model. As a general rule, the quantity of goods and services purchased correlated with the economic activity; these factors in turn correlate with the magnitude of the multiplier.

Specific patient observations included information about socioeconomic status and demographics, occupation, education, and place of residence, which along with personal income and absenteeism data (as compared with normal weight persons) estimates lost work days attributable to obesity-related problems. The lost work days were then converted to full-time job equivalents, i.e., the *jobs* lost due to obesity, which are then entered into the IMPLAN model. Estimates are computed for over 500 subsectors (based on the North American Industrial Classification System, NAICS).

EXPECTED RESULTS AND REMARKS

If an obese worker had one more day of absence or other downtime per month than a normal weight worker, 2002 economic data suggest the region experienced a loss in total output of $9.65 million per year. This loss estimates the economic impact of obesity on the regional economy and takes into account both direct and secondary impacts. The loss represents how much more the economy would produce if these workers followed the average absence/downtime patterns of normal weight workers. To put the loss in perspective, the loss in potential output from obesity is equivalent to slightly more than $500 per person and, in total, is about 1.8% of the total gross state product.

To date, no study has specifically estimated the impact of obesity on a regional economy.[40] The study now under way will estimate lost jobs, income (in dollars), and output (in dollars) attributable to obesity-related illnesses. The findings may aid public policy decision making in regard to the designing and implementation of health-care policy. For example, finding substantial economic impacts from obesity might suggest that employers implement work-site health promotion programs, as some evidence indicates such treatment programs reduce health-related absenteeism.[27,29] More patients are looking for surgery and some of them are ready to pay out of their own pocket,[41] decreasing the health-care costs.

CONCLUSION

The cost of surgery and the impact of the expenses on surgeons, the hospital, health care, and the government are delineated in this chapter. More research and papers need to be developed to obtain a better idea of our progress in halting the spread of morbid obesity nationally and worldwide and to determine the cost to the world economy. As we have seen in this chapter, obesity is a pervasive problem that has a profound impact on the health-care system. Collection of economic data will permit the development of an economic model capable of evaluating the cost effectiveness of obesity surgery. Evaluating the costs and benefits of obesity surgery will aid policymakers, health-care professionals, and organizations in making decisions about the allocation of resources for the treatment of morbid obesity and the role of bariatric surgery.

Acknowledgments

We would like to thank Brad Ewing, PhD, for his economic insights and help, June Wagner for her editing job, and Lisa Bruster for her typographical assistance.

References

1. Albert M: Morbid obesity: The value of surgical intervention. *Clin Fam Pract* 4:447–451, 2002.
2. Angus LD, Cottam DR, Gorecki PJ, Mourello R, Ortega RE, Adamski J: DRG, costs and reimbursement following Roux en-Y gastric bypass: An economic appraisal. *Obes Surg* 13(4):591–595, 2003.
3. Baum C, Ford W: The wage effects of obesity: A longitudinal study. *Health Econ* 13:885–899, 2004.
4. Berke EM, Morden NE: Medical management of obesity. *Am Fam Physician* 62:419–426, 2000.
5. Birmingham CL, Muller JL, Palepu A, et al.: The cost of obesity in Canada. *CMAJ* 160:483–488, 1999.
6. Cawley J: The impact of obesity on wages. *J Hum Resour* 34:451–474, 2004.
7. Colditz GA: Economic costs of obesity. *Am J Clin Nutr* 55:503S–507S, 1992.
8. Colditz GA: Economic costs of obesity and inactivity. *Med Sci Sports Exerc* 31(Suppl 11):S663–S667, 1999.
9. Finkelstein MM: Obesity, cigarette smoking and the cost of physicians' services in Ontario. *Can J Public Health* 92:437–440, 2001.
10. Fisher BL, Schauer P: Medical and surgical options in the treatment of severe obesity. *Am J Surg* 184:S9, 2002.
11. Flum DR, Salem L, Elrod JA, Dellinger EP, Cheadle A, Chan L: Early mortality among Medicare beneficiaries undergoing bariatric surgical procedures. *JAMA* 294(15):1903–1908, 2005.
12. Frezza EE: A plan to establish a private-pay bariatric surgery in the U.S.A. *Obes Surg* 16(1):110–111, 2006.
13. Frezza EE, Wachtel MS, Ewing BT: Bariatric surgery costs and implications for hospital margins: Comparing laparoscopic gastric bypass and laparoscopic gastric banding. Surg Laparosc Endosc Percutan Tech, 2006.
14. Frezza EE: How to improve office collection in a bariatric practice. *Obes Surg* 15:1352–1354, 2005.
15. Goldblatt PB, Moore ME, Stunkard AJ: Social factors in obesity. *JAMA* 192:1039–1044, 1965.
16. Gorstein J, Grosse R: The indirect costs of obesity to society. *Pharmacoeconomics* 5(Suppl 1):58–61, 1994.
17. Jeffrey RW, Forster JL, Dunn BV, French SA, McGovern PG, Lando HA: Effects of work-site health promotion on illness-related absenteeism, *Am College Occup Environ Med* 35(11):1142–1146, 1993.
18. Krott MA, Langley PC, Cox ER: A review of cost-of-illness studies on obesity. *Clin Ther* 40:772–779, 1998.
19. Levy E, Levy P, Le Pen C, et al.: The economic cost of obesity: The French situation. *Int J Obes* 19:788–792, 1995.
20. Narbro K, Agren G, Jonsson E, et al.: Pharmaceutical costs in obese individuals. *Arch Intern Med* 162:2061–2069, 2002.
21. National Institutes of Health. Gastrointestinal surgery for severe Obesity: National Institutes of Health Consensus Development Conference Statement. *Am J Clin Nutr* 55(Suppl 2):S582–S585, 1992.
22. Olson D, Lindall S: *IMPLAN User's Guide*. Minnesota: Minnesota IMPLAN Group 2002, published by State of Minnesota.
23. Oster G, Thompson D, Edelsberg J, et al.: Lifetime health and economic benefits of weight loss among obese persons. *Am J Public Health* 89:1536–1542, 1999.
24. Philipson T: The world-wide growth in obesity: An economic research agenda, *Health Econ* 10:1–7, 2001.
25. Potteiger CE, Prokash RP, Inverso NA, et al.: Bariatric surgery: Shedding the monetary weight of prescription cost in the managed care arena. *Obes Surg* 14:725–730, 2004.
26. Rous L, Donaldson C: Economics and obesity: Costing the problem or evaluating the solutions? *Obes Res* 12(2):173–179, 2004.

27. Sampalis JS, Liberman M, Auger S, Christou NV: The impact of weight reduction surgery on health-care costs in morbidly obese patients. *Obes Surg* 14:939–947, 2004.

28. Seidell JC: Societal and personal costs of obesity. *Exp Clin Endocrinol Diabetes* 106(Suppl 2):7–9, 1998.

29. Sorensen TI: Socio-economic aspects of obesity: Causes or effects? *Int J Obes* 19(Suppl 6):S6–S8, 1995.

30. Oster G, O'Sullivan A, Edelsberg J, et al.: The clinical and economic cost of obesity in a managed care setting. *Am J Manag Care* 6:681–689, 2000.

31. Sturm R: The effects of obesity, smoking, and drinking on medical problems and costs. *Health Aff* 21:245–253, 2002.

32. Swinburn B, Ashton T, Gillespie J, et al.: Health care costs of obesity in New Zealand. *Int J Obes* 21:891–896, 1997.

33. Thompson D, Edelsberg J, Colditz GA, et al.: Lifetime health and economic consequences of obesity. *Arch Intern Med* 159:2177–2183, 1999.

34. Thompson D, Wolf AM: The medical-care cost burden of obesity. *Obes Rev* 2:189–197, 2001.

35. Wang G, Zheng ZJ, Heath G, et al.: Economic burden of cardiovascular disease associated with excess body weight in U.S. adults. *Am J Prev Med* 23:1–6, 2002.

36. Weintraub M: Long-term weight control study conclusions. *Clin Pharmocol Ther* 51:642–646, 1992.

37. Wittgrove AC, Clark GW: Laparoscopic gastric bypass, Roux-en-Y—500 patients: Technique and results, with 3–60 month follow up. *Obes Surg* 10:233–239, 2000.

38. Wolf AM: What is the economic case for treating obesity? *Obes Res* 6(Suppl 1):2S–7S, 1998.

39. Wolf AM, Colditz GA: Social and economic effects of body weight in the United States. *Am J Clin Nutr* 63:466S, 1996.

40. Wolf AM, Colditz GA: Current estimates of the economic cost of obesity in the United States. *Obes Res* 6:97–106, 1998. www.cureyourpractice.com

48

Adolescent Bariatric Surgery

Venita Chandra, MD • Sanjeev Dutta, MD, MA, FRCSC

BACKGROUND

Obesity is rapidly becoming a problem of epic proportions in the adolescent patient population. The implications of this profound health crisis are clearly recognized as serious and immediate, and long-term physical and psychological consequences are being identified. Childhood and adolescent obesity are now considered independent risk factors for adult morbidity and premature mortality.[1,2]

Resorting to bariatric surgery to address these issues in morbidly obese adolescents who have life-threatening comorbidities is a radical concept demanding increasing attention, particularly given the growing amount of data demonstrating positive outcomes after bariatric surgery in the adult population. Adolescence represents a period of significant growth and maturation both physically and emotionally, thus issues unique to this patient population exist, which must be addressed when considering bariatric surgery. This chapter focuses on aspects of bariatric surgery unique to the adolescent population, including the health consequences of obesity in this age group, the indications for bariatric surgery, preoperative and postoperative management, as well as a review of current outcomes.

Epidemiology

In the United States, obesity has far surpassed malnutrition as the most pressing nutritional disorder.[3] Children are the fastest growing segment of the population afflicted by this disorder. The proportion of children and adolescents who are obese tripled between 1980 and 2002.[4,5] Recent prevalence studies in the United States estimate 17.1% of children and adolescents to be overweight.[6] Clear ethnic and racial disparities are also noted with especially high rates of obesity in the Hispanic and African American communities.[6–9] A recent study in a New York City elementary school reviewed over 3,000 students' demographic data and demonstrated the prevalence of overweight in young children to be 43% (more than half of whom were obese) with significantly higher levels among Hispanic and Black children.[10]

This problem of obesity is not isolated to the United States, rising trends in overweight and obesity both in adults and children are apparent in both developed and developing countries worldwide.[11–15] In China, for example, the prevalence of obesity in school children increased from 1.5% in the late eighties to 12.6% in 1997.[16]

Definition of Obesity

Throughout childhood, dramatic changes in adiposity, height, and weight occur; thus, the exact definition of obesity in children and adolescents is subject to much debate. In general, it can be defined as an excess of body fat. Accurate assessment of body fat requires underwater weighing, dual energy x-ray absorptiometery, or bioelectric impedance, all of which are not practical for everyday use.[17]

Body mass index (BMI, kg/m^2) is widely used as a surrogate measure of adiposity, particularly in the adult populations. An adult with a BMI $\geq$ 30 kg/m^2 is considered obese.[18] In children and adolescents who are still growing and have changing body shapes, BMI can be less accurate, particularly as it fails to distinguish between fat and fat-free mass.[17,19] Thus, the application of growth charts and multiple percentiles is necessary to determine overweight and obesity for age and sex in this group.[18,20,21] Pediatric obesity is now generally defined as a BMI greater than the ninety-fifth percentile and pediatric overweight with a BMI greater than the eighty-fifth percentile.[22]

Risk Factors

The extent and impact of today's obesity epidemic both on children and adults demands the question "why?" The answer to this is not straightforward. Overweight and obesity are complex multifactorial phenotypes influenced by an interaction of genetic, behavioral, and environmental factors. An in-depth discussion of this is beyond the scope of this chapter; however, some basic observations can be made.

Risk factors for the development of obesity in childhood or adolescence are multifactorial, although the overall risk accumulates with age. There are robust data demonstrating an association between higher birth weight and higher attained BMI in childhood and early adulthood.[23–28] Interestingly, lower birth weight has also been associated with increased risk of later central obesity,[26,29–32] insulin resistance, and the metabolic syndrome.[26,33–37] Several studies have assessed intrauterine environment and determined maternal obesity and gestational diabetes to be strong predictors of childhood and adolescent obesity.[23,27,38] These risk factors have also been shown, when paired, to be associated with an increased risk of metabolic syndrome during childhood.[27]

Parental BMI is also a significant risk factor for obesity. Parental obesity more than doubles the risk of adult obesity among both obese and nonobese children under the age of 10.[39] Other variables that are shown to be risk factors include duration of breastfeeding, socioeconomic status, maternal smoking status, and hours spent watching television.[25]

Long-Term Effects

Multiple studies suggest that long-term health is significantly compromised due to persistence of adolescent overweight into adulthood.[40–44] This persistence of obesity results in a broad range of adverse health effects.[41] In addition to physical health, overweight in adolescents has harmful effects on their subsequent self-esteem and social and economic characteristics. For example, Gortmaker and colleagues[45] looked at a cohort of 370 overweight adolescents and found that obese young women were less likely to marry, had lower incomes, and had completed less schooling than did nonobese women and that obese young men were less likely to marry than were nonobese men.

CONSEQUENCES AND COMORBIDITIES OF ADOLESCENT OBESITY

With the epidemic of obesity in children, we are seeing an emergence of traditionally adult diseases in this younger population. In addition to medical issues, the psychological sequelae of obesity during some of the most formative years of life have significant impact on how these children and adolescents adapt as effective members of society (Table 48–1). The potential ramifications of these issues on our country's health-care system and on the future health of our nation are quite alarming.

Medical Impact

As in adults, obesity in adolescents is associated with a large number of health consequences. Although these obesity-related comorbidities occur more frequently in adults, significant consequences of obesity as well as the antecedents of adult disease occur in obese children and adolescents.

Metabolic Syndrome and Cardiac Risk Factors

The *metabolic syndrome* is a cluster of risk factors that links insulin resistance, hypertension, dyslipidemia, type 2 diabetes, and other metabolic abnormalities with an increased risk of

Table 48–1.

Consequences and Comorbidities of Adolescent Obesity

Psychosocial	Gastrointestinal
Low self-esteem	Gallstones
Depression	Steatohepatitis
Eating disorders	Gastroesophageal reflux disease
Discrimination, prejudice, social marginalization	**Endocrine**
Poor quality of life, impairment of activities of daily living	Type 2 diabetes mellitus
Neurological	Insulin resistance
Pseudotumor cerebri	Metabolic syndrome
Pulmonary	Precocious puberty
Obstructive sleep apnea	Polycystic ovary syndrome
Asthma and exercise intolerance	**Musculoskeletal**
Cardiovascular	Slipped capital femoral epiphysis
Dyslipidemia	Blount's disease
Hypertension	Forearm fractures
Coagulopathy	Flat feet
Chronic inflammation	Osteoarthritis
Endothelial dysfunction	Scoliosis
Venous stasis disease	Spondylolisthesis
Renal	**Dermatologic**
Glomerulosclerosis	Intertriginous soft-tissue infections Acanthosis nigricans

modified criteria, suggest that the metabolic syndrome is far more common (nearly 50%) among overweight children and adolescents and that its prevalence increases directly with the degree of obesity.[48]

Obese children and adolescents have increased blood lipids as well as glucose intolerance and diabetes.[49–51] Although thought to be a traditionally "adult" disease, type 2 diabetes is becoming shockingly more common in obese children and adolescents. The incidence among adolescents has increased 10-fold since 1982 and is felt to account for one-third of all new cases of diabetes in children,[52] these numbers being even higher in women and Hispanics.[53]

Hypertension is yet another example of a predominantly adult disease, with a rising incidence in the pediatric population.[54–56] The long-term consequences are as yet unknown; however, there is some evidence that childhood hypertension can lead to adult hypertension, and thus the associated development of left ventricular hypertrophy, atherosclerosis, and even early development of coronary artery disease.[44,57–62]

Obstructive Sleep Apnea

Sleep apnea is another significant health consequence of childhood obesity. Symptoms which may include snoring, poor school performance, enuresis, and hyperactivity can have significant effects on quality of life.[63,64] The prevalence of obstructive sleep apnea (OSA) in obese children and adolescents is quoted anywhere from 24% to 59%[65–68]; however, a direct correlation between reduction in OSA indices and reduction in BMI has not been demonstrated.[69]

Pseudotumor Cerebri

Pseudotumor cerebri (PTC) is a rare disorder characterized by increased intracranial pressure. Symptoms include headache, visual field disturbances (the most severe is blindness), and pulsatile tinnitus.[70,71] PTC in adolescents has a direct correlation with obesity.[72,73] Progressive visual impairment indicates the need for aggressive treatment of obesity in patients with this disease.[44] Weight loss is associated with dramatic improvement in symptoms and improvements in objective measures of the disease including visual field abnormalities and lumbar pressures.[74–76]

Musculoskeletal Effects

Overweight children are susceptible to developing orthopedic complications because the tensile strength of bone and cartilage is not evolved to carry substantial quantities of excess weight. As a result, the excess weight carried by obese children is associated with bowing of long bones, which may cause injury to the growth plate and result in slipped capital femoral epiphysis, genu valga, tibia vara (Blount's disease), scoliosis, osteoarthritis, and other injuries.[44,66] Both slipped capital femoral epiphysis and Blount's disease are pediatric orthopedic injuries that are highly associated with obesity in children, and prompt and sustained weight reduction is essential in their treatment.[77,78]

later cardiovascular disease.[46] This syndrome, at first thought to be only an adult phenomenon, is unfortunately becoming more prominent in adolescents and children. Cook and colleagues[47] studied the prevalence of metabolic syndrome in a sample of adolescents from the third National Health and Nutrition Examination Survey (NHANES III) and found the syndrome to be present in 28.7% of overweight adolescents (BMI ≥ 95th percentile). More recent findings, using

Psychosocial Impact

Few problems in childhood have as significant an impact on emotional development as being overweight. Adolescence in and of itself is a tumultuous period of emotional and interpersonal growth and development for children. It is not surprising therefore that the psychosocial consequences of obesity may in fact be the most prevalent of associated comorbidities. Obesity is one of the most stigmatized and least socially acceptable conditions in childhood.[79] Health related quality of life studies document marked impairments in all domains including physical functioning, emotional well-being, social relations, and school functioning in adolescents with severe obesity (BMI > 40 kg/m^2). This level of impairment is even worse than for those youth with chronic disease or cancer.[64,80,81]

Relative to average-weight peers, obese adolescents, particularly females, are socially marginalized and are less likely to be nominated by their peers as a friend.[79] Given the importance of peer acceptance, body image, and physical fitness to social and emotional development, overweight may have lasting implications on child development and adolescent well-being. These adolescents are clearly at considerable risk of continued and mounting psychosocial impairment and poor developmental adaptation.[82] Among severely obese adolescents, there is a high incidence of low self-esteem, sadness, and moderate to severe depressive symptoms. Extreme obesity is associated with an increased risk of suicide and suicidal ideation among adolescents.[66,83,84] The impact of this psychosocial impairment is grand, and some studies even suggest that obesity may be the worst socioeconomic handicap that women who were obese adolescents can suffer.[44,45]

NONSURGICAL THERAPIES

It is evident that the health and psychosocial consequences of child and adolescent obesity are profound, resulting in significant morbidity and increased long-term adult mortality.[41,42,85] Evaluation and treatment of obesity in adolescents and children is imperative in order to avoid later sequelae and requires early multidisciplinary intervention by pediatric care providers.

Obesity results from an imbalance in energy intake and expenditure, thus the ideal treatment for obesity involves decreasing caloric intake while increasing caloric expenditure. Although no evidence-based overweight treatment guidelines exist for adolescent overweight, traditional clinical approaches include combinations of caloric restriction, exercise promotion, and behavior therapy. Considerable evidence shows that behavioral family-based treatment approaches are the most effective nonsurgical methods for the management of childhood obesity.[86–88]

Experience with medication for use in adolescent weight loss is limited. Currently, two medications, orlistat (Xenical, Roche Pharmaceuticals, Nutley, NJ) and sibutramine (Meridia, Knoll Pharmaceutical Company, Bray,

GA), have received FDA approval for long-term use in adolescents. Orlistat inhibits pancreatic lipase and increases fecal losses of triglycerides. Although early evidence showed orlistat use to result in slight improvement in weight control,[89] a recent randomized controlled trial of adolescents using orlistat did not show significant reduction in BMI as compared to placebo at 6 months.[90] In addition, orlistat is associated with high study-dropout rates because of unacceptable flatulence and diarrhea as side effects of the drug.[66,91] Sibutramine is a nonselective inhibitor of serotonin, norepinephrine, and dopamine which acts as an anorectic by stimulating satiety. A randomized controlled trial showed a statistically significant amount of weight loss with sibutramine (10.3 ± 6.6 kg) plus diet and exercise as compared to placebo plus diet and exercise (2.4 ± 2.5 kg)[92]; however, the benefits appear to be only short term.[93]

Successful weight loss and maintenance require great effort and commitment. Although success is possible, most studies show that behavior modification and dieting are associated with poor weight loss, high attrition rates, and high probability of weight regain.[66,94–97] Bariatric surgery appears to be the only intervention with evidence suggesting successful long-lasting (>1 year) effects on body weight in severely obese adolescents.[95] As a result, more and more pediatric providers are considering bariatric surgery for the treatment of obese adolescents.

SURGICAL THERAPIES

Evidence demonstrating the benefit of surgical weight loss in adults is extensive including not only dramatic reductions in BMI but resolution of associated comorbidities, as well as reduced mortality.[98–108] Preliminary experience with bariatric surgery in adolescents suggests efficacy in ameliorating obesity-related morbidities as well.[76,109,110] Thus, for severely obese adolescents who have failed organized attempts at achieving and maintaining weight loss through conventional nonoperative approaches and who have serious or life-threatening conditions, bariatric surgery may provide the only practical alternative for achieving a healthy weight and for escaping the devastating physical and psychological consequences of obesity.[111]

Surgical Options

The goals of surgical therapy for obese adolescents, as for adults, are reduction in excess body weight in addition to reduction or resolution of obesity-related comorbidities and reduction in the risk of early mortality. The National Institutes of Health Consensus Conference has endorsed bariatric surgery as effective in achieving significant and sustained weight reduction as well as ameliorating or resolving most obesity-related comorbidities.[112] The two main bariatric surgical procedures used in the adolescent population today are Roux-en-Y gastric bypass (RYGBP) and adjustable gastric banding. Primarily, malabsorptive procedures such as biliopancreatic bypass with duodenal switch which are occasionally used in adults are not recommended for use in adolescents, given their relative high rate of nutritional sequelae.[21,76,109] No studies to date have compared the efficacy and safety of various bariatric procedures among adolescents; however, both RYGBP and adjustable gastric banding have been effective in treating the medical consequences of severe obesity in adolescence.[76,113–118]

Roux-en-Y Gastric Bypass

The gold standard bariatric surgical procedure in the United States is the RYGBP procedure.[111] The basic principles of this procedure are the same in adolescents as for adults: (1) Creation of a restrictive component (i.e. gastric pouch) and (2) reestablishment of intestinal continuity and creation of a malabsorptive component (i.e., Roux limb bypass of stomach, duodenum, and portion of jejunum). Though it can be done via laparotomy, recent data suggest that the laparoscopic approach has advantages over the open when done by experienced surgeons.[119,120]

The advantages of gastric bypass include excellent largely sustainable excess weight loss, inherent deterrence to the ingestion of sweets, and enhanced satiety. Disadvantages include a greater risk of perioperative mortality demonstrated among adults with gastric bypass (0.5%) compared to those with adjustable gastric banding (0.05%) as well as number of complications such as intestinal leakage, thromboembolic disease, marginal ulcers, dumping syndrome, gastrojejunal stomal stenosis, gastric distension, small bowel obstruction, incisional hernia, symptomatic cholelithiasis, protein calorie malnutrition, and micronutrient deficiencies, especially of iron, calcium, and vitamin B_{12}.[102,109,111,116]

Restrictive Procedures

This category includes both vertical banded gastroplasty and laparoscopic adjustable gastric banding (LAGB). Although the vertical banded gastroplasty has been used in the past in both adult and adolescent populations, it has been largely replaced by the adjustable balloon gastric band and is now only of historic significance.[21] LAGB consists of a laparoscopically placed adjustable balloon band encircling the most proximal stomach creating a very small proximal gastric reservoir. The main advantage of LAGB is its ease and safety of placement, and the lack of an anastomosis results in less morbidity and mortality associated with anastomoses. In addition, weight loss tends to be more gradual and the adjustable band reduces the potential for adverse nutritional consequences.[21,121] Disadvantages include device malfunctions or malposition, slippage, foreign-body infection, and band erosion into the stomach or esophagus.[122] Furthermore, the mechanical devices have a finite lifetime, and thus adolescent patients may need to undergo replacement of the device during their lifetimes.[111]

LAGB is not currently approved by the FDA in the United States for use in adolescents. Studies from Europe and Australia, where the technique has gained significant popularity, show excellent outcomes in adults, with

lower complication rates as compared to those resulting from RYGBP, although preliminary US studies show mixed results.[102,121,123–129] Some data suggest less total excess weight loss in LAGB patients as compared to that in RYGBP patients, although this does not appear to affect resolution of comorbidities.[127,130] In addition, current literature demonstrates similar effectiveness of LAGB in adolescents as for adults in terms of weight loss and resolution of comorbidities,[113,118,131,132] including the most recent publication by Horgan and colleagues[118] reviewing four adolescents (age, 17–19) who underwent the procedure in the United States.

Compared to RYGBP, the LAGB is a particularly attractive option in adolescents as it does not require anatomic rearrangement and is reversed with much greater ease. However, the placement of a foreign body at such an early age raises concerns over the potential for long-term morbidity, such as erosion, and the eventual need to replace the prosthesis due to its limited lifespan. Long-term studies are necessary to better understand these issues.

GUIDELINES FOR BARIATRIC SURGERY IN ADOLESCENTS

In 1991, the National Institutes of Health published consensus guidelines for bariatric surgery in adults. On the basis of these recommendations bariatric surgery is commonly performed in adults with BMI values of ≥ 35 kg/m^2 with comorbidities and for BMI values of ≥ 40 kg/m^2 with or without comorbidities. However, simple adoption of these guidelines for use in younger age groups is generally not felt to be appropriate.[133]

Recommendations specific for bariatric surgery in adolescents have since been proposed by a panel of experts in the field of pediatric obesity.[111] Given the unique metabolic, developmental, and psychological needs of adolescents, bariatric surgery in this population should only be performed at specialized centers under the supervision of multidisciplinary teams of experts experienced in meeting these distinct needs. These teams should include specialists in adolescent obesity evaluation and management, psychology, nutrition, physical activity instruction, and bariatric surgery.[111,134] Depending on the needs of the individual patients, other pediatric experts in fields such as gynecology, endocrinology, pulmonology, gastroenterology, cardiology, anesthesiology, or orthopedics may be consulted.

It is imperative that pediatric surgical specialists performing minimally invasive bariatric procedures have specialized training. There is substantial data showing that minimally invasive bariatric surgery is one of the more technically difficult operations to perform, with a steep learning curve and demonstrated differences in outcome depending on training background of the surgeons.[135] Pediatric surgeons involved in bariatric surgery should pursue advanced training and credentialing as recommended by the American Society for Bariatric Surgery. In addition, initially they should begin to work with an experienced bariatric surgical specialist.[136]

Table 48–2.

Criteria for Adolescent Bariatric Surgery

Failure of ≥6 months of organized weight loss attempts

Attainment of physiologic maturity

BMI ≥ 40 kg/m² with serious obesity-related comorbidities[a]

BMI ≥ 50 kg/m² with less serious obesity-related comorbidities[b]

Commitment to comprehensive medical and psychologic evaluations before and after surgery

Commitment to medical and nutritional requirements postoperatively

Ability to provide informed assent for surgical treatment

Demonstrate cognitive maturity and decisional capacity

Supportive family environment

[a] *Serious comorbidities: Type 2 diabetes mellitus, obstructive sleep apnea, or pseudotumor cerebri.*
[b] *Less serious comorbidities: Hypertension, dyslipidemia, nonalcoholic steatohepatitis, venous stasis disease, significant impairment in activities of daily living, intertriginous soft-tissue infections, stress urinary incontinence, gastroesophageal reflux disease, weight-related arthropathies that impair physical activity, and psychosocial distress.*

Adolescents who have failed multiple nonsurgical weight loss attempts may be considered candidates for surgical intervention. Table 48–2 lists the criteria recommended by Inge and colleagues[111] for patients being considered for bariatric surgery. In general, bariatric surgery is considered an appropriate option for those adolescents with very severe obesity (BMI ≥ 40 kg/m²) along with the presence of serious comorbidities as well as for patients with higher BMI values (≥50 kg/m²) and less serious obesity-related comorbid conditions (Table 48–2).[111] Contraindications to surgery are outlined in Table 48–3.

Preoperative Evaluation

Intensive patient and family preoperative education and evaluation is imperative for the success of bariatric surgery programs. Medical evaluations should include investigation into possible endogenous causes of obesity that may be amenable to treatment as well as identification of any obesity-related health complications, as is done in the adult population. Preoperative evaluation at our institution involves some or all of the procedures listed below as indicated for each individual patient:

- A consistent primary care provider (≥1-year relationship)
- evaluation by pediatric weight clinic

Table 48–3.

Contraindications to Adolescent Bariatric Surgery

Medically correctable cause of obesity

Substance abuse problem within preceding year

Medical, psychiatric, or cognitive condition that would impair the patient's ability to adhere to dietary or medication regimen

Current lactation

Current pregnancy or planned pregnancy within 2 years after surgery

Inability to comprehend or refusal to participate in lifelong medical surveillance

- evaluation by dietician
- evaluation by psychiatrist
- evaluation by physical therapist
- completion of a detailed health questionnaire
- electrocardiogram
- echocardiogram
- ultrasound (to assess for steatohepatitis and cholelithiasis)
  - patients with symptomatic gallstones should have a cholecystectomy before the bariatric procedure.
- bone age study (when indicated)
- polysomnography (sleep study)
- pulmonary function test and/or indirect calorimetry
- endoscopy
- attendance of support groups and education session
- blood tests:
  - complete blood count
  - serum electrolytes, renal and liver function tests
  - calcium and phosphate levels and uric acid levels
  - fasting lipids
  - insulin, blood sugar, hemoglobin A1 C
  - thyroid function tests
  - blood coagulation studies (PT, PTT, INR)

Physiologic maturity must be established prior to consideration of bariatric surgery, as the dietary complexities and potential nutritional consequences following surgery can stunt completion of growth. Physiologic maturation usually occurs along with sexual maturation (Tanner) stage 3 or 4. Most often skeletal maturation (>95% of adult stature) is attained by age 14 in girls and 16 in boys.[137] Obesity is usually associated with precocious puberty, and thus overweight children are often taller and have advanced bone age compared with age-matched nonoverweight children.[138–140] If there is uncertainty about whether adult stature has been attained, skeletal maturation (bone age) can be assessed objectively using a radiograph of the hand and wrist.[137,141]

In addition to undergoing medical assessment, comprehensive psychological evaluations of both potential candidates for bariatric surgery and their parents should be performed.[111,142] This involves assessment of the family unit; determination of coping skills; assessment of the severity of psychosocial comorbidities; review of past/present psychiatric, emotional, behavioral, or eating disorders; and evaluation of cognitive development, including determination of decisional capacity.

These evaluations serve to define potential supports and barriers to patient adherence as well as patient and family preparedness for surgery and the required postoperative lifestyle changes. An in-depth understanding, by the team, of the patients' psychological makeup and their family strengths or family dysfunction could have significant effects on the overall success of bariatric surgery. In addition, although legally consent for the surgical intervention must be obtained by the parents, ethically, the decisional capacity of the adolescent and their ability to give assent for surgery are of utmost importance and need to be clarified prior to proceeding with bariatric surgery.

Postoperative Management

Postoperative follow-up is generally quite intensive in order to verify adherence to diet and vitamin guidelines, ensure optimal postoperative weight loss, and avoid nutritional complications. Often programs establish follow-up visits in the following manner: Weekly for 1 month, monthly until 6 months, quarterly until first 12 months, biannually until 24 months, and yearly thereafter.[140] It is strongly encouraged that all patients have lifelong follow-up in order to ensure optimal weight maintenance and overall health. In addition, the long-term affects of bariatric surgery in this patient population are still unknown, thus ongoing rigorous clinical data collection will allow for structured clinical trials and observations to assist in our understanding and improve patient care.

Adolescents, like adults, are at increased risk of gallstone formation and peptic ulcer development following gastric bypass; therefore, usually ursodiol and proton-pump inhibitors are prescribed. Nonsteroidal anti-inflammatory medications should also be avoided to reduce the risk of intestinal ulceration and bleeding. Expected weight loss after laparoscopic gastric bypass surgery is 20–30 lb in the first month and approximately 10 lb/month until the weight loss plateaus after 12–18 months for a total excess weight loss of approximately 60–70%.[66]

RYGBP necessitates very low calorie, low-carbohydrate dietary intake; thus, attention to ensuring adequate daily protein intake (0.5–1.0 g/kg per day) is important to maintain lean body mass. Vitamin and mineral supplementation is required in order to optimize bone growth in growing adolescents and to avoid nutritional consequences discussed more in detail below. This usually includes chewable or soluble multivitamins, calcium citrate (1200–1500 mg/day), as well as B-complex supplements to reduce the risk of beriberi, which has been documented in adolescents after gastric bypass surgery.[143] Menstruating females should also take iron supplements. Bariatric surgery does not appear to affect the outcome of subsequent pregnancies as long as the period of rapid weight loss has passed; thus, pregnancy is contraindicated for 2 years after surgery.[144]

Nutritional Consequences

Both gastric restrictive and bypass procedures carry an associated risk of macronutrient as well as micronutrient deficiency.[145] In adolescents, the long-term risk of mineral or micronutrient deficiency, though not well defined, is a legitimate concern. Vitamin and mineral deficiencies, including hypovitaminosis A, B_{12}, C, D, E, folic acid, and iron, have all been reported.[143,146,147] The presumed mechanism for these deficiencies is thought to be malabsorption along with decreased oral intake, including poor compliance with medications postoperatively. Given the exponential skeletal growth that occurs during adolescence, it is unclear whether or not the current recommended amount of calcium supplements will be adequate to optimize bone growth. The decrease in bone density that occurs after surgical weight loss, combined with potential vitamin D and calcium deficiencies, may put adolescent bariatric patients at greater risk for fractures later in life.[148]

Compliance

Adolescence is often regarded as a period of experimentation, rebellion, risk taking, and egocentrism. All of these make surgical preparation and adolescent compliance to recommended health behaviors uniquely challenging, particularly when pursuing life-altering procedures like bariatric surgery. Compliance with health-care recommendations in adolescents is shown to be disappointingly low. Adolescents with chronic medical conditions such as cystic fibrosis, cancer, diabetes, and asthma have compliance rates of approximately 40–50%.[149–152] Rand and Macgregor[116] reported poor compliance by adolescents following gastric bypass surgery, with less than 15% of adolescents demonstrating compliance to postoperative dietary multivitamin and nutrient supplementation.

Noncompliance is often associated with such psychosocial factors as low self-esteem, poor cognitive abilities, and insufficient family support.[148] Several studies suggest that behavioral therapy can improve adolescent adherence to strict medical and dietary regimens.[21,153–155] Continued support by behavioral psychologists with expertise in enhancing adherence is essential for success in dietary compliance and long-term follow-up after bariatric procedures in adolescents. With the alterations in eating patterns that are required after bariatric surgery, repetitive reinforcement with structured family involvement and continued support is needed to facilitate the formation of lifelong health-promoting habits.[109]

Outcomes

There is currently a paucity of literature on long-term outcomes of bariatric surgery in adolescents. The majority of recent studies do, however, demonstrate the safety and efficacy of bariatric surgery in adolescent patients in achieving durable weight loss and amelioration of obesity-related comorbidities.[19,66,109,111,114,115,127,132,140,156,157]

In the largest long-term series to date, Sugerman and colleagues[158] reviewed their 20-year experience with RYGBP surgery in adolescents. The vast majority of their procedures were done open. They demonstrated results similar to adult patients, including sustained weight loss, correction of comorbidities, and improved self-image. More recent experience with laparoscopic RYGBP also demonstrates excellent excess weight loss and resolution of comorbidities, although long-term data is still pending.[109,114,157]

Perhaps even more reassuring than the amount of excess weight loss is the dramatic improvement in most obesity-related comorbidities after bariatric surgery. These have been very clearly demonstrated in adults and early reports in adolescents are also showing this to be true.[69,74,76,100,106] Lawson and colleagues[114] recently published the first outcome report from the Pediatric Bariatric Study Group, with their retrospective review of 12 morbidly obese adolescents who underwent RYGBP. In addition to a mean reduction in BMI of 37%, they demonstrated significant improvements in triglycerides, total cholesterol, fasting blood glucose, and fasting insulin after 1 year. Rand and Macgregor[116] reported excellent psychosocial adjustment 6 years after bariatric surgery with patients reporting increased self-esteem, improved social relationships, and feeling more attractive.

Late weight gain remains a potential concern and is still unclear given the limited long-term data. Recidivism in the form of weight gain is estimated at 20–30% in adults. Durable weight loss occurs in most adolescents, yet up to 15% of these patients appear to have late weight regain.[106] This occurrence may be avoided with a behavioral management program specifically designed for adolescents.[87,109] More long-term studies are necessary to further clarify this risk.

SUMMARY

Adolescent obesity is quickly becoming an epidemic worldwide. The impact of its attendant comorbidities will undoubtedly prove devastating to the health of populations across the globe unless practical solutions can be achieved. Programs aimed at prevention clearly must form the cornerstone of this effort. However, effective treatment for those adolescents already suffering from obesity cannot be delayed. There is substantial evidence supporting the benefits of bariatric surgery in this group in terms of excess weight loss and resolution of comorbidities.

The indications for bariatric surgery in adolescents are currently more conservative than those for adults. It may soon become clear, however, that surgical intervention earlier in the course of extreme obesity provides the best opportunity to reverse the debilitating cardiovascular, metabolic, and psychosocial sequelae of this disease.[159,160] The development of multidisciplinary adolescent bariatric teams, both at individual hospitals and on a national and international level, will aid in further clarifying the best treatment strategies.

References

1. Reilly JJ, Methven E, McDowell ZC, et al.: Health consequences of obesity. *Arch Dis Child* 88(9):748, 2003.
2. Freedman DS, Khan LK, Dietz WH, et al.: Relationship of childhood obesity to coronary heart disease risk factors in adulthood: The Bogalusa Heart Study. *Pediatrics* 108(3):712, 2001.
3. Baron M: Trends in pediatric nutrition. *Health Care Food Nutr Focus* 23(4):9, 2006.
4. Hedley AA, Ogden CL, Johnson CL, et al.: Prevalence of overweight and obesity among US children, adolescents, and adults, 1999–2002. *JAMA* 291(23):2847, 2004.
5. Ogden CL, Flegal KM, Carroll MD, Johnson CL: Prevalence and trends in overweight among US children and adolescents, 1999–2000. *JAMA* 288(14):1728, 2002.
6. Ogden CL, Carroll MD, Curtin LR, et al.: Prevalence of overweight and obesity in the United States, 1999–2004. *JAMA* 295(13):1549, 2006.
7. Dwyer JT, Stone EJ, Yang M, et al.: Prevalence of marked overweight and obesity in a multiethnic pediatric population: Findings from the Child and Adolescent Trial for Cardiovascular Health (CATCH) study. *J Am Diet Assoc* 100(10):1149, 2000.
8. Kimm SYS, Barton BA, Obarzanek E, et al.: Obesity development during adolescence in a biracial cohort: The NHLBI Growth and Health Study. *Pediatrics* 110(5):e54, 2002.
9. Freedman DS, Khan LK, Serdula MK, et al.: Racial and ethnic differences in secular trends for childhood BMI, weight, and height. *Obesity* 14(2):301, 2006.
10. Thorpe LE, List DG, Marx T, et al.: Childhood obesity in New York City elementary school students. *Am J Public Health* 94(9):1496, 2004.
11. Wang Y, Monteiro C, Popkin BM: Trends of obesity and underweight in older children and adolescents in the United States, Brazil, China, and Russia. *Am J Clin Nutr* 75(6):971, 2002.
12. Silventoinen K, Sans S, Tolonen H, et al.: Trends in obesity and energy supply in the WHO MONICA Project. *Int J Obes* 28(5):710, 2004.
13. Salazar-Martinez E, Allen B, Fernandez-Ortega C, et al.: Overweight and obesity status among adolescents from Mexico and Egypt. *Arch Med Res* 37(4):535, 2006.
14. Musaiger AO: Overweight and obesity in the Eastern Mediterranean Region: Can we control it? *East Mediterr Health J* 10(6):789, 2004.
15. Wong JPS, Ho SY, Lai MK, et al.: Overweight, obesity, weight-related concerns and behaviours in Hong Kong Chinese children and adolescents. *Acta Paediatr* 94(5):595, 2005.
16. Luo J, Hu FB: Time trends of obesity in pre-school children in China from 1989 to 1997. *Int J Obes* 26(4):553, 2002.
17. Dehghan M, Akhtar-Danesh N, Merchant AT: Childhood obesity, prevalence and prevention. *Nutr J* 4(1):24, 2005.
18. Cole TJ, Bellizzi MC, Flegal KM, Dietz WH: Establishing a standard definition for child overweight and obesity worldwide: International survey. *BMJ* 320(7244):1240, 2000.
19. Inge TH, Zeller MH, Lawson ML, Daniels SR: A critical appraisal of evidence supporting a bariatric surgical approach to weight management for adolescents. *J Pediatr* 147(1):10, 2005.
20. Himes JH, Dietz WH. Guidelines for overweight in adolescent preventive services: Recommendations from an expert committee.

The Expert Committee on Clinical Guidelines for Overweight in Adolescent Preventive Services. *Am J Clin Nutr* 59(2):307, 1994.

21. Nadler EP, Kane TD: Bariatric surgery. In: Langer JC, Albanese CT, (eds.): *Pediatric Minimal Access Surgery*. Boca Raton, Taylor & Francis, 2005; pp. 319–330.

22. Barlow SE, Dietz WH: Obesity evaluation and treatment: Expert Committee recommendations. The Maternal and Child Health Bureau, Health Resources and Services Administration and the Department of Health and Human Services. *Pediatrics* 102(3):E29, 1998.

23. Gillman MW, Rifas-Shiman S, Berkcy CS, et al.: Maternal gestational diabetes, birth weight, and adolescent obesity. *Pediatrics* 111(3):e221, 2003.

24. Singhal A, Wells J, Cole TJ, et al.: Programming of lean body mass: A link between birth weight, obesity, and cardiovascular disease? *Am J Clin Nutr* 77(3):726, 2003.

25. Burke V, Beilin LJ, Simmer K, et al.: Predictors of body mass index and associations with cardiovascular risk factors in Australian children: A prospective cohort study. *Int J Obes* 29(1):15, 2005.

26. Oken E, Gillman MW: Fetal origins of obesity. *Obes Res* 11(4):496, 2003.

27. Boney CM, Verma A, Tucker R, Vohr BR: Metabolic syndrome in childhood: Association with birth weight, maternal obesity, and gestational diabetes mellitus. *Pediatrics* 115(3):e290, 2005.

28. Malina RM, Katzmarzyk PT, Beunen G: Birth weight and its relationship to size attained and relative fat distribution at 7 to 12 years of age. *Obes Res* 4(4):385, 1996.

29. Law CM, Barker DJ, Osmond C, et al.: Early growth and abdominal fatness in adult life. *J Epidemiol Community Health* 46(3):184, 1992.

30. Barker M, Robinson S, Osmond C, Barker DJ: Birth weight and body fat distribution in adolescent girls. *Arch Dis Child* 77(5):381, 1997.

31. Loos RJ, Beunen G, Fagard R, et al.: Birth weight and body composition in young adult men—a prospective twin study. *Int J Obes* 25(10):1537, 2001.

32. Loos RJF, Beunen G, Fagard R, et al.: Birth weight and body composition in young women: A prospective twin study. *Am J Clin Nutr* 75(4):676, 2002.

33. Stern MP, Bartley M, Duggirala R, Bradshaw B: Birth weight and the metabolic syndrome: Thrifty phenotype or thrifty genotype? *Diabetes Metab Res Rev* 16(2):88, 2000.

34. Rich-Edwards JW, Colditz GA, Stampfer MJ, et al.: Birthweight and the risk for type 2 diabetes mellitus in adult women. *Ann Intern Med* 130(4 Pt 1):278, 1999.

35. Poulsen P, Vaag A: The intrauterine environment as reflected by birth size and twin and zygosity status influences insulin action and intracellular glucose metabolism in an age- or time-dependent manner. *Diabetes* 55(6):1819, 2006.

36. Bavdekar A, Yajnik CS, Fall CH, et al.: Insulin resistance syndrome in 8-year-old Indian children: Small at birth, big at 8 years, or both? *Diabetes* 48(12):2422, 1999.

37. Damm P: Gestational diabetes mellitus and subsequent development of overt diabetes mellitus. *Dan Med Bull* 45(5):495, 1998.

38. Vohr BR, McGarvey ST, Tucker R: Effects of maternal gestational diabetes on offspring adiposity at 4–7 years of age. *Diabetes Care* 22(8):1284, 1999.

39. Whitaker RC, Wright JA, Pepe MS, et al.: Predicting obesity in young adulthood from childhood and parental obesity. *N Engl J Med* 337(13):869, 1997.

40. Freedman DS, Shear CL, Burke GL, et al.: Persistence of juvenile-onset obesity over eight years: The Bogalusa Heart Study. *Am J Public Health* 77(5):588, 1987.

41. Must A, Jacques PF, Dallal GE, et al.: Long-term morbidity and mortality of overweight adolescents. A follow-up of the Harvard Growth Study of 1922 to 1935. *N Engl J Med* 327(19):1350, 1992.

42. Must A: Morbidity and mortality associated with elevated body weight in children and adolescents. *Am J Clin Nutr* 63(Suppl 3):445S, 1996.

43. Srinivasan SR, Bao W, Wattigney WA, Berenson GS: Adolescent overweight is associated with adult overweight and related multiple cardiovascular risk factors: The Bogalusa Heart Study. *Metabolism* 45(2):235, 1996.

44. Dietz WH: Health consequences of obesity in youth: Childhood predictors of adult disease. *Pediatrics* 101(3 Pt 2):518, 1998.

45. Gortmaker SL, Must A, Perrin JM, et al.: Social and economic consequences of overweight in adolescence and young adulthood. *N Engl J Med* 329(14):1008, 1993.

46. Reaven GM: Banting lecture 1988. Role of insulin resistance in human disease. *Diabetes* 37(12):1595, 1988.

47. Cook S, Weitzman M, Auinger P, et al.: Prevalence of a metabolic syndrome phenotype in adolescents: Findings from the third National Health and Nutrition Examination Survey, 1988–1994. *Arch Pediatr Adolesc Med* 157(8):821, 2003.

48. Weiss R, Dziura J, Burgert TS, et al.: Obesity and the metabolic syndrome in children and adolescents. *N Engl J Med* 350(23):2362, 2004.

49. Sinha R, Fisch G, Teague B, et al.: Prevalence of impaired glucose tolerance among children and adolescents with marked obesity. *N Engl J Med* 346(11):802, 2002.

50. Duncan GE: Prevalence of diabetes and impaired fasting glucose levels among US adolescents: National Health and Nutrition Examination Survey, 1999–2002. *Arch Pediatr Adolesc Med* 160(5):523, 2006.

51. Ehtisham S, Barrett TG: The emergence of type 2 diabetes in childhood. *Ann Clin Biochem* 41(Pt 1):10, 2004.

52. Pinhas-Hamiel O, Dolan LM, Daniels SR, et al.: Increased incidence of non-insulin-dependent diabetes mellitus among adolescents. *J Pediatr* 128(5 Pt 1):608, 1996.

53. Narayan KMV, Boyle JP, Thompson TJ, et al.: Lifetime risk for diabetes mellitus in the United States. *JAMA* 290(14):1884, 2003.

54. Luma GB, Spiotta RT: Hypertension in children and adolescents. *Am Fam Physician* 73(9):1558, 2006.

55. Stabouli S, Kotsis V, Papamichael C, et al.: Adolescent obesity is associated with high ambulatory blood pressure and increased carotid intimal-medial thickness. *J Pediatr* 147(5):651, 2005.

56. Sorof JM, Lai D, Turner J, et al.: Overweight, ethnicity, and the prevalence of hypertension in school-aged children. *Pediatrics* 113(3 Pt 1):475, 2004.

57. Berenson GS, Srinivasan SR, Bao W, et al.: Association between multiple cardiovascular risk factors and atherosclerosis in children and young adults. The Bogalusa Heart Study. *N Engl J Med* 338(23):1650, 1998.

58. Lauer RM, Clarke WR, Mahoney LT, Witt J: Childhood predictors for high adult blood pressure. The Muscatine Study. *Pediatr Clin North Am* 40(1):23, 1993.

59. Hanevold C, Waller J, Daniels S, et al.: The effects of obesity, gender, and ethnic group on left ventricular hypertrophy and geometry in hypertensive children: A collaborative study of the International Pediatric Hypertension Association. *Pediatrics* 113(2):328, 2004.

60. McGill HC, Herderick EE, McMahan CA, et al.: Atherosclerosis in youth. *Minerva Pediatr* 54(5):437, 2002.

61. McGill HC, McMahan CA, Herderick EE, et al.: Obesity accelerates the progression of coronary atherosclerosis in young men. *Circulation* 105(23):2712, 2002.

62. Gidding SS, Nehgme R, Heise C, et al.: Severe obesity associated with cardiovascular deconditioning, high prevalence of cardiovascular risk factors, diabetes mellitus/hyperinsulinemia, and respiratory compromise. *J Pediatr* 144(6):766, 2004.

63. Styne DM: Childhood and adolescent obesity. Prevalence and significance. *Pediatr Clin North Am* 48(4):823, 2001.

64. Schwimmer JB, Burwinkle TM, Varni JW: Health-related quality of life of severely obese children and adolescents. *JAMA* 289(14):1813, 2003.

65. Marcus CL, Curtis S, Koerner CB, et al.: Evaluation of pulmonary function and polysomnography in obese children and adolescents. *Pediatr Pulmonol* 21(3):176, 1996.

66. Helmrath MA, Brandt ML, Inge TH: Adolescent obesity and bariatric surgery. *Surg Clin North Am* 86(2):441, 2006.

67. Silvestri JM, Weese-Mayer DE, Bass MT, et al.: Polysomnography in obese children with a history of sleep-associated breathing disorders. *Pediatr Pulmonol* 16(2):124, 1993.

68. Mallory GB, Fiser DH, Jackson R: Sleep-associated breathing disorders in morbidly obese children and adolescents. *J Pediatr* 115(6):892, 1989.

69. Kalra M, Inge T, Garcia V, et al.: Obstructive sleep apnea in extremely overweight adolescents undergoing bariatric surgery. *Obes Res* 13(7):1175, 2005.

70. Friedman DI: Pseudotumor cerebri. *Neurol Clin* 22(1):99, 2004.

71. Friedman DI, Jacobson DM: Idiopathic intracranial hypertension. *J Neuroophthalmol* 24(2):138, 2004.

72. Cinciripini GGS, Donahue SS, Borchert MMS: Idiopathic intracranial hypertension in prepubertal pediatric patients: Characteristics, treatment, and outcome. *Am J Ophthalmol* 127(2):178, 1999.

73. Baker RRS, Baumann RRJ, Buncic JJR: Idiopathic intracranial hypertension (pseudotumor cerebri) in pediatric patients. *Pediatr Neurol* 5(1):5, 1989.

74. Chandra V, Dutta S, Albanese CT, et al.: Clinical resolution of severely symptomatic pseudotumor cerebri after gastric bypass in an adolescent: A case report. *Surg. Obes Relat Dis*, 2007 Feb 24.

75. Nadkarni TT, Rekate HL, Wallace DD: Resolution of pseudotumor cerebri after bariatric surgery for related obesity. Case report. *J Neurosurg* 101(5):878, 2004.

76. Sugerman HJ, Sugerman EL, DeMaria EJ, et al.: Bariatric surgery for severely obese adolescents. *J Gastrointest Surg* 7(1):102, 2003.

77. Dietz WH, Gross WL, Kirkpatrick JA: Blount disease (tibia vara): Another skeletal disorder associated with childhood obesity. *J Pediatr* 101(5):735, 1982.

78. Kelsey JL, Acheson RM, Keggi KJ: The body build of patients with slipped capital femoral epiphysis. *Am J Dis Child* 124(2):276, 1972.

79. Strauss RS, Pollack HA: Social marginalization of overweight children. *Arch Pediatr Adolesc Med* 157(8):746, 2003.

80. Zeller MH, Roehrig HR, Modi AC, et al.: Health-related quality of life and depressive symptoms in adolescents with extreme obesity presenting for bariatric surgery. *Pediatrics* 117(4):1155, 2006.

81. Swallen KC, Reither EN, Haas SA, Meier AM: Overweight, obesity, and health-related quality of life among adolescents: The National Longitudinal Study of Adolescent Health. *Pediatrics* 115(2):340, 2005.

82. Bagwell CL, Newcomb AF, Bukowski WM: Preadolescent friendship and peer rejection as predictors of adult adjustment. *Child Dev* 69(1):140, 1998.

83. Eisenberg ME, Neumark-Sztainer D, Story M: Associations of weight-based teasing and emotional well-being among adolescents. *Arch Pediatr Adolesc Med* 157(8):733, 2003.

84. Dong C, Li WD, Li D, Price RA: Extreme obesity is associated with attempted suicides: Results from a family study. *Int J Obes* 30(2):388, 2006.

85. Fontaine KR, Redden DT, Wang C, et al.: Years of life lost due to obesity. *JAMA* 289(2):187, 2003.

86. Jelalian E, Saelens BE: Empirically supported treatments in pediatric psychology: Pediatric obesity. *J Pediatr Psychol* 24(3):223, 1999.

87. Epstein LH, Myers MD, Raynor HA, Saelens BE: Treatment of pediatric obesity. *Pediatrics* 101(3 Pt 2):554, 1998.

88. Kirk S, Zeller M, Claytor R, et al.: The relationship of health outcomes to improvement in BMI in children and adolescents. *Obes Res* 13(5):876, 2005.

89. Chanoine J-P, Hampl S, Jensen C, et al.: Effect of orlistat on weight and body composition in obese adolescents: A randomized controlled trial. *JAMA* 293(23):2873, 2005.

90. Maahs D, de Serna DG, Kolotkin RL, et al.: Randomized, double-blind, placebo-controlled trial of orlistat for weight loss in adolescents. *Endocr Pract* 12(1):18, 2006.

91. Ozkan B, Bereket A, Turan S, Keskin S. Addition of orlistat to conventional treatment in adolescents with severe obesity. *Eur J Pediatr* 163(12):738, 2004.

92. Godoy-Matos A, Carraro L, Vieira A, et al.: Treatment of obese adolescents with sibutramine: A randomized, double-blind, controlled study. *J Clin Endocrinol Metab* 90(3):1460, 2005.

93. Reisler G, Tauber T, Afriat R, et al.: Sibutramine as an adjuvant therapy in adolescents suffering from morbid obesity. *Isr Med Assoc J* 8(1):30, 2006.

94. Tsai AG, Wadden TA: Systematic review: An evaluation of major commercial weight loss programs in the United States. *Ann Intern Med* 142(1):56, 2005.

95. Yanovski JA: Intensive therapies for pediatric obesity. *Pediatr Clin North Am* 48(4):1041, 2001.

96. Figueroa-Colon R, Franklin FA, Lee JY, et al.: Feasibility of a clinic-based hypocaloric dietary intervention implemented in a school setting for obese children. *Obes Res* 4(5):419, 1996.

97. Methods for voluntary weight loss and control. NIH Technology Assessment Conference Panel. Consensus Development Conference, 30 March to 1 April 1992. *Ann Intern Med* 119(7 Pt 2):764, 1993.

98. McTigue KM, Harris R, Hemphill B, et al.: Screening and interventions for obesity in adults: Summary of the evidence for the U.S. Preventive Services Task Force. *Ann Intern Med* 139(11):933, 2003.

99. Sjöström CD, Lissner L, Wedel H, Sjöström L: Reduction in incidence of diabetes, hypertension and lipid disturbances after intentional weight loss induced by bariatric surgery: The SOS Intervention Study. *Obes Res* 7(5):477, 1999.

100. Buchwald H, Avidor Y, Braunwald E, et al.: Bariatric surgery: A systematic review and meta-analysis. *JAMA* 292(14):1724, 2004.

101. Buchwald H, Buchwald JN: Evolution of operative procedures for the management of morbid obesity 1950–2000. *Obes Surg* 12(5):705, 2002.

102. Chapman AE, Kiroff G, Game P, et al.: Laparoscopic adjustable gastric banding in the treatment of obesity: A systematic literature review. *Surgery* 135(3):326, 2004.

103. MacDonald GJ, Long GJ, Swanson GJ, et al.: The gastric bypass operation reduces the progression and mortality of non-insulin-dependent diabetes mellitus. *J Gastrointest Surg* 1(3):213, 1997.

104. Flum DR, Dellinger EP: Impact of gastric bypass operation on survival: A population-based analysis. *J Am Coll Surg* 199(4):543, 2004.

105. Dixon JB, Dixon AF, O'Brien PE: Improvements in insulin sensitivity and beta-cell function (HOMA) with weight loss in the severely obese. Homeostatic model assessment. *Diabet Med* 20(2):127, 2003.

106. Sugerman HJ, Fairman RP, Sood RK, et al.: Long-term effects of gastric surgery for treating respiratory insufficiency of obesity. *Am J Clin Nutr* 55(Suppl 2):597S, 1992.

107. Dymek MP, Le Grange D, Neven K, Alverdy J: Quality of life after gastric bypass surgery: A cross-sectional study. *Obes Res* 10(11):1135, 2002.

108. Christou NV, Sampalis JS, Liberman M, et al.: Surgery decreases long-term mortality, morbidity, and health care use in morbidly obese patients. *Ann Surg* 240(3):416, 2004.

109. Garcia VF, Langford L, Inge TH: Application of laparoscopy for bariatric surgery in adolescents. *Curr Opin Pediatr* 15(3):248, 2003.

110. Strauss RS, Bradley LJ, Brolin RE: Gastric bypass surgery in adolescents with morbid obesity. *J Pediatr* 138(4):499, 2001.

111. Inge TH, Krebs NF, Garcia VF, et al.: Bariatric surgery for severely overweight adolescents: Concerns and recommendations. *Pediatrics* 114(1):217, 2004.

112. Health implications of obesity: National Institutes of Health Consensus Development Conference Statement. *National Institutes of Health Consensus Development Conference Consensus Statement* 5(9):1, 1985.

113. Dolan K, Creighton L, Hopkins G, Fielding G: Laparoscopic gastric banding in morbidly obese adolescents. *Obes Surg* 13(1):101, 2003.

114. Lawson ML, Kirk S, Mitchell T, et al.: One-year outcomes of Roux-en-Y gastric bypass for morbidly obese adolescents: A multicenter study from the Pediatric Bariatric Study Group. *J Pediatr Surg* 41(1):137, 2006.

115. Anderson AE, Soper RT, Scott DH: Gastric bypass for morbid obesity in children and adolescents. *J Pediatr Surg* 15(6):876, 1980.

116. Rand CS, Macgregor AM: Adolescents having obesity surgery: A 6-year follow-up. *South Med J* 87(12):1208, 1994.

117. Soper RT, Mason EE, Printen KJ, Zellweger H: Gastric bypass for morbid obesity in children and adolescents. *J Pediatr Surg* 10(1):51, 1975.

118. Horgan S, Holterman MJ, Jacobsen GR, et al.: Laparoscopic adjustable gastric banding for the treatment of adolescent morbid obesity in the United States: A safe alternative to gastric bypass. *J Pediatr Surg* 40(1):86, 2005.

119. Nguyen NT, Ho HS, Palmer LS, Wolfe BM: A comparison study of laparoscopic versus open gastric bypass for morbid obesity. *J Am Coll Surg* 191(2):149, 2000.

120. Podnos YD, Jimenez JC, Wilson SE, et al.: Complications after laparoscopic gastric bypass: A review of 3464 cases. *Arch Surg* 138(9):957, 2003.

121. O'Brien PE, Dixon JB, Brown W, et al.: The laparoscopic adjustable gastric band (Lap-Band): A prospective study of medium-term effects on weight, health and quality of life. *Obes Surg* 12(5):652, 2002.

122. Chevallier J-M, Zinzindohoué F, Douard R, et al.: Complications after laparoscopic adjustable gastric banding for morbid obesity: Experience with 1000 patients over 7 years. *Obes Surg* 14(3):407, 2004.

123. Nguyen NT, Silver M, Robinson M, et al.: Result of a national audit of bariatric surgery performed at academic centers: A 2004 University HealthSystem Consortium Benchmarking Project. *Arch Surg* 141(5):445, 2006.

124. DeMaria EJ, Jamal MK: Laparoscopic adjustable gastric banding: Evolving clinical experience. *Surg Clin North Am* 85(4):773, 2005.

125. O'Brien PE, Dixon JB, Laurie C, et al.: Treatment of mild to moderate obesity with laparoscopic adjustable gastric banding or an intensive medical program: A randomized trial. *Ann Intern Med* 144(9):625, 2006.

126. Ren CJ, Horgan S, Ponce J: US experience with the LAP-BAND system. *Am J Surg* 184(6B):46S, 2002.

127. Angrisani L, Furbetta F, Doldi SB, et al.: Results of the Italian multicenter study on 239 super-obese patients treated by adjustable gastric banding. *Obes Surg* 12(6):846, 2002.

128. Weiner R, Blanco-Engert R, Weiner S, et al.: Outcome after laparoscopic adjustable gastric banding—8 years experience. *Obes Surg* 13(3):427, 2003.

129. Parikh MS, Laker S, Weiner M, et al.: Objective comparison of complications resulting from laparoscopic bariatric procedures. *J Am Coll Surg* 202(2):252, 2006.

130. Mognol P, Chosidow D, Marmuse J-P: Laparoscopic gastric bypass versus laparoscopic adjustable gastric banding in the super-obese: A comparative study of 290 patients. *Obes Surg* 15(1):76, 2005.

131. Dolan K, Fielding G: A comparison of laparoscopic adjustable gastric banding in adolescents and adults. *Surg Endosc* 18(1):45, 2004.

132. Abu-Abeid S, Gavert N, Klausner JM, Szold A: Bariatric surgery in adolescence. *J Pediatr Surg* 38(9):1379, 2003.

133. Gastrointestinal surgery for severe obesity. Proceedings of a National Institutes of Health Consensus Development Conference. March 25–27, 1991, Bethesda, MD. *Am J Clin Nutr* 55(Suppl 2):487S, 1992.

134. Recommendations for facilities performing bariatric surgery. *Bull Am Coll Surg* 85(9):20, 2000.

135. Hsu GP, Morton JM, Jin L, et al.: Laparoscopic Roux-en-Y gastric bypass: Differences in outcome between attendings and assistants of different training backgrounds. *Obes Surg* 15(8):1104, 2005.

136. Lublin M, Lyass S, Lahmann B, et al.: Leveling the learning curve for laparoscopic bariatric surgery. *Surg Endosc* 19(6):845, 2005.

137. Tanner JM: Normal growth and techniques of growth assessment. *Clin Endocrinol Metab* 15(3):411, 1986.

138. Leonard MB, Shults J, Wilson BA, et al.: Obesity during childhood and adolescence augments bone mass and bone dimensions. *Am J Clin Nutr* 80(2):514, 2004.

139. Wang Y: Is obesity associated with early sexual maturation? A comparison of the association in American boys versus girls. *Pediatrics* 110(5):903, 2002.

140. Inge TH, Zeller M, Garcia VF, Daniels SR: Surgical approach to adolescent obesity. *Adolesc Med Clin* 15(3):429, 2004.

141. Gilli G: The assessment of skeletal maturation. *Horm Res* 45(Suppl 2):49, 1996.

142. Dziurowicz-Kozlowska AH, Wierzbicki Z, Lisik W, et al.: The objective of psychological evaluation in the process of qualifying candidates for bariatric surgery. *Obes Surg* 16(2):196, 2006.

143. Towbin A, Inge TH, Garcia VF, et al.: Beriberi after gastric bypass surgery in adolescence. *J Pediatr* 145(2):263, 2004.

144. Sheiner E, Levy A, Silverberg D, et al.: Pregnancy after bariatric surgery is not associated with adverse perinatal outcome. *Am J Obstet Gynecol* 190(5):1335, 2004.

145. Xanthakos, I: Nutritional consequences of bariatric surgery. *Curr Opin Clin Nutr Metab Care* 9(4):489, 2006.

146. Boylan LM, Sugerman HJ, Driskell JA: Vitamin E, vitamin B-6, vitamin B-12, and folate status of gastric bypass surgery patients. *J Am Diet Assoc* 88(5):579, 1988.

147. Halverson JD: Vitamin and mineral deficiencies following obesity surgery. *Gastroenterol Clin North Am* 16(2):307, 1987.

148. Garcia V, Inge T: Bariatric surgery in adolescents. In: Grosfeld JL (ed.): *Pediatric Surgery*. Nashville, TN, Mosby, 2006.

149. Inge TH, Garcia V, Daniels S, et al.: A multidisciplinary approach to the adolescent bariatric surgical patient. *J Pediatr Surg* 39(3):442, 2004.

150. Phipps S, DeCuir-Whalley S: Adherence issues in pediatric bone marrow transplantation. *J Pediatr Psychol* 15(4):459, 1990.

151. Buston KM, Wood SF: Non-compliance amongst adolescents with asthma: Listening to what they tell us about self-management. *Fam Pract* 17(2):134, 2000.

152. Tamaroff MH, Festa RS, Adesman AR, Walco GA: Therapeutic adherence to oral medication regimens by adolescents with cancer, II: Clinical and psychologic correlates. *J Pediatr* 120(5):812, 1992.

153. Wysocki T, Harris MA, Greco P, et al.: Randomized, controlled trial of behavior therapy for families of adolescents with insulin-dependent diabetes mellitus. *J Pediatr Psychol* 25(1):23, 2000.

154. Lemanek KL, Kamps J, Chung NB: Empirically supported treatments in pediatric psychology: Regimen adherence. *J Pediatr Psychol* 26(5):253, 2001.

155. Fielding D, Duff A: Compliance with treatment protocols: Interventions for children with chronic illness. *Arch Dis Child* 80(2):196, 1999.

156. Breaux. Obesity surgery in children. *Obes Surg* 5(3):279, 1995.

157. Stanford A, Glascock JM, Eid GM, et al.: Laparoscopic Roux-en-Y gastric bypass in morbidly obese adolescents. *J Pediatr Surg* 38(3):430, 2003.

158. Sugerman HJHJ, Sugerman ELEL, DeMaria EJEJ, et al.: Bariatric surgery for severely obese adolescents. *J Gastrointest Surg* 7(1):102, 2003.

159. Capella JF, Capella RF: Bariatric surgery in adolescence. Is this the best age to operate? *Obes Surg* 13(6):826, 2003.

160. Garcia VF, DeMaria EJ: Adolescent bariatric surgery: Treatment delayed, treatment denied, a crisis invited. *Obes Surg* 16(1):1, 2006.

Index